NP320

D1685835

Female Pelvic Medicine and Reconstructive Pelvic Surgery

Springer

London
Berlin
Heidelberg
New York
Hong Kong
Milan
Paris
Tokyo

H.P. Drutz, S. Herschorn and N.E. Diamant (Eds)

Female Pelvic Medicine and Reconstructive Pelvic Surgery

With 252 Figures

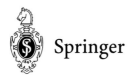

Springer

H.P. Drutz, BA, MD, FRC(C), FACOG, FSOGC
Urogynecology Unit, Mount Sinai Hospital,
Toronto, Ontario, Canada,

S. Herschorn, BSc, MDCM, FRCSC
Division of Urology, University of Toronto,
Sunnybrook and Women's College Health Science Centre,
Toronto, Ontario, Canada,

N.E. Diamant, MD, FRCP(C)
Division of Gastroenterology, Department of Medicine,
University of Toronto, Toronto Hospital,
Toronto, Ontario, Canada

British Library Cataloguing in Publication Data
Female pelvic medicine and reconstructive pelvic surgery
1. Urogynecology   2. Pelvis – Surgery
I. Drutz, H.P. Herschorn, Sender   III. Diament, N.E.
617 .4'6'0082
ISBN 1852334797

Library of Congress Cataloging-in-Publication Data
A catalog record for this book is available from the Library of Congress

ISBN 1-85233-479-7 Springer-Verlag London Berlin Heidelberg
a member of BertelsmannSpringer Science+Business Media GmbH
http://www.springer.co.uk

Typeset by EXPO Holdings, Malaysia
Printed and bound at the Cromwell Press, Trowbridge, Wiltshire, UK
28/3830-543210 Printed on acid-free paper SPIN 10567931

To our wives and our children, whom life is really all about.

and

To present and future generations of urologists, urogynecologists, gynecologists, gastroenterologists, colorectal surgeons, neurologists and all health care providers for women who will work collegially and collaboratively to improve the quality of life for women with pelvic floor disorders.

Foreword

During the last decade we have gained a better understanding of the function of the pelvic floor as a unit.

The most common cause of insufficiency of the pelvic floor and its sphincters is the normal aging of its connective tissue, especially the collagen. It seems that this process can be counteracted by the influence of certain foreign bodies.

Professor Chassar Moir of Oxford was one of the gynecologists who started using synthetic material in the slings at the Aldridge operation. He once told me that in some patients where he later had to make a laparotomy because of other diseases, he had found that the sling's fixation at the aponeurosis had ruptured but the patient still was continent. To me it seemed very likely that it had been some type of action between the sling and the surrounding tissue which strengthened its structure.

Instead of laying a muscle sling over the anterior parts of the divided muscle pubococcygeus at the levator plastic, I therefore tried to put a piece of nylon tissue over the sutured pubocervical ligaments. The result was that the nylon was expelled in single threads, but the patient became continent. After that I placed a piece of Marlex mesh as big as an ordinary postage stamp over the sutured pubocervical ligaments after the continence had been controlled with the bladder filled with 200 ml saline. With this technique five cases with stress incontinence were operated and cured at 5-year follow up. Unfortunately, I could not operate more patients with this technique because I had retired. One patient I had the possibility to control after 25 years. She was still continent at the age of 93 years.

In 1957 I published the vaginal sling operation (J Obstet Gynaecol Br Emp 64:849).

About 40 years later Papa Petros and Ulmsten modified the procedure by using artificial material in the sling, usually polypropylene, and called it TVT (tension free vaginal tape operation) which gives as good results as the levator plastic.

The common genital prolapse is often, even after 100 years, operated according to the "Manchester technique". The rate of recurrence is about 20% or perhaps more in prolapse following hysterectomy.

The new methods of sacrospinous vault suspension and abdominal colposacropexy give better results. Addition of artificial nets such as Marlex mesh will probably improve the results further.

This book gives an excellent description of the anatomy, physiology and pathophysiology of the female pelvic organs as well as conservative and modern operative treatment of their diseases.

A book of this type has not as far as I remember been published before. It is recommended to urologists, urogynecologists, gynecologists, colorectal surgeons and gastroenterologists but also general surgeons, who have to perform acute surgery in the pelvis.

A. Ingelman-Sundberg

Through the last two decades the education, training and practice of pelvic medicine and reconstruction was fragmented, with two specialties pulling in different directions. Female urology was defined by urologists dedicated to pelvic dysfunction and reconstruction. Gynecologists dedicated to the same field defined urogynecology. Both specialties were split with each separately creating its own terminology, its own diagnostic and surgical approach and leaving the rest of the medical community and patients in an undetermined state.

In the last years the Board of Obstetrics and Gynecology and the Board of Urology decided to embark on a joint training program in the field. Not only did they create a new name, Female Pelvic Medicine and Reconstructive Surgery, but they also laid the foundation for a renewed cooperation between the fields.

The publication of *Female Pelvic Medicine and Reconstructive Pelvic Surgery* represents a major attempt to solidify the change. This book brings together the two specialties and creates a first line resource for the specialist as well as the general urologist or gynecologist. The walls between the specialties have fallen and the reader will find a modern and integrated approach to the medical and surgical conditions that encompass pelvic medicine and reconstructive pelvic surgery.

The first group of chapters on anatomy, physiology and diagnosis provide the scientific basis and understanding of the principles of normal and abnormal voiding, anatomical support and a clear description of the different diagnostic procedures important in planning adequate therapy.

In between other important chapters, the reader will find a comprehensive coverage of inflammatory conditions, conservative and surgical treatment of pelvic floor disorders, urinary and fecal incontinence as well as fistula and trauma.

This new book represents an important addition to the practice of pelvic medicine and reconstructive pelvic surgery and should be in the library of every urologist and gynecologist.

Shlomo Raz

I am pleased to be asked to write a foreword to this text on the newest advances in urogynecology. This subject was much neglected a very few years ago, but now, at last, is receiving the attention of some of the best medical minds of our time.

Ancient medical writings describe urinary problems in women. The mummy of Queen Henhenit, who lived around 2050 BC in Egypt, was radiographed in 1935 to reveal a large urinary fistula. Physicians in Europe devised various instruments, using the technologies of their time, trying to solve this miserable condition. In the United States, J. Marion Sims spent his medical career finding ways to cure vesicovaginal fistulas. Howard A. Kelly was appointed the first professor of gynecology at Johns Hopkins Medical School. In 1893 he invented a female cystoscope, using air for insufflation, and became the first person to place a urethral catheter under direct vision. Kelly trained residents in gynecology and female urology. He felt that obstetrics and gynecology should not be combined. Richard TeLinde, Johns Hopkins emeritus professor of gynecology, wrote in 1978 that programs in both fields had not been pursued in most medical centers. He hoped that the trend would reverse itself. Unfortunately it did not. The great technological advances in obstetrics have overwhelmed the trainings in gynecology, and certainly urogynecology.

After my residency and fellowship under Conrad Collins, an advocate of Kelly's views at Tulane Medical School, Department of Obstetrics and Gynecology, in 1956, I found, in clinical practice, that many hysterectomy patients became incontinent of urine. The problem was diagnosis. These women had had uterine prolapse, which kinked the urethra. There was a failure in diagnosing this preoperatively; then with hysterectomy, they became incontinent.

Women were second-class citizens medically. Male instruments were used to examine them. Urologists had focused their expertise on males, and used the female urethra on which to rest their water cystoscopes. A forward-thinking endoscope maker in Germany,

Karl Storz, quickly grasped the concept, and made the first fiberoptic female urethroscope for me, using carbon dioxide for insufflation. The female urethra, less than an inch long, was the neglected site, where so many problems went undiagnosed. Now, at last it was possible to actually see problems, such as the previously rarely diagnosed, urethral diverticula.

There was an overwhelming response from gynecologists and a great many urologists, who realized their training had lacked focus on the delicate balance between the genital and urinary tracts in women. The defining moment came when the American College of Obstetrics and Gynecology issued a directive requiring all residents to learn urogynecology in their programs in order to become Board Certified.

Harold Drutz saw the need for urogynecologists in 1975, and began postgraduate training under great physicians: Axel Ingelman-Sundberg in Sweden, Eric Glen and David Rowan in Scotland; Peter Donker in the Netherlands; urodynamics with Richard Turner-Warwick in England; and surgery to repair vesicovaginal fistulas with Reginald and Catherine Hamlin in Addis Ababa, Ethiopia. In the United States he studied with Emil Tanagho, Paul Hodgkinson, and Alain Rossier. He came to work with me when I was running the first urogynecologic clinic at Women's Hospital, University of Southern California Medical Center, which was a continuation of my good friend, Arnold Kegel's clinic.

By co-editing this volume with a well-known urologist, Professor Sender Herschorn, Chairman of Urology at the University of Toronto, and a noted gastroenterologist, Professor Nicholas Diamant, head of Toronto Western Hospital's Anorectal Motility Laboratory, the editors have bridged the gap of politics of the pelvis, and have successfully compiled a textbook that treats the whole pelvis and not just a pelvis full of holes.

We all stand on the shoulders of pioneers before us, and pray that our work will be continued by new, enthusiastic, capable physicians. The real value of this book is to help those doctors who are seeking to help women.

Jack R. Robertson

Preface

By the turn of the nineteenth century medicine had become so complicated that there started to emerge physicians who were medical doctors and those who were surgical doctors. Further divisions rapidly ensued.

In the twentieth century, and particularly by the completion of the two great World Wars, medical physicians had expanded to include general practitioners, pediatricians, internists, psychiatrists, neurologists, cardiologists, respirologist, rheumatologists, endocrinologists, nephrologists, gerontologists, gastroenterologists, etc, etc. Similarly, the concept of a surgeon had expanded to include general surgeons, neurosurgeons, ophthalmologists, otolaryngologists, cardiovascular, thoracic, urologic, colorectal, obstetric and gynecologic, urogynecologic surgeons etc., etc.

Although this subdivision of the human body has produced tremendous advances in our scope of medical knowledge it has also led to political turfs and the ultimate fractionation of health care for women with pelvic floor disorders. There evolved the pelvis full of "holes" treated by different groups, rather than the "whole" pelvis treated by an integrated multidisciplined approach.

The editors of this textbook have attempted to bring together authors and topics which span the entire range of pelvic floor disorders in women. The content of each chapter represents the views of the author(s). The editors have confined their assistance to review and minor suggestions.

At the dawn of a new century and a new millennium, we have the tools to produce evidence based medicine to answer unsolved problems. It is the hope of all the contributors to this textbook, that all physicians and health care providers for women will work collaboratively and collegially to meet these objectives.

Respectfully submitted,
Harold P. Drutz, MD
Sender Herschorn, MD
Nicholas E. Diamant, MD

Contents

Section 4: Inflammatory Conditions, Painful Bladder and Pelvic Syndromes, Common Bowel Problems

Section 5: Conservative Treatment for Pelvic Floor Disorders

Section 6: Surgical Approaches to Urinary and Fecal Incontinence

Section 7: Surgery for Disorders of Pelvic Support

Section 8: Fistulas, Operative Trauma, Postoperative Problems

Section 9: Training Guidelines

Contributors

Dr **Bunan Alnaif**, Assistant Professor, Department of Obstetrics and Gynecology, Eastern Virginia Medical School, Norfolk, Virginia, USA

Professor **Karl-Erik Andersson**, Department of Clinical Pharmacology, University Hospital of Lund, Lund, Sweden

Dr **Lisa Aptaker-Stirling**, Gynecology, Department of Obstetrics/Gynecology and Reproductive Sciences, UMDNJ-Robert Wood Johnson Medical School, Clinical Academic Building, New Brunswick, NJ, USA

Professor **Said A. Awad**, Department of Urology, Queen Elizabeth II, Health Sciences Centre, Halifax, Nova Scotia, Canada

Professor **Gloria A. Bachmann**, Division Director, Gynecology, Department of Obstetrics/Gynecology and Reproductive Sciences, UMDNJ-Robert Wood Johnson Medical School, New Brunswick, NJ, USA

Professor **Mohamed H. Baghdadi**, Department of Anatomy, Dalhousie University, Halifax, Nova Scotia, Canada

Dr **Philip Scott Bagnell**, Dalhousie University, Halifax, Nova Scotia, Canada

Dr **Kevin R. Baker**, Assistant Professor, Department of Obstetrics and Gynecology, Riverside Medical Centre, Ottawa, Ontario, Canada

Dr **Frederick D. Brenneman**, Trauma Program, Sunnybrook Health Science Centre, North York, Ontario, Canada

Dr **Marcus J. Burnstein**, Associate Professor, Department of Surgery, University of Toronto, St Michael's Hospital, Toronto, Ontario, Canada

Dr **Lesley K. Carr**, Division of Urology, University of Toronto, Sunnybrook and Women's College Heath Science Centre, Toronto, Ontario, Canada

Dr **Patrick J. Culligan**, Assistant Professor, University of Louisville Health Sciences Center, Department of Obstetrics, Gynecology and Women's Health, Division of Urogynecology and Reconstructive Pelvic Surgery, Louisville, Kentucky, USA

Mr **Ian Currie**, Department of Obstetrics and Gynaecology, Stoke Mandeville Hospital, Aylesbury, Buckinghamshire, UK

Professor **Nicholas E. Diamant**, Division of Gastroenterology, Department of Medicine, University of Toronto, Toronto Hospital, Toronto, Ontario, Canada

Professor **Harold P. Drutz**, Professor and Head, Section of Urogynecology, Department of Obstetrics and Gynecology University of Toronto, Mount Sinai Hospital, Lawrence and Frances Bloomberg Department of Obstetrics and Gynecology, Toronto, Ontario, Canada

Dr **Scott A. Farrell**, Professor, Department of Obstetrics and Gynecology, IWK Health Center, Halifax, Nova Scotia, Canada

Dr Donna M. Fedorkow, Department of Obstetrics and Gynecology, McMaster University, Hamilton, Ontario, Canada

Dr Catherine G. Flood, Associate Professor, Urogynecology Clinic Women's Health Clinic, Royal Alexandra Hospital, Edmonton, Alberta, Canada

Dr Martin Friedlich, Colon and Rectal Surgery Resident, University of Toronto, St Michael's Hospital, Toronto, Ontario, Canada

Dr Alan H. Gerulath, Associate Professor, Director of Vulvar Clinic, St Michael's Hospital, Toronto, Ontario, Canada

Wilma M. Greston, MD, Principal Associate, Department of Obstetrics and Gynecology, Chief of Urogynecology, Albert Einstein College of Medicine, Montefiore Medical Center, Bronx, NY, USA

Lesley-Ann M. Hanson RN BSc, Urogynecology Clinic Women's Health Clinic, Royal Alexandra Hospital, Edmonton, Alberta, Canada

Dr Marie-Andrée Harvey, Assistant Professor, Department of Obstetrics and Gynecology, Kingston General Hospital, Kingston, Ontario, Canada

Dr Magdy M. Hassouna, Associate Professor of Surgery (Urology), University of Toronto, The Toronto Hospital, Toronto, Ontario, Canada

Professor Sender Herschorn, Division of Urology, University of Toronto, Sunnybrook and Women's Health Science Centre, Toronto, Ontario, Canada

Mr Steven Heymen, Director of Biofeedback Services UNC-CH, Research Instructor in Medicine, UNC-CH, Chapel Hill, NC, USA

Professor Emeritus Axel Ingelman-Sundberg, Djursholm, Sweden

Dr Corrine F.I. Jabs, Urogynecology, Obstetrics and Gynecology, Regina, Saskatchewan, Canada

Dr Shawna Lee Johnston, Assistant Professor, Department of Obstetrics and Gynecology, Queen's University, Kingston, Ontario, Canada

Dr Martine Jolivet-Tremblay, Division of Urology, University of Montreal, Hospital Maisonneuve-Rosemont, Montreal, Quebec, Canada

Dr Kenneth R. Jones, Clinical Psychologist, Advanced Pain Center of Alaska, Anchorage, AK, USA

Dr Margie A. Kahn, Director of Urogynecology, Assistant Professor, Department of Obstetrics and Gynecology, The University of Texas, Galveston, TX USA

Dr Kathleen C. Kobashi, Co-Director, Continence Center at Virginia Mason, Seattle, USA

Professor Heinz A. Koelbl, 2nd Department of Obstetrics and Gynecology, University Hospital of Vienna, Vienna, Austria

Dr Rose C. Kung, Women's College Hospital, Burton Hall, Toronto, Ontario, Canada

Dr George Lazarou, Assistant Professor, Department of Obstetrics and Gynecology, Chief of Urogynecology, Albert Einstein College of Medicine, Montefiore Medical Center, Bronx, NY, USA

Dr Gary E. Leach, Director, Tower Urology Institute for Continence, Los Angeles, CA, USA

Dr Patricia E. Lee, Department of Obstetrics and Gynecology, University of Toronto, Sunnybrook and Women's Health Sciences Centre, Toronto, Ontario, Canada

Dr Raymond A. Lee, Emeritus Consultant, Departments of Obstetrics and Gynecology and Surgery, Mayo Clinic; Professor of Obstetrics and Gynecology, Mayo Medical School; Rochester, MN, USA

Dr Marie-Claude Lemieux, Department of Obstetrics and Gynecology, Hôpital Maisonneuve-Rosemont, Montréal, Québec, Canada

Dr Constance Ling, The Ottawa Hospital, Ottawa, Ontario, Canada

Dr James A. Low, Professor Emeritus, Department of Obstetrics and Gynecology, Queen's University, Kingston, Ontario, Canada

Dr J. Barry MacMillan, St Joseph's Health Center, London, Ontario, Canada

Dr Thomas C. Mainprize, Associate Professor, Calgary Regional Health Authority, Department of Obstetrics and Gynecology, University of Calgary, Foothills Hospital, Calgary, Alberta Canada

Dr Katherine N. Moore, Assistant Professor, Faculty of Nursing, University of Alberta, Edmonton, Alberta, Canada

Dr J. Edwin Morgan, Women's College Hospital, Toronto, Ontario, Canada

Dr Gillian D. Oliver, Assistant Professor, Head, Division of Pediatric Oncology, Department of Obstetrics and Gynecology, The Hospital for Sick Children, Toronto, Ontario, Canada

Dr Stéphane Ouellet, Department of Obstetrics and Gynecology, Hôpital St-Luc, Montréal, Québec, Canada

Professor C. Lowell Parsons, Division of Urology, UCSD Medical Center, San Diego, CA, USA

Dr Gary Peers, Queen's Medical Center, Honolulu, Hawaii, USA

Dr Sidney B. Radomski, Associate Professor of Surgery, Director of Urodynamics Laboratory, Toronto Western Hospital (University Health Network) Toronto, Ontario, Canada

Professor Shlomo Raz, Professor of Urology, Department of Urology, University of California, Los Angeles School of Medicine, Los Angeles, CA, USA

Dr Magali Robert, Calgary Regional Health Authority, Department of Obstetrics and Gynecology, University of Calgary, Foothills Hospital, Calgary, Alberta, Canada

Professor Jack R. Robertson, Santa Ynez, CA, USA

Dr Theodore M. Ross, Associate Professor, Department of Surgery, Women's College Hospital, Toronto, Ontario, Canada

Anita Saltmarche, RN Faculty of Nursing, University of Alberta, Edmonton, Alberta, Canada

Dr Peter K. Sand, Professor of Obstetrics and Gynecology, Northwestern University; Director, Urogynecology Division; Director, The Evanston Continence Center, Evanston, IL, USA

Dr Abheha Satkunaratnam, Clinical Fellow, Department of Obstetrics and Gynecology, University of Toronto, Toronto, Ontario, Canada

Dr Jane A. Schulz, Assistant Professor, Royal Alexandra Hospital, Department of Obstetrics and Gynecology, University of Alberta; Edmonton, Alberta, Canada

Dr Richard J. Scotti, Professor, Drew University and UCLA, USA

Mr Kevin M. Smith, Specialist Registrar, Royal Berkshire Hospital, Reading, Berkshire, UK

Dr Dana Soroka, Senior Clinical Research Fellow, Division of Urogynecology, Department of Obstetrics and Gynecology, University of Toronto, Mount Sinai Hospital, Toronto, Ontario, Canada

Mr Abdul Sultan, Consultant Obstetrician and Gynecologist, Mayday University Hospital, Thornton Heath, UK

Dr Taryn N. Tang, Research Associate, Women's Mental Health Research Section, Centre for Addiction and Mental Health, Department of Psychiatry, University of Toronto, Toronto, Ontario, Canada

Dr Brenda B. Toner, Professor and Head, Women's Mental Health Research Section, Centre for Addiction and Mental Health, Department of Psychiatry, University of Toronto, Toronto, Ontario, Canada

Dr Eboo Versi, Clinical Associate Professor, OBGYN, UMDNJ, Robert Wood Johnson Medical School, New Brunswick, NJ, USA

Professor William E. Whitehead, Division of Digestive Diseases, University of North Carolina at Chapel Hill, Chapel Hill, NC, USA

Dr David H.L. Wilkie, CUN., Associate Professor Obstetrics and Gynecology, University of British Columbia, Vancouver General Hospital, Vancouver British Columbia, Canada

1 Introduction

1 Urogynecology and Reconstructive Pelvic Surgery: Past, Present and Future

Harold P. Drutz and J. Edwin Morgan

Introduction

Urogynecology, gynecological urology, or female urology is probably as old as medicine itself. The ancient Egyptians, who laid the foundation of medical knowledge, appreciated the close relationship between diseases of the female genital and urinary systems.

For the purpose of major periods of development we will divide our discussion in this chapter into three sections. We will consider the *past* under: (1) prior to the nineteenth century; (2) progress in the nineteenth century. The *present* will review the tremendous progress made during the twentieth century, and for the *future* we will look to the 21st century and a new millennium with suggestions for future initiatives and directions.

Past

Prior to the Nineteenth Century

The Kahun papyrus, written about 2000 BC, was devoted to diseases of women and includes diseases of the female genital organs as well as problems of the urinary bladder [1]. The Ebers papyrus (year 1550 BC) included disorders of micturition as well as gynecological and obstetric problems [2].

In the eighteenth century the Scottish Enlightenment especially had a profound effect on educational institutions in colonial America. Many of the leading colonial universities were led by Scots educated at the University of Edinburgh [3].

A significant number of the founders of medical schools on the Atlantic coast went abroad to receive an MD from the University of Edinburgh and to work in the London anatomical schools, of which the most famous was Great Windmill Street founded by William Hunter (1718–1783) with his brother John Hunter (1728–1793).

Progress in the Nineteenth Century

Garrison's *History of Medicine* states "Operative gynecology, which had no special existence before the beginning of the 19th century, was largely the creation of certain surgeons from the southern states" [4]. Ephraim McDowell was the first to successfully perform ovariotomy an became known as the founder of abdominal surgery. James Marion Sims (Figure 1.1) became known as the father of modern gynecologic surgery with his pioneering work in repairing vesicovaginal fistula. After 29 previous attempts, he achieved his first success with the slave woman Anarca in 1849, using fine silver wire sutures.

The nineteenth century was characterized by attempts to devise some type of instrument by which the interior of the bladder might be observed. In 1806, Bozzini [5] of Frankfurt described a hollow specula for use in the throat, vagina, and female bladder using a mirror for light reflection. The first actual use of any type of cystoscope was described by Segalas of Paris in 1828 [6].

In 1875, G. Simon of Rostock was the first to catheterize the ureters. Rutenberg, 1876, and Grunfield, 1881, both of Vienna, used air distension of the bladder and reflected light from a head mirror. In 1893, Dr Howard A. Kelly (Figure 1.2) announced a method for "The Direct Examination of the Female Bladder with Elevated Pelvis" which became known as the "Kelly open air" method of cystoscopy.

In 1867, Julius Bruck of Breslau devised an instrument with a platinum loop heated by electricity. In

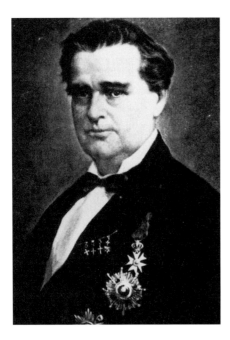

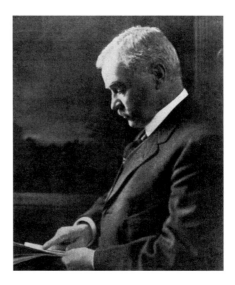

Figure 1.2 Howard Kelly. (Reproduced from the Library of the Academy of Medicine of Toronto, with permission).

Figure 1.1 J. Marion Sims (1813–1883). (Reproduced from page 7 in *Genitourinary Problems in Women*, by Jack R. Robertson, MD. Published by Charles C. Thomas Publishers, Springfield, Illinois, with permission.)

1879, Max Nitze of Berlin added a lens system designed by Leiter of Vienna to the platinum loop. In 1886, Dittel of Vienna adopted the Edison electric lamp to this type of instrument. In 1887 Nitze produced an indirect instrument with sheath and telescope [7].

In 1882, Mosso and Pellacani [8] described cystometry using a smoked drum and water manometer. Poussan [9] in 1892 proposed the concept of urethral advancement to treat stress incontinence.

Howard Kelly's active interest in the urologic phase of gynecology resulted in the inclusion of female urology as an integral part of the Gynecological Department at the Johns Hopkins Hospital. James Brown was the first Chief of Urology at Hopkins. To Dr. Guy L. Hunner fell the lot of healing this subdivision of the Gynecologic Department and his contributions were numerous [7].

Present

Twentieth Century [10]

Reviewing the past century of progress in a new subspecialty entitled Urogynecology and

Reconstructive Pelvic Surgery (URPS) is a daunting task. The quotation that best summarizes this period is the opening sentence from Charles Dickens, *A Tale of Two Cities*, which says: "It was the best of times, it was the worst of times". It was the best of times because undoubtedly we have made tremendous progress in this burgeoning new field; however, it was also the worst of times because of the politics of the female pelvis, where we have had urologists, gynecologists and now, more recently urogynecologists, surgeons and colorectal surgeons, arbitrarily dividing the female pelvis for political, financial and turf reasons, the end result of which is that we have done women a tremendous disservice by fractioning health care for women with pelvic floor disorders.

The politics of the pelvis can be well illustrated by the drawing (Figure 1.3) from the excellent article by Louis Wall and John Delancey on the "politics of the pelvis", showing the territorial imperatives that work on the pelvic floor. This issue is further shown by the cartoon, which shows two surgeons, one saying, "Gee that was close, an inch either way and I would have been out of my specialty."

Voltaire (1694–1788), the French philosopher of the Age of Enlightenment said, "these truths are not for all men, nor for all times". Alphonse Karr (1808–1890), the French critic and novelist, in 1849

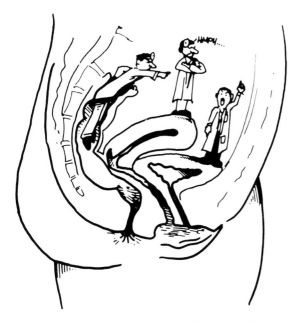

Figure 1.3 Politics of the Pelvis. Territorial imperatives at work on the pelvic floor. A gynecologist, a urologist, and a colorectal surgeon quarrel with each other while ignoring the common ground on which they all stand. (Wall and Delancey (1991) Perspec Biol Med, 34:486–96, University of Chicago Press, with permission.)

wrote "plus ça change, plus c'est la même chose" (the more things change, the more they stay the same). These statements reflect the fact that some of the practices that became ensconced in twentieth-century practice may not withstand the scrutiny of true evidence-based medicine.

A century ago, four main types of treatment for stress urinary incontinence were outlined:

1. Injection of paraffin into the region of the urethra.
2. Massage and electricity.
3. Torsion of the urethra.
4. Advancement of the external urethral meatus.

Almost a hundred years later we are still trying to identify the best bulking agent for periurethral injections, and although it is no longer paraffin we have yet to prove that Teflon, silicone, collagen and/or autologous fat is the best agent.

In 1911, Howard Kelly summarized the known operations that would correct urinary incontinence.

1. Puncture of the bladder and insertion of a catheter.
2. Close the urethra and create a vesicoabdominal fistula.

3. Close the vagina and create a rectovaginal fistula.
4. Simple compression of the urethra by anterior colporrhaphy.
5. Periurethral injection of paraffin.
6. Advancement of the urethral meatus to the clitoris.

Kelly suggested that "the torn or *relaxed* tissues of the vesical neck should be sutured together using two or three mattress sutures of fine silk linen passed from side to side" and reported an initial 80% success rate.

It soon became apparent that anterior colporrhaphy often did not produce long-term results, which led to the evolution of sling procedures. Three Europeans pioneered sling operations: (1) in 1910, Gobell suggested transplantation of the pyramidalis muscle: (2) in 1914 Frankenheim recommended the pyramidalis be attached to strips of the rectus muscle; (3) in 1917 Stoeckel suggested combining the Gobell and Frankenheim procedures with plication of the vesical neck.

Further sling variations included those by Giordano, 1907, who suggested the gracilis muscle be wrapped around the urethra' and Souier, 1911, who recommended that the levator ani muscles be placed between the vagina and the urethra. In 1923 Thompson recommended the use of strips of rectus muscle in fascia in front of the pubic bones and underneath the urethra. In 1929, Martius described the bulbocavernosus muscle fat pad graft which we continue to use today.

In 1923 Victor Bonney (Figure 1.4) stated: "Incontinence depends in some way upon a sudden and abnormal displacement of the urethra and urethrovesical junction immediately behind the symphysis".

In 1924, B. P. Watson, originally from Edinburgh and latterly at the university of Toronto' stated: "So far as the incontinence of urine is concerned, the important sutures are those which overlap the fascia at the neck of the bladder and so restore it to its normal position". He reported 65.7% cure rate, 21.9% improvement, and 12.4% failure rate.

A landmark in genitourinary surgery occurred in 1949 when Marshall, Marchetti and Krantz (MMK) published their paper on "The correction of stress incontinence by simple vesicourethral suspension". They suggested that "this operation was particularly valuable for patients whose first procedure failed". In their first 44 patients they described 82% excellent results, 7% improvement and 11% failure.

In 1950 H.H. Fouracre Barns described the round ligament sling operation for stress incontinence, which was also popularized by Paul Hodgkinson.

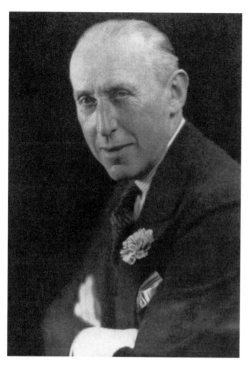

Figure 1.4 Victor Bonney. (Reproduced from the Library of the Academy of Medicine of Toronto, with permission.)

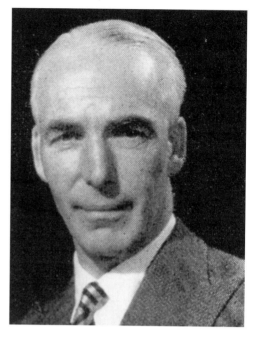

Figure 1.5 Norman Jeffcoate. (Reproduced from the Library of the Academy of Medicine of Toronto, with permission.)

In the twentieth century dramatic leaps forward were made in diagnostic procedures. In 1939, Lewis introduced the use of an aneroid barometer for cystometry. In 1952, Jeffcoate (Figure 1.5) and Roberts introduced the concept of radiographic changes in the posterior urethrovesical angle. In 1953, Hodgkinson (Figure 1.6) described lateral bead chain cystography to identify the posterior urethrovesical angle. In 1956 Bailey in England described seven variations in the urethrovesical angle, and this concept was further modified in 1962 by Tom Green in the United States who described Green type I and type II incontinence.

The concept of uroflowmetry was introduced by Von Garrelts in 1956. In 1964, Enhorning, Miller and Hinman combined cystometry with radiographic screening of the bladder. In 1969, Brown and Wickham described the concept of urethral pressure profilometry. Another landmark occurred in 1971, when Patrick Bates, Sir Richard Turner-Warwick and Graham Whiteside introduced synchronous-cine-pressure-flow cystography, with pressure and flow studies, and so the field of videourodynamics came into its own.

In 1974, James, Flack, Caldwell and Smith introduced the Urilos monitor for evaluation pelvic floor

dampness and determining whether or not the fluid was urine. In 1975, Asmussen and Ulmsten described the use of microtip transducers for measuring urethral closure pressures. In 1981, Sutherst, Brown and Shawer introduced the pad-weighing test as an objective measurement of the severity of urinary incontinence.

A landmark contribution was made by Goran Enhorning, who in 1961 suggested that "Surgical treatment for stress incontinence is probably mainly beneficial because it restores the neck of the bladder and the upper part of the urethra to the influence of intra-abdominal pressure". This laid the foundation for the concept of pressure-transmission ratios and the idea that successful operations for stress incontinence work by restoring the urethrovesical junction to an intra-abdominal position.

By 1956, Jeffcoate had attempted to caution gynecologists, stating the "the absence of the posterior urethrovesical angle is merely a sign of incompetence of the internal sphincter. The presence of an angle is a function of the involuntary muscle at the urethrovesical junction, not the muscle of the pelvic floor", and so the simplistic approach of static cystourethrograms began to be questioned. Green had attempted to simplify radiographic diagnosis into

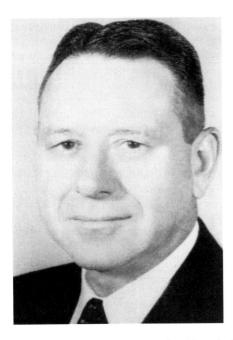

Figure 1.6 Charles Paul Hodgkinson. (Reproduced from the Library of the Academy of Medicine of Toronto, with permission.)

type I' which he suggested could be repaired with anterior colporrhaphy, and type II stress incontinence, which required a retropubic urethropexy. In the unit in Toronto, Drutz showed the limited accuracy of static cystourethrograms and this work was confirmed by numerous other investigators.

In 1959, Jim Low, originally at the University of Toronto and subsequently at Queens University in Kingston, Ontario' proposed the concept of barium paste to further identify the urethrovesical junction and he felt that this technique improved "demonstration of the precise anatomical defect in the closure mechanism of the urethra".

In 1961, John Burch first reported on his modification of the MMK procedure and described a retropubic colpourethropexy using the anterolateral aspects of the vault of the vagina and the bladder neck and elevating them to Cooper's ligament. Burch recognized the potential complication of his procedure when done by itself, as the recurrence or creation of rectocele, enterocele, uterine or vault prolapse. He listed ventral hernia and vesicovaginal fistula as potential complications.

In 1963, Paul Hodgkinson described the concept of detrusor dyssynergia, a term later referred to as the unstable bladder and more recently as the overactive bladder. Hodgkinson recognized the importance of discovering and treating this condition prior to undertaking any surgery for so-called stress urinary incontinence.

In 1968, John Chassar Moir introduced the concept of the gauze hammock operation as a modification of the Aldridge sling procedure described in 1942. Chassar Moir recognized that "Operations of this type do no more (although no less) than support the bladder neck and vesicourethral junction and so prevent the undue descent of the parts when the woman strains of coughs".

The more things change, the more they stay the same.

By the 1970s Hodgkinson advocated the operative failures in the treatment of stress urinary incontinence involved mainly three areas:

1. Incorrect diagnosis and the fact that bladder instability may have been the cause of the incontinence and not simple stress incontinence.
2. That the wrong operation may have been chosen and that some operations gave better long-term results than others.
3. The concept of technical failure, in that an appropriate operation may have been chosen, but was not performed technically well and/or the wrong suture material may have been used.

Therefore, by the 1970s genitourinary surgeons began to recognize that the vaginal approach to primary stress incontinence probably gave less than 50% success rates whereas the suprapubic approach gave success rates more commonly in the 80% or higher range. Consequently, gynecologists began to question the old adage: "Do vaginal plastic procedure first; if this fails go from above". In 1973, J. E. Morgan introduced indications for primary retropubic urethropexy: minimal pelvic floor relaxation; chronic chest disease; occupations involving lifting; patients who were heavily involved in athletics that often caused incontinence; and obesity.

In the 1970s urologists and gynecologists made a major move towards endoscopic bladder neck suspensions, with variations on the theme being basically those of Pereyra, Raz and Stamey; numerous other variations such as Gittes, Cobb – Raagde etc. appeared in the literature. By the 1990s urologists have recognized that the long-term results of these endoscopic bladder neck procedures have not provided the enduring results that were initially cited.

The more things change, the more they stay the same.

The 1990s have brought tremendous advances in the role of minimally invasive techniques. The Americans have shown a significant interest in the use of bone anchoring devices as "stabilizing" procedures. The long-term durability of these procedures needs to be determined.

Future

At the dawn of the twenty-first century and a new millennium, the obvious question is "Where do we go from here?" We feel that the main fields of activity and responsibility for urogynecologists and reconstructive pelvic surgeons (URPS) will fall into the following seven areas:

1. Education
2. Surgery
3. Uropharmacology
4. Neurophysiology
5. Bahaviour modification
6. Collagen
7. Ultrasound and other new technologies

Education

In education we must set international standards for what constitutes acceptable postgraduate training in URPS. We need increasing dialogue, not monologue, between urologists, gynecologists, and colorectal surgeons. We need more interaction between international societies such as the International Urogynecological Association (IUGA) and the International Continence Society (ICS). We need strong national societies to collaborate with these international societies who in turn can influence groups such as the Federation International of Gynecology and Obstetrics (FIGO) and the World Health Organization (WHO).

With our colleagues in obstetrics and gynecology, endocrinology, rheumatology, and cardiology we must emphasize the fact that menopause research does not just involve general menopause symptoms, osteoporosis, and cardiovascular disease, but also the role of urogenital aging.

We need to work to dispel myths of primary health care providers that incontinence is an inevitable part of aging and that nothing can be done to help it, or that all patients will require surgery. We need to review our undergraduate medical school curricula to ensure that primary care physicians can manage common genitourinary problems such as the use of pessaries for supporting pelvis floor weakness.

We must educate other health care workers about the prevalence of incontinence as a health care problem, and we need to train continence nurse supervisors who in turn will train other colleagues in the management of both the institutionalized and non-institutionalized patient with urinary and/or fecal incontinence. We have to create effective continuing medical education (CME) events to disseminate this knowledge to health care providers.

The lay population, individual families and caregivers need to be educated about the prevalence of incontinence. We have to work with the media to promote education, and we must attempt to gain government and international support to reach these goals. Urinary incontinence is now the commonest cause of admission to long-term institutionalized centers in the United States and Canada. We must show the lay population that diapers for adults are not a treatment for urinary incontinence. Urogynecology societies (both national and international) must play a pivotal role in this process.

We need to educate government and health care providers about just how expensive a health care problem incontinence is. In 1995, estimates in the US were $26.5 billion per year or $3565.00 per individual older than 65 years. About 50% of these costs are drawn from the economy to diagnose, treat, care for, and rehabilitate patients with urinary incontinence. These costs are increasing rapidly [11]:

1984	$3.94 billion
1993	$10.12 billion
1995	$12.53 billion

Surgery

Within the field of surgery in urogynecology and reconstructive pelvic surgery (URPS) we must honestly evaluate what we do. Over 200 operations have been described for the treatment of stress urinary incontinence. Therefore we must design randomized controlled trials (RCT), which will undoubtedly require multicentered studies in order to have sample sizes large enough to give valid power to the studies. These studies should have a minimum of 2-year, and preferably 5-year, follow-up periods before any valid conclusions can be drawn. Evaluation of these studies must include quality of life assessment and cost effectiveness analysis.

Uropharmacology

Within the field of uropharmacology, we must work with pharmaceutical companies to create more selective drugs for lower urinary tract disorders. Future research on drugs for the overactive bladder (OAB) will look at central nervous system (CNS) drugs that stimulate γ-aminobutyric acid (GABA) receptors. Potentially, drugs that affect GABA, opioid, 5-hydroxytryptamine (serotonin), norepinephrine, dopamine, and glutamic acid receptors and mechanisms can be developed, but a selective action on the lower urinary tract (LUT) maybe difficult to obtain [12].

Peripheral targets or research will include muscarine receptors, adrenoreceptors, tachykinins and vanilloid receptors, prostanoids, and drugs that act to inhibit calcium influx or potassium channel openers [12].

Well-designed prospective RCTs, with placebo groups of sufficient size to produce meaningful data are required in all future drug studies, and need also to be done with respect to the effectiveness of bulking agents.

Neurophysiology

The role of neurophysiologic testing in the evaluation of pelvic floor disorders needs to be clarified. What has happened is that these studies have become an either all or nothing type of situation, where is some centers all patients are evaluated with neurophysiologic testing and in others none of these modalities is available. We need well-designed research to determine whether or not pudendal terminal motor nerve latency (PMTNL) testing is a meaningful predictor of success or failure of an incontinence and/or prolapse operation. Additionally, we need to establish the role of anorectal manometry, defecography, electromyographic studies and ultrasound in the evaluation of fecal incontinence and/or rectal prolapse. Furthermore the use of MRI scanning and other imaging techniques in the diagnosis and evaluation of pelvic floor disorders must be scientifically established as to whether or not they are practical and cost-effective methods of assessment.

Behaviour Modification

We need RCTs with long-term follow-up to assess the effectiveness of functional electrical stimulation (FES), vaginal cones, urethral plugs and other devices now being recommended to treat urinary incontinence and other pelvic floor disorders. We need to convince government and other health-care providers that funding for behavior modification techniques is as important as paying for surgical procedures or other treatments that may not be that highly effective.

Collagen

We need to define the role of collagen in pelvic floor disorders in women. We need effective qualitative and quantitative assays to determine whether or not there are defects of specific types of collagen in patients with these disorders, and we need research to determine whether or not there are potential genetic markers that may be screened by blood testing to identify women who genetically may be at risk for pelvic floor prolapse. We need to look at collagen in is relationship to estrogen and the general effects of urogenital aging to see whether or not these are independent factors.

Ultrasound and Other New Techniques

There will undoubtedly be an increasing use of ultrasonography in the evaluation of the anatomic defects of stress urinary incontinence (SUI) and other pelvic floor disorders. Progress in this field has been hampered by a lack of standardization in urogynecologic sonography. The German Association of Urogynecology has attempted to make recommendations for standardization of methodology. The fact that different methods are used, such as abdominal, perineal, introital, vaginal and rectal has further impeded progress in this field. Recently intraurethral ultrasonography has shown that sphincter measurements can be a prognostic factor in patients who underwent SUI operations. Recently 5 MHz three-dimensional ultrasonography of the urethra has been used to investigate urethral sphincter damage. Doppler and color studies may play an increasing role in the evaluation of urethrovesical disorders.

New directions will evaluate the practicality of fiberoptic catheters and will look at micromotion detection, mathematical equations, and intravesical sensors.

Conclusions

At the ICS (International Continence Society) meeting in Boston in 1986, Sir Richard Turner-Warwick defined the urogynecologist as "neither the general urologist nor the general obstetrician and gynecologist, but someone who has special, training and expertise in genitourinary problems in women". Recently we expanded this definition to include urogynecology and reconstructive pelvic surgery [10]. Such a physician implies "a surgeon with specialized training in the conservative and surgical management of women with urinary and/or fecal incontinence, persistent genitourinary complaints and disorders of pelvic floor supports".

As the French writer Marcel Proust said, "We must never be afraid to go too far, for the truth lies beyond". Thus we must accept that the truths we identify today may well have to be changed in the future. However, if we work collaboratively to produce well-designed scientific research, we should be able to produce evidence-based medicine that will stand the test of time.

In an editorial published in the *International Urogynecology Journal* about "Urogynecology and reconstructive pelvic surgery: alive and well and growing in Canada" I (HPD) drew a conclusion which reflects the philosophy behind this textbook: "We have come a long way, we have only just begun".

References

1. Fischer I. Geschichte Der Gynakologie, in Halban-Seitz: Biologie Und Pathologie des Weibes, Vol. 1. Berlin and Vienna: Urban & Schwarzenberg, 1924.
2. Luring HLE. Du uber die medicinischen Kentnisse der alten Aegypter berichtenden Papyri. Leipzig, 1880.
3. Miller G. European influences in colonial medicine. CIBA Symposia 1947;510–21.
4. Garrison FH. History of Medicine, 4th edn. Philadelphia: Saunders, 1929;507–10.
5. Bozzini P. Journal der praktischen Heilkunde. Berlin: Hufeland, 1806.
6. Segalas PS. Traité des rétentions d'urine et les maladies qu'elles produisent, suivi d'un grand nombre d'observations. Paris: Mequignon-Marvis, 1898.
7. Everett HS. History of female urology. In: Youssef AF, editor, Gynecological Urology Springfield, IL: Charles C. Thomas, 1960; 5–14.
8. Mosso A, Pellacani P. Sur les functions de la vessie. Arch Ital Biol 1882;1:97.
9. Poussan. Arch Clin Bord 1892; No. 1.
10. Drutz HP. The first century of urogynecology and reconstructive pelvic surgery: where do we go from here? Int Urogynecol J 1996;7:348–353. [Contains references for the 'Present' and 'Conclusions' sections of this chapter.]
11. Wagner TH Hu TW. Economic costs of urinary incontinence in 1995. Urology 1998;51:355–61.
12. Andersson KE. The overactive bladder: pharmacologic basis of drug treatment. Urology 1997; 50(Suppl 6A):74–84.

2 Prevalence of Urinary Incontinence, Pelvic Organ Prolapse and Anal Incontinence in Women

Donna M. Fedorkow

Introduction

Typically defined, burden of illness involves the determination of levels of mortality and morbidity. Urogynecologic and related disorders rarely pose a life-threatening illness. However, they often result in significant morbidities. The relevant morbidities have been characterized by Fletcher et al. as the five D's [1]. These are disease (frequency), discomfort, disability, dissatisfaction and destitution (the financial cost of illness). Measures of morbidity must therefore include the full range of manifestations of disease that would be considered important.

Measuring Disease Frequency

The prevalence of a condition is the number of cases of a given condition that exists at a particular time. It is one of the two commonly used evaluations of disease frequency. The other is incidence, which refers to the risk of a condition developing during a defined period of time. In mathematical terms, the prevalence is equal to the incidence multiplied by the duration of the disease [2]. Prevalence data are derived primarily from non-experimental cross-sectional survey design methods. The quality of the estimates produced by such surveys depends upon several factors. These include, the study population, the method for subject selection, the method for data collection and the response rates for those subjects. If these issues are not considered and identified, bias and/or random error may result [3]. Bias refers to a systematic deviation from the true value of a variable, such that the generated value of that variable is distorted in a consistent over- or underestimation. Random error, on the other hand, is a non-systematic deviation of the true value of

the variable. Deviation due to random error can increase or decrease the estimated value of an individual measurement. The effective random error is that the over- and underestimates serve to increase the variability of the variable, but does not affect the value of the variable.

Data from specialized urogynecologic centers, while providing a good estimate of prevalence from their referral populations, probably cannot be used to make inferences about the general population. The estimate provided by the tertiary care center sample will more than likely result in an overestimate of the overall prevalence (a biased estimate). Ideally, in order to interpret prevalence rates, it is necessary to define the denominator (What is the population?). The denominator of a rate should include the population or sample of that population relevant to the question being asked. It is important not to generalize beyond the confines of the population under study.

Equally important in the interpretation of the measure of frequency is the definition of the numerator (the case). It is necessary to know the basis on which a case is defined as the criteria used can strongly influence the rate generated.

In any prevalence study, the subjects should be ideally a random sample of all eligible subjects. This implies that every individual has an equal probability of being selected. The method of "random" selection (phone book, electoral records, etc.) may influence the characteristics of the sample group. More often, a selected sample is chosen. Such a practice is acceptable so long as it understood to whom the results apply.

The study of chronic conditions which often do not come to the attention of specialists or primary care givers can result in an underestimate of prevalence. Urogynecologic and related disorders often go unreported and undetected. Information regarding their prevalence can only be garnered by population-based surveys. Additionally, many such conditions are managed conservatively either by the patient herself or in a primary care setting and may not allow identification in many research strategies.

Similarly, a research question which is too inclusive may generate a prevalence that is an overestimate of the true burden of illness. For example, a question such as "have you ever experienced an incontinence episode?", should exact a 100% prevalence rate as there are no newborns who are born continent. In order to have relevance, such questioning should have an ability to identify clinical relevant problems.

In any measurement, a large proportion of nonresponders may lead to a biased estimate. This could represent either an over- or underestimate of the true prevalence.

The inclusion of individuals suffering from an acute illness may overestimate the prevalence. Brocklehurst et al. [4] found that of the patients who became incontinent following cerebrovascular accident, 41% has spontaneous resolution of their incontinent symptoms within two weeks. To include this group in an estimate of chronic incontinence would be an overestimate of the true clinical burden.

Other issues which need to be addressed when considering prevalence include the reliability and validity of the measurement. Reliability refers to the ability of the measurement tool under question to generate the same results in different situations, while validity addresses the measurement tools' ability to assess what is intended [5].

Physical and Psychological Burdens of Illness

In addressing the burden of illness, three strata need to be considered. These are, the affected individuals, their care givers and society in general [6]. Burden of illness can also be categorized as avoidable or unavoidable [7]. Avoidable burden includes those symptoms or morbidities for which effective intervention exists, while unavoidable burden refers to symptoms or morbidities for which no effective intervention exists.

As with many chronic conditions, clinical significance is based on the viewpoint of the individual and those associated with the individual. Without a perception of a clinically significant problem, the condition probably does not warrant assessment and treatment [6]. Many sufferers,

however, fail to seek appropriate evaluation or investigation for clinically relevant disease.

Many evaluations of burden have focused on specific aspects of illness such as physical or psychological burdens.

Physical burdens have been studied in the context of urinary incontinence more than other urogynecologic or related problems. Physical burdens cited include skin rashes, breakdown pressure sores and urinary tract infection [8]. In addition, falls with their associated risk of bone fracture, could result from wet floors or a sense of urgency to reach the toilet [9]. With treatment the above burdens can be avoided.

As with physical burdens, psychological impact has received more attention with respect to urinary incontinence. The psychological impact of urinary incontinence is dependent upon attitude and general health. Urinary incontinence implies an indignity to the social integrity of the individual [10]. A sequence of events may occur involving fear, shame or embarrassment [11].

The psychological characteristic of patients with urinary incontinence have been assessed [12]. Those individuals with detrusor instability have been shown to have more somatic manifestations with anxiety than any other group, as measured in descriptive as well as case-controlled studies. It is, however, unclear whether this represents a cause or effect.

Norton attempted to quantify the psychological impact of urinary incontinence in an outpatient group of tertiary care patients [13]. She developed a disease-specific questionnaire. Her conclusions that incontinence predisposed to diminished social and mental well-being, sexual difficulties and embarrassment, although interesting, are difficult to interpret as the measurement has not undergone any validity or reliability testing.

A further study designed to look at the number of incontinence episodes per week and the quantity of fluid lost in relation to Norton's questionnaire demonstrated little correlation between the number of episodes (R = 0.06) and the fluid loss (R = 0.23). This study of highly motivated, well-educated, middle-class women showed that self-perception and daily activities were affected to a greater extent than social interactions [14]. These results, however, cannot be generalized to include all incontinent women.

The Incontinent Stress Questionnaire (ISQ-P) was developed at the Pennsylvania State University for the evaluation of the psychologic impact of urinary incontinence in an institutionalized geriatric population [15]. The scale was developed from many items, resulting in a 20-item scale. Internal consistency was determined using an appropriate statistical analysis [16]. The reliability of the measurement was assessed using the test–retest reliability, which is a measure of the stability of the measurement over time [17]. The preliminary analysis indicated that patients demonstrated motor retardation and agitated symptoms, as well as feelings of abandonment, and showed somatic concerns associated with the urinary incontinence as related to accepted measurement scales [15].

The York Incontinence Perception Scale (YIPS) is another domain-specific tool focusing on the psychological aspects of urinary incontinence [18]. The 26-item scale was used to evaluate community-dwelling women in Toronto, Ontario, measuring the influence of urinary incontinence on a person's ability to participate in activities. The study demonstrated a positive psychosocial impact of their treatment regimen when compared to non-treatment controls.

Care givers, whether family or professionals, are adversely affected when caring for incontinent individuals. Care givers are most often involved with incontinent individuals because of another affliction which has rendered the individuals incapable of managing their incontinence themselves. Noelker demonstrated a perceived care burden, doubts about care giving and reported negative effects on family and other social relationships on the part of the family care giver [19]. Urinary incontinence has been identified as a frequent reason for institutionalization among the elderly [11]. Although most studies have not adequately addressed the relative influence of urinary incontinence on admission to long-term care facilities, it has been cited along with confusion and difficulties in ambulation as one of the three main precipitators [19–21]. Furthermore, family members often regard an incontinent individual as a source of stress and economic concern [21].

Once institutionalized, patient care may be influenced by incontinence. Nurses often have negative feelings towards urinary incontinence that can be displaced to the incontinent person [20–22]. Spiro has identified the increased level of care required for the care of incontinent people (changing wet clothing and bed linen, and the care of decubitus ulcers) as a source of frustration to the nursing staff [23]. In a survey of 156 professional health care givers in a long-term care facility, Yu et al. found that over 50% of the staff felt frustrated, tired, discouraged and irritable over having to look after patients with incontinence [15]. Additionally, one third expressed guilt at their negative feelings towards their patients.

Presently interest has focused on the development of refined quality of life measurement tools.

Health-related quality of life (HRQL) tools have been developed to measure individuals' physical, social and emotional status as well as their overall life satisfaction. These skills can be generic or condition specific. Generic tools are designed to assess the HRQL across a wide range of health conditions. Such tools can be used not only to assess the impact of a particular disease on a population, but to compare the impact of different disease states and different populations. Condition-specific instruments are designed to determine the impact of a particular condition, such as urinary incontinence [24].

Generic tools which have been used in the study of urogynecologic disorders include the Nottingham Health Profile (NHP) [25], Sickness Impact Profile (SIP) [26], and the Short Form-36 (SF-36) [27].

Naughton and Wyman used the NHP to compare women with urinary incontinence to age-matched controls [25]. They found that there is considerable variability among individuals in their perceptions and responses to urinary symptoms.

A study of 36 community-living women used the SIP to characterize the impact of urinary incontinence on HRQL and found that the impact of urinary incontinence on everyday behavior is age and symptom dependent [26].

These nonspecific tools, although effective, are often cumbersome to administer and require that women focus on the disease under discussion.

In 1992, the SF-36, a generic HRQL tool, was published [27]. Since then it has been expanded through the International Quality of Life Assessment Project [28]. This questionnaire has gained popularity because of it ease of administration and its ability to compare HRQL impact between disease states, as well as monitoring effect of treatment [27]. The SF-36 has been used to study many conditions and now hosts its own website [28]. Sand et al. have used this scale to assess the efficacy of transvaginal electrostimulation in treating genuine stress urinary incontinence [29]. They did not find a difference in the change of SF-36 scores between the treatment and control groups. Kutner et al. have used the SF-36 scale to investigate variations in older adults' perceived health and functioning [30]. They found that depressive symptomatology and ambulation difficulty were related to sleep disturbance, falling and urinary incontinence.

Hopefully, such generic tools will continue to be used in urogynecologic studies.

Condition-specific tools pertaining to urogynecology include the Incontinence Impact Questionnaire (IIQ), Urogenital Distress Inventory (UDI) [31], and the Kings Health Questionnaire [32].

The IIQ is a 30-item analogue scale which considers activities such as shopping and entertaining as well as emotions such as anger and fear, while the UDI concentrates on measuring the degree to which symptoms associated with urinary incontinence are troubling to women [31].

The Kings Health Questionnaire was developed as an HRQL to assess the quality of life of women with specific urodynamic diagnosis [32]. This 4-point analogue scoring tool measures eight different domains. These include limitations, emotional problems, sleep disturbances, and severity measurements. The questionnaire has been shown to be reliable and valid with good stability over time. This is a relatively recent questionnaire which shows great promise. With wider application, the generalized ability of the tool should be established.

HRQL is an important measurement in evaluating urogynecologic disorders and treatment. Their increased use can only help in our understanding of the related conditions.

Economics

The Consensus Development Conference on Urinary Incontinence in Adults (1990) has stated that a highly conservative estimate of the national direct costs of managing urinary incontinence in the community is US$7 billion annually in the United States [8]. The additional direct costs of institutionalized patients have been reported by the same group to be approximately US$3.3 billion annually [8].

Little information on the health care sector costs of urinary incontinence exists prior to 1980. Most available studies focus on the care of incontinent elderly people in nursing homes [33]. Few studies consider the community-dwelling patient. Borrie and Davidson estimated that in their chronic care center, with their prevalence of urinary incontinence (62%) and fecal incontinence (46%), the total annual costs of nursing time devoted to the care of incontinence per patient was $9771 (Canadian dollars) based on 1986 dollars [34].

Wagner and Hu performed an economic analysis on the cost of urinary incontinence (both male and female) using 1993 US dollars. They estimate that the economic costs of urinary incontinence totals US$26.3 billion or US$3565 per individual aged 65 and older with the condition. This is considerably higher than a previous estimate by Hu, when the total costs of urinary incontinence in the elderly in the USA using 1984 US dollars were estimated to exceed US$8 billion per year [35]. They estimate that this increase in costs is partly due to increases in

medical and routine care as well as the growing population of aging adults. They estimate that US$13.1 billion dollars per year go towards treating the consequences of urinary incontinence such as urinary tract infection or skin breakdown [36].

The fiscal burden to the individual with urinary incontinence involves the direct costs of urinary applications, laundry and other supplies. In some settings, the cost of diagnostic evaluation, surgery and pharmacotherapy are directly incurred by the individual. Additionally, the cost of the treatment and physical burdens may fall on the individual. Indirectly, the condition and its consequences may result in a loss of earnings by an affected individual. Precise estimates of the cost to the individual are unknown and depend upon the severity of the conditions.

Prevalence of Urinary Incontinence

Urinary incontinence is defined as the involuntary loss of urine, which is perceived to be a social and hygienic problem [37]. Many studies have been designed to estimate the prevalence of the problem. Estimates in the literature have varied from 4% to 50% [38]. This variation is explained by differences in population being sampled (denominator) and a lack of consistency in the definitions of urinary incontinence employed (numerator). Table 2.1 outlines the wide variation in definitions of urinary incontinence used in clinical studies. These differences in thresholds for identification of cases can lead to a biased estimate which can serve to over- or underestimate the true prevalence.

Mohide [6], in a review of the existing prevalence studies, provided issues to be considered in the review of such studies. She emphasized that prevalence rates varied both within and between study settings. Her conclusion was that even after critical review of the literature, it is difficult to be precise about the prevalence of urinary incontinence [6]. She provided strategies to use when reviewing prevalence studies (Table 2.2).

Table 2.1 Variety of definition of urinary incontinence used in prevalence studies

Any episode at any time
Any episode in last six months
Any episode in last year
At least once per month
At least twice per month
A problem to the patient

Table 2.2 Some issues to consider when reviewing prevalence and descriptive studies of urinary incontinence

1. Was the definition of urinary incontinence specified?
   - Was an operational level of clinical significance included?
   - Did the definition include the types or patterns or incontinence that are relevant to the population under study?
2. Was the method of sampling documented?
3. Did the study include sufficient information about the demographic and functional status of the subjects as well as relevant medical data?
4. Did the investigators describe the study setting in sufficient detail?
5. Was the data sources(s) likely to minimize underreporting?
6. Was the measurement instrument shown to have adequate scientific properties such as reliability and validity?
7. Were data collection method(s) and procedures used that would minimize or avoid biases?
8. Was a response rate of 75% or greater achieved?

Estimates based on individuals with occasional or transient incontinence episodes exceed 50% in several studies [39,40]. Yarnell et al. reported on 1060 women over the age of 18 using a geographic register [41]. Overall, 45% of the participants claimed to have had at least one incontinent episode during adult life. Of the groups reporting incontinence, only 5.6% reported urine leakage sufficient to wet clothing with a frequency of at least once per week. This group represents 2.3% of the total sample surveyed [41].

The prevalence of urinary incontinence in community-dwelling women over 60 years of age was reported by Doikno et al. as 37.7% [42]. The definition of urinary incontinence used was any uncontrolled loss occurring in the previous 12 months without regard to severity. However, considering the number of days with urine loss, 145 of the 1150 patients surveyed (12.6%) experienced involuntary urinary loss on 50 or more days in the studied year.

A report of community women by Jolleys [43] found that 343 of 833 women surveyed (41%) had at least one episode of incontinence. Forty-eight (5.8%) of the total sample needed to wear protection against leakage.

From this information, it is apparent that if individuals with transient incontinence are included and not identified, the overall estimate of prevalence may be exaggerated. This suggests that studies that do not define a measurement of clinically relevant incontinence run the risk of an overestimated prevalence.

Thom, in a systematic review of the literature using strict definitions for inclusion, stratified the prevalence data by frequency of incontinence episodes [38]. He limited the review to the community population-based studies and stratified for frequency and age (Table 2.3). Intuitively, one would expect prevalence to decrease with increasing definitions of severity. This appears to be borne out in younger women. However, this trend is less

Table 2.3 Aggregate prevalence of urinary incontinence in population-based studies

Frequency of incontinence	No. of studies	Range (%)	Aggregate prevalence
Women >50 years:			
Ever	7	16.8–50.7	24.3 (23.4–25.3)
1+ /year	4	16.9–49.6	36.2 (34.0–38.5)
1+ /2 months	1	—	10.2 (8.3–12.4)
1+ /months	2	21.7–41.3	38.9 (37.9–39.9)
2+ /months	3	10.2–21.5	11.7 (10.5–13.0)
1+ /week	4	6.3–27	13.6 (12.4–14.9)
2+ /week	1	—	22.9 (14.9–26.1)
3+ /week	1	—	5.2 (2.9–8.0)
>1+ /day	7	5.2–16.7	11.3 (10.8–11.8)
Women <64 years:			
Ever	7	12.1–37.4	24.1 (23.4–24.8)
1+ /12 months	3	5.7–42.3	22.5 (21.0–24.1)
2+ /months	2	8.5–15.5	9.2 (8.6–9.9)
> 1+ /week	3	4.0–7.7	5.4 (4.5–6.4)

obvious from the literature addressing older women.

In 1997, a Canadian polling company conducted a telephone survey of a random and representative sample of 1500 community-dwelling adults regarding urinary incontinence [44]. The respondents were asked if they had ever been diagnosed by a physician as having urinary incontinence and whether, in the past year, they had had an involuntary loss of urine. Five percent of women surveyed had been diagnosed by a physician as having urinary incontinence. Of these, 41% reported a diagnosis of stress incontinence, 12% urgency incontinence, 15% overflow incontinence and 26% mixed incontinence. Seven percent of respondents reported an involuntary loss of urine within the previous year, translating to a prevalence of urinary incontinence of 8.8% or approximately 1.9 million Canadians. This study found that over half of the incontinent population (56%) is under 55 years of age. Only half of the respondents (55%) have ever spoken to a physician about their incontinence.

Urinary incontinence has been cited as a major reason for nursing home admission, with the American NIH Consensus Statement estimating that 50% of nursing home residents are incontinent [8]. Kralj in a review of the literature concluded that 57.2% of women living in nursing homes suffered from urinary incontinence, compared with 41.6% of elderly women residing in the community [45]. He also demonstrated an increase in prevalence with increasing age from 16% in the 20–29-year-old age group to 40% in those aged 45–64. Age as an associated variable in increasing prevalence of urinary incontinence has not been universally accepted. Jolleys [43] demonstrated a peak prevalence of 45–54 years with a gradual decrease with advancing age. Similar findings were reported by Yarnell et al. [41] and Brocklehurst et al. [46]. Doikno et al., [42] failed to find a statistical significant difference in prevalence across all age groups.

Rekers et al. [47] used a mailed questionnaire to 1920 Dutch women to assess the prevalence of incontinence. With their 68% response rate, they found that approximately 26.5% of the study population reported urinary incontinence. Although the overall prevalence of incontinence did not differ between age groups, there was a trend towards a higher proportion of women reporting larger losses in the older ages [47].

The stability of prevalence measurement has not been carefully studied. Milne and colleagues reported on 10 patients and found that only four admitted to urinary incontinence at baseline measurement and two months later [48]. The variation of self-reporting tools has been studied by Resnick et al. [49]. They found that in a structured questionnaire, self-reporting of prevalence estimates of urinary incontinence are stable over a two-week period. Some variability in the measurement may be accounted for by remission or treatment of symptoms. Nygaard and Lemke reported a remission rate for urinary incontinence of 22.1% and 25.1% at three- and six-year follow-up respectively [50]. These findings have implications when comparing studies and assessing treatments.

Because not all incontinent individuals seek medical attention, the true extent and impact of the problem are not known [8]. In a large study of patients presenting to a tertiary care referral center, 60% had delayed seeking medical help for more than one year from the onset of symptoms [51]. Half of these patients claim to be too embarrassed to approach their physician with their complaints while 17% felt that incontinence was a normal function of aging.

Similarly, Holst and Wilson, found that in a community-based group of incontinent women, 81% did not seek medical attention because they did not regard their condition as abnormal [52]. A further 10% has not sought help because of low expectations of the benefit of treatment.

The poor self-reporting of urinary incontinence was further explored by Roberts et al. in a cohort of women 50 years of age or over [53]. They found a prevalence of urinary incontinence of 49%. Of these only 13% had sought care for urinary symptoms.

The perceived impact of urinary incontinence has been addressed earlier in this chapter. However, Foldspang and Mommsen evaluated the impact of urinary incontinence on specific social interactions [54]. In their survey of 2613, women aged 30–59, they found that of the 388 women reporting urinary incontinence, 21.9% abstained from social activities because of the incontinence (Table 2.4).

The prevalence of urinary incontinence remains difficult to estimate. Available information suggests that despite prevalence rates consistently in the 10–20% range, underreporting of the condition by the patient remains a problem. A clear increase in disease prevalence with increasing age does not appear to be a consistent feature of urinary incontinence.

Prevalence of Pelvic Organ Prolapse

Pelvic organ prolapse (POP) represents a weakening of the pelvic floor which results in descended pelvic organs with downward pressure [55]. Defects are

Table 2.4 Frequency of reported abstention from social activity due to urinary incontinence

Activity	Frequency (388 women)	Percent
Work	5	1.3
Visiting friends	10	2.6
Sport	70	18.0
Shopping	13	3.4
Sexual intercourse	27	7.0

Source: Foldspang and Mommsen [54].

characterized as cystocele, urethrocele, enterocele, rectocele, and uterine prolapse depending on the organs involved. Despite the fact that POP represents the admitting diagnosis of 20% of women undergoing major abdominal surgery [56], little is known of the prevalence of the condition.

Table 2.5 outlines existing studies on the prevalence of POP in which populations and proportions could be determined. The different prevalences noted are best explained by the vastly different populations and the different endpoints studied. The majority of studies do not consider those women who do not seek treatment or who are managed conservatively and therefore would serve to underestimate the true burden.

The Oxford Family Planning Association Study represents one of the few population-based studies [57]. The authors concede that the sample differs from the general UK population in that the women at entry to the study were less likely to have chronic disease, smoke heavily, to be obese or be of lower socioeconomic class. They suspect that the 3.9% incidence seen in their group may underestimate of the true risk of prolapse. Not surprisingly the highest rate of prolapse was found in older women undergoing major gynecologic surgery.

Although the etiology of POP remains under discussion, numerous authors have noted certain trends. Strohbehn has noted that young women with prolapse have a high proportion of connective tissue

Table 2.5 Studies assessing prevalence of pelvic organ prolapse

Author	Year	Population	Proportion	Prevalence (95% CI)
Mant et al. [57]	1997	Hospital admissions, family planning clinics	597/15292	0.039 (0.036–0.042)
Kjerulff et al. [70]	1996	NIH survey	658/31617	0.021 (0.019–0.022)
Younis et al. [71]	1993	Women undergoing medical examination	258/509	0.51 (0.46–0.55)
Dudkiewicz et al. [72]	1983	Women employed in cement industry	86/218	0.39 (0.33–0.46)
Mant et al. [57]	1997	Women attending family planning clinics post-hysterectomy admissions	63/2233	0.028 (0.022–0.035)
Harris et al. [62]	1998	Nulliparous women, incontinence clinic	62/748	0.082 (0.064–0.10)
Mattox and Bhatia [65]	1996	Incontinence clinic – referrals	31/171	0.18 (0.13–0.24)
Norton et al. [60]	1995	Women attending gynecology clinic		
		Cystocele	73/106	0.69 (0.60–0.77)
		Rectocele	65/107	0.61 (0.51–0.70)
		Uterus/vault	45/107	0.42 (0.33–0.51)
Peacock et al. [64]	1994	Black women referred to urogynecologic clinic		
		Cystocele	116/159	0.73 (0.65–0.80)
		Rectocele	88/159	0.55 (0.46–0.63)
		Uterus/vault	41/159	0.26 (0.19–0.33)
Pepe et al. [73]	1988	Postmenopausal gynecologic admissions	31/330	0.094 (0.065–0.13)
Olsen et al. [61]	1997	Surgery for POP in HMO	395/149554	0.0026 (0.0024–0.0029)
Brieger et al. [74]	1996	Gynecologic surgery	578/2313	0.25 (0.23–0.27)
Naylor et al. [75]	1984	Major gynecologic surgery	841/2901	0.29 (0.27–0.31)
Jaluvka [76]	1977	Women >79 years age, major gynecologic surgery	59/662	0.089 (0.069–0.11)
Vuroma et al. [77]	1998	Hysterectomy	37409/89069	0.42 (0.42–0.42)
Luoto et al. [78]	1994	Hysterectomy	675/9000	0.075 (0.069–0.080)
Allard and Rochette [79]	1991	Women undergoing hysterectomy >50 years	4695/36107	0.13 (0.13–0.13)

disorders, congenital anomalies and neuromuscular disease compared to older women [58]. The association between joint hypermobility and genital tract prolapse was explored by Al-Rawi and Al-Rawi [59]. In their study of 76 women with a prolapse, compared to age- and parity-matched controls without prolapse, there was a statistically significant increase in joint hypermobility in those women with POP compared to those without. These findings were confirmed by Norton et al., who concluded that women with joint hypermobility have a significantly higher prevalence of POP than women with normal joint mobility [60].

Olsen et al. demonstrated that the lifetime risk of undergoing an operation for prolapse increases with increasing age to a rate of 11% by age 80 [61]. This may indicate an increased risk with advancing age or may represent a higher threshold for operating on older women with prolapse.

Although parity is often cited as an etiologic factor in the development of POP, Harris and colleagues have reported that 62 out of 748 patients (8.3%) in their sample of women with POP were nulliparous [62].

The majority of studies have not considered racial differences in the prevalence of POP. Bump, in a study of 200 consecutive referrals, found that the prevalence of severe prolapse was the same for blacks as for whites (24% and 23%) [63]. Peacock in a descriptive study of a black inner city population found prolapse rates similar to those found in a study by Norton and colleagues in a primarily white population [64]. Mattox and Bhatia compared the prevalence of prolapse in a referral group of Hispanic and white women [65]. They found that although presenting symptoms differed between the groups, ethnic group was a poor predictor of prevalence.

Prolapse and urinary incontinence problems are known to be related. Women who have severe genitourinary prolapse, although continent, may have underlying stress urinary incontinence. Benson reported that of 100 women presenting with urinary incontinence, 51 demonstrated genitourinary relaxation [66]. In a series of ten patients having complete prolapse of the genitourinary tract, with no complaints of incontinence, Richardson and colleagues found that nine (90%) were subsequently found to have sphincter weakness and incontinence following reduction of the procidentia [67]. Rosenzwerg et al. found that significant genitourinary prolapse was coupled with a 44% rate of underlying occult stress incontinence [68].

Significant POP can cause tension on the ureters resulting in hydronephrosis and, potentially, kidney damage. Beverly and colleagues have assessed 375 patients undergoing surgery for POP [69]. Thirteen

of these patients (4.0%) had mild hydronephrosis, 9 (2.8%) had moderate hydronephrosis and 3 (0.9%) had severe hydronephrosis. Not surprisingly, they found an increasing risk of hydronephrosis with increasing severity of prolapse. They concluded that the risk of hydronephrosis is real, if low, in women with POP.

The community prevalence of POP is likely in the 4–5% range of adult women. It represents a significant proportion of gynecologic surgical procedures done on women. Nulliparous women are not immune to the development of POP. To date, no obvious interracial differences have been noted. Latent stress urinary incontinence and hydronephrosis remains a concern in those individuals with severe POP and should be part of the overall evaluation.

Prevalence of Anal Incontinence

Studies assessing the prevalence of anal incontinence suffer from inconsistent and non-standardized definitions. The condition can involve the involuntary passage of gas, liquid or solid stool. The sensitive nature of the problem begets underreporting in the physician's office. Enck et al. reported that only 5% of patients with fecal incontinence will volunteer the problem [80]. The accuracy and reliability of reporting mechanisms for fecal incontinence, particularly in community-based studies, have been questioned. Resnick and colleagues have shown 90% agreement in a small telephone survey in the self-reporting of fecal incontinence [81]. This suggests that such a survey method yielded stable results over the two-week study period.

Current prevalence studies have three main foci: community-based studies, institutionalized patients, and the community-dwelling elderly,.

A loss of anal control with increasing age has been the conclusion of many community-based studies. Thomas and colleagues estimated a prevalence of fecal incontinence of 0.42% in men and 0.17% in women aged 15–64 years of age [82]. This is compared to 1.09 for men and 1.233% for women over the age of 65 years. Despite the known risk of obstetric trauma, the higher prevalence of fecal incontinence in men compared to women found by Thomas et al. was confirmed by Johanson and Lafferty, who reported that the prevalence of fecal incontinence was 1.3 times greater in men than in women [83].

The greater prevalence in men has not been confirmed in other studies. Drossman et al., in a nationally based US household survey, found a prevalence of fecal incontinence of 7.8% (424/5430). The male-to-female ratio was similar, with 7.9% (208/2639) of men and 7.7% of (215 /2791) of women reporting fecal incontinence [84]. They confirmed an increasing prevalence with increasing age. Additionally, they reported that fecal incontinence caused an average 11.7 days missed from work or school because of illness in the previous year.

A state-wide sample of 6959 individuals was undertaken by Nelson et al. in Wisconsin [85]. An overall prevalence of 2.2% across all age groups was reported. Thirty percent of positive respondents were over the age of 65 years and 63% were women.

Giebel and colleagues surveyed a select sample of Germans over 18 years of age [86]. They found that 4.8% had difficulty controlling the passage of solid stool, while close to 20% experienced difficulty in the control of liquid stools or flatus. Of those with incontinence, 8.5% reported that they use protective underclothing because of their problem.

Community-based studies provide a wide range of prevalence estimates. These differences are most likely due to differences in the definition of focal incontinence used rather than a true population-based difference in prevalence. There is a consistent trend to support an increasing prevalence of fecal incontinence with increasing age regardless of sex. The reported increased prevalence in men compared to women is not a universally appreciated finding. Additional well-designed population-based studies, using consistent definitions, are necessary before the true prevalence is known. It is apparent that those individuals suffering from fecal incontinence experience burden from their condition. These burdens include losing time from work and school. The scope of the physical, emotional and economic burden of fecal incontinence has yet to be determined.

The higher prevalence of fecal incontinence in men compared to women noted by Thomas et al., in their community-based study [82], was not borne out in their evaluation of institutionalized individuals [87]. They found, in a 1987 study of London region old people's homes, that 15.7% of male and 16.7% of female residents experienced two or more anal incontinence episodes per week. The low prevalence noted may reflect the strict definition used to identify subjects.

Johanson et al. evaluated fecal incontinence in a nursing home population [88]. They found that of the 388 residents studied, 46% were incontinent of feces. This incontinence was found to be 1.5 time more common in males than in females.

Nelson and colleagues, in a large state-wide assessment of nursing home dwellers, reported on the prevalence of fecal incontinence for 1992 and 1993 [89]. They found that in both years studied, an equal proportion of males and females were noted to have fecal incontinence. In 1992, they reported that 46.5% (2457/5285) of males and 46.5% (6014/12 939) of females had any history of fecal incontinence. The figures changed little in 1993 with 46.9% (2247/4796) of men and 45.5% (5613/12331) of women noted to have fecal incontinence.

Read and colleagues reported that constipation and fecal incontinence frequently coexist in the institutionalized elderly [90]. They cited common causes as overflow incontinence secondary to fecal impaction, with pudendal neuropathy, remote obstetric trauma and spinal disease as contributory factors. This may help explain a prevalence of at least one fecal incontinence episode per week in 30% of patients on geriatric wards reported by Barrett et al. [91].

The association between urinary and fecal incontinence in the institutionalized elderly has been reported by Ouslander and colleagues [92]. They reported that 64% of individuals with urinary incontinence had concomitant fecal incontinence. Cognitive impairment and mobility problems were identified as significant contributors to the dual incontinence. Similar findings were reported by Borrie and Davidson in 1992, with 46% of patients studied having fecal incontinence and 44% demonstrating both fecal and urinary incontinence [34].

Fecal incontinence appears to be a large problem amongst the institutionalized elderly. With the exception of the study by Thomas et al. [82], prevalence estimates are consistently in excess of one-third of the sample studied. Like the previously mentioned population-based studies, differences in prevalence between men and women are not consistent findings.

The reported prevalence of fecal incontinence in the community-dwelling elderly is, not unexpectedly, lower than that in institutions. Campbell et al. found a prevalence of 3.1% (17/559) in a random sample of subjects over 65 years of age [93]. A similar prevalence of 3.7% was found in an age- and sex-stratified random sample of non-institutionalized Olmstead County, Minnesota residents [94]. In a Japanese study of community-dwelling people aged 65 years or older, Nakanishi and colleagues found a fecal incontinence prevalence of 2.1% (30/1405) [95]. These prevalence findings are remarkably similar across cultures and nationalities. This suggests that factors relating to the aging process itself are responsible for the prevalence noted.

The above studies included both men and women in their analyses. Kok and colleagues reported on a sample of Dutch women aged 60 years and over

[96]. They found a prevalence of fecal incontinence of 4.0% (19/472) in women between 60 and 84 years of age and 17.0% (26/153) for women over the age of 85 years. This study suggests an increasing prevalence of fecal incontinence with increasing age. The findings in this women-only study demonstrate a prevalence rate very similar to that found in studies addressing the community-dwelling geriatric population of both sexes.

Fecal incontinence is a condition which has begun to receive attention from the public and medical profession. Prevalence rates are inconsistent. Much of this inconsistency has to do with a lack of standardized definitions and reporting. A consistent feature of the reported literature is an increase in prevalence with increasing age regardless of the population studied.

References

1. Fletcher RH, Fletcher SW, Wagner EH. Introduction, health outcomes. In: Satterfield TS, editor. Clinical Epidemiology – the Essentials, 3rd edn. Baltimore, MD: Williams & Wilkins, 1996; 5.
2. Fletcher RH, Fletcher SW, Wagner EH. Frequency, bias in prevalence outcomes. In: Satterfield TS, editor. Clinical Epidemiology – the Essentials, 3rd edn. Baltimore, MD: Williams & Wilkins, 1996; 85.
3. Fletcher RH, Fletcher SW, Wagner EH. Introduction, Bias. In: Satterfield TS, editor. Clinical Epidemiology – the Essentials, 3rd edn. Baltimore, MD: Williams & Wilkins, 1996; 7.
4. Brocklehurst JC, Andrews K, Richards B, Laycock PJ. Incidence and correlates of incontinence in stroke patients. J Am Geriatr Soc 1985;33:540–2.
5. Fletcher RH, Fletcher SW, Wagner EH. Abnormality, performance of measurements. In: Satterfield TS, editor. Clinical Epidemiology – the Essentials, 3rd edn. Baltimore, MD: Williams & Wilkins, 1996; 23
6. Mohide EA. The prevalence and scope of urinary incontinence. Clin Geriatr Med 1986;2:639–55.
7. Tugwell P, Bennett KJ, Sackett DL. The measurement of iterative loop: A framework for the critical appraisal of needs, benefits and costs of health interventions. J Chron Dis 1985;38:339–351.
8. Urinary Incontinence in Adults, NIH Consensus Statement (1988) Oct 3–5;7(5):1–32.
9. Ashley MF, Gryfe CI, Aimes A. A longitudinal study of falls in the elderly: II. Some circumstances of falling. Age Ageing 1977;6:211–20.
10. Wilson T. Incontinence of urine in the aged. Lancet 1948;347–77.
11. Ory MG, Wyman JF, Yu L. Psychosocial factors in urinary incontinence. Clin Geriatr Med 1986;2:657–71.
12. Drutz HP, Doody K, Gilbey P. The role of psychological screening tests in the evaluation of women with persistent lower urinary tract problems: A prospective, blinded study. Int Urogynecol J 1995;9(1):21–30.
13. Norton C. The effects of urinary incontinence in women. Int Rehabil Med 1982;4:9–14.
14. Wyman JF, Harkins SW, Choi SC, Taylor JR, Fantl JA. Psychosocial impact of urinary incontinence in women. Obstet Gynecol 1987;70:378–81.
15. Yu LC, Kaltrieder DL, Hu T, Igou JF, Craighead WE. Measuring stress associated with incontinence: The ISW-P tool. J Gerontol Nurs 1989;15:9–15.
16. Yu LC. Incontinence stress index: Measuring psychological impact. J Gerontol Nurs 1987;13:18–25.
17. Applegate WB. Use of assessment instruments in clinical settings. J Am Geriatr Soc 1987;35:45–50.
18. Roberts RO, Jacobsen SJ, Rhodes T, et al. Urinary incontinence in a community-based cohort: Prevalence and health-care-seeking. J Am Geriatr Soc 1998;46:467–72.
19. Noelker LS. Incontinence in the aged cared for by family. Gerontology 1983;23:258.
20. Patterson RL, Jackson GM. Behavioral modifications with the elderly. In: Hersen M, Eisler RM, Miller P, editors. Progress in Behavioral Modifications. Academic Press, 1980.
21. Wells T. Social and psychological implications of incontinence. In: Brocklehurst JC, editor. Urology in the Elderly. Edinburgh: Churchill Livingstone, 1984.
22. Bartol M. Psychosocial aspects of incontinence. In: Burnside I, editor. Psychosocial Nursing, McGraw Hill, 1980.
23. Spiro L. Bladder training for the incontinent patient. J Gerontol Nurs 1978;4:28–35.
24. Ware JEJ, Sherbourne CD. The MOS 36 item Short Form Health Survey (SF-36). I. Conceptual framework and item selection. Med Care 1992;30:473–83.
25. Naughton MJ, Wyman JF. Quality of life in geriatric patients with lower urinary tract dysfunction. Am J Med Sci 1997;314:219–27.
26. Hunskaar S, Vinsnes A. The quality of life in women with urinary incontinence as measured by the sickness impact profile. J Am Geriatr Soc 1991;39:378–82.
27. Ware JEJ, Sherbourne CD. The MOS 36 item Short Form Health Survey (SF-36). I. Conceptual framework and item selection. Med Care 1992;30:473–83.
28. Ware Jr JE, Gandek B. Overview of the SF-36 Health Survey and the International Quality of Life Assessment (IQOLA) Project. J Clin Epidemiol 1998;51(11):903–12.
29. Sand PK, Richardson DA, Staskin DR et al. Pelvic floor electrical stimulation in the treatment of genuine stress incontinence: A multicenter, placebo-controlled trial. Am J Obstet Gynecol 1995;173(1):72–9.
30. Kutner NG, Schechtman KB, Ory MG et al. Older adults' perceptions of their health and functioning in relation to sleep disturbance, falling and urinary incontinence. J Am Geriatr Soc 1994;42:757–62.
31. Shumaker SA, Wyman JR, Uebersax JS et al. Health related quality of life measures for women with urinary incontinence: the Incontinence Impact Questionnaire and the Urogenital Distress Inventory. Quality of Life Research 1994;3:291–306.
32. Kelleher CJ, Cardozo LD, Khullar V, Salvatore S. A new questionnaire to assess the quality of life of urinary incontinent women. Br J Obstet Gynaecol 1997;104:1374–9.
33. Ouslander JG, Kane RL. The costs of urinary incontinence in nursing homes. Med Care 1984;22:69–79.
34. Borrie MJ, Davidson HA. Incontinence in institutions: costs and contributing factors. Can Med Assoc J 1992;147(3):322–8.
35. Wagner TH, Hu T-W. Economic costs of urinary incontinence in 1995. Urology 1998;51:355–61.
36. Wagner TH, Hu T-W. Economic costs of urinary incontinence. Int Urogynecol J 1998;9:127–8.
37. Abrams P, Blavais JG, Stanton SL, Anderson JT. The standardization of terminology of lower urinary tract function recommended by the International Continence Society. Int Urogynecol J 1990;1:45–8.
38. Thom D. Variation in estimates of urinary incontinence prevalence in the community: Effects of differences in

definition, population characteristics and study type. J Am Geriatr Soc 1998;46:473–80.

39. Nemir A, Middleton RP. Stress incontinence in young nulliparous women. Am J Obstet Gynecol 1954;68:1166–8.

40. Wolin LH. Stress incontinence in young, healthy nulliparous female subjects. J Urol 1969;101:545–9.

41. Yarnell JWG, Richard CJ, Stephenson TP. The prevalence and severity of urinary incontinence in women. J Epidemiol Community Health 1981;35:71–4.

42. Doikno AC, Brock BM, Brown MB, Herzog AR. Prevalence of urinary incontinence and other urological symptoms in the non-institutionalized elderly. J Urol 1986;136:1022–5.

43. Jolleys JV. Reported prevalence of urinary incontinence in women in a general practice. Br Med J 1988;296:1300–2.

44. Angus Reid Group. Urinary incontinence in the Canadian adult population. Submitted to Veritas Communications 1997; 1–13.

45. Kralj B. Epidemiology of female urinary incontinence, classification or urinary incontinence, urinary incontinence in elderly women. Eur J Obstet Gynecol Reprod Biol 1994;55:39–41.

46. Brocklehurst JC, Dillane JB, Griffiths L, Fry L. The prevalence and symptomatology of urinary infection in an aged population. Gerontol Clin 1968;10:242–53.

47. Rekers H, Drogendijk AC, Valkenburg H, Riphagen F. Urinary incontinence in women from 35 to 79 years of age: prevalence and consequences. Eur J Obstet Gynecol Reprod Biol 1992;43:229–34.

48. Milne JS, Hope K, Williamson J. Variability in replied to a questionnaire on symptoms of physical illness. J Chron Dis 1970;22:805–10.

49. Resnick NM, Beckett LA, Branch LG, Scherr PA, Wetle T. Short-term variability of self report of incontinence in older persons. J Am Geriatr Soc 1994;42:202–7.

50. Nygaard IE, Lemke JH. Urinary incontinence in rural older women: Prevalence, incidence and remission. J Am Geriatr Soc 1996;44:1049–54.

51. Norton PA, MacDonald L, Stanton S. Distress associated with female urinary complaints and delay in seeking treatment. Neurourol Urodyn 1987;6:170–6.

52. Holst K, Wilson PD. The prevalence of female urinary incontinence and reasons for not seeking treatment. NZ Med J 1988;101:756–8.

53. Roberts RO, Jacobsen SJ, Rhodes T et al. Urinary incontinence in a community-based cohort: Prevalence and health-care seeking. J Am Geriatr Soc 1998;46:467–72.

54. Foldspang A, Mommsen S. The International Continence Society (ICS) Incontinence Definition: Is the social and hygienic aspect appropriate for etiologic research? J Clin Epidemiol 1997;50(9):1055–60.

55. Fergusson ILC. Genital prolapse. Br J Hosp Med 1981;26:67–72.

56. Cardozo L. Prolapse. In: Whitfield CR, editor. Dewhurst's Textbook of Obstetrics and Gynaecology for Postgraduates. Oxford: Blackwell Science, 1995; 642–52.

57. Mant J, Painter R, Vessey M. Epidemiology of genital prolapse: observations from the Oxford Family Planning Association study. Br J Obstet Gynaecol 1997;104:579–85.

58. Strohbehn K, Jakary, JA, Delancey JOL. Pelvic organ prolapse in young women. Obstet Gynecol 1997;90(1):33–6.

59. Al-Rawi ZS, Al-Rawi ZT. Joint hypermobility in women with genital prolapse. Lancet 1982;i:1439–41.

60. Norton PA, Baker JE, Sharp HC, Warenski JC. Genitourinary prolapse and joint hypermobility in women. Obstet Gynecol 1995;85(2):225–8.

61. Olsen AL, Smith VJ, Bergstron JO, Colling JC, Clark AL. Epidemiology of surgically managed pelvic organ prolapse and urinary incontinence. Obstet Gynecol 1997;89(4):501–6.

62. Harris RL, Cundiff GW, Coates KW, Bump RC. Urinary incontinence and pelvic organ prolapse in nulliparous women. Obstet Gynecol 1998;92(6):951–4.

63. Bump RC. Racial comparisons and contrasts in urinary incontinence and pelvic organ prolapse. Obstet Gynecol 1993;81(3):421–5.

64. Peacock LM, Wiskind AK, Wall LL. Clinical features of urinary incontinence and urogenital prolapse in a black inner-city population. Am J Obstet Gynecol 1994;171(6):1464–71.

65. Mattox TF, Bhatia NN. The prevalence of urinary incontinence or prolapse among white and Hispanic women. Am J Obstet Gynecol 1996;174(2):646–8.

66. Benson JT. The history and physical examination in women with urinary incontinence. Am Urogynecol Soc Quart Report 1989;7:1.

67. Richardson DA, Bent AE, Ostergard DR. The effects of uterovaginal prolapse on urethrovesical pressure dynamics. Am J Obstet Gynecol 1983;146:901–5.

68. Rosenzweig BA, Pushkin S, Blumenfeld D, Bhatia NN. Prevalence of abnormal urodynamic test results in continent women with severe genitourinary prolapse. Obstet Gynecol 1992;79(4):539–42.

69. Beverly CM, Walters MD, Weber AM, Piedmonte MR, Ballard LA. Prevalence of hydronephrosis in patients undergoing surgery for pelvic organ prolapse. Obstet Gynecol 1997;90(1):37–41.

70. Kjerulff KH, Erickson BA, Langenberg PW. Chronic gynecological conditions reported by US women: Findings from the National Health Interview Survey, 1984 to 1992. Am J Publ Health 1996;86(2):195–9.

71. Younis N, Khattab H, Zurayk H, el-Mouelhy M, Amin MF, Farag AM. A community study of gynecological and related morbidities in rural Egypt. Stud Fam Plann 1993;24(3):175–86.

72. Dudkiewicz J, Kaminski K, Rybczynska A. Preventative gynecologic examinations of women employed in the cement industry. Med Pr 1983;34(1):89–94.

73. Pepe F, Panella M, Pepe G, Panella P, LaSpina E, Sala C. Current aspects of gynecological pathology in post-menopause. Clin Exp Obstet Gynecol 1988;15(3):80–3.

74. Brieger GM, Yip SK, Fung YM, Chung T. Genital prolapse: A legacy of the West? Aust NZ J Obstet Gynaecol 1996;36(1):52–4.

75. Naylor AC. Hysterectomy – analysis of 2901 personally performed procedures. S Afr Med J 1984;65:242–5.

76. Jaluvka V. Major gynecological operations on women of 80 years of age or more. Arch Gynakol 1977;222(1):73–93.

77. Vuroma S, Teperi J, Hurskainen R, Keskimaki I, Kujansuu E. Hysterectomy trends in Finland in 1987–1995 – a register based analysis. Acta Obstet Gynecol Scand 1998;77(7):770–6.

78. Luoto R, Kaprio J, Keskimaki I, Pohjanlahti JP, Rutanen EM. Incidence causes and surgical methods for hysterectomy in Finland 1987–1989. Int J Epidemiol 1994;23(2):348–58.

79. Allard P, Rochette L. The descriptive epidemiology of hysterectomy, Province of Quebec, 1981–1988. Ann Epidemiol 1991;1(6):541–9.

80. Enck P, Beilefeldt K, Rathmann W et al. Epidemiology of faecal incontinence in selected patient groups. Int J Colorectal Dis 1991;6(3):143–6.

81. Resnick NM, Beckett LA, Branch LG, Scherr PA, Wetle T. Short-term variability of self report of incontinence in older persons. J Am Geriatr Soc 1994;42(2):202–7.

82. Thomas TM, Egan M, Walgrove A, Meade TW. The prevalence of faecal and double incontinence. Community Med 1984;6:216–20.

83. Johanson JF, Lafferty J. Epidemiology of fecal incontinence: the silent affliction. Am J Gastroenterol 1996;91(1):33–6.

84. Drossman DA, Li Z, Andruzzi E et al. U.S. Householder survey of functional gastrointestinal disorders. Prevalence, sociodemography, and health impact. Dig Dis Sci 1993;38(9):1569–80.

85. Nelson R, Norton N, Cautley E, Furner S. Community-based prevalence of anal incontinence. JAMA 1995;274(7):559–61.

86. Giebel GD, Lefering R, Troidl H, Blochl H. Prevalence of fecal incontinence: what can be expected? Int J Colorectal Dis 1998;13:73–7.

87. Thomas TM, Ruff C, Karran O, Mellows S, Meade TW. Study of the prevalence and management of patients with faecal incontinence in old people's homes. Community Med 1987;9(3):232–7.

88. Johanson JF, Irizarry F, Doughty A. Risk factors for fecal incontinence in a nursing home population. J Clin Gastroenterol 1997;24(3):156–60.

89. Nelson R, Furner S, Jesudason V. Fecal incontinence in Wisconsin nursing homes. Dis Colon Rectum 1998;41:1226–9.

90. Read NW, Celik AF, Katsinelos P. Constipation and incontinence in the elderly. J Clin Gastroenterol 1995;20(1):61–70.

91. Barrett JA, Brocklehurst JC, Kiff ES, Ferguson G, Faragher EB. Anal function in geriatric patients with faecal incontinence. Gut 1989;30:1244–51.

92. Ouslander JG, Kane RL, Abrass IB. Urinary incontinence in elderly nursing home patients. JAMA 1982;248(10):1994–8.

93. Campbell AJ, Reinken J, McCosh L. Incontinence in the elderly: prevalence and prognosis. Age Ageing 1985;14(2):65–70.

94. Talley NJ, O;Keefe EA, Zinsmeister AR, Melton LJ 3rd. Prevalence of gastrointestinal symptoms in the elderly: a population-based study. Gastroenterology 1992;102(3):895–901.

95. Nakanishi N, Tatara K, Naramura H et al. Urinary and fecal incontinence in a community-residing older population in Japan. J Am Geriatr Soc 1997;45:215–19.

96. Kok ALM, Voorhorst FJ, Burger CW et al. Urinary and faecal incontinence in community-residing elderly women. Age Ageing 1992;21:211–15.

2 Anatomy, Physiology and Neurophysiology

3 Anatomy of the Pelvic Floor

Richard J. Scotti, George Lazarou and Wilma Markus Greston

Anatomy is to pelvic surgery as vocabulary is to language: The more detailed one's knowledge is in anatomy, the more fluent and facile one becomes in the operating room.

Introduction

A knowledge of the anatomy of the pelvis is essential to the education of all obstetrician-gynecologists, especially those engaged in reconstructive and urogynecologic surgery. Indeed, with the exception of the brain and cranial base, the anatomy of the pelvis is perhaps the most complicated in the body, since lying within it, passing through it, attaching to it, and bifurcating or synapsing within it are multiple muscles, nerves, vessels and organs which support the important functions of ambulation, reproduction, sexuality and elimination of liquid and solid waste. Considering these diverse activities, it is astounding how wonderfully compact and functionally streamlined the human pelvis actually is! Since there are so many structures within the pelvic cavity, operating within it carries certain risks, as the pelvic surgeon attempts to restore anatomy while respecting the structures which support these diverse functions.

Since form follows function, the urogynecologic/reconstructive pelvic surgeon needs to consider both anatomic and functional components. Preoperatively, intraoperatively and postoperatively, these components can be measured by various functional (urodynamic, anal physiologic, neurophysiologic, etc.) tests and anatomic (site specific assessment, urethral axis determination imaging studies, etc.) outlined in other chapters of this text. The responsible pelvic surgeon also must be willing to retest anatomic and functional variables postoperatively to ensure that the anatomic correction(s)

have not compromised function of the various structures in the pelvis.

The goal of this chapter is to discuss anatomy in a very simple and practical way, i.e., how it relates to function and how to negotiate the anatomy in order to optimally execute urogynecologic and pelvic surgical procedures without compromising other anatomic structures or their functions. For more detailed anatomy, the reader is referred to the excellent resources cited in the references.

Although pelvic anatomic structures had been described by Andreas Vesalius [1], who performed meticulous dissections categorizing and labeling each structure, it is only recently that anatomists have studied the dynamic functional aspects of the anatomy of the pelvic floor and continence mechanisms. Of modern anatomists writing in the English language, it was Nichols and Randall [2] who gave us an indication that studying anatomy in fixed cadavers did not actually illustrate the changing anatomy of the pelvis during various activities, particularly standing and straining. Dynamic magnetic resonance imaging (MRI) and other imaging studies have recently revealed the changing anatomic relationships during defecation and micturition as well [3,4]. Therefore, understanding the anatomy of a functional living being is of great importance to the pelvic surgeon whose mission is to restore anatomy while preserving or improving function.

Basic Considerations

An explanation of basic anatomic and functional principles will aid in our understanding of the basic anatomy. These concepts are: (1) the overall structure and function of the pelvic floor, (2) the vaginal-uterine axis, and (3) the circumferential attachment sites of the vagina and uterus.

Structure and Function of the Pelvic Floor

The assumption of the upright posture brought with it certain adaptive anatomic and functional evolutionary changes. Let us consider for a moment the anatomy of animals which walk on all fours (*quadrupeds*). They have no pelvic floor. The muscle groups which comprise the pelvic floor in primates are present in these lower mammals but turn backwards to wag the tail. The abdominal contents in these animals are supported by the abdominal wall which, in most of their functional activities, is parallel to the ground, bearing the effects of gravity.

In primates, particularly humans, who spend most of their waking hours in the upright position, the pelvic floor evolved. It is basically a sling of several muscle groups and ligaments connected at the perimeter to the 360∞ ovoid shape of the bony pelvis. The pelvic floor supports the abdominal and pelvic organs, preventing them from descending out of the pelvic and abdominal cavities. It is slightly concave, funneling in a downward direction. The muscles of the pelvic floor are also in a tonic state of contraction, but the same coordinated activity can cause the muscles to contract and shorten, reducing the degree of concavity of the pelvic floor.

The pelvic floor contains three principal perforations that allow the urethra, vagina, and rectum to pass through it (Figure 3.1). Some anatomic dissections illustrate that the urethra passes between the pubic symphysis and the pelvic floor; this point of difference is not of great functional significance, since the urethral opening is the smallest of the three and rarely a portal for prolapse. Other smaller perforations of insignificant pathologic importance allow vessels and nerves to pass through and around the pelvic floor.

The largest of the openings in the pelvic floor, the perforation through which the vagina passes, the *genital hiatus*, is of paramount importance to the gynecologist since it is the site of pelvic organ prolapse. This hiatus is stretched during childbirth. The muscles of the pelvic floor can also become partially denervated, increasing the size of the genital hiatus as well as the concavity of the downward funneling of the pelvic floor. Since the genital hiatus is the weakest point in the pelvic floor support mechanism, it is the most frequent site of pelvic organ prolapse. The additive effects of aging, declining quality of connective tissue and collagen, estrogen withdrawal [6] (estrogen receptors are present in the

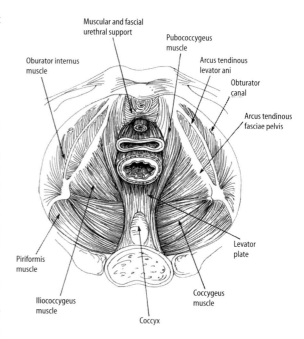

Figure 3. 1   The pelvic floor (as viewed from above). Scotti RJ, Lazarou G. Abdominal approaches to uterine suspension. *Operative Techniques in Gynecologic Surgery* 2000;5(2):90. [5]

muscles of the pelvic floor [6]), and constipation with straining at stool, create ideal conditions for the development of pelvic organ prolapse. Furthermore, detachment of the vagina and uterus from their lateral apical and posterior supports favors downward descent and eversion of the vagina. These support structures are discussed in more detail below.

The Vaginal-Uterine Axis

Another important basic consideration is the vaginal-uterine axis. Many anatomy texts are based on dissections done on fixed cadavers in the supine position; thus, for many years, no attention was paid to the vaginal axis. It was thought to be more or less parallel to the long axis of the body. Understanding the biaxial orientation of the vagina and uterus is critical to proper anatomic and functional restoration of pelvic support. In the supine position, the vagina may appear to be uniaxial, conforming more or less to the long (vertical) axis of the body. However, when a person stands, the axis appears to change: the lower one-third of the vagina remains parallel to the long axis of the body, while the upper two-thirds of the vagina and uterus dip backward, becoming more perpendicular to the long axis (Figure 3.2a). When the woman is asked to strain, this change becomes more marked as the angle of the upper vagina approaches more closely the per-

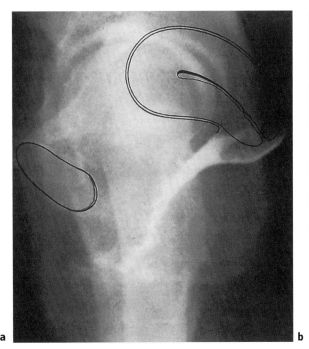

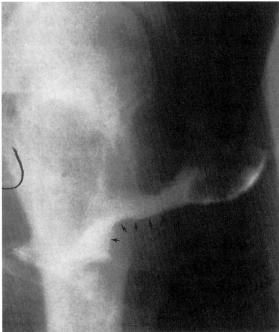

a   b

Figure 3.2 The vaginal axis in the standing position both resting (a) and straining (b). Barium paste has been placed in the vagina. Nichols DH, Randall CL. *Vaginal Surgery*, 4th edn. Baltimore: Lippincott Williams & Wilkins; 1996; 3-18. [2]

pendicular plane with respect to the long axis of the body and the upper vagina rests on the pelvic floor. Barium mold radiographic studies of Nichols and Randall [2] and Funt and associates [7] were milestones in our understanding of this important functional anatomic relationship.

As we review the anatomy of vaginal and uterine attachment points below, we will understand why the concept of the vaginal axis or "axes" (as the vagina is really biaxial) is so important. During straining, the vagina actually becomes parallel to the pelvic floor (Figure 3.2b), providing a second barrier (in addition to the pelvic muscles, pelvic diaphragm and ligaments) to further downward descent of pelvic and visceral organs through the genital hiatus. This additional barrier, the upper vagina, tends to close the opening in the levator plate by sitting over it like a flap valve mechanism preventing other abdomino-pelvic organs from prolapsing through the genital hiatus (Figure 3.3).

Circumferential Support of the Vagina and Uterus

The vagina and uterus are supported circumferentially by bridges of intervening connective tissue to the bony pelvis, just as the hub of a wheel (the vagina and uterus) is attached to the rim (the bony

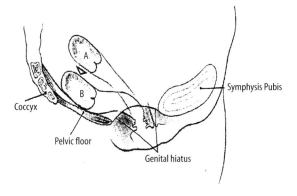

Figure 3.3 The upper vagina at rest (A) is reflected posteriorly during straining (B) and covers over the genital hiatus like a flap valve, preventing prolapse of other abdominal organs. Scotti RJ et al. In: Rosenthal RA, Zenilman ME, Kathick MK, editors. *Principles and Practice of Geriatric Surgery*. New York: Springer, 2001; 824. [8]

pelvis) by intervening spokes (the connective tissue bridges) (Figures 3.4 and 3.5).

Anterior Support

The lower one-third of the vagina is supported anteriorly by the muscular and fascial urethral supports (pubourethral and urethropelvic ligaments) as seen in Figures 3.4 and 3.5. These ligaments run from the posterior pubic bone and fuse laterally to the urethra and anterior lateral vagina. They are of vari-

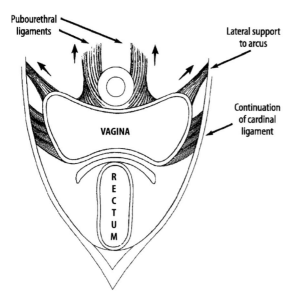

Figure 3.4 Anterior and lateral supports of the vagina. The lower anterior vagina is supported by the pubourethral ligaments, as well as the lateral attachments to the arcus tendineus. Nichols DH, Randall CL. *Vaginal Surgery*, 4th edn. Baltimore: Lippincott Williams & Wilkins; 1996; 3-18. [2]

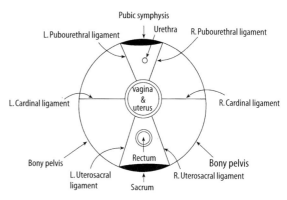

Figure 3.5 Figurative illustration of pelvic supports based on the analogy of a bicycle wheel with a hub (vagina and uterus), spokes (pelvic support structures), and rim (bony pelvis). Scotti RJ et al. In: Rosenthal RA, Zenilman ME, Kathick MK, editors. *Principles and Practice of Geriatric Surgery*. New York: Springer, 2001; 824. [8]

able strength containing much elastin and collagen but with variable amounts of smooth muscle [9]. Although this hypothesis has never been tested, the pubourethral ligaments alone probably could not support the entire lower vagina because of their small size and because of the variable amount of muscle contained within them, which has a tendency to stretch. Fortunately, the lower anterior vagina is also supported laterally by fascial bands connected to the fibromuscular coat of the vagina (part of the endopelvic fascial circular investment of vagina and cervix) which attach laterally to the arcus tendineus fascia pelvis, a thick fibrous band which runs obliquely from the pubic bone to the ischial spine (Figures 3.1, 3.4, 3.5).

Lateral Support

The anatomic design of the arcus tendineus is nearly functionally perfect. When intact, not only does it support the lateral vagina, but because of its oblique orientation, it allows the upper vagina to turn posteriorly, such that during standing and straining the upper vagina and uterus become parallel to and sit upon the levator plate (the pelvic floor) as described above (Figures 3.2a, 3.2b, 3.3). The arcus and the vaginal fascial attachment to the arcus have a certain degree of mobility which allows the vagina, particularly the upper two-thirds, to assume this orientation parallel to the pelvic floor (and perpendicular to the long axis of the body). In addition to the arcus tendineus, the upper vagina

and uterus are also supported laterally to the cardinal (Mackenrodt's) ligament (Figures 3.4, 3.5).

Posterior Support

The principal posterior supports of the vagina are the uterosacral ligaments (Figure 3.5). These tend to pull the cervix and upper vagina posteriorly, toward the sacrum, helping to maintain the posterior inclination of the upper vagina. Mengert, in his classical studies, was able to demonstrate the strong holding power of the lateral (cardinal ligaments) and posterior (uterosacral ligaments) support of the vagina and uterus [10].

Apical Support

The apex of the vagina is also supported by the uterosacral ligaments. The uterus and cervix and the upper lateral supports of the arcus tendineus also provide further apical support.

It can generally be stated that all the support to the vagina and uterus are additive and interlock and coordinate with each other, like a well-organized mesh or network.

Anatomy of the Pelvic Floor Support

Now that these basic concepts have been covered and understood from a functional standpoint, the detailed anatomy makes perfect sense. In order to understand the structural anatomy, we will consider building the pelvis beginning with the bony framework, in the same way as an engineer or contractor would build an edifice starting with the strong framing (the bones), its hardware and fasteners (the ligaments), its electrical plumbing and supply systems (the nervous and vascular components) and its various floors and walls.

The Bones

The bones of the pelvis give shape to the lower body and, most importantly, provide both strong attachment and articulation for the lower extremities and their important functions. Hence, the bony pelvis by design is made of large bones which are fused together by collagen matrix, and reinforced for added stability by cross struts comprised of several ligaments.

The bony pelvis is composed of the sacrum, coccyx and two bilaterally symmetrical innominate hip bones. The innominate bone on each side is divided into the pubis, ileum and ischium. The bony pelvis is illustrated in Figure 3.6 with the interconnecting ligaments. These ligaments act as braces to limit the mobility of the bones and to add stability. They also serve as excellent reattachment points for prolapsed pelvic organs, and are of great importance to pelvic surgeons. The sacrospinous ligament runs from the ischial spine to the lateral body of the sacrum. The sacrotuberous ligament runs from the ischial tuberosity to the sacrum, partially fusing at the sacrum with the sacrospinous ligament medially (Figure 3.6). The lacunar ligaments (not pictured) run from the medial end of the inguinal ligament and attach to the pectineal line beyond the pubic tubercle forming a pseudo-foramen which allows the femoral vessels and nerves to leave the pelvis.

The inguinal ligament (not pictured) extends from the anterior superior iliac spine to the pubic

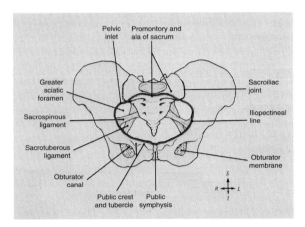

Figure 3.6   The bony pelvis and ligaments. Gosling JA, Harris PF, Humpherson JR, Whitmore I, Willan PLT. *Atlas of Human Anatomy*, 2nd edn. Philadelphia: Lippincott Williams and Wilkins, 1985. [11]

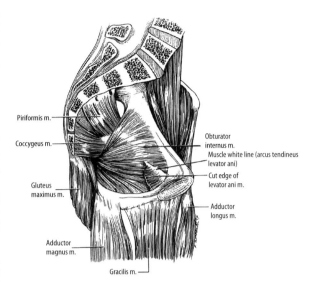

Figure 3.7   Left lateral pelvis. The obturator internus muscle lines the inner pelvis. It then exits the pelvis through the lesser sciatic foramen. The piriformis passes through the greater sciatic foramen. The coccygeus attaches to the medial surfaces of the ischial spine and the sacrospinous ligament. Retzky SS, Rogers RM Jr, Richardson AC. In: Brubaker LT, Saclarides TJ, editors. *The Female Pelvic Floor. Disorders of Function and Support*. Philadelphia: FA Davis Company, 1996;3-21. [12]

tubercle. The greater sciatic foramen transmits the piriformis muscle, sciatic nerve, superior and inferior gluteal nerves and vessels, pudendal nerve and vessels and the nerve of the obturator internus muscle, as seen in Figures 3.7 and 3.8. The internal pudendal nerves and vessels pass through the greater sciatic foramen behind the ischial spine through Alcock's canal (Figure 3.8). The pudendal nerve, vessels and nerve of the obturator internus then re-enter the pelvis through the lesser sciatic foramen.

These landmarks, particularly the ischial spines, sciatic foramina and the sacrospinous ligaments, are of paramount importance to pelvic surgeons, since the ischial spine, the iliococcygeus muscle attaching to it, and the sacrospinous ligament are key pelvic reattachment sites, in close proximity to the pudendal nerve. Of obstetric interest, it is also thought that the area of vulnerability to partial denervation of the pudendal nerve during childbirth occurs at this very point where it is compressed against the relatively unyielding bony pelvis by the descending fetus [13]. This denervation may put patients at risk for urinary incontinence, fecal incontinence and pelvic organ prolapse.

Obturator Internus and Externus Muscles

The next layer, attached directly to bone, is the obturator internus muscle. The obturator internus muscle

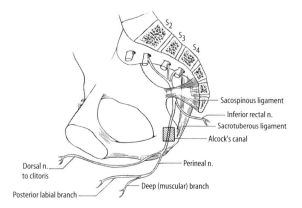

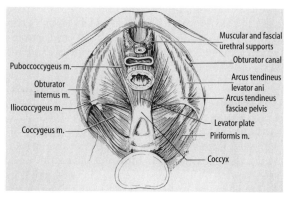

Figure 3.8 Right hemipelvis. The pudendal nerve, artery, and vein exit the pelvis through the greater sciatic foramen posterior to the sacrospinous ligament, and re-enter the pelvis through the lesser sciatic foramen, passing through Alcock's canal. Retzky SS, Rogers RM Jr, Richardson AC. In: Brubaker LT, Saclarides TJ, editors. *The Female Pelvic Floor. Disorders of Function and Support.* Philadelphia: FA Davis Company, 1996;3-21. [12]

Figure 3.9 The levators originate from the arcus tendineus. Both pairs of these muscles fuse in the midline. Note the posterior triangles of the pelvic floor. The paired coccygeus and piriformis muscles also fuse in the midline. Retzky SS, Rogers RM Jr, Richardson AC. In: Brubaker LT, Saclarides TJ, editors. *The Female Pelvic Floor. Disorders of Function and Support.* Philadelphia: FA Davis Company, 1996;3-21. [12]

is a much more important structure for reconstructive pelvic surgeons since it lines the inner surface of the ischium, ileum and pubic bones and also is the attachment point for the muscles of the pelvic floor, as well as the all-important arcus tendineus fascia pelvis. The arcus tendineus fascia pelvis or "white line", the lateral attachment point for the muscles of the pelvic floor and lateral vagina, arises directly from the surface of the obturator internus muscle (Figure 3.1). Fibers of this band are also attached to the obturator membrane, the thick fibrous sheath which covers most of the obturator foramen. In fact, the obturator foramen is practically covered by this membrane and the obturator internus and externus muscles on either side. A small perforation in the membrane (the obturator canal), at its antero-superior border, admits the obturator neurovascular bundle to supply the adductors of the leg (Figure 3.9). The remainder of obturator membrane is nerve and vessel free and serves as an attachment point for the muscles lining the inner pelvis (the obturator internus) and, to a variable degree, the arcus tendineus fascia pelvis which arises both from the surface of the obturator internus but also sends some fibers to the obturator membrane. It may also be used as a pelvic reattachment point during paravaginal repair. The fibers of the obturator internus muscle converge as they travel inferiorly, forming a small band of tendons which exit the lesser sciatic foramen and attach to the greater trochanter of the femur.

The obturator externus muscle lines the outer surface of the pelvis and is of functional significance to pelvic support.

The Anterior Pelvic Floor Triangle (Levator Group)

Three muscles form the levator group which comprise the layer overlying the obturator internus. They form roughly the anterior half (triangle) of the pelvic floor. These three muscles are perhaps the most important to the gynecologist. They provide the principal support of the pelvic organs and they are frequently stretched, injured or denervated in childbirth. Anteriorly, as seen in Figures 3.1 and 3.9, are the pubococcygeus and the iliococcygeus muscles, which act as one unit and have several functions. The fibers of the muscle run obliquely from the inner surface of the pubic bone following the course of the "white line" and, joining their contralateral counterparts in the midline, are fused together at the median raphe. They are perforated by urethra, vagina and rectum. The fibers of the puborectalis and the pubococcygeus also attach to the lateral vagina, with some passing around the posterior vagina. The puborectalis and pubococcygeus also pass posteriorly around the rectum. Contraction of these muscles (the Kegel pelvic floor exercise) pulls the rectum anteriorly and upwardly and has some function in the maintenance of urinary and fecal continence. The levator group muscles involuntary contract during a cough, compressing the urethra, vagina and rectum. They serve as the principal support of the anterior half of the pelvic floor.

The Posterior (Anal) Pelvic Floor Triangle – the Coccygeus and Piriformis Muscles

The coccygeus originates from ischial spines and the lateral pelvic sidewall posterior to the ischial spine to which it is attached by fascial bands. This muscle is fused with the iliococcygeus at its posterior border, and forms one functional sheet of muscle. These muscles are joined to their contralateral counterparts through an intervening median raphe and also fuse posteriorly with the coccyx (Figures 3.1, 3.9). The paired iliococcygeus muscles also contract in concert with the muscles of the anterior triangle (levator group) of the pelvic floor, helping to support the vagina and rectum. The coccygeus muscles also assist in maintaining the normal uterine and vaginal axis.

The most posterior muscles of the pelvic floor, which fill in the last gap of space, are paired piriformis muscles. These thick muscles arise from anterior sacrum and greater sciatic notch bilaterally (Figures 3.1, 3.7 and 3.9). Since these muscles are very thick, they serve as the bulk which fills in the posterior triangles. They appose each other in the midline and are bulkier than the other muscles of the pelvic floor. The piriformis muscles support the more anterior vagina or rectum anatomically, but do not have as much of a functional role as do the anterior pelvic floor muscles. They functionally complete the posterior sling of the pelvic floor. The belly of each muscle turns downward as the fibers converge to form tendons, and exit the pelvis through the greater sciatic foramen to insert onto the greater trochanter of the femur (Figure 3.7). Their principal function, besides lending posterior support to the pelvic floor, is to abduct and laterally rotate the thighs. In this respect, they are functionally similar to obturator internus muscles. Both obturator internus and piriformis line the inner pelvis and support viscera, but exit the pelvis to aid in ambulation.

Endopelvic Fascia

This layer is a fibromuscular tissue consisting of collagen, elastin and smooth muscle. It is a continuation of the abdominal transversalis fascia and includes a parietal and a visceral component. The visceral fascia lies immediately beneath the peritoneum and attaches to and joins the bladder, vagina, uterus and rectum. The parietal fascia has areas of condensation, ligaments and septa, which provide fixation of the pelvic floor. The parietal fascial supports the viscera and defines the anatomic location of the pelvic viscera, by giving them adequate fixation (e.g., uterosacral and cardinal liga-

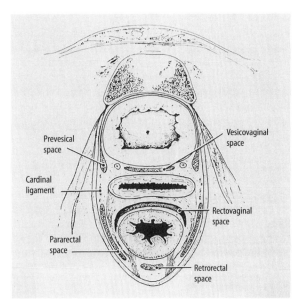

Figure 3.10   The endopelvic fascia provides septation (rectovaginal, vesicovaginal septae) and defines spaces (prevesical, vesicovaginal and rectovaginal). DeLancey JOL. In: Rock JA, Thompson JD, editors. Te Linde's Operative Gynecology, 8th edn. Philadelphia: Lippincott Williams & Wilkins, 1997, 77. [14]

ments), septation (e.g., rectovaginal and vesicovaginal septae) and definition of pelvic spaces (e.g., prevesical, vesicovaginal, and rectovaginal) as seen in Figure 3.10. The endopelvic fascia serves to suspend the viscera over the levator plate and provides physical support to neurovascular channels.

The Parametrium

Anatomically, the cardinal ligament lies directly lateral to the cervix and vagina and the uterosacral ligament lies posterolateral. These structures are not separate, but are discrete condensations of the endopelvic fascia, providing further support and holding the cervix and upper vagina over the levator plate. The cardinal ligaments contain vascular pedicles supplying the uterus and upper vagina while the uterosacral ligaments restrict downward prolapse of the uterus and upper vagina. Detachment of these structures can cause uterovaginal prolapse [15].

Broad and Round Ligaments

These structures form lateral attachments of the uterus cephalad to the cardinal ligaments. They are probably unimportant in providing pelvic support.

The Midline Fasciae

The muscular and fascial urethral supports (pubourethral ligament) distal to the levators run between the pubis and the urogenital diaphragm, enveloping and suspending the mid-urethra (Figures 3.1, 3.2, 3.5, 3.9). DeLancey has demonstrated the functional role of these ligaments in micturition [9]. Damage to these ligaments causes posterior and inferior movement of the mid-urethra without hypermobility at the bladder neck and has been associated with stress urinary incontinence [16].

The urethropelvic ligaments are slightly cephalad to the level of the pubourethral ligaments and envelop the proximal urethra. These ligaments, along with fibers from the pubococcygeus muscle, travel from the anterior aspect of the tendinous arch to the anterior vaginal wall, bladder neck, and proximal urethra. This specialized portion of the endopelvic fascia provides the major musculofascial support of the bladder neck and proximal urethra and may assist in opening of the urethra during voiding.

The Superficial Compartment of the Urogenital Triangle

Anterior Triangle/Perineal Membrane
The perineal membrane (urogenital diaphragm) is a fibrous layer composed of smooth and striated muscles providing further anterior pelvic outlet support (Figure 3.11). Laterally, it attaches to the ischiopubic ramus while fusing medially with the perineal body and the sidewalls of the vagina. The perineal membrane tightens to prevent further downward descent of the lateral vaginal walls and perineal body when the levator ani muscles relax. Also, during sudden increases in intra-abdominal pressure, fibers from the perineal membrane contract to steady the perineum.

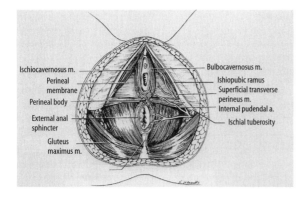

Figure 3.11 An inferior view of the pelvic floor. The superficial compartment of the urogenital triangle surrounds the vagina and urethra. The perineal membrane is labeled. Retzky SS, Rogers RM Jr, Richardson AC. In: Brubaker LT, Saclarides TJ, editors. *The Female Pelvic Floor: Disorders of Function and Support*. Philadelphia: FA Davis Company, 1996;3-21.[12]

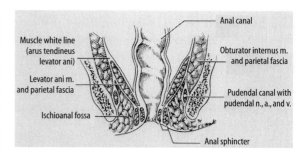

Figure 3.12 Coronal section of the ischiorectal fossa illustrating pudendal canal Retzky SS, Rogers RM Jr, Richardson AC. In: Brubaker LT, Saclarides TJ, editors. *The Female Pelvic Floor: Disorders of Function and Support*. Philadelphia: FA Davis Company, 1996;3-21.[12]

Posterior Triangle/Ischiorectal Fossa
The ischiorectal (ischioanal) fossa lies in the posterior triangle of the pelvis between the pelvic walls and the levator ani muscles (Figure 3.12). It is a space filled with adipose tissue which can be the site of hematoma formation, especially after obstetrical trauma. Anteriorly, the fossa lies above the perineal membrane. Medially, the space is bounded by the levator ani muscles and anterolaterally by the obturator internus muscle. Posteriorly, the space is bounded by the gluteus maximus. The pudendal neurovascular plexus traverses this space at its lateral margins and is prone to injury during vaginal reconstructive and operative obstetrical procedures.

Perineal Body
The perineal body or central perineal tendon (Figure 3.11) is formed by the convergence of the tendinous attachments of the bulbocavernosus, the external anal sphincter, and the superficial transverse perineal muscle. The contribution of the perineal body to pelvic support is minimal, as support of the pelvic outlet is maintained by continuity of the perineal membrane and the upward traction exerted by the levator ani muscle. Nonetheless, it represents an important anatomic central connection between the pelvic and urogenital diaphragm.

Pelvic Vasculature

The knowledge of the vasculature of the pelvis is essential to pelvic surgeons, as lacerations of pelvic vessels can result in severe hemorrhage. At the level of the fourth lumbar vertebra, the aorta bifurcates and the right and left common iliac arteries arise. The common iliac vessels bifurcate at the level of the fifth lumbar vertebra to form the internal and external iliac vessels. Each external iliac vessel exits the pelvis below the inguinal ligament to become the femoral artery and vein, while in the vicinity of the inguinal ligament, the external iliac artery gives off

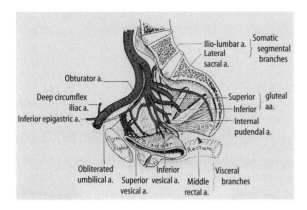

Figure 3.13 The blood supply of the pelvis. Anderson JE. *Grant's Atlas of Anatomy*, 8th edn. Baltimore: Williams & Wilkins, 1983. [17]

the inferior epigastric artery and the deep iliac circumflex artery (Figure 3.13).

The internal iliac artery supplies the pelvic viscera, walls of the pelvis and the perineum. The posterior trunk of the internal iliac artery is composed of the iliolumbar artery, the lateral sacral artery and the superior gluteal artery. Such vasculature supplies somatic musculature. There is an extensive network of anastomoses with collateral circulation about the hip. Anomalies are common.

The anterior trunk of the internal iliac artery supplies both somatic and visceral structures. As depicted in Figure 3.13, the inferior gluteal artery in the pelvis supplies portions of the coccygeus, piriformis and levator ani muscles. The internal pudendal artery supplies the perineum as it enters the pelvis via the lesser sciatic foramen traversing the ischiorectal fossa (Figure 3.8). The obturator artery supplies somatic structures in the anteromedial thigh. The vessel runs ventrally along the pelvic side wall, medial to the obturator fascia, and exits the pelvic cavity via the obturator canal to supply the adductor muscles. Both the obturator artery and vein have many anomalies which can be troublesome in reconstructive pelvic surgery, especially when reattaching the prolapsed vagina to the pelvic sidewall and arcus tendineus [18].

The umbilical artery is another branch of the anterior division of the hypogastric artery. Prior to its obliteration, it gives off vascular supply to the bladder, specifically the superior vesical artery, the middle vesical arteries, and medial umbilical ligaments.

The uterine artery travels medially on the superior surface of the levator ani and passes superior to the ureters and the cardinal ligament and then ascends between the layers of the broad ligament to supply the uterus. The middle rectal artery supplies part of the rectum and the inferior vesical artery supplies the neck of the bladder.

There are also extensive venous plexuses within the pelvic cavity. The principal drainage of the pelvis is into the internal iliac vein. However, abundant anastomoses connect the systemic drainage with the hepatic portal system.

The Nerve Supply to the Pelvis

The lumbosacral plexus provides somatic innervation to the pelvis and the lower extremities (Figure 3.14). The lumbar plexus (T12–L4) lies in the posterior abdominal wall and iliac fossa. The lumbosacral trunk (L4–L5) contributes to the sacral plexus (L4–S3). Knowledge of the specific sensory and motor nerve contributions is essential for evaluating nerve injuries that may occur in complicated pelvic surgery. Also, these nerves can be injured by errant sutures or instruments placed on the pelvic sidewall superior to the ischial spines.

The major nerves of interest in the lumbar plexus include the iliohypogastric, ilioinguinal, lateral cutaneous, genitofemoral, femoral and obturator nerves. The iliohypogastric nerve (T12, L1) supplies sensory fibers to the suprapubic region. The lateral femoral cutaneous nerve (L2, L3) supplies sensory fibers to the lateral thigh.

The genitofemoral nerve (T11, L2) innervates the skin overlying the labia and a small region of the superior thigh. The femoral nerve (L2–L4) has motor function assisting in hip flexion and leg extension while the sensory component provides innervation to the anterior and medial thigh and medial leg. The obturator nerve (L2–L4) supplies

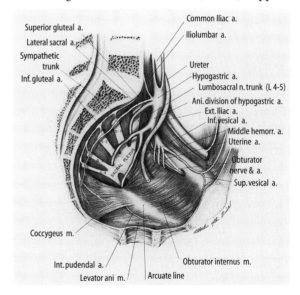

Figure 3.14 Left hemipelvis showing major neurovascular components to the pelvis. Mattingly RF. *Te Linde's Operative Gynecology*, 6th edn. Philadelphia: JB Lippincott, 1977, 32. [19]

motor innervation to the adductor muscles of the thigh and sensory innervation to the upper thigh.

The anterior division of the lumbosacral trunk contributes the tibial portion of the sciatic nerve while the posterior division contributes the superior and inferior gluteal nerves and the common peroneal nerve. The sacral plexus (L4–S3) lies in the minor pelvis and supplies the gluteal region, posterior thigh, leg, foot and perineum. The pelvic plexus arises from spinal nerves S2–S3 or S3–S4 and consists of parasympathetic fibers as well as visceral afferent fibers from portions of the pelvic viscera.

The sacral plexus (Figure 3.5) has five major branches: (1) The superior gluteal nerve (L4–S1) exits the pelvis superior to the piriformis portion of the greater sciatic foramen. (2) The inferior gluteal nerve (L5–S2) exits the pelvis inferior to the piriformis of the greater sciatic foramen. Damage to either of the two branches, which may occur during pelvic surgery, causes weakness in abducting the hip, resulting in a rolling gait. (3) The common peroneal nerve (L4–S2) exits the pelvis inferior to the piriformis of the greater sciatic foramen. Nerve injury results in foot drop and inability to evert the foot. (4) The tibial nerve (L4–S3) exits from the infra-piriform region of the greater sciatic foramen. (5) The pudendal nerve (S2–S4), whose anatomical course was described above, supplies motor and sensory innervation to the perineum via the inferior hemorrhoidal and perineal nerve. Any of the above nerves can be injured during reconstructive pelvic surgical procedures near the greater sciatic foramen, sacrospinous ligament or iliococcygeus fascia. The femoral nerve is subject to stretch injury if the hips are hyperflexed or outwardly rotated during surgical procedures.

Ureter

The anatomic proximity of the urinary and genital tract puts both the ureter and bladder at risk during gynecologic surgery. Although full consideration of urologic complications is given Section 8, a few important anatomical landmarks will be reviewed here.

The ureter is about 25 to 30 cm long and is divided anatomically into abdominal and pelvic components. In the abdomen, the ureter travels along the anterior aspect of the psoas muscle and enters the pelvic inlet and passes over the bifurcation of the internal and external iliac arteries medial to the ovarian vessels [20].

The pelvic portion of the ureter passes along the postero-lateral pelvic wall anterior to the internal iliac artery and descends further in the pelvis lateral to the uterosacral ligaments, entering into the base

of the broad ligament. At the level of the internal os, it crosses under the uterine artery, approximately 1.5 cm lateral to the cervix, and then crosses medially over the anterior fornix of the vagina to enter the wall of the bladder at the vesical trigone (Figures 3.15, 3.16). The ureteral blood supply is variable, with contributions from the renal, ovarian, common iliac, internal iliac, uterine and vesical arteries, while the innervation is via the ovarian and vesical plexus. These intricate neurovascular tissues may be damaged from extensive pelvic dissection and ultimately present with postoperative complications. It is extremely important to avoid stripping or injury to the serosa investment of the ureter (Waldeyer's sheath) to avoid injury to small vessels and nerves supplying the ureter. Inadvertent ligation, crushing

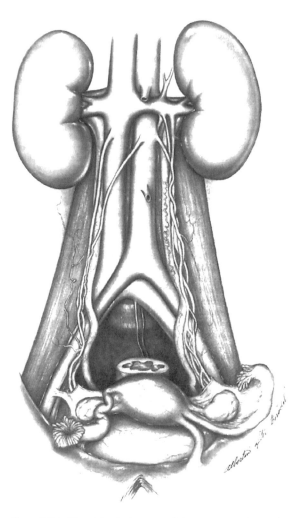

Figure 3.15 The abdominal course of the ureter anterior to the common iliacs. The ureter deviates posteriorly at the pelvic brim, passes under the uterine arteries and courses just lateral to the uterosacral ligaments. Rock JA, Thompson JD, editors. *Te Linde's Operative Gynecology*, 8th edn. Philadelphia: Lippincott-Raven Publishers, 1997, 1138. [21]

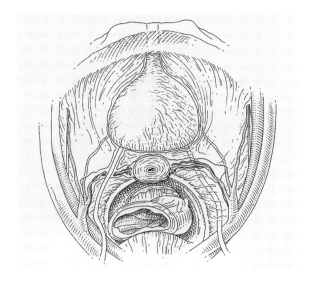

Figure 3.16 The course of the pelvic portion of the ureter, which courses along the sidewall of the pelvis over (anterior to) the common iliac, then medial to the hypogastric and over (anterior to) the uterine artery. Of significance is its proximity to the ovarian vessels, the uterine vessels, and the uterosacral ligament. Rock JA, Thompson JD, editors. *Te Linde's Operative Gynecology*, 8th edn. Philadelphia: Lippincott-Raven Publishers, 1997, 1139. [21]

or severance of the ureter are the most common injuries. Since complex reconstructive surgery, particularly high uterosacral ligament fixation, carries even greater risk for ureteral injury than other benign or oncologic surgery, many experts advocate confirming ureteral patency preoperatively and intraoperatively by cystoscopic examination.

Summary and Key Points

A thorough knowledge of anatomic relationships affords the pelvic surgeon the comfort of eliminating guesswork while repairing defects in the pelvis with confidence. With practice, persistence, and meticulous observational skills, anatomic structures can be seen and palpated during surgical procedures. The most important structures to be avoided are the ureters, the obturator vessels and nerves, and the pudendal vessels and nerves. To avoid sacral plexus injuries, one must never place sutures near the pelvic sidewall superior to the ischial spines. Lengthy procedures also subject the patient to the risk of nerve stretch injury and increased blood loss.

Since many anomalies exist in the pelvis, the surgeon must exercise constant attention and vigilance. Moreover, pelvic organ prolapse predisposes for both distortion and displacement of normal structures, especially the ureter. The pelvic surgeon must also be aware of distorted anatomy and attempt to avoid errant structures.

The study of anatomy requires meticulous attention to detail and repetitious exercises to commit it to memory. Yet, when confronted with challenging dilemmas in the operating room, the surgeon's knowledge of anatomy can provide confidence and ease to overcome these difficulties.

References

1. O'Malley CD. Andreas Vesalius of Brussels. Berkeley, CA: University of California Press, 1964; 1514–64.
2. Nichols DH, Randall CL. Vaginal Surgery, 4th edn. Baltimore: Williams & Wilkins, 1996; 1–42.
3. Healy JC, Halligan S, Reznek RH et al. Dynamic MR imaging compared with evacuation proctography when evaluating anorectal configuration and pelvic floor movement. AJR Am J Roentgenol 1997;169:775–9.
4. Kirschner-Hermanns R, Wein B, Niehaus S, Schaefer W, Jakse G. The contribution of magnetic resonance imaging of the pelvic floor to the understanding of urinary incontinence. Br J Urol 1993;72:715–18.
5. Scotti RJ, Lazarou G. Abdominal approaches to uterine suspension. Operative Techniques in Gynecologic Surgery 2000;5:88–99.
6. Smith P, Heimer G, Norgren A, Ulmsten U. Localization of steroid hormone receptors in the pelvic muscles. Eur J Obstet Gynecol Reprod Biol 1993;50:83–5.
7. Funt MI, Thompson JD, Birch H. Normal vaginal axis. South Med J 1978;71:1534–5.
8. Scotti RJ, Hutchinson-Colas J, Budnick LE, Lazarou G, Greston WM. Benign gynecologic disorders in the elderly. In: Rosenthal RA, Zenilman ME, Kathick MK, editors. Principles and Practice of Geriatric Surgery. New York: Springer, 2001; 817–33.
9. DeLancey JOL. The pubovesical ligament: a separate structure from the urethral supports ("pubo-urethral ligaments"). Neurourol Urodyn 1989;8:53–61.
10. Mengert WF. Mechanics of uterine support and position. I. Factors influencing uterine support (an experimental study). Am J Obstet Gynecol 1936;31:775–82.
11. Gosling JA, Harris PF, Humpherson JR, Whitmore I, Willan PLT. Atlas of Human Anatomy. Philadelphia: JB Lippincott Company, 1985.
12. Retzky SS, Rogers RM, Jr, Richardson AC. Anatomy of female pelvic support. In: Brubaker LT, Saclarides TJ, editors. The Female Pelvic Floor: Disorders of Function and Support. Philadelphia: FA Davis Company, 1996; 3–21.
13. Smith ARB, Hosker GL, Warrell DW. The role of partial denervation of the pelvic floor in the etiology of genitourinary prolapse and stress incontinence of urine. A neurophysiological study. Br J Obstet Gynaecol 1989;96:24–8.
14. DeLancey JOL. Surgical anatomy of the female pelvis. In: Rock JA, Thompson JD, editors. Te Linde's Operative Gynecology, 8th edn. Philadelphia: Lippincott-Raven, 1997.
15. DeLancey JOL. Anatomic aspects of vaginal eversion after hysterectomy. Am J Obstet Gynecol 1992;166:1717–24.
16. Milley PS, Nichols DH. The relationship between the pubo-urethral ligaments and the urogenital diaphragm in the human female. Anat Rec 1971;170:281–3.
17. Anderson JE. Grant's Atlas of Anatomy, 8th edn. Baltimore: Williams & Wilkins, 1983.

18. Scotti RJ, Garely A, Greston WM, Flora RF, Olson TR. Paravaginal repair of lateral vaginal wall defects by fixation to the ischial periosteum and obturator membrane. Am J Obstet Gynecol 1998;179:1436–445.

19. Mattingly RF. Te Linde's Operative Gynecology, 5th edn. Philadelphia: JB Lippincott, 1977.

20. Woodburne RT. Essentials of Human Anatomy, 8th edn. New York: Oxford University Press, 1988.

21. Thompson JD. Operative injuries to the ureter: prevention, recognition, and management. In: Rock JA, Thompson JD, editors. Te Linde's Operative Gynecology, 8th edn. Philadelphia: Lippincott-Raven Publishers, 1997.

4 Neurophysiologic Control of the Lower Urinary Tract and Anorectum

Marie-Claude Lemieux and Stéphane Ouellet

Continence and appropriate evacuation of urine and stool is the result of coordinated action of the skeletal and smooth muscles of the lower urinary tract and the anorectum. The neural control of these muscles is complex, not fully understood and mostly studied in animals although valuable information has been derived from the observation of the effects of neurological injury or disease in humans. Full understanding of the neurophysiologic control of micturition and defecation is therefore not the goal of the chapter but rather an review of known information regarding the integration of autonomic and somatic nervous systems in regulating these functions.

The Lower Urinary Tract

Both central and peripheral nervous systems interact to control lower urinary tract function (Figure 4.1). The peripheral nervous system is composed of both autonomic nerves (sympathetic and parasympathetic) and somatic nerves. Regulation of involuntary activity (smooth muscle, visceral functions) is the role of the autonomic system whereas somatic nerves control voluntary activity (skeletal muscles).

Preganglionic parasympathetic efferents originate in the intermediolateral cell columns of the sacral spinal cord at the level of S2 through S4 and travel through the the pelvic nerve synapsing on cholinergic neurons in the pelvic plexus or on intramural ganglia located directly within the bladder or urethral wall [1, 2]. Detrusor smooth muscle cells are densely innervated [3]. The majority of these nerve endings are considered excitatory cholinergic (parasympathetic) in type and promote bladder contraction via muscarinic receptor stimulation [4, 5]. Many different muscarinic receptors types are identified in the bladder wall but the M3 subtype is

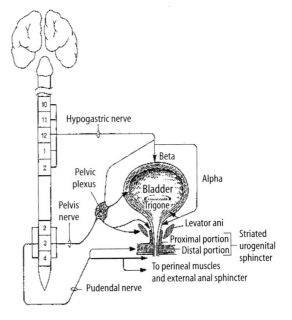

Figure 4. 1 Innervation of the urethra and bladder. (Walters MD, Karram MM, *Urogynecology and Reconstructive Pelvic Surgery*, 2nd Edition, Mosby, pp 16, 1999.)

believed responsible for this activity [6]. Histochemical studies show that cholinergic nerves are abundant in all parts of the bladder but less extensive in the urethra [7]. The effect of parasympathetic stimulation on the urethra is controversial but likely results in urethral relaxation, which is mediated by nonadrenergic-noncholinergic neurotransmitters [8].

Sympathetic preganglionic efferents arise from the thoracolumbar region of the spinal cord between the levels of T10 to L2. The preganglionic efferents travel in the hypogastric nerve and synapse on the postganglionic neurons in the sympathetic chain but can also course through the sympathetic chain and synapse on postglanglionic neurons in the pelvic plexus . These neurons then synapse either on noradrenergic neurons in the pelvic plexus or within the bladder wall and urethra [9, 10]. Sympathetic innervation (via alpha and beta receptors)predominates in the urethra and is by comparison relatively sparse to the detrusor cells, mostly located in the trigone area [11]. In the bladder, beta adrenergic receptor stimulation of the detrusor will result in smooth muscle relaxation but this is likely of little clinical significance . The sympathetic nerves may also act on the parasympathetic terminals, modulating them to inhibit cholinergic excitation of the bladder [12]. Alpha adrenergic receptor stimulation (predominant in the bladder base and the urethra) will cause urethral smooth muscle contraction [3] but, as for the bladder, there is little evidence that beta adrenoreceptor stimulation will result in clinically evident relaxation of the urethra [8].

Skeletal muscles are found in the urethra and the pelvic floor. Their activity is coordonated with that of the smooth muscles of the bladder and urethra allowing the storage and evacuation of urine. The female urethra has two muscular coats: an outer sleeve of circumferential striated muscles (the rhabdosphincter) and an inner coat of smooth muscle fibers . Motor cell bodies of nerves supplying the rhabdosphincter lie in the ventral horn of the 2nd, 3rd and 4th sacral segment of the spinal cord (Onuf's nucleus). These fibers travel through the pudendal nerve, but there may also be some innervation of the urethral sphincter through the pelvic nerve [12]. The rhabdosphincter contains striated muscle fibers that are predominantly slow-twitch (type 1 muscle fibers) in nature; it has therefore the characteristic of being able to continuously contract and consequently contribute to the baseline tone of the urethra, particularly in its middle third where the muscle is at its thickest. There is additional striated muscle periurethrally (fast-twitch or type 2), originating from the medial part of the levator ani (pubococcygeus), which aids in providing additional occlusive force on the urethral wall with increases in intra-abdominal pressure [6, 12].

The pelvic nerve, the pudendal nerve and the hypogastric nerve not only transmit efferent impulses to the bladder wall and urethra but also afferent information from the lower urinary tract to the lumbosacral spinal cord [12]. Most of the afferent supply of the bladder and urethra travels through the pelvic nerve; these afferents are the most important for initiating storage and voiding reflexes in the lower urinary tract [8]. Some afferent input is also received through the hypogastric nerve [8] which may explain why presacral neurectomy does not seem to cause alteration in bladder or urethral sensation [13]. Pelvic afferent nerves have been further described in animal studies to be myelinated (A-delta) or unmyelinated (C-fiber) and convey information regarding bladder distension or pain [6]. Based on studies of the effects of lesions on humans, sensory afferents from the lower urinary tract are believed to travel in the dorsal, lateral and ventral columns of the spinal cord to the thalamus, brainstem and other rostral locations. The dorsal columns transmit information about sensation of touch and pressure in the urethra and innocuous sensations from the pelvic floor muscles [14]. The lateral columns (spinothalamic tract) convey information concerning temperature sensation in the urethra and sensation of bladder fullness and desire to void as well as pain sensation from skin, bladder, urethra [15]. The central projections of these afferents overlap in the spinal cord, where information is relayed either to other regions of the spinal cord or to the brain, suggesting an intricate level of coordination between the lower urinary tract and upper neurological centers which results in the coordination of the visceral smooth muscle activity of the bladder and urethra with the activity of the urethral rhabdosphincter [6, 10]. Central neural modulation of the lower urinary tract is important for the storage and elimination fonctions of the lower urinary tract. This modulation may be under either voluntary or involuntary control. Supraspinal modulation of autonomous nerve function has been found to originate from medulla, pons, hypothalamus and cerebral cortex [16]. The frontal cortex and septal areas of the brain exert inhibitory control of the detrusor in the human [10]. A discrete area in the pons (the pontine micturition center) also appears necessary for micturition; when stimulated it will cause bladder contraction and synchronous urethral sphincter relaxation [10]. Voiding reflexes detailing the supraspinal control of micturition have been derived principally from brain-lesioning experiments in cats [16]. In essence, to promote urine storage, spinal reflex activity through efferent pathways will maintain pudendal nerve stimulation of the external urethral sphincter as well as adrenergic stimulation of the internal urethral sphincter, while enhancing detrusor inhibition through sympathetic nerves and inhibiting parasympathetic stimulation of the bladder. On the other hand, when bladder fullness is expressed by increasing afferent vesical activity, the spinobulbospinal voiding reflexes initiated, if a decision has been made to void, will inhibit the pudendal stimulation of the external urethral sphincter as well as inhibiting sympathetic outflow to the internal urethral sphincter and simultaneously stimulate parasympathetic efferents to the detrusor and urethra thus resulting in bladder emptying [8].

Anorectum

Anorectal control ressembles that of the lower urinary tract since it is also regulated by interactions between the autonomic and somatic nervous systems, and may be under reflex or voluntary control. But, fecal continence differs from urinary continence since it is also dependant upon stool consistency (solid, liquid or gas). In a way similar to the bladder and urethra, the rectum and anus depend on coordinated action of both smooth and squeletal muscles for proper function but the physiology of the anorectum is complex and not completely understood. Whereas the rectum contains only smooth muscle (arranged in an inner circular layer and a longitudinal outer layer), the activity of the anal canal results from the action of both smooth muscle (the internal anal sphincter) and skeletal muscle (the external anal sphincter) [18, 19].

Both parasympathetic and sympathetic efferents innervate the rectum [20] (Figure 4.2). Sympathetic stimulation (from the inferior mesenteric plexus for the distal part of the rectum and the hypogastric plexus for the more proximal part) causes inhibition of rectal smooth muscle activity . Parasympathetic efferents from the pelvic nerve result in contraction of the rectal wall. As far as afferent information, the rectal wall is only sensitive to stretch, this information being transmitted by the parasympathetic nerve; it is insensitive to pain, touch, cold or pressure [21]. Sensation from the rectum initiate from parasympathetic nerve receptors for rectal distension, located on the outside of the rectal wall itself in the pelvic fascia or musculature, and travel to the sacral cord (mostly S2 and S3), in the pelvic visceral nerve and then to higher centers [22, 23]. Some afferent information may also be relayed in the hypogastric nerve [24].

The anal canal has a rich sensory nerve supply. Both an inner internal anal sphincter, made of smooth muscles continuous with the smooth muscle layer of the rectum, and an outer squeletal muscle layer, the external anal sphincter, are resposible for anal canal function(Figure 4.3). The internal anal smooth muscles are different from other smooth muscles in that they are under constant intrinsic tonic activity. The internal anal sphincter is responsible for 85% of the resting pressure in the anal lumen, whereas the external anal sphincter accounts mostly for demands of additional increases in squeeze pressure. The role of the parasympathetic innervation to the internal anal canal is not well defined but believed to be inhibitory [25, 26].

Sympathetic innervation is the dominant autonomic innervation to the internal anal sphincter. Alpha adrenergic receptors are excitatory but there

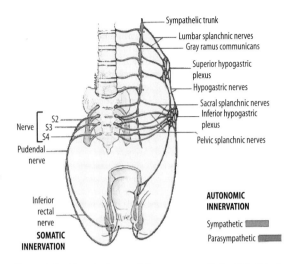

Figure 4. 2 Muscular layers of the anorectum (Netter F. H., Colacino S., Atlas of Human Anatomy, Ciba-Geigy, pp. 370, 1989)

may also be a contribution made by inhibitory beta adrenergic stimulation resulting in a dual action [18, 26]. But even though sympathetic nerves are in majority responsible for the enhanced activity of the internal anal sphincter, when sympathetic stimulation is abolished, the internal anal sphincter retains some of its basal tone [25]. A contribution to this anal sphincter tone is also provided by the submucosal vascular plexus (anal cushions)since it is readily distensible and will therefore hold the anal mucosa in apposition during abdominal straining by increasing vascular congestion [24]. Sensation from the urethral mucosa, the skin of the genital area and the anal canal travel through the pudendal nerve [27]. The very sensitive anal epithelium will be able to discriminate between solid, liquid or gas content in the anal canal.

The striated anal sphincter and the puborectalis muscle (the most medial part of the levator ani) are the squeletal muscles involved in fecal continence. The external anal sphincter is the continuation of the puborectalis (Figure 4.3) and it is innervated by the inferior rectal branch of the pudendal nerve [27]. In some cases, a additional input from a direct branch of the fourth sacral nerve has been described [26]. Like the striated muscle sphincter of the urethra, the external anal sphincter and the puborectalis contain a predominance of type 1 fibers and therefore maintain a tonic continuous activity, even at rest, but are also capable of short periods of additional phasic activity [28]. When stimulated by a sharp increase in abdominal pressure, the external anal sphincter will contract but, in addition, the contraction of the puborectalis also displaces the anorectum anteriorly therefore narrowing the anorectal angle and obstructing the

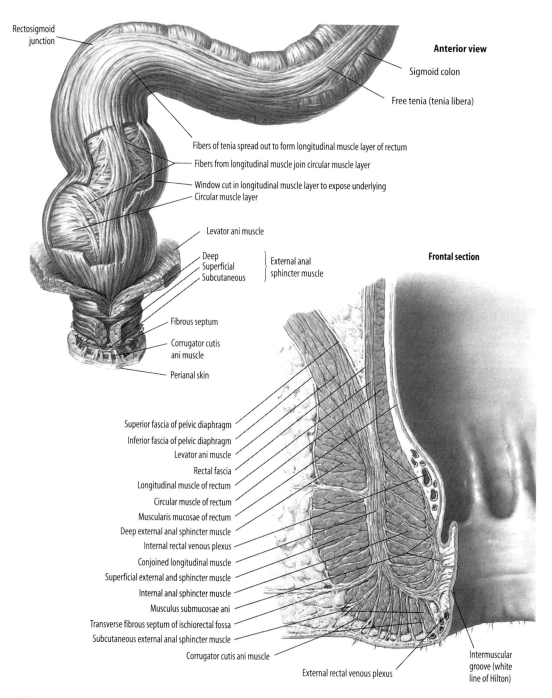

Rectosigmoid junction

Anterior view

Sigmoid colon

Free tenia (tenia libera)

Fibers of tenia spread out to form longitudinal muscle layer of rectum

Fibers from longitudinal muscle join circular muscle layer

Window cut in longitudinal muscle layer to expose underlying

Circular muscle layer

Levator ani muscle

Deep
Superficial
Subcutaneous

External anal sphincter muscle

Frontal section

Fibrous septum

Corrugator cutis ani muscle

Perianal skin

Superior fascia of pelvic diaphragm
Inferior fascia of pelvic diaphragm
Levator ani muscle
Rectal fascia
Longitudinal muscle of rectum
Circular muscle of rectum
Muscularis mucosae of rectum
Deep external anal sphincter muscle
Internal rectal venous plexus
Conjoined longitudinal muscle
Superficial external and sphincter muscle
Internal anal sphincter muscle
Musculus submucosae ani
Transverse fibrous septum of ischiorectal fossa
Subcutaneous external anal sphincter muscle
Corrugator cutis ani muscle

External rectal venous plexus

Intermuscular groove (white line of Hilton)

Figure 4. 3 Innervation of the anal sphincter (Moore K. L., Satter eld S., Clinically Oriented Anatomy, 3rd Edition, Lippincott Williams & Wilkins, pp. 290, 1992

passage of stool. The importance of this contribution of the puborectalis to fecal continence remains controversial. The puborectalis and the external anal sphincter share the same innervation [27]. The pudendal nerve, via its inferior rectal branch, also conveys proprioceptive impulses from the striated muscles of the pelvic floor.

Reflex and voluntary activation of smooth and squeletal muscles of the anorectum and pelvic floor will integrate to either allow defecation or favor rectal storage in the normal individual. The complete neural pathway involved in control of the anorectum is complex. There is evidence that a neural reflex pathway is located at the sacral spinal cord level, since it has been observed that there remains residual autonomous function of bladder and rectum in suprasacral cord transection patients [29]. Although most work has been done in animals, experiments in humans have revealed that part of the superior frontal gyrus and anterior cingulate gyrus along with the adjacent white matter are important for conscious awareness and control of anal sphincter function [30]. Upon rectal filling, the activity of the smooth muscle of the anal canal is completely inhibited (the rectoanal inhibitory reflex) [31]. This relaxation of the internal anal sphincter is a reflex likely mediated by an intrinsic intramural plexus since this reflex is preserved after high cord compression, resection of the rectum, spinal anasthesia and pudendal block [32]. Relaxation of the proximal anal canal will allow the rectal contents to come into contact with the very sensitive anal mucosa of the mid anal canal during what is called the sampling reflex [32]. Once the bolus is recognized (solid, liquid or gas), the external anal sphincter and puborectalis either relax, therefore normal defecation occurs, or they contract, thus forcing the fecal material back into the rectum. In order to maintain fecal continence the following elements are necessary: consistency of stool, capacity of rectum, normal sampling reflex, normal anorectal sensation, normal anal resting tone, intact innervated puborectalis and external anal sphincter muscles and volitional control. In contrast to urinary continence where urine remains the only medium, in the rectum, stool consistency may greatly vary (solid, liquis, flatus) thus affecting continence control in an otherwise competent sphincter. To complicate matters further, there appears to be controversy about whether the anal and urethral sphincters are activated separately or if they function together [25].

In recent years there has been an increasing interest into fecal and urinary incontinence fueled by a greater awareness of these issues from physicians and patients. A better understanding of the neurophysiological basis of voiding and fecal dysfunction, can be instrumnental in helping those affected by these disturbing problems and clearly justifies ungoing research in this field.

References

1. Gilpin CJ, Dixon JS, Gilpin SA, Gosling JA (1983) The fine structure of autonomic neurons in the wall of the human urinary bladder. J Anat 137:705–713
2. Crowe R, Burnstock G, Light JK (1988) Intramural ganglia in the human urethra. J Urol 140:183–187
3. Chai TC, Steers WD (1996) Neurophysiology of micturition and continence. Urologic Clinics of North America 23(2):221–236
4. Daniel EEL, Cowan W, Daniel VP (1983) Structural bases for neural and myogenic control of human detrusor muscle. Can J Physiol Pharmacol 61:1247–1273
5. Ek A, Alm P, Andersson KE, Persson CGA (1977) Adrenergic and cholinergic nerves of the human urethra and urinary bladder. A histochemical study. Acta Physiol Scand, 99:345–352
6. de Groat WC (1999) Basic neurophysiology and neuropharmacology. In Abrams P, Khoury S, Wein A (eds)Proceedings 1st International Consultation on Incontinence, Health Publications Ltd, p107–154
7. de Groat WC (1993)Anatomy and physiology of the lower urinary tract. Urologic Clinics of North America 20(3)383–401
8. Hoyles CHV, Lincoln J, Burnstock G (1994) Neural control of pelvic organs. In Rushton DN (eds) Handbook of neuro-urology, MDI, p1–54
9. Lincoln J, Burnstock G (1993) Autonomic innervation of the urinary bladder and urethra In: Maggi CA (ed) Nervous control of the urogenital tract. Harwood Academic Publishers, pp33–68
10. de Groat WC, Booth AM (1980) Physiology of the urinary bladder and urethra. Ann Intern Med, 92:312–315
11. Gosling JA (1979) The structure of the bladder and urethra in relation to function. Urologic Clinics of North America (6):31–38
12. Sundin T, Dahlstrom A, Norten L, Svedmyr N (1977) The sympathetic innervation and adrenoreceptor function of the human lower urinary tract in the normal state and after parasympathetic denervation. Invest Urol (14), 322–328
13. Dixon J, Gosling J. (1987) Neuromorphology:Structure and Innervation in the Human. In: Torrens M, Morrison JFB (eds)The Physiology of the Lower Urinary Tract, Springer-Verlag, pp3–22
14. Nathan PW (1956) Sensations associated with micturition. Br J Urol, 28:126–131
15. Morrison JFB(1987)Bladder control:role of higher levels of the central nervous system. In:Torrens M, Morrison JFB(eds)The physiology of the lower urinary tract, Springer-Verlag, pp. 193–236
16. de Groat WC, Booth AM, Yoshimura N(1993) Neurophysiology of micturition and its modification in animal models of human disease In Maggi CA(eds) The autonomic nervous system:nervous control of the urogenital system, vol 3, Harwood Academic Publishers, London p. 227
17. Nathan PW(1952) Thermal sensation in the bladder J Neurol Neurosurg Psychiatr 15:148–149
bladder. A histochemical study. Acta Physiol Scand, 99:345–352
17. Learmont JR (1931) A contribution to the neurophysiology of the urinary bladder in man, Brain (54) 147–176
18. Gordon PH (2001) Anorectal anatomy and physiology, Gastroenterology Clinics of North America,30(1), 1–13
19. Keighley MR(1993) Faecal incontinence in:Keighley MRB, Williams NS (eds)Surgery of the anus, rectum and colon, Vol 1, pp. 516–608
20. Wood JD (1981) Physiology of the enteric nervous system. In: MI Grossman, ED Jacobson, SG Schultz(eds) Physiology of the gastrointestinal tract. Raven press, New York, pp1–37
21. Gordon PH (1987) The anorectum:anatomic and physiologic considerations in health and disease, Gastroenterology clinics of north america, 16(1):1–15
22. Duthie HL, Gairns FN(1960) Sensory nerve-endings and sensation in the anal canal region of man. Br Surg 47:585

23. Lane RHS, Parks AG(1977) Function of the anal sphincter following colo-anal anastomosis. Br J Surg. 64:596–599
24. Haas P, Fox TA, Haas GP (1984) The pathogenesis of haemorrhoids, Dis Colon Rectum, 27:442–450
25. Burleigh DE(1992) Pharmacology of the internal anal sphincter. In: Henry MM, Swash M (eds) Coloproctology and the pelvic floor 2nd edition, Butterworth-Heinemann, p37–53
25. Lestar B, Pennickx F, Kerremans RP(1989) The composition of anal basal pressure. An in vivo and in vitro study in man, Int J Colorectal Dis, 4:118–122
26. Rasmussen O (1994) Anorectal function, Dis Colon Rectum, 37:386-403
27. Uher EM, Swash M (1998) Sacral reflexes: physiology and application, Dis Colon Rectum, 41, 1165–1177

28. floyd WF, Walls EW (1953) Electromyography of the sphincter ani externus in man. Journal of Physiology, 122, 599–609
29. Vodusek DB, Janko M, Loker J(1983) Direct and reflex responses in perineal muscles on electrical stimulation, J of Neurology, Neurosurgery, and Psychiatry (46) 67–71
30. Andrew J, Nathan P(1964) Lesions of the anterior frontal lobes and disturbances of micturition and defecation, Brain, 87:233–262
31. Lestar B, Pennick F, Kerremans RP(1989) The composition of anal basal pressure. An in vivo and in vitro study in man, Int J Colorectal Dis, 4:118–122
32. Schuster MM, Hookman P, Hendrix TR, Mendeloff AI(1965) Simultaneous manometric recording of internal and external anal sphincter reflexes. Bull Johns Hopkins Hosp, 116, 79–88

5 Clinical Aspects of Urinary, Genital and Lower Bowel Anomalies and Ambiguous Genitalia

Gillian D. Oliver

Introduction

This chapter endeavors to provide the necessary background in congenital anomalies of the urogenital system and lower bowel for the pelvic surgeon. Incorporated in this synopsis is a brief review of embryology, sexual development, and intersex disorders. Surgical principles in restoring anatomy are discussed.

Embryology of the Urogenital System

A through understanding of the development of the urogenital system is essential for the pelvic surgeon to accurately diagnose a presenting anomaly. A full appreciation of the potential variations in anatomy will enable the surgeon to anticipate surgical challenges, and thereby achieve superior postoperative results.

Formation of the Urologic System

The urogenital system begins as the cloaca at week 4 of embryogenesis [1]. The cloaca arises from the yolk sac as a union of the hindgut, allantois and wolffian duct. In week 7, the urorectal septum forms, and fuses with the cloacal membrane, thereby bisecting the cloaca into the dorsal hindgut and ventral urogenital sinus. At the same time, the urogenital membrane dissolves, creating an opening in the urogenital sinus (Figure 5.1).

The mesonephric duct contributes to the adult ureter and urethra [1]. In week 5, the mesonephric duct gives rise to the ureteric bud. Both enter the cloaca together at the dorsomedial aspect of the

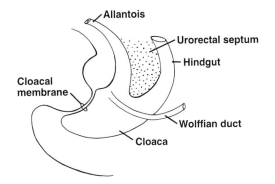

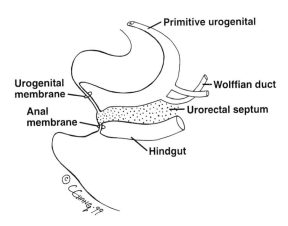

Figure 5.1 Formation of the primitive urogenital system: weeks 4–7 embryogenesis.

cloaca (week 7). The mesonephric duct divides the urogenital sinus into a cranial urethrovesical canal and caudal definitive urogenital sinus. With growth, the mesonephric bud migrates superiolaterally to the eventual location of the ureter, while the original mesonephric duct migrates inferiomedially to form the trigone and proximal urethra. The most caudal portion of the mesonephric duct can persist in adulthood as Gartner's duct [2]. The urethrovesical canal is destined to form the bladder, part of the urethra (prostatic) in males and the entire urethra in females. By the twelfth week of embryogenesis, splanchnopleuric mesoderm surrounds the bladder to provide smooth muscle. Eventually, the allantois regresses, and is identified as a remnant known as the urachus (Figure 5.1).

Gonadal Development

At week 4 of development, the embryo's gonads begin to form. Initially, a gathering of biopotential primordial germ cells, mesenchyme and coelomic epithelium identified as the genital ridge, the gonadal tissue demonstrates its potential under the influence of the organism's sex chromosomes [3]. The gonads are destined to become ovaries, unless influenced by the sex-determining region, a segment of genes located on the short arm of the Y chromosome. This gene sequence directs production of testicular determinant factor (TDF), which is essential to the development of the male testes. In the male, the medulla of the gonad proliferates, and the cortex regress. In the female, the cortex proliferates and the medulla regresses to form ovaries. It is felt that regulatory genes, located on the autosomal chromosomes, also make a significant contribution to testicular development [4].

By week 5, under the influence of TDF, the coelomic epithelium proliferates and penetrates the underlying mesenchyme, giving rise to the primitive sex cords [2]. At the same time, a mesenchymal band forms at the caudal end of the gonad as a precursor of the gubernaculum. This is followed in week 6 by migration of the primordial germ cells into the primitive testes. In the testes, Sertoli cells are evident by week 6 of embryogenesis. These cells produce mullerian inhibiting factor (MIF), a parahormone which actively suppresses the formation of the paramesonephric (mullerian) system ipsilateral to the gonad in which MIF is produced. This is known as the Jostian principle [5]. In 1947, Jost eloquently demonstrated the local parahormone effect of MIF in an experiment using embryological rabbits. He castrated male rabbits at progressively later stages of development, and demonstrated the importance of testes to ipsilateral duct development.

At 8 weeks, Leydig cells are developed and under the influence of placental hCG begin to produce testosterone [3]. Testosterone actively stimulates the evolution of the wolffian system, eventually giving rise to the vas deferens, epididymis, and seminal vesicles. Dehydrotestosterone (DHT) is detectable by 14 weeks and it is this testosterone derivative that is

responsible for virilization of the external genitalia [3] (Figure 5.2).

Formation of the Female Internal Genitalia

At week 6, the paramesonephric duct evolves from the coelemic epithelium of the urogenital ridge near the third thoracic somite [1]. The wolffian duct lies just under the coelemic epithelium. It is thought the wolffian duct may act as a trigger to the formation of the paramesonephric duct and as a guide for its caudal growth [1]. The paramesonephric duct grows lateral to the wolffian duct, crossing medially within the pelvic brim to fuse with its counterpart from the other side, thus forming the uterovaginal primordium. This structure will eventually give rise to the uterus, cervix and upper vagina, as the dividing septum dissolves by the end of embryonic week 11. The cranial portion of the paramesonephric ducts remains unfused, forming the left and right fallopian tubes (Figure 5.3).

The uterovaginal primordium approaches the urogenital sinus at the mullerian tubercle, which lies between the two orifices of the laterally placed wolffian ducts [1]. This meeting of the uterovaginal primordium and the mullerian tubercle stimulates development of two endodermal invaginations termed sinovaginal bulbs. These bulbs grow until approximately week 16 to create the solid primitive vaginal plate. The primitive vaginal plate canalizes to create a tubular structure, the vaginal canal, by 20 weeks of gestation. Therefore, the vaginal canal is derived from the urogenital sinus but the surrounding fibromuscular wall is from the paramesonephric duct. The surrounding mesenchyme condenses, and transforms into the uterine stroma and myometrium. The cervix is formed at 20 weeks of gestation by condensation of the stromal cells between the uterine and vaginal structures (Figure 5.3).

It is important to remember that without TDF, the gonads develop into ovaries in which the cortex of the structure proliferates and the medulla regresses. Note that unless suppressed by MIF, the paramesonephric (mullerian) system will spontaneously develop and become the fallopian tubes, uterus, cervix, and upper vagina. Furthermore, without testosterone, the wolffian system will spontaneously regress or fail to develop beyond primitive structures. It is of note that the evolution of the paramesonephric duct starts 2 weeks behind Sertoli cell MIF production. It is therefore possible for the Sertoli cells to exert their suppressive influence on

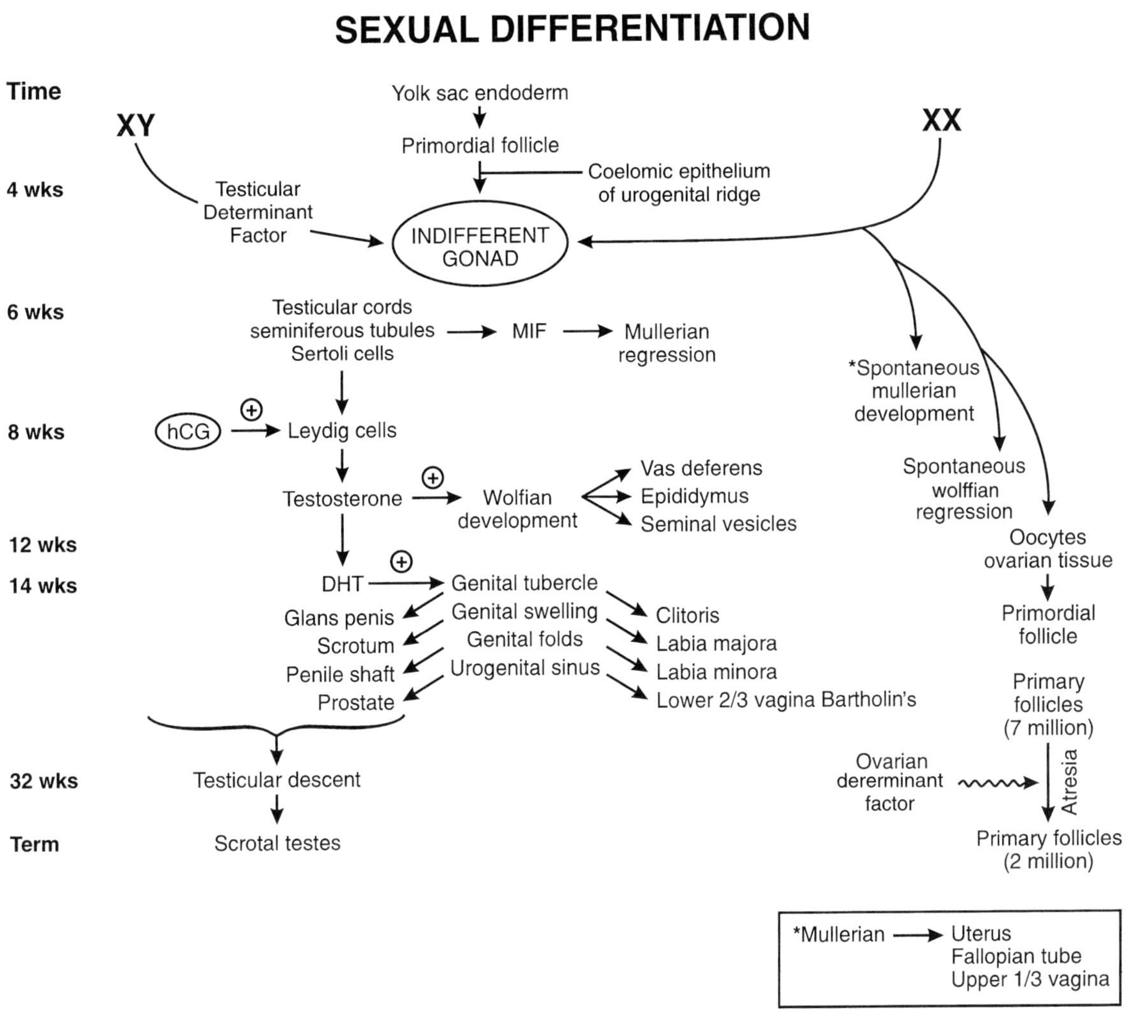

SEXUAL DIFFERENTIATION

Figure 5.2 Sexual differentiation.

the paramesonephric duct before an arrest in the testicular development. This is known as Swyer's syndrome (XY female without internal genitalia, but no testes or testosterone production).

Formation of External Genitalia

The external genitalia begins at 6 weeks of embryogenesis, when the mesenchyme surrounding the cloaca proliferates, giving rise to the genital tubercle, and more lateral cloacal folds [2]. By week 7, labioscrotal swellings, lateral to the cloacal folds, can be identified. The endoderm of the cloaca thickens to form the urethral plate. The ectoderm of the genital tubercle is in contact with the endoderm of the urethral plate. The cloacal folds infold to create a "primitive urethral groove", and the urogenital sinus advances along this tract to provide an endodermal lining in all but the most superficial part of the adult urethra.

The common anlagen are the genital tubercle, urethral folds and labioscrotal swellings [2]. In the male, the genital tubercle becomes the corpora cavernosa and glans penis. The urethral folds form the urethra, and the labioscrotal swellings fuse to form the scrotum. In the female, the genital tubercle forms the clitoris, the labioscrotal swellings form the labia majora, and the urethral folds form the labia minora (Figure 5.4).

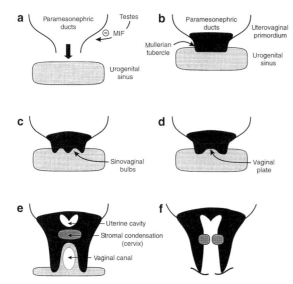

Figure 5.3   Evolution of the mullerian system.

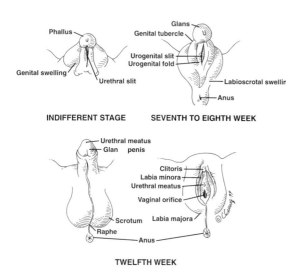

Figure 5.4   Development of the external genitalia.

Clinical Aspects of Congenital Anomalies

Development of the urogenital structures evolves over a period of 20 weeks, and there are a multitude of opportunities to disrupt the process giving rise to an array of potential anomalies. These anomalies can be seen in isolation or as part of a more complex picture. The earlier the assault to the developing embryo, the more extensive the anomaly. For example, disruption of the formation of the cloaca or

urogenital sinuses can impact on the subsequent development of the paramesonephric ducts. This is an important point to be remembered by all pelvic surgeons, whether urologist, general surgeon, or gynecologist. Recognizing the distinction between development of the urinary, alimentary, and genital systems is artificial. Such categorization facilitates understanding of the various anomalies encountered, their potential etiology, and therefore an organized approach to management. However, all surgeons experienced in dealing with congenital anomalies of the urogenital system appreciate the value of a multi-disciplined approach in restoring their patient to as near as possible normal anatomy and function.

Cloacal Deformities

This defect represents a failure of the septation of the cloaca leading to persistence of the rudimentary midgut, and imperforate anus [6]. It is reported to occur in 1/200 000 to 1/250 000 newborns [7]. The precipitating insult occurs early in embryogenesis at approximately week 4 [6]. The resultant disruption in pelvic anatomy can also lead to gender ambiguity [8]. Therefore, gender assignment must also be established early in the diagnosis.

Initially, these newborns require a diverting colostomy [9]. Anal pull-through and reconstruction of the bladder conduit and drainage should be coordinated as a single procedure [9]. Otherwise, performing an anal pull-through in isolation can lead to obstruction of the urinary outflow via the rectovaginal fistula and its sequelae [8]. Vesicoureteral reflex is common in these individuals, and reimplantation is often necessary at the same time [8]. Reconstruction of the genitalia is entertained in later infancy after the integrity of the alimentary and urinary systems has been preserved [10].

Normalization as much as possible of the external anatomy to assigned gender is usually achieved in early childhood. Although vaginal drainage must be established in the newborn phase, creation of a functional vaginal passage should be delayed until after puberty [10]. If the vagina enters the urogenital sinus low, it can be mobilized and exteriorized by a transperineal approach [9]. However, if the vagina fuses high in the urogenital sinus, a diverting vaginoplasty with grafting is required, leaving the urogenital sinus to function as the urethra [9].

Imperforate Anus

The high imperforate defect results from disruption of formation of the urorectal septum at approximately week 7 of embryogenesis [1]. Agenesis of the anorectal canal is usually associated with a rectovaginal fistula. A lower imperforate anus can result from either persistence of the anal membrane, or excessive fusion of the genital folds [1]. In Hall's series of 162 cases of imperforate anus, 79% had rectovaginal fistulas [11]. Of these, 22 had associated vaginal anomalies other than rectovaginal fistula. These defects included vaginal septum, agenesis, partial agenesis, and imperforate hymen. In 51 patients whose upper genital tracts were investigated, 18 had anomalies including uterine didelphys, bicornuate uterus or hypoplastic uterus.

Bladder Exstrophy

A relatively uncommon congenital anomaly, bladder exstrophy occurs in approximately 1/50 000 newborn females [12]. It is more common among males, at 1/30 000 to 1/40 000 [13]. A proportion of these males will have associated genital disfiguration such that sex reassignment might have to be considered.

Classically, the defect includes the absence of the lower anterior abdominal wall with protrusion of the internal bladder mucosa to the external environment [10]. The bladder neck is poorly defined, and the urethra is short and dilated. Pubic bones are splayed, causing the mons to be split. Also, the phallus is bifid, splayed or only a rudimentary structure. The vagina is usually short, horizontal, and stenosed. Lateral fusion defects of the mullerian system are common. The anus is usually displaced anteriorly.

The etiology of the diagnosis has two theories. Patton and Barry theorize that this defect is due to the caudal displacement of the genital tubercle which allows persistence of the cloacal membrane [14]. Marshall and Muecke claim there is overdevelopment of the cloacal membrane, preventing the migration of the mesenchyme tissue between the endodermal and ectodermal layers [15]. This results in a larger than usual defect for the anal and urogenital orifices.

Clearly, the primary goal in management of this anomaly is preservation of renal function, followed by reconstruction of the bladder to gain urinary continence [10]. If continence is not achievable, then socially acceptable urinary division is the next acceptable alternative. Surgical reconstruction favors a two-stage procedure. Initial closure of the bladder and abdominal wall within 48 hours of life is performed (Figure 5.5a). Follow-up continence surgery is attempted at around age three (Figure 5.5b) [16]. Penile reconstruction can also be done

around this time. Vaginal and perineal reconstruction is best delayed until after puberty [12].

From a gynecologic perspective, these individuals are at risk for vaginal stenosis and dyspareunia [12,17,18]. Uterine prolapse is also seen as a result of the splayed pelvis and lack of urogenital support [12,17]. Uterine anomalies and their associated outflow concerns are common [12]. Fertility can be compromised as a result of the mullerian anomalies as well as postoperative intra-abdominal adhesions and consequent fallopian tube injury. Recurrent and chronic vulvitis can result from incomplete urinary continence. Prophylactic urinary antisepsis predisposes these women to recurrent yeast vulvovaginitis.

In pregnancy, these women face an even greater risk of ascending urinary infection, and should be vigilantly monitored for this complication [12,18,19]. There is no evidence, however, of deterioration in renal function [12]. Those with stomal sites for intermittent catheterization report increased risk of stomal prolapse [19]. There has been no reported increase in obstructive complications from ileal conduits or ureterosigmoid transplant [12].

Fetal risk of bladder exstrophy is not increased [12]. Early ultrasound and maternal alpha-fetoprotein screening will help diagnose bladder exstrophy prenatally [20]. Intrauterine growth restriction due to uterine anomalies is a concern, as is prematurity and fetal malpresentation.

At delivery, consideration should be given to protecting and preserving prior continence surgery, as damage is unlikely to be as successfully repaired with subsequent surgery. Patients with bladder neck surgery or ureterosigmoidostomy should undergo elective cesarean section, although Krisiloff would suggest delivery for obstetric indications only [12,19]. Those without significant uterine prolapse should also be counseled for cesarean section delivery to prevent subsequent prolapse after vaginal delivery [12,19]. Blakeley and Mills suggest patients with ileal conduits should deliver vaginally, if at all possible, as previous surgery leaves a high risk of difficult bowel dissection at the time of cesarean section [12]. It is the author's opinion that this is the very situation one wishes to avoid, an emergency procedure where minutes count, and would therefore support elective cesarean sections in these patients as well. Of course, cesarean section delivery for the usual obstetrical indications is also appropriate. Ideally, cesarean sections should aim for a lower segment incision, but a classical incision may be preferable or necessary to preserve the reconstructed bladder and the patient should be made aware of this possibility.

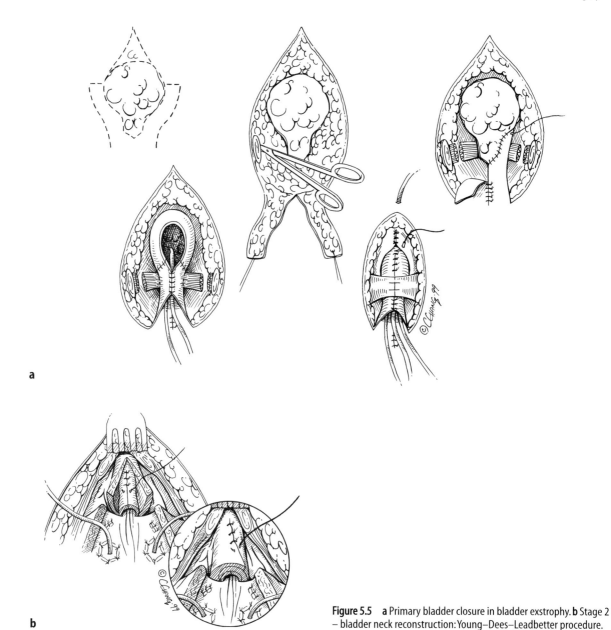

a

b

Figure 5.5 **a** Primary bladder closure in bladder exstrophy. **b** Stage 2 – bladder neck reconstruction: Young–Dees–Leadbetter procedure.

Ectopic Ureter

This uncommon anomaly is highly associated with duplication of the ureters [1]. Ectopic ureter is the abnormal position of the ureter outside the bladder such as the urethra, vestibule, or vagina. These individuals present with urinary incontinence or persistent watery vaginal discharge. Diagnosis is usually made by high index of suspicion on history and confirmatory intravenous pyelogram. Surgery involves isolation of the ectopic ureter and reimplantation in the appropriate bladder trigone.

Prune Belly

An extremely rare condition estimated to be present in 1/35 000 to 1/50 000 live births, this defect is due to failure of development of the secondary mesenchyme at week 12 of embryogenesis [21]. It is exceedingly rare in females. These individuals have megabladder, along with absence of urethra, vagina, and rectum. Surgery aims to provide appropriate drainage of bowel and bladder. In the rare cases of females with prune belly syndrome, mullerian defects are reported [21]. The surgeon should

Table 5.1 AFS classification of uterovaginal anomalies (modified)

Class I	Dysgenesis
Class II	Disorders of vertical fusion
Class III	Disorders of lateral fusion
Class IV	Unusual configurations (mixed)

endeavor to create a functional vagina and preservation of fertility if at all possible.

Uterovaginal Anomalies

The true incidence of anomalies of the mullerian system is probably under-represented as the spectrum of defects can span from minor clinically inconsequential fusion defects to complete failure of the process. The modified American Fertility Society (AFS) classification system offers a useful approach to organizing the potential variations in paramesonephric (mullerian) development [22] (Table 5.1).

Class I – Mullerian Duct Dysgenesis

Failure of the paramesonephric ducts to develop (mullerian agenesis) is also known as Mayer–Rokatansky–Kuster–Hauser syndrome after the various gynecologists who describe this condition [23]. Mayer was the first to recognize this anomaly in 1829 [24]. Mullerian agenesis is thought to show autosomal dominant inheritance, with an incidence estimated to be 1/4000 to 1/5000 female births [25].

These women usually present in teen years with primary amenorrhea, having gone through an apparently otherwise normal puberty. Clinical examination is entirely normal except for the finding of an absent vaginal opening, or vaginal dimple in the otherwise normal external female genitalia (Figure 5.6). The major differential diagnosis is complete androgen insensitivity syndrome. However, women with mullerian agenesis have a normal XX karyotype and intact ovarian function. Ultrasound will confirm the absence of or rudimentary upper vaginal and uterine structures with normally placed ovaries, possessing evidence of follicle development. Other differential diagnoses include imperforate hymen, transverse vaginal septum, and partial vaginal agenesis, all of which can be excluded by presence of a functional uterus and hematocolpos on ultrasound.

It is important to remember the close association of the paramesonephric and mesonephric duct during embryogenesis. It is not surprising then to learn that 30% of individuals with mullerian agene-

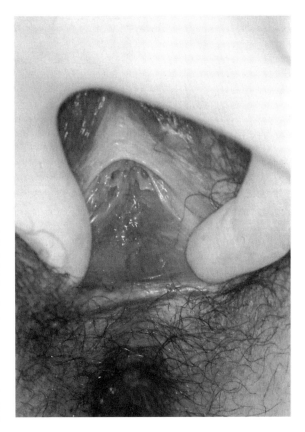

Figure 5.6 Vaginal agenesis.

sis have associated renal anomalies, such as unilateral renal aplasia, pelvic kidney, or renal ectopia [26]. Interestingly, these women also have approximately 10% incidence of minor skeletal anomalies such as spina bifida occulta and absent ribs [27].

Once the diagnosis of mullerian agenesis has been confirmed, treatment goals should include appropriate patient education regarding her condition [26]. It is important she understand that she will never menstruate or carry a pregnancy, but that she can expect to attain normal sexual function and has the potential to reproduce with use of in vitro fertilization and surrogacy.

Approaches to the creation of a neo-vagina in this condition have been widely and extensively published [17,22–25,27–32,36,38–44,46]. In assessing the various techniques, the surgeon should always bear in mind that the goal is to create a female vagina, rather than a receptacle for a penis. There are several surgical techniques which will be discussed shortly, but there is also a growing recognition of the success and advantages of progressive dilating in developing the endogenous vaginal tissue into a very acceptable vaginal canal.

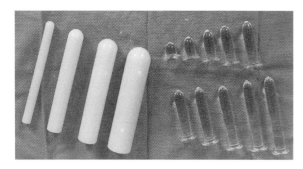

Figure 5.7 Vaginal dilators. Left: Frank dilators. Right: Ingram dilators.

Initially described by Frank in 1938, pressure dilation of the vaginal remnant has regained prominence as a preferable approach in the motivated patient [28]. Using sequentially larger dilators, the patient actively stretches the incumbent vaginal skin by daily exercises (Figure 5.7). Pressure dilation requires patience, persistence, and determination on the part of the patient along with a supportive health care team to provide ongoing education and monitoring of progress. Given the above conditions, one could expect to see an acceptable vaginal canal in 3–9 months of daily dilating. Ingram introduced the concept of self-dilation using sequential dilators mounted strategically on a bicycle seat [29]. Using the patient's own body weight to provide a more aggressive dilation, Ingram reported quicker results than seen by the Frank method.

Pressure dilation spares the patient major surgery, its inherent risks and resultant tell-tale scar. It also is a more forgiving approach to the non-compliant patient who might be at risk for not maintaining postoperative dilating and subsequently develop a vaginal stricture. Since progressive dilating creates no scars, there is no risk of stricture, only recoverable loss of length from sexual inactivity or non-compliance with dilation. Complications of pressure dilation include inappropriate dilation of other orifices such as urethra or rectum, inadequate progress due to discomfort or aversion to dilating and prolapse of the stretched vaginal skin [27].

Surgical Approaches to Creation of a Neovagina. The surgical creation of a vagina is often necessary in complex anomalies where anatomy is not conducive to self-dilation. Other indications for a surgical approach include patient inability to self-dilate or the patient's unwillingness to wait the average 3–9 months required for self-dilation to achieve an acceptable vaginal canal. It is important, however, to counsel the patient that surgery itself is not a quick and easy solution, and to emphasize that ongoing

life-long dilation of the vaginal canal will often still be required even after surgery.

The timing of neovaginoplasty remains somewhat controversial. The gynecologic literature would favor waiting until the patient is physically and emotionally mature enough to understand the goals and complications of surgery, as well as comply with postoperative dilation and care of the neovagina [9,12,26,30]. This would certainly be true in mullerian agenesis, in which the diagnosis is not commonly made until late puberty anyway. In more complex anomalies, there is a growing popularity among pediatric surgeons to perform a one-step reconstruction in the early childhood years, citing the reduced numbers of procedures and the restoration to "normal" anatomy as quickly as possible [31,32]. Literature examining long-term follow-ups of this early reconstruction is lacking, particularly regarding sexual function and performance, as the majority of these patients are just now entering puberty. Anecdotal experience of the author would suggest that while the resulting anatomy is cosmetically acceptable, the potential function of the neovaginal passage is questionable. Given that repeated surgery on the vagina leads to increased risk of fistula, stenosis, graft sloughing, and infection, and long-term data supporting a one-step surgery clearly is lacking, the author recommends caution in embracing this trend.

Skin Graft Vaginoplasty. Introduced by McIndoe in 1938, this technique involves developing the potential space between the urethra and rectum where the vaginal canal would normally be placed [33]. A split thickness skin graft is then harvested from the patient's buttock or thigh, placed over a soft inflatable phallic-shaped mold and placed in this potential space. The graft is then secured in place with a series of interrupted sutures at the vulvovaginal verge. The upper graft is held in place by the pressure of the inflated mold which is secured in place by retaining sutures until such time as the surgeon removes the mold. Firm plastic molds have also been used; however, there is an associated increased risk of hematoma, fistulas, and graft sloughing (Figure 5.8) [23,30,33,34].

The length of time until removal of the mold is variable, dependent on individual surgeons' preferences. This can range from 7 days to 6 months. However, most agree that nightly insertion of the mold and daily vaginal dilation are needed to maintain canal length and caliber during the healing phase of up to 3–6 months. Subsequently, the frequency of dilating and use of a night mold is again subject to individual surgeon preference. In general, ongoing monitoring against shortening and stric-

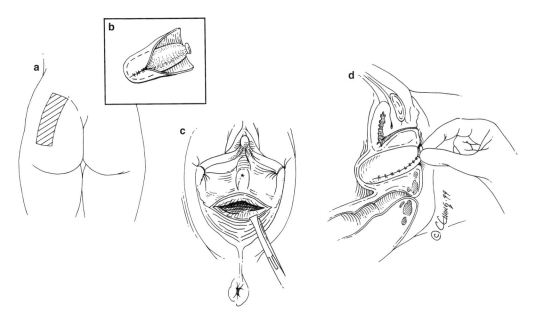

Figure 5.8 The McIndoe procedure for vaginoplasty.

ture formation is a common concern [23,30,33–35]. In spite of this issue, the skin graft vaginoplasty remains one of the most popular approaches to a neovagina. The technique generally has a high success rate with relatively minimal risk to the patient. Surgical risks include intraoperative bleeding, injury to the urethra or rectum, and inadequate skin graft harvest [23,30,33–35]. Postoperative complications include infection, graft shortening, stenosis, dyspareunia, and graft site cheloid formation [23,33,34,49]. Modifications in this technique have been offered, including use of amnion for graft tissue, thereby avoiding the graft site scarring. The use of amnion carries the risk of transmittable blood-borne diseases such as HIV, hepatitis B or C, leaving this variation less desirable for a young, otherwise healthy patient.

Skin Flap Vaginoplasty. Skin flaps in vaginal reconstruction have received great attention, and a number of techniques have been described [9]. The perineal flap, in which an inverted U-flap is created on the perineum and placed into the vaginal canal to bridge the lower vagina, is a commonly used technique [9]. This is an effective approach when a majority of the vaginal tract is formed, and only the lower one-third of the vagina is stenosed, or absent, such as in mild virilizing syndromes [9].

In situations where the vagina is absent or a significant portion is deficient, a number of flap designs have been used [36–40]. These include: the vulvovaginal (Williams) pouch; myocutaneous groin or gluteal flaps; gracilis flap; transpelvic rectus abdominis flap; and expanded vulvar flaps. These techniques can be helpful in bringing additional blood supply to the area such as in post-irradiation cancer cases, but is generally not the procedure of choice in congenital anomalies (Figure 5.9).

Colononeovagina. The use of the bowel to act as a vaginal canal was first described by Baldwin in 1904 using ileum [23]. Pratt, in 1972, repopularized the role of bowel using the lower colon [23]. In this approach, a segment of sigmoid colon is isolated via laparotomy. More recently, laparoscopic bowel harvest has been described [41]. The blood supply to the segment is maintained and the segment transplanted to the potential vaginal space which has been developed from below. The segment of colon used is then closed superiorly, creating a blind-ended neovagina. This technique offers the advantage of using the patient's own tissue (no transmittable infection), reduced risk of stricture (inherently tubular tissue), and bringing a good blood supply to the operative field (less risk of infection or graft failure). However, this technique also has significant risks in addition to the previously stated surgical risks, such as postoperative peritonitis and sepsis, bowel stricture, obstruction and death [42]. Inflammation and ulceration of the neovagina has also been reported [42].

The use of colonic tissue brings a naturally secretory tissue to the neovagina. The discharge is often copious, foul smelling, and quite distressing to the

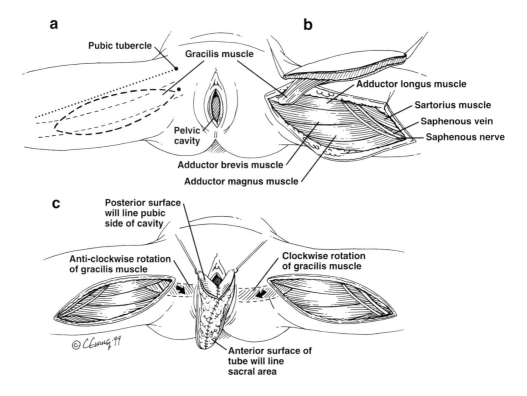

Figure 5.9 Vaginal reconstruction with bilateral gracilis myocutaneous flaps.

patient. Regular douching can help control this problem, but it remains a significant postoperative issue [43]. In the past, the risk of serious complications has made colonovaginoplasty less popular for creation of a neovagina in an otherwise healthy young woman [44]. However, improved surgical techniques are challenging this perspective [24,41,43,45]. The use of a colononeovagina in developing a passage in younger children requiring earlier surgery for the drainage of a functional uterus (mucocolpos or hematocolpos) deserves consideration as freedom from postoperative dilating for the very young and emotionally immature patient makes this approach an appealing option [9].

Class II – Disorders of Vertical Fusion

This classification includes a spectrum of defects resulting in blockage of the genital outflow tract including (a) imperforate hymen, (b) transverse vaginal septum, (c) partial vaginal agenesis, and (d) cervical agenesis.

Imperforate Hymen. A common anomaly, this defect usually presents in late puberty as a visible fluctuate membrane bulging at the introitus in an adolescent with abdominal pain, amenorrhea and possibly a pelvic mass (hematocolpos). It can also present in

the neonate as a mass protruding at the introitus (mucocele) which regresses over the first 6 weeks of life as the effects of maternal estrogen decrease [9]. Imperforate hymen represents failure of the canalization process of the vaginal plate at the extreme caudal aspect, the urogenital sinus (Figure 5.10) [1].

The major differential diagnosis is a lower transverse vaginal septum. Repair of the imperforate hymen involves a simple cruciate incision of the hymen and evacuation of the hematocolpos under anesthetic. It is prudent to perform a speculum examination to ensure the remainder of the vagina is patent and normal with a visible cervix.

Transverse Vaginal System. The transverse septum is a blockage of the vaginal tract between the cervix and the hymen. Incidence of this disorder is reported in a range of 1/2000 to 1/70 000, dependent on the population studied [46]. In the Amish population, for example, it appears to demonstrate an autosomal recessive pattern, and owing to increased consanguinity is much more common [47]. However, in the majority of cases, the defect is felt to be idiopathic. Although the septal length is variable, it is generally thicker the more superior in the vagina. Upper vaginal septa are more common (46%), versus middle (35%) and lower vaginal septa

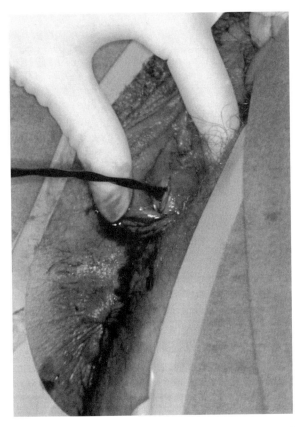

Figure 5.10 Incision of imperforate hymen and release of hematocolpos.

(19%) [48]. It is reported that the higher the septum, the greater its impact on subsequent pregnancy rates, suggesting an influence on cervix anatomy or function [48]. It is the author's opinion that higher septa are often thicker and more difficult to repair surgically. Subsequent pregnancy rates might reflect postoperative stenosis and impaired sexual function, leading to decreased sperm deposition at the cervical verge. A good postoperative result should alleviate these concerns in reproductive performance and studies controlling for these variables need to be completed.

These individuals usually present in mid to late puberty, with pelvic pain and amenorrhea. The author has, however, experienced a presentation of life-threatening bilateral uteric obstruction due to a higher transverse vaginal septum and mucocele in the neonate. Endometriosis is associated with this defect, thought to be due to reversed menstrual regress. Earlier studies suggesting this relationship to endometriosis commonly made the diagnosis at time of presentation and surgical repair when hematocolpos was present [49]. This is a questionable diagnosis under these conditions. The author

would suggest the diagnosis be entertained and confirmed if necessary, should the patient return with associated symptomatology. Laparoscopy at the time of septal repair should be reserved for cases suggesting additional upper tract anomalies.

Differential diagnosis of the transverse system includes partial vaginal agenesis, obstructive longitudinal vaginal system, and imperforate hymen. The possibility of a partial vaginal agenesis should always be ruled out prior to surgical repair of a transverse vaginal system, as partial vaginal agenesis will often require skin grafting to alleviate the obstruction and maintain a patent canal. This can be achieved by a detailed assessment of the septal thickness prior to surgery. One should be able to feel a bulging mass anteriorly on rectal examination, up to the level of the septum identified on vaginal examination. Transvaginal or labial ultrasound will help confirm one's clinical impression. An obstructed longitudinally vaginal septum is commonly mistaken for a transverse vaginal septum, as the obstructed canal fills and blocks the entire vaginal passage. A history of painful menses with a finding of upper tract duplication should alert the surgeon to this possibility.

The surgical approach to correction of a transverse vaginal system involves resection of the entire septum, and reattachment of the upper to lower vagina. If the septum is relatively thin, reattachment can easily be accomplished by a series of interrupted radial sutures at the site of resection. However, in the thickened septum in which this defect is larger, mobilization of the usually distended upper vaginal cuff may be necessary. Alternatively, a Z-plasty approach to the edges of the upper and lower vagina may be necessary to bridge the defect. This involves suturing the upper and lower vagina cuffs to the lateral underlying paravaginal tissue to provide a continuous path of endovaginal tissue and hemostasis. Some secondary epithelialization is sought in this situation. Alternatively, preoperative dilation of the septum can be done using menstrual suppression to gain the necessary time to stretch the tissue [50]. The immediate complications of repair of this defect include injury to urethra or rectum, hemorrhage and poor visibility. Long term, the issue of contracture of the surgical scar leading to vaginal stenosis, and recurrent obstruction is a major concern [49]. Proper initial resection and repair along with early and aggressive postoperative dilation can minimize this risk.

Partial Vaginal Agenesis. This defect involves the partial absence of the vaginal canal with an intact upper genital tract. Consequently, these individuals present with abdominal pain and primary amenorrhea in mid to late puberty. The major differential diagnosis is transverse vaginal septum. The key difference between these two conditions is the extent of the blockage. In partial vaginal agenesis, the extent of the defect is such that skin grafts are required to bridge the defect between the upper and lower vagina. In addition, there is an increased risk of fistula formation to either the urethra or rectum as the paravaginal plane is absent. Preoperative preparation and informed consent are clearly important.

Cervical Agenesis. This defect represents the failure of stromal condensation and canalization of the mullerian tubercle in formation of the cervix. These individuals present much like other disorders of vertical fusion with abdominal pain and primary amenorrhea in mid to late puberty. Preoperative diagnosis of this defect is paramount as the patient counseling, and surgical management, is quite different than other vertical fusion defects. Unless there is clearly an identifiable cervix and endocervical canal on ultrasound, the author highly recommends preoperative magnetic resonance imaging (MRI). Again, not only should a cervical structure be identifiable, but also a patent endocervical canal. This is a reliable finding on MRI with an experienced radiologist. Failure to identify these structures should raise significant concern for a diagnosis of cervical agenesis.

Management of cervical agenesis remains disappointing. Attempts at fertility preservation by creation of the cervix and canalization of the passage from uterus to vagina have been fraught with failure. Neovaginoplasty can be used to recreate the upper vagina but not to replicate the cervix in terms of uterine continence, mucus production, and a physiologic barrier to ascending infection. The resulting cervix is always stenotic and at risk for reobstruction. Although patency may be established, subsequent reproductive performance remains compromised with risk of cervical factor infertility, incompetent cervix, recurrent pelvic inflammatory disease, and its resultant upper tract damage [51]. Traditionally, cases of cervical agenesis have been managed by hysterectomy for relief of the hematocolpos [51]. However, in spite of these concerns, in selected cases, there is renewed optimism for surgical correction of this anomaly [52]. Success rates in terms of fertility and fecundity with this technique remain yet to be determined.

Disorders of Lateral Fusion
These anomalies can be classified as either obstructive or non-obstructive. Non-obstructive lateral

fusion defects range from the T-shaped uterus, classically associated with diethylstilbestrol (DES) exposure, to complete uterine and vaginal duplication, dependent on the time of the insult. For example, an insult at 6–7 weeks will result in uterine didelphys, whereas a later insult at 11–12 weeks gives rise to a septate uterus [1].

Although it is often sought as a cause for habitual abortion, less than 10% of women with recurrent pregnancy loss have abnormal anatomy on hysterosalpingogram (HSG) [53]. The septate uterus is associated with a term pregnancy rate of between 5 and 10% with a known risk of prematurity, malpresentation and cesarean section [53]. Metroplasty can improve term pregnancy rates to as much as 80–90% in cases of septate uterus [53]. Hysteroscopic septal resection should be considered as the surgery of choice if one is certain to be dealing with a septate uterus, rather than bicornuate uterus.

The impact of metroplasty on bicornuate uterus is less clear. There is a known tendency to improve gestational age at delivery with each subsequent pregnancy [53]. This is felt to be a result of increased uterine capacity with subsequent pregnancies. Reliable data is therefore not available on surgical intervention in cases of bicornuate uterus. The surgeon should be reasonably comfortable that he or she is truly improving the uterine environment by metroplasty if improved reproductive outcome is the goal.

Complete genital tract duplication can also be associated with prematurity, malpresentation and cesarean section, but generally surgical correction is not indicated. On occasion, the patient can present with dyspareunia, difficulty with use of tampons or chronic vaginal discharge from a poorly draining, narrow vaginal passage. In these situations, resection of the vaginal septum may be indicated [48].

Obstructive lateral fusion defects usually present shortly after menarche as severe dysmenorrhea. The pain is a result of uterine distension of the obstructed horn. If the obstructed passage can be alleviated, then facilitating drainage is the main goal of the surgery. In some cases, however, permanent drainage cannot be achieved, and the mullerian remnant must then be excised by either laparoscopy or laparotomy.

Mixed Fusion Defects
This category includes combined complex fusion defects often resulting from an earlier developmental insult such as bladder exstrophy or cloacal defect. These complex anomalies are detailed elsewhere.

Ambiguous Genitalia

The external genitalia is destined to become female unless actively influenced by the presence and ability to respond to DHT [3]. The term male pseudohermaphroditism is applied to chromosomal males (XY) who are undervirilized. Female pseudo-hermaphroditism refers to genetic XX females who have virilized genitalia. True hermaphroditism is applied to individuals with XX and XY cell lines expressed with evidence of both ovarian and testicular tissue present.

Determination of an individual's sex is a culmination of four factors (Table 5.2) [3]. One's chromosomal pattern determines one's potential biologic sex. The phenotype of an individual reflects the impact of the chromosomes on that individual's development. Chromosomal sex and phenotypic sex may or may not be congruent. The psychological makeup of the individual then overlays on the phenotypic sex, which again may or may not be congruent. Commonly, all three of these factors are in agreement. Finally, socialization to gender influences one's sexual identity and behavior. Obviously, this arrangement does not always evolve so harmoniously, leading to conflicts in chromosomal, phenotypic, and psychological sexual identity.

Ambiguous genitalia is an emotionally charged diagnosis that can incite great distress among medical people who are unfamiliar with such conditions. This anxiety is transmitted to the parents of the unclassifiable newborn. Societal norms, bigotry, and ignorance add to the crisis, bringing a sense of shame and fear of the unknown for the family.

The first task of the attending physician is to reassure all present at delivery that while uncommon, ambiguous genitalia is a diagnosis that is both well recognized and manageable. If the physician is inexperienced with the condition, it is not unreasonable to acknowledge one's own limitations, reassure the concerned parents that experts in the field are available and then facilitate a prompt referral to these resources. It is best to avoid guessing the sex of the child based on the ambiguous genitalia and risk creating bias in the minds of the caregivers [3].

As this condition is commonly part of a syndrome, the next task is to rule out more extensive congenital anomalies that may be more serious in terms of impacting on the newborn's health and potential [3]. Once it is certain that the newborn's problem is limited to ambiguous genitalia, the physician can begin to clarify its etiology.

The decision on sex of rearing is a complex and recently controversial issue [54]. Traditionally, there are three aspects to consider. Firstly, does the individual have any reproductive potential based on their genetic sex? If this potential is evident, sex assignment is typically based on genetic sex. Secondly, will the individual have the potential anatomically to function sexually? Thirdly, the parental preferences and cultural influences must be considered. For example, a male child with inadequate external anatomy for sexual function or reproductive capacity may still be preferable in some cultures to a surgically converted "female" with normalized genitalia, and capable of normal sexual function but sterile.

In recent years, challenges have been made against the use of "normal" or mainstream heterosexual behavior as the gold standard in surgery and decision-making in this population [56]. The medical establishment has been criticized for intervening on behalf of the newborn. It has been suggested that these individuals be left untouched until adulthood, at which time decisions of sexual identity and corrective surgery can be made by the individual themselves. Proponents of this philosophy cite the dysphoria reported by some of the sex reassigned individuals as support for their argument [54]. Given the greater majority of these reassigned individuals who are not even aware of their "true" genetic gender, or if aware, do not choose to vocalize their opinion on this debate, it is questionable that this issue will ever be resolved by proper scientific study. However, the overwhelming range of experience by physicians involved with individuals born with ambiguous genitalia produces an inherent bias towards providing these newborns with a definitive gender and normalization on which to begin life [55].

True Hermaphrodite

These individuals possess both ovarian and testicular tissue. Approximately 60% actually have ovotestes which rarely produce spermatozoa, but commonly do produce oocytes [3]. They frequently have a uterine structure. Several cases of pregnancy have been reported in true hermaphrodites in which the testicular tissue has been removed. The etiology can be 46XX/46XY chimerism or 46XX undiagnosed chimerism. Other etiologies include translocation of

Table 5.2 Factors contributing to sexual identity

Genetic sex (chromosome)
Phenotype (anatomy)
Psychologic (gender identity)
Sociologic (external appearance)

testicular determining factor from the Y to the X chromosome or an autosome. Alternately, true hermaphroditism can be rarely seen when there is expression of the autosomal sex reversal gene [3].

Male Pseudohermaphroditism

Mixed Gonadal Dysgenesis
These individuals possess a combination of both male and female chromosomes. They present with a range of expression from a male with cryptorchism and hypospadias to a female with pubertal failure or pubertal virilization. The dysgenetic gonads are known to have a lifetime risk of 30% malignant transformations such as dysgerminoma or gonadoblastoma [3]. In individuals raised as females, the gonads cannot be accurately monitored due to their internal location. This, plus the risk of virilization at puberty, support the early removal of the gonads by minimally invasive techniques. In those raised as males, where the gonads are placed in the scrotum and are more easily monitored for malignant transformation, the gonads can be maintained. Infertility is common in these males [4].

Deficiency of Testosterone Biosynthesis
A defect in the ability to produce testosterone will inhibit the full expression of the XY potential, leading to ambiguous genitalia. These are generally autosomal recessive conditions causing defective or inadequate production of enzymes required in the production of testosterone and include:

- 17-α-hydroxylase deficiency
- 3-β-ol dehydrogenase deficiency
- 17 ketosteroid reductase deficiency
- 17–20 desmolase deficiency
- congenital adrenal lipoid hyperplasia

These individuals are able to produce MIF, and therefore develop normal internal male anatomy. The inadequate testosterone production and therefore inadequate DHT leads to under-virilization of the external anatomy. The extent of this under-virilization is dependent on the severity of the enzyme deficiency. Challenging the newborn with weekly injections of human chorionic gonadotropin (HCG) to stimulate Leydig cell testosterone production can be used to help determine if the individual possesses any capacity to further virilize and improve penile length at puberty [3].

Complete Androgen Insensitivity (AIS)
This is an X-linked inherited disorder in which there is no ability for peripheral tissue to respond to androgens. The incidence is quoted as 1/20 000 to

1/64 000 [4]. Consequently, these "XY girls" are born with entirely normal appearing female external genitalia. They typically present in late puberty with primary amenorrhea, and at this time are discovered to have absent internal female anatomy and a blind ended vagina. More careful physical assessment will reveal an absence of axillary or pubic hair, yet well-developed breasts with somewhat pale areola. Chromosome testing confirms an XY pattern, differentiating this diagnosis from mullerian agenesis (XX). The gonads are normal testes, producing high levels of testosterone which can be detected in peripheral blood samples. These testes have approximately a 30% risk of malignant transformation and therefore should be removed laparoscopically at the time of diagnosis and age-appropriate hormone replacement therapy (HRT) instituted [3]. The major differential diagnosis for AIS includes incomplete AIS, 5-a-reductase deficiency and mullerian agenesis.

Incomplete Androgen Insensitivity
Also an X-linked recessive disorder, incomplete AIS is a condition in which there are defective or diminished numbers of androgen receptors in peripheral tissue. Individuals with incomplete AIS can present with a range of findings from azospermic males to females indistinguishable from those with complete AIS, depending on the density and effectiveness of the androgen receptors. In those assigned to the female gender, gonadectomy is recommended, along with the appropriate reconstruction of the anatomy. Again, age-specific HRT is indicated.

5-α-Reductase Deficiency
This is an autosomal recessive condition. These individuals are born with a defective 5-α-reductase enzyme and therefore do not efficiently convert testosterone to 5-DHT [3]. 5-DHT is essential for virilization of the external genitalia. Depending on the degree of the enzyme defect, these individuals can be born with normal external female genitalia. Inguinal hernias with undescended testes are common and often the first hint of the diagnosis in a "female" newborn.

In 5-α-reductase defect there are, however, normal peripheral androgen receptors. Therefore, at puberty with the increase in testosterone production, some further virilization can occur. With the higher testosterone levels yet normal peripheral receptors, breast tissue is suppressed and therefore there is no breast development in these patients. In those born with ambiguous genitalia, a challenge with HCG will reveal an increased testosterone to DHT ratio for diagnosis of this defect [3].

Agonadia

More commonly associated with multiple congenital anomalies, agonadia involves the failure of the XY gonad to evolve beyond early embryogenesis. Depending on the timing of failure, internal anatomy can be mixed with either wolffian or mullerian structures, or both present. External anatomy can also be indeterminate. The infant has very low testosterone levels, undetectable gonads and an XY chromosomal pattern. Pelvic ultrasound usually shows no identifiable internal anatomy or rudimentary mullerian structures only. Sex of rearing is usually female.

Leydig Cell Agenesis

An early embryological insult results in failure of the formation of Leydig cells in an XY individual and therefore no testosterone production. As a result, they are born with female external genitalia. Since MIF is produced by the Sertoli cells, internal female development is suppressed. The wolffian structures develop internally, but these individuals have no reproductive potential.

Cloacal Defects

Although not classifiable as an intersex disorder, cloacal defects commonly result in disfigurement of the external genitalia. In male infants, this can result in ambiguous genitalia and gender confusion. This anomaly is discussed in more detail elsewhere.

Female Pseudohermaphroditism

Congenital Adrenal Hyperplasia (CAH)

By far the most common cause of female virilization, CAH is the result of an inherited defect of one of the enzymes in the conversion of cholesterol to cortisol by the adrenal gland [57]. A complex pathway, there are several enzymes which can be affected which will lead to excessive production of androgens resulting in virilization of the developing female fetus. The three enzyme defects virilizing females are: (a) 21-hydroxylase defect, (b) 11-β-hydroxylase defect, and (c) 3-β-ol dehydrogenase defect (Figure 5.11). A deficiency in 17-α-hydroxylase is also recognized. This blocks production of androgens, thereby leading to under-virilization or male pseudohermaphrodites (see "Deficiency of Testosterone Biosynthesis", above).

21-Hydroxylase Deficiency. The most common form of CAH, 21-hydroxylase deficiency is seen in over 95% of cases. The incidence is 1/5000 to 1/25 000 in Caucasian populations, yet as frequent as 1/700 among Yupik Eskimos [57]. There are two forms of

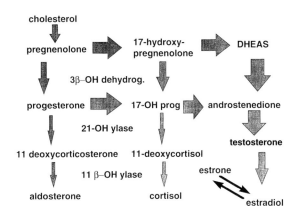

Figure 5.11 CAH: steroid pathways affected.

21-hydroxylase deficiency, the simple (salt sparing), and the salt wasting form. The difference in these two types reflects the severity of the enzyme defect.

Located on chromosome 6p, there are six alleles involved in production of this enzyme, and therefore, variable expression [58]. The 21-hydroxylase enzyme is also involved in production of aldosterone, which modulates the renal control of potassium and sodium losses. The salt wasting form leads to altered fluid and electrolyte balances. Consequently, these individuals tend to present with more virilized anatomy, along with dehydration, hyperkalemia, hyponatremia, and the sequelae including seizures, shock and death. Approximately 60% of 21-hydroxylase CAH are of the salt wasting variety [57].

Simple CAH represents a less severe form of the condition. These females usually have clitoromegaly, mild labioscrotal fusion and rugation, a normally placed urethra, and some hyperpigmentation of the genitalia. Work-up confirms XX chromosomes, normal internal anatomy, with elevated 17-hydroxyprogesterone levels and normal electrolytes. Medical management includes cortisol replacement and careful monitoring of growth and development. Inadequate cortisol replacement can lead to excessive endogenous androgen production, premature epiphyseal closure and short stature. Counseling regarding increased cortisol needs in times of stress or infection is vital [57].

Surgical management includes clitoroplasty, usually prior to graduation from diapers, and perineoplasty or lower vaginoplasty if necessary after menarche to facilitate use of tampons and sexual function [39,59]. At puberty, monitoring for virilization is heightened, specifically looking for hirsutism, acne and oligomenorrhea. Although fertility is compromised due to anovulation and oligomenorrhea,

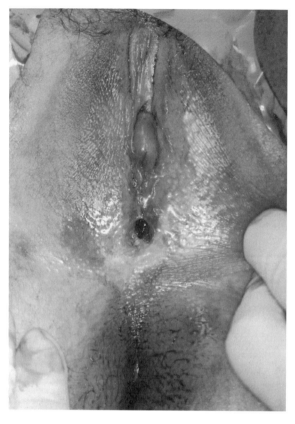

Figure 5.12 CAH (salt wasting): common urogenital opening, prior clitoroplasty.

correction of this problem can result in restored fertility, conception and delivery.

While there is no evidence these women have altered ability to deliver vaginally, it may be preferable to perform elective cesarean sections if there has been excessive perineal reconstruction in the past [18,39]. During pregnancy, careful monitoring of cortisol replacement needs is important as is prophylactic coverage for the stress of labor. Preconceptual counseling as to the genetics of CAH is helpful [58]. Testing of the partner for carrier status is recommended. Management of the potentially affected fetuses is outlined later.

Salt wasting CAH is a much more challenging situation [58]. Inadequate cortisol replacement or aldosterone supplementation can be life-threatening. Parental and patient education and compliance is essential. From a gynecologic perspective, the genitalia tend to be much more virilized with marked clitoromegaly, fusion of the urethra and vagina leading to a common urogenital opening and extensive posterior labioscrotal fusion (Figure 5.12) [59]. The urethrovaginal fusion can be variable and it is vital this anatomy be delineated preoperatively

[60]. Fusion at the lower third requires perineoplasty and a lower mobilizing vaginoplasty [59]. Alternatively, fusion can be at the internal bladder sphincter, requiring complete vaginoplasty including skin grafting [9].

Timing of surgical correction is dependent on the extent of the anatomical distortion. Clitoroplasty is usually performed in early childhood, leaving the common urogenital opening to be dealt with at puberty or later when patient compliance can greatly assist with the postoperative results [61]. Proper menstrual egress can be a concern if the urethral fusion is high. In this situation, surgery in early puberty in anticipation of obstructive hematocolpos may be necessary. However, if possible, it is preferable to delay surgery until the genitalia have evolved through puberty, are well vascularized, estrogenized, and the patient is fully comprehensive and compliant with the goals of surgery.

11-β-hydroxylase CAH. This autosomal recessive (chromosome 8) condition involves a defect in production of 11-β-hydroxylase [58]. It is seen in approximately 5% of cases of CAH. It has an incidence of 1/100 000 white births, particularly in Moroccan Jews [58]. This enzyme converts 11-deoxycorticosterone to corticosterone, and converts 11-deoxycortisol to cortisol. Consequently, a block at this level also results in elevated 11-deoxycorticosterone, which causes salt retention, leading to hypertension in these individuals.

3-β-ol dehydrogenese CAH. This enzyme converts dehydroepiandrosterone sulfate (DHEAS) to androstenedione, 17-hydroxypregnenalone to 17-hydroxyprogesterone, and pregnenalone to progesterone. Consequently, these affected individuals cannot produce aldosterone, and are therefore also salt wasters. DHEA is androgenic, and so the increased levels virilize the female fetus. The lack of testosterone production, for which androstenedione is a precursor, also leads to male pseudohermaphroditism.

Clitoroplasty. Clitoral reduction is best performed in early childhood, while the individual is still diapered, and not yet toilet trained. Evidence suggests gender identity is not solidified until after age 18 months; therefore efforts to establish the phallic structure as a clitoris should be made by this time [55]. Clitorectomy or amputation of the clitoris is no longer acceptable [39]. Preservation of the dorsal vessels and nerves is essential to maintaining normal clitoral sensation and sexual response.

A semicircular incision is made between the shaft and glans, allowing dissection and retraction of the overlaying skin. The dorsal artery, vein and nerve are identified and dissected free of the lateral crura. The crura are then isolated bilaterally, ligated at each end, and excised. The remaining pedicle of dorsal vessels, nerve and glans are then accordioned to the subpubic arch and secured with sutures bilaterally. On occasion, bilateral wedging of the glans itself may be necessary to achieve a cosmetically acceptable clitoris. The previously retracted skin can then be used to fashion labia minora bilaterally.

Pregnancy and CAH. CAH is an autosomal recessive trait that is common. It is estimated that 1/20 to 1/250 people in the North American population are carriers [57]. Preconceptual counseling and screening is valuable in families known to have this gene defect. In women known to be at risk for a fetus with CAH, either due to family history or a previously affected child, early diagnosis of pregnancy is essential. Proper treatment can prevent genital disfigurement in the affected female child [62]. These women are initially placed on dexamethasone (dose: 1.5 mg/day in divided doses) in an effort to provide transplacental cortisol replacement to the fetus and prevent excessive androgen production. Risks with dexamethasone therapy include excessive maternal weight gain, hypertension, gestational diabetes, and gastrointestinal upset [63].

At approximately 11 weeks gestation, chorionic villus sampling is done to identify the sex of the fetus, and if the fetus is affected with CAH. If there is an affected female fetus, treatment is maintained throughout pregnancy. If there is an affected male fetus, treatment is usually discontinued as genitalia are not disfigured for males and the known risks of maternal steroid ingestion outweigh the theoretical fetal benefits of continued steroid support. Of course, in the unaffected fetus, treatment is discontinued [64].

Teratogenic

Exposure to a virilizing agent can result in ambiguity of the female genitalia. The impact is dependent on the androgen strength, dose, and timing. Exposure at 5–12 weeks gestation impacts on the vaginal tube and labioscrotal anatomy [1]. After 12 weeks, exposure impacts only on the clitoris [1]. Endogenous androgen sources are rare, but include ovarian tumors in pregnancy such as an arrhenoblastoma, Leydig cell tumor, or luteoma of pregnancy. External androgen sources such as medroxyprogesterone acetate and norethindrone rarely impact as the placenta acts as a barrier to these molecules.

Conclusion

This chapter has reviewed the embryology of the female urogenital system in the context of congenital anomalies encountered by the clinician. The intent of this approach is to give the pelvic surgeon a greater understanding of the spectrum of variability in the anatomy of the female reproductive system and the impact of one anomaly on associated structures. A basic review of sexual development of the fetus is provided. The management issues of abnormal anatomy and ambiguous genitalia are discussed. Finally, a discourse on the surgical aspects of these clinical challenges is presented with the hope that the reader gains a better appreciation of the complexity and controversies of pelvic reconstruction for the child or adult regardless of the surgeon's background training in this field.

References

1. Marshall FF. Embryology of the lower genitourinary tract. Urol Clin North Am 1978;5(1):3–15.
2. Baramki TA. Embryology of the urogenital system in man and genetic factors in intersex problems and transexualism. Clin Plast Surg 1974;1(2):01–213.
3. Saenger P. Abnormal sexual differentiation. J Pediatr 1984;104(1):1–17.
4. Blyth B, Churchill BM, Houle AM, McLorie GA. Intersex. In: Gillenwater JY, Grayhack JT, Howard SS, Duckett JW, editors. Adult & Pediatric Urology, Vol. 2, 2nd edn. Year Book Medical Publishers, 1987; 1916–31.
5. Jost A. Recherches sur la différenciation sexuelle de l'embryon de Lapin. III. Rôle des gonades foetales dans la différenciation sexuelle somatique. Arch Anat Micr Morph Exp 1947;36:271.
6. Smith DW. Recognizable Patterns of Human Malformation. Philadelphia: WB Saunders, 1976; 350.
7. Soper RT, Kilger K. Vesico-intestinal fissure. J Urol 1964;92:490–501.
8. Hendren WH. Cloacal malformations: experienced with 105 cases. J Pediatr Surg 1992;27(7):890–901.
9. Hendren RH. Reconstructive problems of the vagina and female urethra. Clin Plastic Surgery 1980;7(2):207–34.
10. Jeffs, RD. Exstrophy and cloacal exstrophy. Urol Clin North Am 1978;5(1):127–40.
11. Hall R, Fleming S, Gysler M, McLorie G. The genital tract in female children with imperforate anus. Am J Obstet Gynecol 1985;151:169–71.
12. Blakeley CR, Mills WG. The obstetric and gynaecologic complications of bladder exstrophy and epispadias. Br J Obstet Gynaecol 1981;88:167–173.
13. Stanton, SL. Gynecologic complications of epispadias and bladder exstrophy. Am J Obstet Gynecol 1974;119:749–54.
14. Patton JF, Barry A. The genesis of exstrophy of the bladder and epispadias. Am J Anat 1952;90:35–9.
15. Marshall VF, Muecke EC. Variations in exstrophy of the bladder. J Urol 1962;88:766–96.
16. Stein R, Fisch M, Bauer H, Friedberg V, Hohenfellner R. Operative reconstruction of the external and internal genitalia in female patients with bladder exstrophy or incontinent epispadias. J Urol 1995;154:1002–7.

17. Stein R, Stockle M, Fisch M, Nakai H, Muller SC, Hohenfellner R. The fate of the adult exstrophy patient. J Urol 1994;152:1413–16.

18. Burgige KA, Hensle TW, Chambers WJ, Leb R, Jeter KF. Pregnancy and sexual function in women with bladder exstrophy. Urology 1986;28:12–14.

19. Krisiloff M, Puchner P, Tretter W, Macfarlane M, Lattimer J. Pregnancy in women with bladder exstrophy. J Urol 1978;119:478–9.

20. Gosden C, Brock DJH. Prenatal diagnosis of exstrophy of the cloaca. Am J Med Genet 1981;8:95–109.

21. Woodward J. The prune belly syndrome. Urol Clin North Am 1978;5(1):75–93.

22. American Fertility Society Classification of Mullerian Anomalies. Fertil Steril 1988;49:952.

23. DeSouza AZ, Maluf M, Perin PM, Filho FM, Perin L. Surgical treatment of congenital uterovaginal agenesis: Mayer–Rokitansky–Kuster–Hauser Syndrome. Int Surg 1987;72:45–7.

24. Dean GE, Hensle TW. Neovaginal construction in children with Mayer-Rokitansky syndrome in vaginal reconstruction of the absent vagina. Dialogues Pediatr Urol 1994;17(7):2–3.

25. Golditch IM. (1969) Vaginal aplasia. Surg Gynecol Obstet 129:361–5.

26. Harkins JL, Gyster M, Cowell CA. Anatomical amenorrhea: The problems of congenital vaginal agenesis and its surgical correction. Pediatr Clin North Am 1981;28(2):345–353.

27. Altcheck A. What to do when there is no vagina. Contemp OBGyn 1988;August:50–68.

28. Wabrek AJ, Mullard PR, Wilson WB, Pion RJ. Creation of a neovagina by the Frank non-operative method. Obstet Gynecol 1971;37(3):418–13.

29. Ingram, JM. The bicycle seat stool in the treatment of vaginal agenesis and stenosis: A preliminary report. Am J Obstet Gynecol 1981;140:867–71.

30. Buss JG, Lee RA. McIndoe Procedures for vaginal agenesis: results and complications. Mayo Clin Proc 1989;64:758–61.

31. Hinderer UT. Reconstruction of the external genitalia in the adrenogenital syndrome by means of a personal one-stage procedure. Plast Reconstr Surg 1989;84(2):325–37.

32. Oesterling JE, Gearhart JP, Jeffs RD. A unified approach to early reconstructive surgery of the child with ambiguous genitalia. J Urol 1987;138:1079–84.

33. McIndoe AM, Banister JB. An operation for the cure of congenital absence of the vagina. J Obstet Gynaecol Br Emp 1938;45:490–4.

34. Hojsgaard A, Villadsen I. McIndoe procedure for congenital vaginal agenesis: Complications and results. Br J Plast Surg 1995;48:97–102.

35. Rock JA, Reeves LA, Retto H, Baramki TA, Zucur HA, Jones HW. Success following vaginal creation for Mullerian agenesis. Fertil Steril 1983;39:809–13.

36. Okada E, Iwahira Y, Maruyama Y. Treatment of vaginal agenesis with expanded vulval flap. Plast Reconstr Surg 1996;98(3):530–3.

37. Velidedeoglu HV, Coskunfirat OK, Bozdogan MN, Sahin U, Turkguven Y. The surgical management of incomplete testicular feminization syndrome in three sisters. Br J Plast Surg 1997;50:212–16.

38. O'Brien BM, MacIssac IA, Maher PJ, Barbaro C. Treatment of vaginal agenesis with a new vulvovaginoplasty. Plast Reconstr Surg 1990;85(6):942–8.

39. Spence HM, Allen TD. Genital reconstruction in the female with adrenogenital syndrome. Br J Urol 1973;45:126–30.

40. Wan T, Whetzel T, Mathes SJ, Vasconez LO. A fasciocutaneous flap for vaginal and perineal reconstruction. Plast Reconstr Surg 1987;80(1):95–102.

41. Jordan GH, Winslow BH. Grafting techniques for vaginal reconstruction. Dialogues Pediatr Urol 1994;17(7):6–7.

42. Hensle TW, Reiley EA. Vaginal replacement in children and young adults. J Urol 1998;159:1035–8.

43. Atala A, Hendren WH. Reconstruction with bowel segments. Dialogues Pediatr Urol 1994;17(7):4–6.

44. Baskin LS, Duckett JW. Complete vaginal reconstruction. Dialogues Pediatr Urol 1994;17(7):3–4

45. Lenaghan R, Wilson N, Lucas C, Ledgerwood A. The role of rectosigmoid neocolporrhaphy. Surgery 1997;122:856–60.

46. Mattingly RF, editor. Telinde's Operative Gynecology, 6th edn. Philadelphia: JB Lippincott, 1977; 347.

47. McKusick VA, Weiboecher RG., Gragg GW. Recessive inheritance of a congenital malformation syndrome. JAMA 1968;204:113–14.

48. Rock JA, Zacur HA, Dlugi AM. Pregnancy success following surgical correction of imperforate hymen and complete transverse vaginal septum. Gynecology 1982;59:448–51.

49. Sanfilippo JS, Wakim NG, Schikler KN, Yussman MA. Endometriosis in association with uterine anomalies. Am J Obstet Gynecol 1986;154:39–43.

50. Hurst BS, Rock JA. Preoperative dilation to facilitate repair of the high transverse vaginal septum. Fertil Steril 1992;57:1351–3.

51. Rock JA, Jones HW Jr. Reparative and Constructive Surgery of the Female Generative Tract. Baltimore: Williams & Wilkins, 1983.

52. Ade-ajayi AM, Malene PS. Colonovaginoplasty for cervicovaginal atresia. J Urol 1997;157:333–4.

53. Tjaden BL, Rock JA. Uterovaginal anomalies. In: Carpenter SE, Rock JA, editors. Pediatric and Adolescent Gynecology. New York: Raven Press, 1992; 313–40.

54. Recommendations for Treatment: Intersex Infants and Children. Intersex Society of North America, 1995.

55. Diamond M, Sigmundsen M. Sex reassignment at birth: Long term review and clinical implications. Arch Pediatric Adolesc Med 1997;151:298–303.

56. Reiner W. To be male or female: That is the question. Arch Pediatr Adolesc Med 1997;151:224–5.

57. White P, New M, Dupont B. Congenital adrenal hyperplasia. Part I. N Engl J Med 1987;316(24):1519–24.

58. White P, New M, Dupont B. Congenital adrenal hyperplasia. Part II. N Engl J Med 1987;316(25):1580–6.

59. Donahue PK, Hendren WH. Perineal reconstruction in ambiguous genitalia infants raised as females. Ann Surg 1984;200(3):363–71.

60. Verkauf BS, Jones HW. Masculinization of the female genitalia in congenital adrenal hyperplasia: Relationship to the salt losing variety of the disease. South Med J 1970;63:634–8.

61. Hendren WH, Atala A. Repair of the high vagina in girls with severely masculinized anatomy from adrenogenital syndrome. J Pediatr Surg 1995;31(1):91–4.

62. Pang S, Pollack M, Marshall R, Immmken L. Prenatal treatment of congenital adrenal hyperplasia due to 21-hydroxylase deficiency. Medical Intelligence 1990;32(2):111–15.

63. Levine LS, Pang S. Prenatal diagnosis and treatment of congenital adrenal hyperplasia. J Pediatr Endo 1994;7(3) 193–200.

64. Speiser PW, New MI. Prenatal diagnosis and treatment of congenital adrenal hyperplasia. J Pediatr Endo 1994;7(3):183–91.

6 Classification of Disorders of Female Pelvic Support and the Role of Collagen

Jane A. Schulz and Harold P. Drutz

Background

Pelvic floor dysfunction (encompassing genital prolapse, urinary, and fecal incontinence) is very common but our epidemiological studies are poor. Not only is our literature on prevalence and incidence inadequate, but we have not come to a universal consensus on assessment of the pelvic floor.

History and physical examination are key components in our patient assessment. As part of this, a detailed pelvic examination is important in developing a comprehensive management plan. If treatment strategy focuses exclusively on the support or function of one compartment or organ system, long-term success is unlikely. This has been shown in previous work of both Burch and Wiskind et al. Burch, in a review of patients who had had his retropubic suspension, showed 100% of the women were symptomatically relieved but 8% developed a postoperative enterocele [1]. In the review by Wiskind et al., 82% of women were dry following a Burch retropubic suspension but 27% required subsequent surgery for prolapse [2].

In their 1972 paper, Baden and Walker recognized that there was "an inability to communicate meaningful information about a common gynecologic problem" and created the vaginal profile [3] (Figure 6.1). However, almost 30 years later, Brubaker and Norton reviewed the clinical classification and nomenclature for pelvic support defects (presented at the ICS meeting, Rome 1993) [4] and concluded that there was still no universally accepted method for performing pelvic examinations and reporting physical findings. Terminology that has commonly been used to refer to pelvic organ prolapse includes urethrocele, cystocele, enterocele, uterine descensus or prolapse, procidentia, vault prolapse and rectocele.

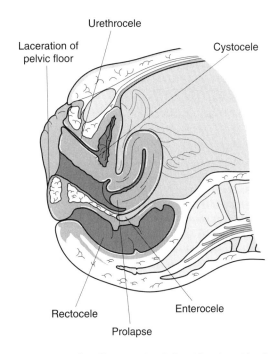

Figure 6.1 Vaginal profile: 0-0–0-0–0-0. Normal vagina with adequate support of all six components. Note sites of the six potential lesions of vaginal relaxation. This figure represents a patient with no prolapse according to Baden and Walker's original six-point classification system in the vaginal profile. (Reproduced from Baden and Walker [3]; copyright Baden and Walker.)

However, it is often not clear exactly what the examiner is describing.

The International Continence Society has been at the forefront in the standardization of terminology of lower urinary tract function since the establishment of the Committee on Standardization of Terminology in 1973 [5]. The committee's efforts over the last two decades have led to worldwide

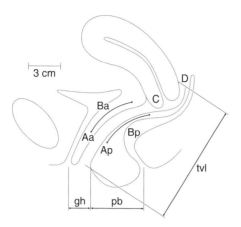

Figure 6.2 Six sites (points Aa, Ba C, D, Bp, and Ap), genital hiatus (gh), perineal body (pb), and total vaginal length (tvl) used for pelvic organ support quantitation. (Reproduced from Bump et al. [6] with permission.)

acceptance of terminology standards, allowing efficient and precise communication among physicians. Although prolapse and pelvic floor dysfunction are closely related to urinary tract function, accurate communication has not been possible due to the absence of a universally accepted system for describing pelvic organ position. The grading systems in existence have not been validated for reproducibility or the clinical significance of different grades. We have all seen patients with large prolapse and minimal symptoms, and also the patient with significant pelvic pressure but minimal demonstrable prolapse. The absence of standard, validated definitions has prevented comparison between institutions and longitudinal comparison within institutions [6].

Following the review by Brubaker and Norton, a multidisciplinary committee from the International Continence Society (ICS), American Urogynecologic Society (AUGS), and the Society of Gynecologic Surgeons (SGS) drafted a standardization document in 1993. Reproducibility studies were done in Europe and the USA that showed good inter-observer and intra-observer reproducibility [7]. The document was accepted by the ICS, AUGS, and SGS in 1995/6. This led to the creation of the pelvic organ prolapse quantification examination (POPQ) (Figure 6.2).

Difficulties with Pelvic Organ Prolapse Grading

There are a number of areas of confusion that arise when discussing pelvic organ prolapse. The main factor is that the terminology used is often inconsis-

tent. Other factors that vary and lead to variations in description of findings include: the position of the examination, the volume in the bladder, whether the patient is asked to strain, and whether traction is applied to the uterus. There are multiple grading systems that can be used; these will be described later in this chapter.

Objective classification of pelvic organ prolapse presupposes a knowledge of normal pelvic support. However, at present there is no objective data regarding "normal support" in women of different ages, childbearing history, or surgical history. Also, there is no information directly correlating physical findings with subjective or objective measurements of pelvic organ function.

Terminology

The following terms are currently widely accepted in the urogynecologic community.

- *Urethrocele*: a protrusion of the urethra into the vagina signifying loss of fascial supports of the urethra

- *Cystocele*: a protrusion of the bladder into the vagina signifying loss of fascial supports of the bladder

- *Uterine prolapse*: a protrusion of the cervix and uterus into the barrel of the vagina (also referred to as descensus or procidentia)

- *Enterocele*: herniation of the pouch of Douglas (cul-de-sac) between the uterosacral ligaments into the rectovaginal septum (often contains small bowel)

- *Rectocele*: protrusion of the rectum into the vagina signifying loss of fascial supports of the rectum

Assessment of the Pelvic Floor

Position of the Examination

There is general consensus that the assessment of pelvic organ prolapse should be performed such that support in all parts of the vagina can be evaluated. Various positions have been used including supine lithotomy, 45° lithotomy, a birthing chair, the left lateral position, and standing. It may be useful to ask the patient to point out what they are feeling as abnormal or to use a mirror to confirm the correlation of physical findings with patient symptoms. The standing position is helpful to demonstrate prolapse that may not be obvious with the patient recumbent; however, it is often difficult to assess certain areas with the patient standing, so this should certainly be combined with some form of assessment with the patient lying down.

Comparisons have been done between different positions of patient assessment. In 1998 Swift and Herring reported on 51 women examined both in the dorsal lithotomy position and standing; they found no statistically significant difference in the stages assigned between the two groups [8]. The American College of Obstetricians and Gynecologists has recommended examining women in lithotomy, sitting, and standing [9]. At the American Urogynecologic Society (AUGS) Meeting in 1995, Montella and Cater reported on the difference between examinations done in the dorsal lithotomy position versus the birthing chair; they found greater protrusion of the prolapse in the sitting position but never by more than one stage [10]. In Walters and Karram's 1992 AUGS report on enterocele, a recommendation was made to perform routine examinations in the lithotomy position, and then standing if the symptoms did not correlate with the physical findings [11].

Methods of Grading

Multiple methods of prolapse grading have been described. Most are modifications of Baden and Walker's original vaginal profile, with four degrees of prolapse described [3]. In the popular gynecologic text by Mishell et al., pelvic examination in the lithotomy position is recommended, with examination of the anterior vaginal wall with speculum blade retraction of the posterior vaginal wall, and examination of the posterior vaginal wall with speculum blade retraction of the anterior vaginal wall. They recommended rectal examination to help detect an enterocele. Degrees of prolapse are described as first degree with descent of the prolapse into the upper vagina, second degree is prolapse to the introitus, and third degree (complete) is prolapse through the introitus [12]. Shull recommended examination recumbent with straining and then repeated standing, with the patient's foot on a stool, and straining if needed. Also recommended, was retraction of the vaginal walls with speculum blades and description of findings as clearly as possible, by specifying the site being examined and describing the support in relation to fixed points in the pelvis, such as the ischial spines. In this review, it was suggested that a mid-vaginal axis should be used as a point of reference; there is no loss of support if structures fail to cross the axis with strain. The cervix or cuff has no loss of support if it

fails to descend past the spines with strain [13]. Raz acknowledged the existence of many grading systems, but used a description that was slightly different. For cystocele, Raz labeled grade 1-2 as mild to moderate hypermobility of the anterior vaginal wall with strain, grade 3 as descent of the vaginal wall through the introitus, and grade 4 as descent of the bladder base through the introitus. Uterine prolapse was described by Raz as grade 1 with minimal mobility, grade 2 with descent to the mid-vagina, grade 3 as descent to the introitus and grade 4 (procidentia) as prolapse through the introitus. Raz's description of rectoceles was grade 1 for a saccular protrusion of the posterior vaginal wall, grade 2 for a bulge at the introitus, and grade 3 as a protrusion beyond the introitus [14]. Nicholls and Randall recommended examination in lithotomy and then standing (relaxed and straining in both positions). They used a modification of the system described by Beecham in 1980 [15].

The POPQ (pelvic organ prolapse quantification) system was developed in 1996. It is an objective, site-specific system for describing, quantifying, and staging female pelvic support. Certain sites along the vaginal wall are the reference points and their descent is measured in centimeters in relation to the hymen. Negative values indicate position above the hymenal ring and positive values denote points of descent below the hymen [6]. Intra- and interobserver reliability has been evaluated and found to be good; this system is now gaining wider acceptance and is allowing enhanced clinical and academic communication regarding individual patients and populations of patients [7].

Collagen and the Pelvic Floor

Pelvic Floor Dysfunction

There is abundant literature on the evaluation and management of stress urinary incontinence and pelvic floor prolapse, but relatively few epidemiological studies exist. Etiology is rarely discussed and causative factors are not well defined. In many cases, including the relationship of childbearing to pelvic floor damage, we have indirect but not direct evidence regarding etiology. Most literature makes references to the effects of pregnancy, childbirth, and increases in intra-abdominal pressure, but clearly each individual responds differently to these factors. Most practitioners have seen patients that have had multiple children, that have chronic chest conditions and have no prolapse; the opposite scenario is a patient that has good health and has only had one child, but has severe pelvic organ prolapse. Clearly, the etiology is multifactorial, and genetic factors, including collagen and other connective tissues, play a role.

Epidemiology

Regarding epidemiological studies, there are many problems with the reporting of pelvic floor problems; these include embarrassment leading to underreporting and previous problems with inconsistencies in description of prolapse. There is no disease model for pelvic floor disorders, as there is for such conditions as cancer; this contributes to some difficulties with the epidemiology. Some studies have reported up to 77% women having some degree of prolapse, but this is not always symptomatic [16]. Some estimates suggest that only 10-20% of patients will seek medical care for their pelvic floor dysfunction due to embarrassment, lack of knowledge about all the treatment options available, and the thought that nothing can be done as this is just a normal part of aging.

Etiologic Factors

The etiologic factors contributing to urinary incontinence and pelvic floor prolapse are probably best described by Peggy Norton as intrinsic or underlying factors versus extrinsic and environmental factors [17]. The intrinsic factors include: race, anatomic differences, connective tissue changes, and neurologic abnormalities. The extrinsic factors include: pregnancy and childbirth, aging, hormone effects, non-obstetric pelvic trauma and radical pelvic surgery, increases in intra-abdominal pressure, and medication effects.

Intrinsic Factors

There is a higher prevalence of stress urinary incontinence in white women [17,18], with less frequent stress urinary incontinence and prolapse in black women [15,18]. The racial differences are believed to be related to differences in pelvic anatomy, connective tissues, and pelvic supports. Zacharin reported in 1977 that cadaveric specimens from Chinese women had thicker pelvic fascia [19]. Prolapse is more frequent among white, Egyptian, and East Indian women, but less common among Orientals, African Americans, South African Bantu, and blacks of West Africa [14].

Anatomic differences are proposed as a causative factor in pelvic floor dysfunction. DeLancey found that the anterior-posterior levator hiatus diameter

was greater in women with prolapse and stress urinary incontinence [20]. Also, the South African Bantu woman's pelvis is small compared to European women, which may protect the Bantu from developing prolapse [15]. The mechanical stability of the genitourinary tract depends on collagen. There is evidence that the underlying connective tissue is insufficient in women with prolapse; also, a decrease in total collagen content has been reported in stress incontinent women [21]. There is certainly a relationship between estrogen and connective tissue; therefore, it is important to consider not only connective tissue content but also metabolic changes. Small case series have reported increased prevalence of prolapse in patients with neurologic disorders, such as spina bifida. This is likely related to some effect at the level of origin of the pudendal nerve supply, (S2,3,4), which contributes significantly to pelvic floor innervation.

Extrinsic Factors

Pregnancy and childbirth remain key factors in the pathogenesis of pelvic floor disorders. Contributing factors include: hormonal effects in pregnancy, the pressure of the uterus and its contents, denervation (especially stretch or crush injury to the pudendal nerve), connective tissue changes or injury, and mechanical disruption of muscles and sphincters. Effects related to aging include gravity, neurologic changes, the loss of estrogen, changes in connective tissue cross-linking, and reduced elasticity.

Because of the common embryonic origin of the bladder, urethra, and vagina from the urogenital sinus, there is a high concentration of estrogen receptors in the tissues of pelvic support. Falconer et al. described a general collagen deficiency state in women due to the lack of estrogen [22]. Urethral coaptation is also affected by the loss of estrogen [23]. Other external factors that may contribute to the development of prolapse include trauma or radical pelvic surgery that affects pelvic floor and urethral supports and the local nerve supply.

Increases in intra-abdominal pressure may result from chronic pulmonary disease, constipation with straining, heavy lifting, high impact exercise (such as parachute jumping or high impact aerobics) [24,25], ascites, or obesity. Any of these put additional pressure on the pelvic floor and may contribute to the development or exacerbation of prolapse. Medications may unmask incontinence, but are unlikely to contribute to prolapse; alpha-blockers used for hypertension may lower urethral closure pressures and benzodiazepines may contribute to smooth muscle relaxation.

Table 6.1 Main types of collagen

Type	Tissue distribution
I	Bone, tendon, skin, dentin, ligament, fascia, arteries, uterus
II	Hyaline cartilage
III	Skin, arteries, uterus
IV	Basement membranes
V	Basement membranes, other tissues

Collagen Types

Collagen is a fibrous protein that accounts for approximately 30% of total body protein. It is produced by fibroblasts and provides tensile strength for skin, tendons and bone. Nineteen different types of collagen have been identified; types I and III comprise the main structural components of epithelial tissue (Table 6.1).

Collagen Metabolism

There is an intricate balance between biosynthesis and degradation. The fundamental collagen unit is tropocollagen; each collagen unit is a triple helix of poypeptide (alpha) chains. The tight helix formation is facilitated by glycine at every third position. Proline and hydroxyproline also form cross-links to stabilize the collagen. Peptidases act on procollagen to form fibrils; lysine oxidation then occurs to form cross-links and provide tensile strength. A maturation and glycation process occurs to give the final product. Acid cathepsins and matrix metalloproteinases contribute to collagen degradation. Therefore, biochemical studies are required in addition to histology to show collagen defects [26].

Collagen Content

In 1987, Ulmsten et al. studied specimens of skin, fat, and round ligament from 15 women (8 who had genuine stress incontinence). They found 40% less collagen in the skin specimens from the incontinent women and 25% less collagen in the round ligament tissue [21]. Falconer et al. in 1994 took skin biopsies from 11 postmenopausal women (7 who had stress urinary incontinence), and found that the skin fibroblasts in the stress incontinent women produced 30% less collagen [22]. This work supports the hypothesis that stress urinary incontinence is due to altered connective tissue metabolism. A reduced type I:III collagen ratio was found by Norton et al. in women with genital prolapse

but not in those with stress urinary incontinence. Collagen synthesis was also found to be altered in patients with recurrent inguinal hernias and recurrent genital prolapse [27,28]. Further work was done by Makinen et al. in 1986 showing decreased fibroblasts and altered collagen fibril orientation in women with prolapse [29]. Rechberger et al. assessed vesicovaginal fascial specimens in 16 women (11 with stress urinary incontinence), and found less collagen in the fascia of the incontinent women [30]. In 1990, Sayer et al. examined women with bladder neck prolapse and stress urinary incontinence and found that they had a cross-link modification of their collagen in the pubocervical fascia, compared to women with only stress urinary incontinence [31]. Keane et al. studied 52 nulliparous women; they found a reduction in collagen content in the stress incontinent group and found a reduced type I:III collagen ratio in those women less than 30 years of age with stress urinary incontinence. This group felt that the composition of vaginal epithelium closely resembles that of endopelvic fascia [32].

Collagen Metabolism and Prolapse

Jackson's group in Bristol, England, has done much of the work on collagen and its metabolism in pelvic organ prolapse. In their 1996 work, they took vaginal epithelial tissue from premenopausal women (eight of whom had prolapse). They found that prolapse was associated with alterations in collagen metabolism; there was also 25% less collagen content in the prolapse specimens and no change in the type I:III collagen ratio. Further, they found the elastin content in these patients was unchanged, and there was increased matrix metalloproteinase 2 and 9 and cathepsin activities. The specimens examined by Jackson's group had an increased concentration of intermediate cross-links, indicating new collagen synthesis, but of an immature type that is easier to degrade. The conclusions of the Bristol group were that the main problem in genitourinary prolapse is increased collagen degradation with decreased tissue strength; they also felt that the increased synthesis of new collagen is overcome by its preferential degradation, and that research should be targeted to inhibition of collagenolytic activity [33].

Nichols stated that there seems to be an increased incidence of prolapse in diabetic patients [34]. This may relate to metabolic factors; in 1996, Cohen felt that protein glycosylation may be a mechanism of acquired collagen weakness in the diabetic patient [35].

Estrogen and Collagen

Collagen is transcribed from mRNA in ribosomes of fibroblasts, which have estrogen receptors. Estrogen may stimulate fibroblasts directly or act via a hormone mediator to influence collagen synthesis. There are certainly cellular changes related to the menopause; these include: a slowing of cell division and growth, a reduced capacity for tissue repair, and degenerative changes in elastic connective tissue. Jackson's group did some additional work with a placebo-controlled trial of estrogen in 33 women. They found that estrogen stimulates synthesis of new collagen, and collagen turnover (through stimulation of matrix metalloproteinases) [36]. Brincat et al. published work in 1983 and 1985; the first study compared skin biopsies in 29 postmenopausal women with no hormone replacement with those from 26 women that had been given estrogen and testosterone. They found that the mean collagen content of skin was 48% greater in the treated women [37]. Not only was skin collagen content and thickness greater in women treated with estrogen and testosterone, but in untreated women, skin collagen content declined in relation to menopausal, not chronological, age [38]. Connective tissue collagen is thought to contribute to the generation of urethral pressure. In 1988 Versi et al. showed a correlation between urethral pressure measurements and skin collagen content, and suggested that the beneficial effect of estrogens on urethral function is mediated via collagen [23]. Further work looking at the effect of local estrogens on the urethra was completed by Hilton and Stanton in 1983; this showed a decrease in stress urinary incontinence with increased maximal urethral closure pressure, functional urethral length, and pressure transmission ratio [39]. In 1989, Bhatia et al. did similar work showing an improvement in stress urinary incontinence, increased maximal urethral closure pressure, increased pressure transmission ratio, but unchanged functional urethral length with vaginal estrogen [40]. Elia and Bergman also did some urethral function work and showed that estrogens increase urethral pressure by up to 30%, with improvement or cure of stress urinary incontinence in many cases. They noted an additive effect on urethral function when estrogens are combined with alpha-adrenergic drugs [41].

Other work looking at the effect of estrogens has not been so encouraging. Fantl did a meta-analysis reviewing 166 articles; this showed a significant overall subjective improvement in all patients and in those with genuine stress incontinence alone. However, there was no significant effect on the quantity of fluid loss, but there was a significant effect on maximal urethral closure pressure [42]. Fantl's further work in 1996 was a randomized, double-blind, placebo-controlled trial in 83 hypoestrogenic incontinent women. The treatment group received three months of cyclic hormone replacement therapy; there was no significant difference in clinical or quality of life variables between the two groups [43]. Emphasis was made about the need for prospective, controlled trials, especially looking at the effects of local estrogen, which may play a greater role than systemic estrogen therapy for the treatment of incontinence. Hilton stated that both endogenous and exogenous estrogens have a positive effect on cell cycle activity in the squamous epithelium of the female lower urinary tract and vagina; this is indicated by Ki67 antigen expression (an indicator of mitotic activity) [44].

Other Affected Organ Systems

Collagen is part of all connective tissues; therefore, the loss of estrogen has impact at multiple sites. Osteoporosis is associated with estrogen deficiency; a decline in collagen likely plays a role in the development of osteoporosis. Brincat et al. in their collagen work showed that the loss of skin thickness and dermal collagen paralleled the loss of bone density in menopausal women [45]. There are estrogen receptors present in the brain; this has led to the suggestion of associations between estrogen deficiency, dementia, and the resulting incontinence.

Connective Tissue Disorders

The first reference to a hypermobility syndrome was made by Hippocrates in the fourth century BC [46]. An association was reported between hypermobility and knee effusions, hip dislocation, osteoarthrosis, chondrocalcinosis, mitral valve prolapse, hernias, striae, and varicose veins. In 1982 Al-Rawi and Al-Rawi reported on 76 Iraqi women with prolapse; of these, 66% had joint laxity compared with 18% of controls [47]. Norton et al. found women with joint hypermobility had a higher prevalence of genital prolapse, but no increase in stress urinary incontinence [27].

The Marfan syndrome is a connective tissue disorder involving an abnormality of the fibrillin gene (chromosome 15). Fibrillin is another component of connective tissue, and is present in ligaments and fascia. Patients with the Marfan syndrome are known to have other manifestations of connective tissue weakness, such as hernias and aneurysms. They have also been shown, in a small case series, to have a higher prevalence of incontinence and prolapse [48]. Ehlers–Danlos syndrome is a connective tissue disorder affecting collagen types I and III. There are ten subtypes of this syndrome with varied manifestations. Stoddart et al. reported a common finding of prolapse in these women [49]; McIntosh et al. showed 59% incontinence and 29% prolapse in a group of 41 women with Ehlers–Danlos syndrome [50].

Clearly, there is a spectrum of genetic connective tissue abnormalities that contribute to the development of pelvic floor dysfunction. There is much need for further research in this area.

Summary

Genitourinary prolapse is perhaps more common than previously thought. Multiple systems of classification exist, but the standardized POPQ evaluation has been developed by the ICS, SGS, and AUGS to allow clarity of description among the medical profession. Childbirth remains the main causative factor in the development of pelvic floor dysfunction, with many other exacerbating factors. However, connective tissue, especially collagen, plays an equally important role. Collagen provides tensile strength to tissue; deficiencies in collagen content and metabolism have been implicated in the pathogenesis of stress urinary incontinence and prolapse. There is evidence that estrogen plays a role in collagen metabolism, and that estrogen is therapeutic in the connective tissue of postmenopausal women. Further research is required regarding minor genetic defects that may be causative of connective tissue defects. Perhaps, in this group of women, pregnancy and labor management should be approached differently to help to prevent defects; also, this group may require a different type of pelvic floor repair, with reinforcement with synthetic materials, to allow a more durable result.

References

1. Burch JC. Urethrovaginal fixation to Cooper's ligament for correction of stress incontinence, cystocele and prolapse. Am J Obstet Gynecol 1961;81:281.
2. Wiskind AK, Creighton SM, Stanton SL. The incidence of genital prolapse after the Burch colposuspension. Am J Obstet Gynecol 1992;167(2):399–404.
3. Baden WF, Walker TA. Genesis of the vaginal profile: A correlated classification of vaginal relaxation. Clin Obstet Gynecol 1972;15:1048–54.
4. Brubaker LT, Norton PA. Proceedings of International Continence Society 23rd annual meeting, Rome, Italy, September 1993; 200.
5. Abrams P, Blaivis JG, Stanton SL, Anderson JT. The International Continence Society Committee on Standardisation of Terminology: the standardisation of terminology of lower urinary tract function. Scand J Urol Nephrol 1988;11(4S): 5–19.
6. Bump RC, Matthiason A, Bø K, Brubaker LP, DeLancey JOL, Klarskov P, Shull BL, Smith ARB. The standardization of terminology of female pelvic organ prolapse and pelvic floor dysfunction. Am J Obstet Gynecol 1996;175:10–17.
7. Hall AF, Theofrastous JP, Cundiff GW et al. Interobserver and intraobserver reliability of the proposed International Continence Society, Society of Gynecologic Surgeons, and American Urogynecologic Society pelvic organ prolapse classification system. Am J Obstet Gynecol 1996;175:1467–71.
8. Swift SE, Herring M. Comparison of pelvic organ prolapse in the dorsal lithotomy compared with the standing position. Obstet Gynecol 1998;91:961–4.
9. Pelvic Organ Prolapse. American College of Obstetricians and Gynecologists. ACOG technical bulletin no. 214. Washington DC: American College of Obstetricians and Gynecologists, 1995.
10. Montella JM, Cater JR. Comparison of measurements obtained in supine and sitting position in the evaluation of pelvic organ prolapse (abstract). In: Proceedings of the Annual Meeting of the American Urogynecologic Society; Oct 1995.
11. Walters MD, Karram MM. Enterocele. American Urogynecologic Society quarterly report. Chicago: American Urogynecologic Society, October 1992; 10.
12. Mishell DR, Stenchever MA, Droegemueller W, Herbst AL, editors. Comprehensive Gynecology, 3rd edn. St Louis, MO: Mosby, 1997; 547–68.
13. Shull BL. Clinical evaluation of women with pelvic support defects. Clin Obstet Gynecol 1993;36(4): 939–51.
14. Raz S, editor. Female Urology, 2nd edn. Philadelphia: WB Saunders Company, 1996; 445–73.
15. Nicholls DH, Randall CL, editors. Vaginal Surgery, 4th edn. Baltimore: Williams & Wilkins, 1996; 101–18.
16. Brubaker LT, Saclarides TJ, editors. The Female Pelvic Floor: Disorders of Function and Support. Philadelphia, PA: FA Davis Company, 1996; 256.
17. Norton PA. Etiology of genuine stress incontinence. In: Brubaker LT, Saclarides TJ, editors. The Female Pelvic Floor: Disorders of Function and Support. Philadelphia, PA: FA Davis Company, 1996; 153–7.
18. Mallett VT, Bump RC. The epidemiology of female pelvic floor dysfunction. Curr Opin Obstet Gynecol 1994;6(4):308–12.
19. Zacharin RG. Chinese anatomy: the pelvic supporting tissues of Chinese and Occidental female compared and contrasted. Aust NZ J Obstet Gynecol 1977;17:11.
20. DeLancey JOL, Hurd WW. Size of the urogenital hiatus in the levator ani muscles in normal women and women with pelvic organ prolapse. Obstet Gynecol 1998;91: 364–8.
21. Ulmsten U, Ekman G, Giertz G, Malmstom A. Different biochemical composition of connective tissue in continent and stress incontinence women. Acta Obstet Gynecol Scand 1987;66:455–7.
22. Falconer C, Ekman G, Malmstom A, Ulmsten U. Decreased collagen synthesis in stress incontinent women. Obstet Gynecol 1994;84:583–6.
23. Versi E, Cardozo L Brincat M, Cooper D, Montgomery J, Studd J. Correlation of urethral physiology and skin collagen in post-menopausal women. Br J Obstet Gynaecol 1988;95:147–52.
24. Bø K, Stien R, Kulseng-Hanssen S, Kristofferson M. Clinical and urodynamic assessment of nulliparous young women

with and without stress incontinence symptoms: a case-control study. Obstet Gynecol 1994;84(6):1028–32.

25. Nygaard IE, Thompwon FL, Svengalis SL, Albright JP. Urinary incontinence in elite nulliparous athletes. Obstet Gynecol 1994;84(3):342.

26. Prokop DJ, Kivirikko KI, Tuderman L, Guzman NA. The biosynthesis of collagen and its disorders. N Engl J Med 1979;301(1):13–23.

27. Norton PA, Baker JE, Sharp HC, Warenski JC. Genitourinary prolapse and joint hyper mobility in women. Obstet Gynecol 1995;85:225–8.

28. Friedman DW, Boyd CD, Norton P, Greco RS, Boyarsky AH, Mackenzie JW, Deak SB. Increases in type III collagen gene expression and protein synthesis in patients with inguinal hernias. Ann Surg 1995;221(1):116–17.

29. Makinen J, Soderstrom KO, Killholm P, Hirvonen T. Histological changes in the vaginal connective tissue of patients with and without uterine prolapse. Arch Gynecol 1986;239:17–20.

30. Rechberger T, Donica H, Baranowski W, Jakowski J. Female urinary stress incontinence in terms of connective tissue biochemistry. Eur J Obstet Gynecol Reprod Biol 1993;49:187–91.

31. Sayer T, Hosker GL, Dixon JS, Warrell DW. A study of paraurethral connective tissue in women with stress incontinence of urine. Neurourol Urodyn 1990;9:319–20.

32. Keane DP, Sims TJ, Bailey AJ, Abrams P. Analysis of pelvic floor electromyography and collagen status in premenopausal nulliparous females with genuine stress incontinence. Neurourol Urodyn 1992;11:308–9.

33. Jackson SR, Avery NC, Tarlton JF, Eckford SD, Abrams P, Bailey AJ. Changes in metabolism of collagen in genitourinary prolapse. Lancet 1996;347:1658–61.

34. Nicholls DH, Randall CL, editors. Vaginal Surgery, 4th edn. Baltimore: Williams & Wilkins, 1996; 536–40.

35. Cohen MP. Diabetes and Protein Glucosylation. New York: Springer Verlag, 1986.

36. Jackson S, Avery N, Shepherd A, Abrams P, Bailey A. The effect of oestradiol on vaginal collagen in post-menopausal women with stress urinary incontinence (Abstract) Neurourol Urodyn 1996;327–8.

37. Brincat M, Moniz CF, Studd JWW, Darby AJ, Magos A, Cooper D. Sex hormones and skin collagen content in post-menopausal women. Br Med J 1983;287:1337–8.

38. Brincat M, Moniz CJ, Studd JWW, Darby AJ, Magos A, Embury G, Versi E. Long-term effects of the menopause and sex hormones on skin thickness. Br J Obstet Gynaecol 1985;92:256–9.

39. Hilton P, Stanton SL. The use of intravaginal oestrogen cream in genuine stress incontinence. Br J Obstet Gynaecol 1983;90:940.

40. Bhatia NN, Bergman A, Karram MM. Effect of estrogen on urethral function in women with urinary incontinence. Am J Obstet Gynecol 1989;160:176–81.

41. Elia G, Bergman A. Estrogen effects on the urethra: beneficial effects in women with genuine stress incontinence. Obstet Gynecol Surv 1993;48(7):509–15.

42. Fantl JA, Cardozo L, McClish DK et al. Estrogen therapy in the management of urinary incontinence in postmenopausal women: A meta-analysis. First report of the hormones and urogenital therapy committee. Obstet Gynecol 1994;83:12–18.

43. Fantl JA, Bump RC, Robinson D, McClish DK, Wyman JF et al. Efficacy of estrogen supplementation in the treatment of urinary incontinence. Obstet Gynecol 1996;88(5):745–9.

44. Blakeman P, Hilton P. Cellular and molecular biology in urogynecology. Curr Opin Obstet Gynecol 1996;8:357–60.

45. Brincat M, Galea R, Baron, Xuereb A. Changes in bone collagen markers and in bone density in hormone treated and untreated post-menopausal women. Maturitas 1997;27(2):171–7.

46. Kirk JA, Ansell BM, Bywaters EGL. The hypermobility syndrome. Ann Rheum Dis 1967;26:419.

47. Al-Rawi ZS, Al-Rawi ZT. Joint hypermobility in women with genital prolapse. Lancet June 1982; 1439–41.

48. Jabs C, Monga AK, Stanton SL, Child AH. Stress incontinence and pelvic organ prolapse in women with Marfan syndrome. Int Urogynecol J 1999;10(suppl 1):S6.

49. Stoddard JF, Myers RE. Connective tissue disorders in obstetrics and gynecology. Am J Obstet Gynecol 1968;102:240–3.

50. McIntosh LJ, Mallett VT, Frahm JD, Richardson DA, Evans MI. Gynecologic disorders in women with Ehlers Danlos syndrome. J Soc Gynecol Invest 1995;2:559–64.

7 The Effect of Pregnancy and Childbirth on the Lower Urinary Tract and Pelvic Floor

Kevin M. Smith and Harold P. Drutz

Introduction

As the perinatal mortality rate has fallen, obstetricians have begun to focus on improving perinatal maternal and fetal morbidity. The relationship between pregnancy, parturition and the pelvic floor is quintessential to the obstetrician and urogynecologist. The lower urinary tract undergoes many physiological changes during pregnancy and these may manifest themselves as urinary symptoms. Also, the pelvic floor undergoes extreme trauma during parturition and this is often cited as a cause of uterovaginal prolapse and bladder symptoms later in life. If this relationship can be established, it may be possible to manipulate parturition to minimize long-term maternal morbidity from pelvic floor damage. The evidence for this will be examined in this chapter.

Mechanical Trauma to Pelvic Structures in Pregnancy and Childbirth

Direct Damage to Pelvic Support and Sphincter Mechanisms

Displacement of the Pelvic Structures

The earliest account of changes in the lower urinary tract as a result of pregnancy and labor comes from anatomical dissections of two women in the nineteenth century [1]. One had died in late pregnancy and the other died in labor. These sagittal dissections showed a change in position of the bladder and urethra. Malpas et al. [2] reviewed these findings and performed radiological studies in pregnancy and childbirth. They found a displacement of the bladder neck and elongation of the urethra during labor. It was postulated that this stretching could cause irreversible damage to the pelvic support structures and sphincter mechanisms and be a contributing factor towards the development of pelvic organ prolapse and urinary incontinence in later life. Although cystoscopic studies [3] have confirmed bladder trauma following vaginal delivery, this is to be expected following such a traumatic event, and in itself does not prove that the damage is irreversible and a precursor of pelvic floor disorders.

Does Pregnancy Cause Anal Sphincter Damage?

It is known that overt lacerations of the anal sphincter caused by childbirth are a major cause of fecal incontinence. Sultan et al. [4] prospectively investigated 20 women who were to deliver by cesarean section, to establish whether pregnancy itself had any effect on the function and morphology of the anal sphincters. Anal endosonography and manometry were performed during pregnancy and six weeks after cesarean section. There was no significant difference in the thickness of puborectalis, the internal nor the external anal sphincter before and after cesarean delivery. The maximum resting pressure and squeeze pressures were not significantly changed. Pregnancy itself does not, therefore, appear to have any significant effect on anal sphincter morphology or function. Any changes in sphincter function are likely to be due to mechanical trauma of labor and/or vaginal delivery rather than hormonal changes in pregnancy.

Does Labor/Childbirth Cause Anal Sphincter Damage?

In 1993, Sultan et al. [5] studied 202 consecutive women prior to delivery, and managed to follow up 150 of them after delivery. Twenty-eight (35%) of the primiparas who delivered vaginally had a new sphincter defect on endosonography at 6 weeks postpartum and these defects persisted in all the women studied at 6 months. Of the 48 multiparous women studied, 19 (40%) had a sphincter defect before delivery and 21 (44%) afterwards. None of the women who underwent cesarean section had a new sphincter defect after delivery. The external sphincter defects noted endosonographically were associated with the more objective finding of significantly lower squeeze pressures (increase above resting pressure, 70 ± 38 versus 44 ± 13 mmHg; p < 0.001). There was also a strong association (p < 0.001) between anal sphincter defects and the development of bowel symptoms. This is direct evidence of labor and/or vaginal delivery causing symptomatic pelvic floor damage, which persists at least until 6 months postpartum.

MacArthur [6], in a study on fecal incontinence following childbirth, noted that some women developed fecal incontinence following emergency cesarean section, but none developed fecal incontinence after an elective cesarean section. This implies that damage to the pelvic floor may be acquired during labor itself and not just during vaginal delivery.

In summary, therefore, the evidence would point to the fact that pelvic floor damage, manifest as either overt or occult anal sphincter damage, is caused by vaginal delivery and possibly by labor itself, although this last point needs further investigation. This sphincter damage has a high correlation with symptoms of fecal urgency and incontinence following delivery. At 6-month follow-up, both the sphincter defects and the related symptoms persisted [5], implying persistence of the pelvic floor damage.

It would appear that most de-novo sphincter damage occurs after the first vaginal delivery. The prevalence of symptoms, however, increases following vaginal delivery in multiparas without a significant increase in the number of new sphincter defects [5] (Figure 7.1). This may indicate that the sequelae of anatomical damage are somehow compounded by subsequent vaginal deliveries. Indeed, Ryhammer et al. [7], in a sample of 304 women who delivered vaginally without overt sphincter damage, found that the number of women with permanent incontinence of flatus increased significantly after the third vaginal delivery compared with the first and second deliveries (odds ratio 6.6; 95% confidence interval 2.4–18.3). Persistent urinary incontinence was also significantly increased after

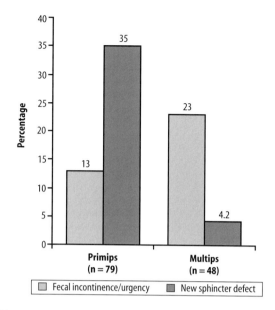

Figure 7.1 Percentage of primiparas and multiparas presenting with new symptoms of fecal urgency or incontinence and those manifesting new anal sphincter damage on endosonography following vaginal delivery (from Sultan et al.[5]).

the third delivery compared with the first and second (odds ratio 3.2; 95% confidence interval, 1.1 – 9.1) – Figure 7.2.

Indirect Damage to the Pelvic Support and Sphincter Mechanisms

Does Labor and/or Vaginal Childbirth Damage the Nerves of the Pelvis?

Overt and occult anal sphincter damage are known to be common after vaginal delivery. Snooks et al. [8], in a study of twenty patients with anterior external anal sphincter division, showed that pudendal

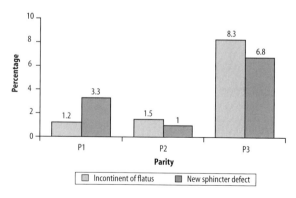

Figure 7.2 Prevalence of incontinence of flatus and urine related to the number of vaginal deliveries (from Ryhammer et al.[7]).

nerve damage coexisted with the overt muscle injury in 60% of these patients. Just as occult sphincter damage is common after vaginal delivery, it is perhaps unsurprising that occult nerve damage can also occur. Allen et al. [9] investigated 96 nulliparous women to establish whether childbirth causes damage to the striated muscles and nerve supply of the pelvic floor. These women were examined at 36 weeks' gestation, at 2–5 days postpartum and again at 2 months after vaginal delivery. They used concentric needle electromyography (EMG), pudendal nerve conduction tests and assessment of pelvic floor muscle strength using a perineometer, and found evidence of pelvic floor denervation in 80% of cases. In severe cases this was associated with incontinence.

Further evidence for vaginal delivery causing nerve injury comes from Snooks et al. [10], who found evidence of pelvic floor denervation in women who delivered vaginally but not in the cesarean section group. The same authors [11] compared similar groups both antepartum and postpartum and confirmed that vaginal delivery results in pelvic floor denervation. Sultan et al. [12], in a prospective study, investigated 128 pregnant women at 34 weeks' gestation or beyond, at 6–8 weeks postpartum and again in a subgroup (n = 24) 6 months following delivery. They found a significant prolongation of the pudendal nerve terminal motor latencies (PNTML), that is the time interval between electrical stimulation of the nerve and induced contraction of the external anal sphincter, in those women who delivered vaginally. The PNTML was not prolonged in those who delivered by elective cesarean section, but was significantly increased in those who underwent cesarean section during labor.

These studies have established that vaginal delivery, and possibly also labor, does cause denervation of the pelvic floor musculature. The question, however, is whether or not the direct damage to the muscles, sphincters and nerves of the pelvic floor, persists and forms the basis of uterovaginal prolapse and incontinence problems later in life. Indeed, Sultan et al. [12] reported that 75% of women with a significantly prolonged PNTML at 6 weeks, had normal measurements when restudied 6 months after delivery.

Is Pelvic Floor Denervation Associated with Long-term Problems?

There is good evidence that vaginal childbirth, and possibly labor with subsequent cesarean section, can cause a degree of denervation of the pelvic floor musculature. Is there any evidence, however, that such damage is associated with symptoms in the patient?

The association of partial denervation of pelvic floor musculature with fecal and urinary incontinence has been made by Snooks et al. [10,13]. They investigated 40 women with idiopathic fecal incontinence, 20 of whom also had stress urinary incontinence and found the terminal motor latencies in the pudendal and perineal nerves were significantly increased when compared with 20 controls. The perineal nerve terminal latency was more markedly increased in the 20 patients with double incontinence than those with fecal incontinence alone.

Further evidence comes from Smith et al. [14], who performed single fiber electromyography on the pubococcygeus muscle in 69 asymptomatic women and 105 women with urinary stress incontinence of urine, genitourinary prolapse or both. The symptomatic women had a significant increase in denervation of the pelvic floor compared with asymptomatic women. The results also suggested that partial denervation of the pelvic floor is a normal accompaniment to aging and is increased by childbirth. The results of these two studies provide direct evidence of damage to the innervation of the pelvic floor musculature in urogenital prolapse and incontinence of feces and urine.

Does the Neurological Damage Caused Specifically by Childbirth Have Long-term Sequelae?

It is reasonably well established that childbirth causes damage to the nerves in the pelvis and that nerve damage is found in patients with urogenital prolapse and incontinence or both. Is there any evidence, however, that the nerve damage sustained specifically in childbirth has any of these long-term sequelae?

The fact that neurological damage due to childbirth can be long-standing and associated with incontinence has been established by Snooks et al. [15]. They conducted a 5-year follow-up on 14 of 24 multiparous women (58%) who had delivered vaginally. Five of these women had developed clinical symptoms of stress incontinence during the 5-year period. There was manometric and neurophysiological evidence of muscle weakness due to partial denervation of the pelvic floor with pudendal neuropathy, which was more marked in those women with incontinence. Although this study suffers from small numbers and lack of control group, it does provide some evidence that pudendal neuropathy due to vaginal delivery persists and may form the basis of incontinence later in life.

It is possible that the direct trauma sustained by the urethral and anal sphincters during labor and vaginal delivery is compounded by damage to the nerves supplying the pelvic floor musculature in the first and subsequent deliveries. This would explain why the number of patients with incontinence of flatus or urine increases, particularly after the third vaginal delivery [7] – see Figure 7.2), and yet the majority of the detectable trauma to the sphincters is sustained during the first vaginal delivery [5] – see Figure 7.1).

Which Aspects of Labor and Delivery Cause Pelvic Floor Damage?

The evidence presented so far supports the following points:

- Vaginal delivery, and possibly also labor, causes *direct* damage to the pelvic musculature including support structures and sphincters.
- Vaginal delivery, and possibly also labor, causes *indirect* damage to the pelvic muscles and sphincters by causing varying degrees of denervation.
- Both the *direct* and the *indirect* damage sustained during labor and vaginal delivery may be the basis of uterovaginal prolapse and problems of fecal and urinary incontinence in later life.

The big question is whether or not any particular part or type of labor or delivery can be held accountable for the pelvic floor damage. If so, short of performing an elective cesarean section on everyone, it may be possible to manipulate labor and vaginal delivery to minimize pelvic trauma and so reduce the long-term morbidity. The length of labor, instrumental delivery and the size of the baby have all been implicated in worsening the pelvic trauma of vaginal delivery. However, there have been no randomized, controlled trials (RCTs) into this area, so the definitive answers still elude us. In such circumstances, we must base our clinical practice on the best available evidence short of RCTs.

Instrumental Delivery and Pelvic Floor Damage

MacArthur et al. [6], in a retrospective, cohort study, interviewed 906 women for a mean of 10 months following delivery and gathered information on postpartum fecal incontinence. They found that, among the vaginal deliveries, instrumental delivery, including forceps and vacuum extraction, was the only independent risk factor for the development of fecal incontinence. The data from this study can be expressed in a two-by-two table (Table 7.1) and the number needed to harm (NNH) calculated to be 16

Table 7.1 2×2 table summarizing data from MacArthur et al. [6], on the development of fecal incontinence following spontaneous vaginal delivery and instrumental vaginal delivery

	Instrumental delivery	No instrumental delivery
Fecal incontinence	12	24
No fecal incontinence	114	733

Table 7.2 2×2 table summarizing data from MacArthur et al. [6], on development of fecal incontinence in those delivered instrumentally and those delivered by emergency cesarean section

	Instrumental delivery	Emergency cesarean section
Fecal incontinence	12	6
No fecal incontinence	114	

(95% CI ± 20). In other words, for every 16 instrumental deliveries, a patient is likely to develop fecal incontinence. This study did not differentiate between forceps and vacuum delivery and, interestingly, emergency cesarean section did not seem to confer any protection against developing incontinence (Table 7.2).

In a study into anal sphincter disruption during vaginal delivery in 1993, Sultan et al. [5], noted that eight out of ten patients delivered by forceps sustained sphincter damage, whereas none of the five patients delivered by vacuum extraction sustained any sphincter damage. In a further study [16] to investigate this observation further, the same authors looked at 43 primiparas who had undergone instrumental delivery (17 vacuum and 26 forceps) and compared them with 47 who had normal, vaginal deliveries. The results showed that those delivered by forceps developed significantly more defecatory symptoms than those delivered by vacuum or those in the control group. Those delivered by forceps also sustained significantly more anal sphincter trauma than those delivered by vacuum and those who delivered spontaneously (Table 7.3).

Another study by Sultan et al. [17], in which they retrospectively reviewed the obstetric variables that predisposed to third degree anal sphincter tears, found that third degree tears occurred in 50% of patients undergoing forceps delivery compared to 7% in a matched control group (p = 0.000 01). There were no third degree tears sustained in 351 vacuum deliveries.

Table 7.3 Table summarizing data from Sultan et al. [16], comparing the onset of defecatory symptoms and sphincter defects following different modes of vaginal delivery

	Defecatory symptoms, n (%) *p value*	Sphincter defect, n (%) *p value*
Spontaneous delivery	2 (4)	17 (36)
Forceps delivery	10 (38) *0.003*	21 (81) *0.0005*
Vacuum delivery	2 (12) *NS*	4 (21) *NS*

NS, not significant; p values calculated in comparison with spontaneous delivery group.

Such studies, because they were not randomized, do not exclude selection bias. For example, the selection of forceps instead of a vacuum extractor may be because the operator anticipated a more difficult, and therefore more traumatic, delivery. Interestingly, and once again highlighting the need for RCTs in the field, Allen et al. [9] found that forceps delivery did not increase the degree of pelvic floor denervation when compared with spontaneous, vaginal childbirth. In the absence of an RCT, however, there seems to be some evidence in favor of using a vacuum extractor rather than forceps for instrumental deliveries in order to minimize pelvic floor trauma.

Large Babies and Pelvic Floor Damage
It may be an over-simplification to suggest that larger babies produce more pelvic floor damage when delivered vaginally, as this does not take into account the size of the maternal pelvis. Once again there have been no RCTs into this area, but the available evidence would suggest that vaginal delivery of babies of higher birthweight does cause more pelvic trauma. In 1986, Snooks et al. [11], in their analysis of 122 consecutive deliveries, found worse pelvic floor denervation in women delivering higher birthweight babies. This is a finding common to other, more recent studies: Sultan et al. [17] found that vaginal delivery of a baby of birthweight 4 kg or more was significantly more likely to cause a third degree tear (p = 0.000 02); Allen et al. [9] found that while 80% of women delivering vaginally sustained some degree of pelvic floor denervation, those delivering heavier babies had more damage, and Sultan et al. [12] found the PNTML to be significantly prolonged in women delivering heavier babies.

Length of Labor and Pelvic Floor Damage
During the second stage of labor, the fetal head lies deeply in the pelvis and the pelvic contents are compressed. A longer second stage might be expected, therefore, to produce more pelvic floor damage. Snooks et al. [11] found that pudendal nerve damage was worse following a long second stage and other investigators [9,11] have also shown more severe pelvic floor denervation following a long, active part of the second stage. It is not known whether allowing longer for passive descent in the second stage and curtailing the active pushing phase by vacuum extraction would reduce pelvic floor damage, but one might postulate that this may be the case. Once again, the need for careful, randomized, controlled trials is highlighted.

Episiotomy, Third Degree Tears and Pelvic Floor Damage
In a prospective study, Rockner et al. [18] investigated pelvic floor muscle strength pre- and post-partum in 87 women with uncomplicated pregnancies. In the group of women with vaginal delivery, they identified three subgroups: those with an episiotomy, those who underwent spontaneous laceration and those with an intact perineum. There were no differences in mean birthweight, labor length and mean head circumference of the baby between these groups. Pelvic floor muscle strength, assessed by vaginal cones, was weakest in the episiotomy subgroup, the difference in values between this subgroup and each of the other subgroups and the elective cesarean section group being significant. No difference was evident between the spontaneous lacerations and the intact perineum subgroups. Although third degree tears are associated with more severe pudendal nerve damage and defecatory symptoms [5,11], an episiotomy is not necessarily protective. Sultan et al. [12] found that 44% of women who were delivered without instruments and had a third degree tear had had an episiotomy.

Lower Urinary Tract Symptoms During Pregnancy

Lower urinary tract problems are common during pregnancy and will be of concern to the pregnant women who suffer from them. It is important for obstetricians and gynecologists to be aware of the spectrum of symptoms, their causes and likely outcome in order to give appropriate advice. To date, most studies have looked at the prevalence of abnormal voiding patterns and stress incontinence. More recently, other symptoms, such as urgency and urge incontinence, have been explored.

Voiding Patterns

An increase in diurnal urinary frequency and nocturia is almost ubiquitous during pregnancy. Francis [19] found that 81% of women experienced frequency of micturition at some stage during the pregnancy, and that the prevalence was the same in both nulliparous and multiparous women. A *cross-sectional* study of 181 women by Stanton [20] showed that frequency, defined as seven or more voids a day, and nocturia, defined as two or more voids at night, both increased in prevalence as the pregnancy progressed, but returned to pre-pregnancy levels in the puerperium (Figure 7.3). Cardozo and Cutner [21] performed a *longitudinal* study on 119 pregnant women and confirmed these findings (Figure 7.4). Increased frequency and nocturia started in the first trimester and the prevalence increased as the pregnancy progressed. Parity made no difference to the prevalence of these symptoms. Overall, they found that 91% of pregnant women described an increase in the number of voids in a 24-hour period.

The reason for this change in voiding pattern has not been fully determined, but is probably multifactorial. The bladder is certainly distorted during pregnancy by the enlarged uterus. This seems obvious and has been documented radiologically [2,19] and cystoscopically [22]. It has been shown that patients who have uterine fibroids impingeing on the bladder show an improvement in their symptom of urinary frequency when the fibroids have been shrunk with gonadotropin-releasing

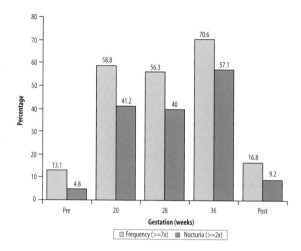

Figure 7.4   Graph summarizing data from Cardozo and Cutner [21], showing prevalence of urinary frequency and nocturia at different stages of pregnancy.

hormone analogues [23]. It is possible, therefore, that extrinsic pressure on the bladder in pregnancy can cause a change in voiding pattern.

Francis [19] and Parboosingh and Doig [24] both performed cross-sectional studies comparing fluid intake and urine output in a series of women at each trimester of pregnancy and compared values to those in non-pregnant, normal controls. They concluded that increased fluid intake and urine output may be sufficient to explain the prevalence of frequency in pregnancy. Cardozo and Cutner [21] found that pregnant women spend more hours in bed, which may account for the nocturia.

Symptoms of frequency and nocturia have certainly not been correlated to cystometric findings during pregnancy. Muellner [25] and Youssef [26] both found a gradual *increase* in bladder capacity as pregnancy progressed, and this was accompanied by a *decrease* in bladder tone. Francis [19] carried out 50 cystometrograms on pregnant women and found no correlation between bladder capacity and frequency. These studies, however, were cross-sectional, and it may be that the relative change in bladder capacity is more important than the absolute value. Cardozo and Cutner [21], however, performed a longitudinal study recording the volume at first desire to void and bladder capacity at 28 weeks' gestation, 36 weeks' gestation and postpartum, and found no significant change in either parameter (Table 7.4).

A change in voiding pattern seems to be almost universal in pregnant women. It begins in the first trimester and the prevalence increases as pregnancy progresses. This change may be due to a combination of extrinsic pressure on the bladder and

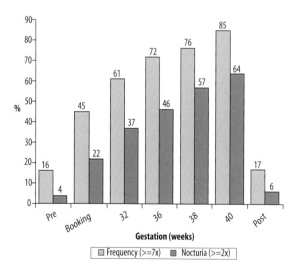

Figure 7.3   Graph summarizing data from Stanton et al. [20], showing the prevalence of urinary frequency and nocturia at different stages of pregnancy.

Table 7.4 Table summarizing data from Cardozo and Cutner [21], showing cystometric changes in pregnancy

	28 weeks' gestation	36 weeks' gestation	Postpartum
Median FDV (ml)	190	250	200
Median bladder capacity (ml)	475	430	440

changes in fluid intake and urine production in pregnancy. The symptoms almost invariably improve postpartum. A pregnant woman presenting with symptoms of frequency and nocturia should, however, be screened for acute cystitis, which occurs in about 1% of pregnancies [27]. If there is no infection, reassurance is all that is required.

Stress Incontinence

Stress urinary incontinence (SUI) is also common during pregnancy. It occurs in 31–67% of pregnant women [19,28] and its onset is likely to occur in any trimester (Figure 7.5). Stanton et al [20] showed, in a cross-sectional study, that there was a significantly higher prevalence of SUI in multiparas than primiparas prior to pregnancy, suggesting, perhaps, some residual effect of previous pregnancies. As pregnancy progresses, the prevalence of SUI increases, with no difference between primiparas and multiparas (Figure 7.6). Postpartum, the symptom of SUI largely resolves, although 6% of primiparas and 11%

of multiparas were found to have persistent SUI in the puerperium.

The reason for SUI in pregnancy in terms of pressure dynamics has been explained by Iosef et al. [29]. They investigated 14 pregnant women *with* SUI and compared the urodynamic findings with those of 12 pregnant women *without* SUI. In all the women, they found an increase in bladder pressure. In those who remained continent this was matched by an increase in maximal urethral closure pressure (MUCP), maximal urethral pressure (MUP), functional urethral length (FUL) and urethral length (UL). Those women with SUI did not show these increases in urethral pressures and urethral length. These findings were reproduced by Cutner [30], who also found improved pressure transmission ratios in the urethra of *continent* pregnant women. These findings do not explain why some women develop symptoms of SUI during pregnancy and others do not. It may be that *relative* changes in bladder and urethral pressures determine the development or otherwise of SUI, with those women with lower pre-pregnancy urethral pressures being more prone to

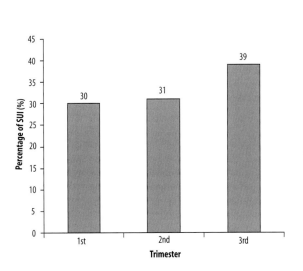

Figure 7.5 Graph summarizing data from Francis [19], showing gestation at onset of symptom of stress urinary incontinence (SUI).

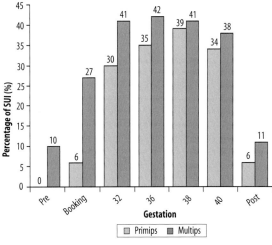

Figure 7.6 Graph summarizing data from Stanton et al. [20], showing prevalence of stress urinary incontinence (SUI) at different gestations of pregnancy.

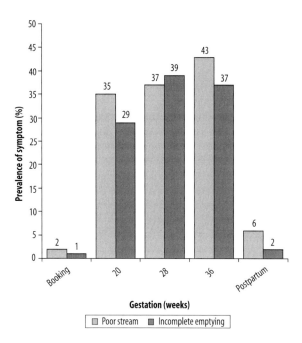

Figure 7.7 Graph summarizing data from Cutner [30], showing the prevalence of symptoms of voiding difficulties during pregnancy.

SUI in pregnancy. Longitudinal studies into this are, as yet, lacking.

The situation is further complicated by the discovery that a proportion of pregnant women with SUI actually has detrusor instability. Clow [31] investigated 25 women, 15 of whom had developed SUI, by subtracted, provocative cystometry. Three of the women with SUI had detrusor instability, which resolved in the puerperium. Detrusor instability in pregnancy has been documented by other groups [32,33], and it has been postulated that it may be related to high progesterone levels [34]. As with non-pregnant women with the symptom of urinary incontinence, one has to question the cause carefully. On the whole, most women who develop SUI during pregnancy can be reassured that the symptom will resolve by the end of the puerperium. In a few, however, this transient symptom may be a marker for long-term problems. The long-term sequelae of childbirth on the pelvic floor have been discussed earlier.

Retention of Urine

Symptoms of voiding difficulties are quite common during pregnancy, with up to 43% of women describing poor stream and 37% describing what they perceive as incomplete emptying, by the end of the third trimester [32] (Figure 7.7). However, once the voided volume had been taken into account, no

difference was found in the peak flow rate or average flow rate between those women with and those without the symptoms of poor stream or incomplete emptying. It would seem, therefore, that these symptoms are a function of the small volumes being voided.

Urinary *retention* during pregnancy is quite rare. It is classically described in some women with a retroverted uterus, which becomes impacted in the pelvis, usually between 8 and 12 weeks' gestation, and causes outflow obstruction. Once the uterus is large enough to become an abdominal organ, the problem resolves spontaneously. In the interim, it may be possible to antevert, and so disimpact the uterus using a lever-type pessary, such as a Smith–Hodge pessary. If this fails, it may be necessary to leave a catheter in place until the uterus rises out of the pelvis [35–37]. There has also been a report of urinary retention caused by impaction of a fibroid during pregnancy [38].

Urinary retention postpartum is more common, with a reported prevalence of between 0.8% [39] and 14.6% [40] of vaginal deliveries. Part of the reason for this broad range in reported prevalence is due to differences in what different investigators consider to be significant post-void residual bladder volume. This varies between 150 ml [40] and 500 ml [39]. Andolf et al. [41] investigated the prevalence of postpartum retention in women after vaginal delivery to determine whether parturients with urinary retention developed voiding problems later in life. Of 539 women, they found 1.5% with a post-void residual bladder volume of more than 150 ml. They found that all symptoms related to this raised residual resolved within a few days of delivery, and at 4-year follow-up they found no difference in the symptoms of these women compared with the general population. Yip et al. [40] studied 691 women who had undergone vaginal delivery and found 9.7% had overt (symptomatic) urinary retention and 4.9% had covert (asymptomatic) urinary retention. They defined urinary retention as a post-void bladder residual of more than 150 ml. All those with covert "urinary retention" resolved within the puerperium. They found, also, that urinary retention was related to the length of labor, whereas Andolf et al. [41] believed that primiparity, instrumental delivery and epidural analgesia were risk factors for postpartum urinary retention. Olofsson et al. [39] found a significant increase in what they described as "clinically significant" urinary retention (>500 ml), in women who had received an epidural. Weissman et al. [42], however, in a study of 106 women who had undergone vaginal childbirth, 68 of whom had an epidural, found no difference in post-void bladder residual between the two groups. The relationship of parturition and epidural analgesia to urinary retention is still unclear. Postpartum urinary retention may be quite common but, on the whole, is self-limiting. Occasionally, however, clinically significant urinary retention may occur and become a more chronic problem, requiring the use of clean, intermittent, self-catheterization or suprapubic catheterization [43].

Lower urinary tract symptoms are almost universal in the antenatal period and in most cases are transient. Retention of urine is one of the few conditions that must be treated, as there may be long-term consequences. The symptoms of frequency and stress incontinence are those which have been most examined in pregnancy. It would appear that the former has no long-term sequelae but the latter may be an indicator of potential sphincter damage during delivery. The recent documentation of detrusor instability antenatally further confuses the picture and demonstrates the need for functional studies to determine the exact significance of these lower urinary tract symptoms.

References

1. Braune W. Atlas of Topographical Anatomy. Leipzig: Veit, 1872.
2. Malpas P, Jeffcoate TNA, Lister UM. The displacement of the bladder and urethra during labour. J Obstet Gynaecol Br Empire 1949;56:949–60.
3. Funnell JW, Klawans AH, Cottrell TLC. The postpartum bladder. Am J Obstet Gynecol 1954;67:1249–56.
4. Sultan AH, Kamm MA, Hudson CN. Effect of pregnancy on anal sphincter morphology and function. Int J Colorectal Dis 1993;4:206–9.
5. Sultan AH, Kamm MA, Hudson CN. Anal sphincter disruption during vaginal delivery. N Engl J Med 1993;23:1956–7.
6. MacArthur C, Blick DE, Keighley MR. Faecal incontinence after childbirth. Br J Obstet Gynaecol 1997;104:46–50.
7. Ryhammer AM, Bek KM, Laurberg S. Multiple vaginal deliveries increase the risk of permanent incontinence of flatus or urine in normal premenopausal women. Dis Colon Rectum 1995;11:1206–9.
8. Snooks SJ, Henry MM, Swash M. Faecal incontinence due to external anal sphincter division in childbirth associated with damage to the innervation of the pelvic floor musculature: a double pathology. Br J Obstet Gynaecol 1985;8:824–8.
9. Allen RE, Hosker GL, Smith AR, Warrell DW. Pelvic floor damage and childbirth: a neurophysiological study. Br J Obstet Gynaecol 1990;9:770–9.
10. Snooks SJ, Swash M, Setchell M, Henry MM. Injury to innervation of the pelvic floor musculature in childbirth. Lancet 1984;ii:546–50.
11. Snooks SJ, Swash M, Henry MM, Setchell M. Risk factors in childbirth causing damage to the pelvic floor innervation. Int J Colorect Dis 1986;1:20–4
12. Sultan AH, Kamm MA, Hudson CN. Pudendal nerve damage during labour: prospective study before and after childbirth. Br J Obstet Gynaecol 1994;1:22–8.
13. Snooks SJ, Barnes PR, Swash M. Damage to the innervation of the voluntary anal and periurethral sphincter muscula-
ture in incontinence: An electrophysiological study. J Neurol Neurosurg Psychiatry 1984;12:1269–73.
14. Smith AR, Hosker GL, Warrell DW. The role of partial denervation of the pelvic floor in the aetiology of genitourinary prolapse and stress incontinence of urine. A neurophysiological study. Br J Obstet Gynaecol 1989;1:24–8.
15. Snooks SJ, Swash M, Mathers SE, Henry MM. Effect of vaginal delivery on the pelvic floor: a five year follow-up. Br J Surg 1990;2:1358–60.
16. Sultan AH, Kamm MA, Bartram CI, Hudson CN. Anal sphincter trauma during instrumental delivery. Int J Gynaecol Obstet 1993;43:263–70.
17. Sultan AH, Kamm MA, Hudson CN, Bartram CI. Third degree obstetric anal sphincter tears: risk factors and outcome of primary repair. BMJ 1994a308:887–91.
18. Rockner G, Jonasson A, Olund A. The effect of mediolateral episiotomy at delivery on pelvic floor muscle strength evaluated with vaginal cones. Acta Obstet Gynecol Scand 1991;70:51–4.
19. Francis WJA. Disturbances in bladder function in relation to pregnancy. J Obstet Gynaecol Br Empire 1960;67:353–66.
20. Stanton SL, Kerr-Wilson R, Harris GV. The incidence of urological symptoms in normal pregnancy. Br J Obstet Gynaecol 1980;87:897–900.
21. Cardozo L, Cutner A. Lower Urinary Tract symptoms in pregnancy. Br J Urol 1997;80(Suppl 1): 14–23.
22. Hundley JM Jr, Siegel IA, Hachel FW, Dumler JC. Some physiological and pathological observations on the urinary tract during pregnancy. Surg Gynecol Obstet 1938;66:360–79.
23. Langer R, Golan A, Neuman M, Schneider D, Bukovsky I, Caspi E. The effect of large uterine fibroids on urinary bladder function and symptoms. Am J Obstet Gynecol 1990;163:1139–41.
24. Parboosingh J, Doig A. Studies of nocturia in normal pregnancy. J Obstet Gynaecol Br Commonw 1973;80:888–95.
25. Muellner SR. Physiological bladder changes during pregnancy and the puerperium. J Urol 1939;41:691–5.
26. Youssef AF. Cystometric studies in gynecology and obstetrics. Obstet Gynecol 1956;8:181–8.
27. Harris RE, Gilstrap LC, Pretty A. A single dose antimicrobial therapy for asymptomatic bacteriuria in pregnancy. Obstet Gynecol 1982;58:546–8.
28. Beck RP, Hsu N. Pregnancy, childbirth and the menopause related to the development of stress incontinence. Am J Obstet Gynecol 1965;91:820–3.
29. Iosef S, Ingemarsson I, Ulmsten U. Urodynamic studies in normal pregnancy and in the puerperium. Am J Obstet Gynecol 1980;137:696–700.
30. Cutner A. The urinary tract in pregnancy. In: Cardozo L, editor. Urogynaecology, 1st edn. Edinburgh: Churchill Livingstone, 1997; 417–42.
31. Clow WM. Effect of posture on bladder and urethral function in normal pregnancy. Urol Int 1975;30: 9–15.
32. Cutner A, Cardozo LD, Benness CJ. Assessment of urinary symptoms in early pregnancy. Br J Obstet Gynaecol 1991;98:1283–6.
33. Cutner A, Cardozo LD, Benness CJ. Assessment of urinary symptoms in the second half of pregnancy Int Urogynecol J 1992;3:30–2.
34. Cutner A, Burton G, Cardozo LD, Wise BG, Abbott D, Studd J. Does progesterone cause an irritable bladder? Int Urogynecol J 1993;4:258–61.
35. Myers DL, Scotti RJ. Acute urinary retention and the incarcerated, retroverted, gravid uterus. A case report. J Reprod Med 1995;40(6):487–90.
36. Silva PD, Berberich W. Retroverted, impacted, gravid uterus with acute urinary retention: report of two cases and a review of the literature Obstet Gynecol 1986;68(1):121–3.

37. Nelson MS. Acute urinary retention secondary to an incarcerated, gravid uterus. Am J Emerg Med 1986;4(3): 231–2.
38. Schwartz Z, Dgani R, Katz Z, Lancet M. Complete urinary retention caused by impaction of leiomyoma in pregnancy. Acta Obstet Gynecol Scand 1986;65(5):525–6.
39. Olofsson CI, Ekblom AO, Ekman-Ordeburg GE. Post-partum urinary retention: a comparison between two methods of epidural analgesia. Eur J Obstet Gynecol Reprod Biol 1997;71(1):31–4.
40. Yip SK, Brieger G, Hin LY, Chung T. Urinary retention in the post-partum period. The relationship between obstetric

41. factors and the post-partum, post-void residual bladder volume. Acta Obstet Gynecol Scand 1997;76(7):667–72.
41. Andolf E, Iosif CS, Jorgensen C, Rydhstrom H. Insidious urinary retention after vaginal delivery: prevalence and symptoms at follow-up in a population-based study. Gynecol Obstet Invest 1994;38(1):51–3.
42. Weissman A, Grisaru D, Shenav M, Peyser RM, Jaffa AJ. Post-partum surveillance of urinary retention by ultrasonography: the effect of epidural analgesia. Ultrasound Obstet Gynecol 1995;6(2):130–4.
43. Watson WJ (1991) Prolonged post-partum urinary retention. Mil Med 156(9):502–3.1

3 Investigation of Pelvic Floor Dysfunction

8 Clinical Evaluation of the Pelvis

Scott A. Farrell

Introduction

A central tenet of the Hippocratic oath is the injunction to do no harm. Patients attend physicians trusting that our knowledge is sufficient and our discretion complete, but above all else, that they will be treated with empathy and judiciousness. If we are to avoid doing harm we must recognize that patients have needs which encompass both the physical and psychological realms.

Patients come to a physician with a set of goals [1]. These goals can be listed in order of priority: (1) to receive an explanation for the cause(s) of their problem(s); (2) to be given effective therapy; and (3) to minimize the inconvenience and discomfort of both the investigation and the treatment. It is possible to provide exemplary care while meeting these goals. The majority of women presenting for the first time with pelvic organ dysfunction have neither significant disease nor uncommon neurologic abnormalities. A comprehensive evaluation which minimizes complex technological investigations is possible and will provide the basis for the first line treatment.

Although at first glance this clinical approach appears to be straightforward, there are several obstacles which lie in the road of the physician who aims to achieve these goals. In their article on the politics of the female pelvis, Wall and DeLancey highlight the problems which can result from the traditional subdivision of the female pelvis into domains reserved for the specialties of urology, gynecology and colorectal surgery [2]. This artificial subdivision of the pelvic structures encourages a form of tunnel vision in which each organ is treated as if it was independent from adjacent organs. It ignores the functional overlap of the pelvic organs. Therapy resulting from this approach, at best, by ignoring this functional overlap, will be incomplete and at worst, may precipitate iatrogenic problems – witness the patient in whom milder degrees of pelvic organ prolapse are transformed by an incontinence procedure into clinically significant pelvic prolapse [3]. Recognition of the limitations inherent in pelvic subdivision has resulted in two thrusts: (1) greater collaboration between the specialties which treat pelvic organ problems and (2) establishment of training programs designed to equip physicians with a comprehensive understanding of the pelvis.

Every clinical evaluation begins with an interaction between a physician who promises to provide advice and care and a patient who attends the physician with a medical problem. If it is to be successful, this interaction should have the following goals:

1. The physician must understand the impact of the problem on the patient's life and the expectations with which the patient enters into their relationship.

2. The patient must be informed about the full spectrum of investigations and treatment options and they must be engaged in the selection process.

3. A contract must be established which represents the consensus of this interaction.

Failure to achieve all of these goals will mean that the interaction is less than fully satisfactory for one or both parties.

The logical order of the steps in this clinical interaction is (1) information gathering and summarization (2) discussion of a differential diagnosis and investigation plan (3) investigations (4) review of findings and (5) development of a treatment plan.

Table 8.1 The components of a basic evaluation of urinary and/or anal incontinence

1. Medical history and symptom review
2. Urinalysis and urine culture
3. 24-hour urolog/anolog
4. Record of dietary intake and bowel evacuation pattern
5. Physical examination
6. Objective demonstration of incontinence

Information Gathering

Although comprehensive evaluation of every patient ensures that nothing will be overlooked, such an unwavering approach is neither cost-effective nor necessary to maintain a standard of exemplary patient care. A triage approach to investigation and management is better suited to the above-mentioned goals [1]. Women complaining of urinary and/or anal incontinence who have not undergone pelvic surgery qualify for a basic evaluation [4]. The components of this basic evaluation are listed in Table 8.1.

Medical Information

A medical history and symptom review permit: (1) the identification of patients who should undergo more extensive investigation; (2) the formulation of a differential diagnosis for the cause of incontinence; and (3) an assessment of the degree of lifestyle impairment caused by incontinence. The traditional medical history relies upon the communication skills of both the physician and their patient for its completeness. In some cases, where both participants in this interaction are fluent and versed in the interpretation of both verbal and non-verbal communication, a clear picture of the clinical problem will emerge. In other circumstances where communication is poor or pressure of time prevails, the clinical picture may be incomplete or distorted. Tables 8.2 and 8.3 illustrate symptoms consistent with certain diagnostic categories of urinary and fecal incontinence. Inquiry concerning these symptoms forms the core of the incontinence history. To improve the chance of achieving a clear and accurate clinical picture, the medical history should be supplemented by two forms of additional information – questionnaires and diaries.

Traditional questionnaires help to fill out and complete the clinical history [5]. By having the patient complete a standardized questionnaire, the physician ensures that no important details of the medical history will be overlooked. While ensuring the comprehensiveness of the medical history, the questionnaire saves time for a busy clinician. But the traditional clinical history, even when it is supplemented by a questionnaire, neglects an equally important component of the patient's history – the impact of the clinical condition on their quality of life. Global quality of life measures look at the total medical picture and its impact upon lifestyle and sense of well-being. Symptom-specific quality of life measures are better able to focus on the symptoms of a particular organ system and measure their impact [6]. They provide insight into the relative importance of the symptoms.

Table 8.2 A urinary tract symptom review

Symptoms suggestive of stress incontinence	Loss of urine with activities producing sudden increases in intra-abdominal pressure (coughing, lifting and jolting physical activities) Urine volume lost with each episode is small (few drops to a tablespoon) Patient able to satisfactorily protect against socially embarrassing incontinence episodes by using menstrual pads
Symptoms suggestive of unstable bladder	Frequent episodes of urgency incontinence Urine volume lost with each episode is often large (tablespoon to greater than one cup) Urinary frequency Incontinence episodes provoked by sensory stimuli (feeling cold temperature, hearing running water) Patient often has to resort to incontinence garments to avoid socially embarrassing incontinence episodes
Symptoms suggestive of an irritative abnormally in the urethra or bladder	Urinary frequency prompted by an inability to tolerate the pain caused by bladder filling. Nocturia Hematuria Dysuria

Table 8.3 Symptoms and findings associated with diagnostic categories of fecal incontinence

Overflow incontinence	*Symptoms*: continuous leakage of liquid stool (often in physically or mentally impaired patients) *Cause*: impairment of anorectal sensation *Physical findings*: rectal examination and/or abdominal X-rays confirm fecal impaction
Reservoir incontinence	*Symptoms*: rectal urgency and incontinence of liquid stool *Causes*: inflammatory bowel disease, radiation proctitis, rectal ischemia, etc. *Physical findings*: vary with the disease process
Recto sphincter incontinence	*Symptoms*: fecal staining, incontinence of liquid or solid stool *Causes*: impairment of anal sphincter function and rectal sensation *Physical findings*: impairment of external anal sphincter and puborectalis muscle function. Decreased rectal sensation

Diaries are a means of obtaining a more objective record of the events of daily life [7]. In the case of the urinary incontinence diary, the urolog (Figure 8.1), the frequency and volume of micturitions and the quality and quantity of fluid consumption are recorded. Incontinence episodes and their precipitating factors are also noted. This objective record provides: (1) a clear reflection of the frequency and severity of incontinence episodes and (2) some clues as to the etiology of the incontinence. This information forms the basis for a number of practical recommendations for lifestyle modification (Table 8.4).

A similar record to document episodes of anal incontinence is useful. Dietary and behavioral modification will help patients with anal incontinence (Table 8.5). Despite the wealth of useful information obtained by using these methods, medical history alone is not sufficient to make a definitive diagnosis and must be supplemented by other investigations [8].

Clinical Examination

The extent of the clinical examination will reflect both the complexity of the presenting clinical picture and the contract established between physician and patient. The clinical evaluation of patients should be tailored to their presenting complaint(s). While many patients will present with a spectrum of interrelated problems, it is helpful to outline the conservative clinical evaluation of three symptom categories – urinary incontinence, anal incontinence and pelvic organ prolapse. Before outlining the investigations specific to these symptom categories, discussion will focus on the investigation common to all, the pelvic examination.

Pelvic Examination

The pelvic examination should be designed to evaluate both the structural and functional integrity of the pelvic structures and organs. Structural integrity is reflected in the quality of the tissues, the location and support of the pelvic organs, and the presence of pelvic organ pathology. Functional integrity is assessed by tests which measure neurologic function, as well as smooth and striated muscle function. A complete pelvic examination can be completed with a few basic pieces of equipment (Figure 8.2).

UROLOG

The urolog is a record of your bladder function for one 24 hour period. You will be asked to record the following information: (1) the volumes you void (2) the volumes you drink and any episodes of leaking. Please follow the instruction carefully and bring this record to your urodynamics clinic appointment.

DATE	TIME	VOLUME VOIDED (ml)	EPISODES OF LEAKING	ACTIVITY AT TIME OF LEAK	FLUID INTAKE

1. Please record the time and volume each time you empty your bladder.
2. Please record the time of any episodes of leaking and indicate what was happening at the time: C - cough
S - sneeze
L - lifting
R - rushing to the bathroom, etc.
3. Please indicate how much you leaked: - small
- medium
- large
4. Please record the volume and type of fluids you drink.

Figure 8.1 The urolog.

Table 8.4   Urinary symptom based lifestyle guidelines

Symptom	Recommendations
1. Urinary frequency and/or urgency	Reduce 24-hour intake to 5–6 cups
	Caffeine containing beverages and foods should be eliminated from the diet
	Avoid or reduce alcohol intake
	Void at regular intervals during the day (at least every 2 hours)
2. Nocturia	Reduce 24-hour fluid intake to 5–6 cups
	Stop drinking after the evening meal
	Avoid caffeinated beverages in the evening
	Identify and eliminate other causes of waking
3. Stress incontinence	Void every 2 hours to keep the bladder volume low
	Void prior to any vigorous physical activity

Table 8.5   Dietary and behavioral modification for patients with anal incontinence

- A low residue diet to improve stool consistency and to decrease colonic pressure
- Avoidance of flatus-producing foods (high fiber) and carbonated beverages
- Decreased air swallowing by the avoidance of sipping hot beverages and chewing gum
- Daily exercise to stimulate bowel function
- A visit to the bathroom within 15 to 30 minutes after each meal will promote regular bowel evacuation by enlisting the natural gastrocolic reflex
- Avoidance of straining at stool which can exacerbate denervation injury by stretching the pudendal nerve
- Regular use of a mild suppository (glycerin) at the same time each day may help to promote regular bowel emptying

Examination for the Structural Integrity of the Pelvis

The examination for the structural integrity of the pelvis includes an estimation of the thickness of the vaginal epithelium, an indirect reflection of exposure of the pelvic organs to estrogen. Adequate amounts of estrogen are essential to the maintenance of (1) thick vaginal and urethral epithelium, (2) normal blood flow to the urethral adventitia and periurethral vascular plexus, and (3) normal pelvic nerve conduction. Deficiency of estrogen clearly compromises the structural integrity of the pelvis [9–11].

Pelvic organ prolapse often accompanies incontinence. Identification and quantification of pelvic organ prolapse is essential for two reasons: (1) pelvic prolapse may compromise the voiding–continence mechanisms and (2) it must be taken into account when developing both conservative and surgical treatment plans. Until recently, a number of semiquantitative systems were used to characterize pelvic organ prolapse [12,13]. The reliability and reproducibility of these systems was not proven. A collaborative effort among a number of surgical societies resulted in the development of a more objective system for quantifying pelvic organ prolapse called the POP-Q [14]. This system relies upon nine site-specific measurements which can also be combined into an ordinal staging system. This

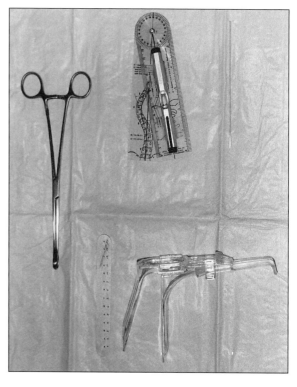

Figure 8.2   Equipment for clinical pelvis examination.

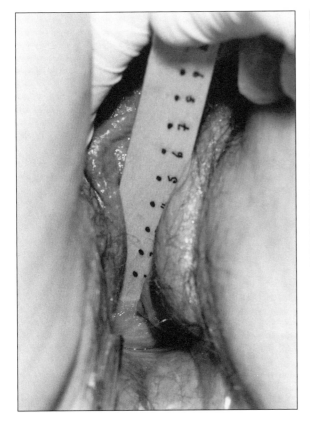

Figure 8.3 Tongue depressor marked in centimeters.

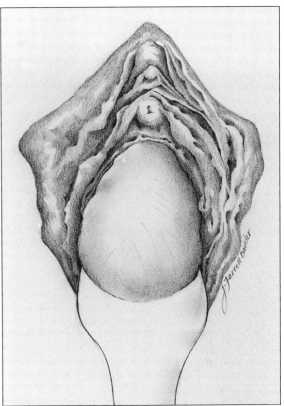

Figure 8.4 Pulsion-type cystocele (central defect).

system has proven to be reproducible [15]. Although a number of measurement tools have been described, a tongue depressor marked with indelible ink works well and is readily available (Figure 8.3). Although a reproducible system should result in greater consistency when research results are reported, any advantages it may offer the clinical process of classification and management of patients remain to be demonstrated. Richardson has demonstrated that the anterior vaginal wall depends for its support not only upon the integrity of the tissues separating the bladder from the vagina, but also upon its attachment to the arcus tendineus fascia pelvis (ATFP) [16]. Examination of the anterior vaginal compartment must be designed to identify specific defects. The two most common findings are central and paravaginal defects. In their classic presentations, cystoceles caused by these two defects have distinct appearances. The pulsion-type cystocele, caused by stretching and attenuation of the anterior vaginal wall tissues (central defect), has a smooth surface devoid of rugae (Figure 8.4) [17]. The traction-type cystocele caused by detachment of the pelvic sidewall support (paravaginal defect),

in contrast, results in preservation of vaginal rugae (Figure 8.5). Support of the vaginal fornices during the examination, while eliminating a traction cystocele due to a paravaginal defect, will have no effect on a pulsion-type cystocele caused by a central defect (Figure 8.6). Some patients will be found to have a combination of both defects.

Pelvic masses, extrinsic to the pelvic organs or arising from them, may be identified during pelvic examination. Extrinsic masses impinging upon pelvic organs, by affecting their function, will produce a variety of symptoms. Intrinsic masses raise the possibility of malignancy and must be considered in the management plan.

Examination of the Functional Integrity of the Pelvis

The functional integrity of the pelvis is primarily dependent upon normal nerve conduction in conjunction with normal function of both autonomically innervated smooth muscle and somatically innervated striated muscle. Although dysfunction of autonomic innervation and smooth muscle sphinc-

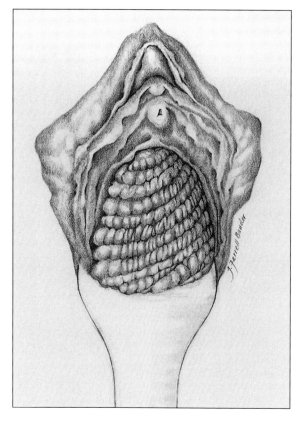

Figure 8.5   Traction-type cystocele (paravaginal defect).

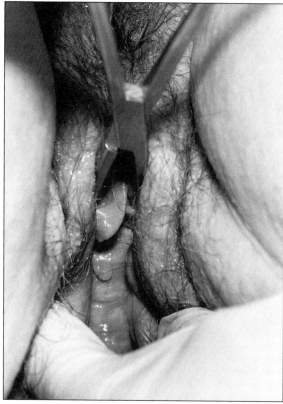

Figure 8.6   Ring forceps supporting the lateral vaginal fornices.

ter function may be inferred from symptoms, there are no tests which can be performed during a pelvic examination to identify these problems. During the pelvic examination, functional integrity is reflected by the normality of a basic neurologic examination (Table 8.6) and by the striated muscle activity. Questions which the examiner should consider during the examination of the functional integrity of the pelvic muscles include: (1) Are the muscles morphologically symmetrical? (2) Are there any defects in the muscle such as hernias or tears from obstetrical trauma? (3) Is there any scarring? (4) What is the volume of the muscles? (5) Is there voluntary symmetrical contraction? (6) Does

contraction elevate the bladder neck and/or anorectal angle? [18]

The examiner uses both inspection and palpation to answer these questions. During inspection when the levator ani muscle group is healthy, voluntary contraction of these muscles will result in a puckering and indrawing of the vaginal introitus, anal sphincter and perineal body. Coughing should produce little or no descent of the perineum either in the supine or standing positions. In the patient whose levator ani muscle function is compromised, voluntary contraction may produce minimal puckering or no movement at all. Coughing will produce perineal descent and gaping of the vaginal introitus with accompanying pelvic organ prolapse. These observations are exaggerated in the standing position.

During palpation, the examiner attempts to evaluate muscle bulk, resting tone, contractile strength and reflex response to cough. Vaginal examination with a gloved index finger (Figure 8.7) permits assessment of the resting bulk and symmetry of the paravaginal muscles, primarily the pubococcygeus

Table 8.6   The elements of a screening neurologic evaluation of the incontinent woman

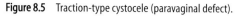

1.	Sensory dermatomes of the lower limbs
2.	Strength in the lower limbs
3.	Sacral nerve reflexes (a) Bulbocavernosus
	(b) Anocutaneous

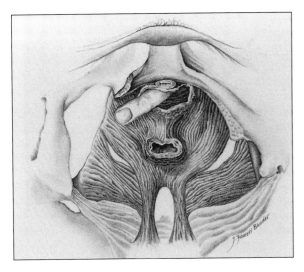

Figure 8.7   Palpation of pubococcygeus muscle.

muscles (PCM). Normally, the PCM is felt as a distinct 1 to 2 cm band which surrounds the vaginal introitus and closes it. A weak or attenuated PCM may be indistinguishable from the surrounding tissues. During rectal examination, the intact external anal sphincter (EAS) grasps the examining finger. The pubococcygeus muscle swings around the anorectal junction and at rest it pulls the junction forward to create an acute angle between the anal canal and rectal ampulla. If there is a deficiency of the anterior EAS it is usually accompanied by a deficient perineal body. By palpation, this area will seem to be composed almost exclusively of skin.

The voluntary function of the pelvic floor muscles can be assessed subjectively. A more sophisticated evaluation of pelvic floor function known as the PERFECT scheme involves assessments of the power (P), the endurance (E) and the number of repetitions (R) which a subject is able to achieve [19]. Every (E) contraction (C) is timed (T) to ensure that progress can be objectively demonstrated. Using this system the power of a muscular contraction is graded from 0 (no movement) to 5 (strong contraction), a system based upon the Oxford grading system. Both slow and fast twitch muscle fibers contribute to power. The endurance, measured in seconds, is the duration of time that a maximum vaginal contraction can be maintained and reflects the activity of slow twitch fibers. The number of maximum vaginal contractions which can be repeated and held for a specified time becomes the patient's baseline "number", forming the basis for her exercise prescription. Re-evaluation of patient performance is recommended once weekly for the first month and every 2 weeks after that for up to 6 months.

Other aspects of pelvic muscle function which can be evaluated include coordination and reflex response. A patient with a healthy functioning pelvic floor should be able to contract and relax the pelvic floor both quickly and slowly on command. An increase in intra-abdominal pressure should result in a reflex contraction of the pelvic floor muscles which can be observed at the introitus and palpated digitally.

Components of the Clinical Examination for Specific Symptom Categories

Urinary Incontinence

Urinalysis and urine culture are essential before beginning a more involved investigation of the urinary tract. Urinary tract infection (UTI) may be responsible for some or all of a patient's symptoms [20]. If UTI is diagnosed, successful treatment should be confirmed before other investigations and therapy are initiated. Symptoms may resolve after successful treatment of UTI. Instrumentation, whether for endoscopic evaluation or urodynamics testing, may exacerbate UTI and lead to iatrogenic complications. Falsely positive urodynamic test results may occur if UTI is present.

The stress test, conducted by having the patient cough in either the supine or standing position, provides objective evidence of urinary incontinence. This test may provide some evidence of the clinical severity of incontinence. Patients who leak, after voiding, while coughing in the supine position probably have a much more compromised continence mechanism when compared to those who leak minimally while coughing in the standing position with a full bladder. A more objective measure of the severity of urinary incontinence can be achieved using a pad test [7]. With a symptomatically full bladder the patient is asked, while wearing a pre-weighed perineal pad, to perform a number of activities which would normally induce incontinence. The post-test pad weight difference is calculated. During stress testing, the ability of the patient to augment the continence mechanism can be assessed. Some patients are able to contract the pelvic floor muscles, thereby elevating the urethrovesical junction (UVJ) and constricting the external urethral sphincter sufficiently to prevent urinary incontinence during coughing.

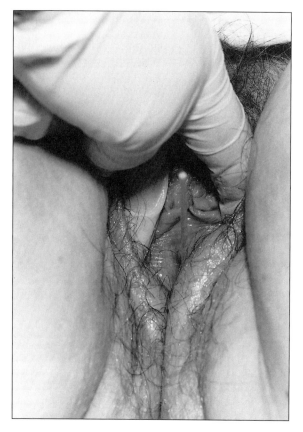

Figure 8.8 Q-tip angle at rest.

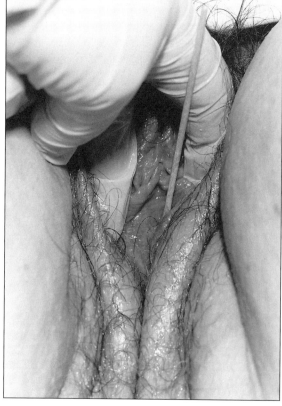

Figure 8.9 Q-tip angle with Valsalva.

UVJ mobility can be assessed clinically by visual inspection of the anterior vaginal wall or by using a lubricated Q-tip inserted to the UVJ – the Q-tip test. If either the resting (Figure 8.8) or straining angles (Figure 8.9) of the Q-tip exceed 30° above the horizontal, the UVJ is hypermobile. UVJ hypermobility should be demonstrated before mechanical (pessary) or surgical support is undertaken.

When symptoms of overactive bladder are prominent in the clinical picture, detrusor instability must be suspected. A simple office (or bedside) testing device involves a 60 ml syringe attached by an adapter to a straight catheter (Figure 8.10). Aliquots of fluid are used to fill the syringe. An elevation of the water level in the syringe accompanied by symptoms of urgency is strongly suggestive of unstable bladder.

Fecal Incontinence

The neurological and functional examinations of the pelvis outlined earlier encompass most of what is necessary for the clinical evaluation of fecal incontinence. Rectal examination rules out impacted stool while assessing the function of the external anal sphincter and the puborectalis muscle.

Pelvic Prolapse

The standard pelvic examination includes an assessment for pelvic organ prolapse. When moderate to severe degrees of prolapse of the anterior and/or central compartments exist, stress urinary incontinence may be masked. In some patients, reduction of the prolapse will reveal this "latent" stress incontinence (Figure 8.11). A finding of latent stress incontinence should prompt a modification of both the conservative and surgical management plan.

Conclusions

Armed with the information gathered from this basic clinical evaluation of the pelvis, the physician is in a position to outline conservative treatment

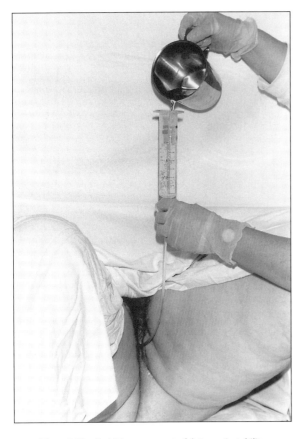

Figure 8.10 Bedside assessment of detrusor instability.

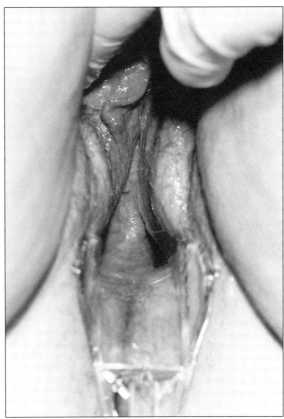

Figure 8.11 Prolapse reduction-test for latent stress incontinence.

options. In some cases more extensive investigation will be warranted, but the majority of patients neither want nor require extensive evaluation prior to a trial of conservative therapy.

References

1. Farrell SA. A triage approach to the investigation and management of urinary incontinence in women. J Soc Obstet Gynaecol Can 1998;20:1153–8.
2. Wall LL, DeLancey JOL. The politics of prolapse: a revisionist approach to disorders of the pelvic floor in women. Int Urogynecol J 1993;4:304–9.
3. Wiskin AK, Creighton SM, Stanton SL. The incidence of genital prolapse following the Burch colposuspension. Am J Obstet Gynecol 1992;167:399–405.
4. Drutz HP, Farrell SA, Mainprize TC. Guidelines for the evaluation of genuine stress incontinence prior to primary surgery. J Soc Obstet Gynaecol Can 1997;19:633–9.
5. McCarthy T. Medical history and physical examination. In: Ostergard DR, Bent AE, editors. Urogynecology and Urodynamics – Theory and Practice, 3rd edn. Philadelphia: Williams & Wilkins, 1991; 99–101.
6. Shumaker SA, Wyman JF, Uebersax JS, McClish D, Fantl IA. Health-related quality of life measures for women with urinary incontinence: the incontinence impact questionnaire and the urogenital distress inventory. Qual Life Res 1994;3:291–306.
7. Pierson CA. Pad testing, nursing interventions and urine loss appliances. In: Ostergard DR, Bent AE editors. Urogynecology and Urodynamics – Theory and Practice, 3rd edn. Philadelphia: Williams and Wilkins, 1991; 209–27.
8. Jensen JK, Neilsen Jr FR, Ostergard DR. The role of patient history in the diagnosis of urinary incontinence. Obstet Gynecol 1994;83:904–10.
9. Fantl JA, Wyman JF, Anderson RL, Matt DW, Bump RC. Postmenopausal urinary incontinence: comparison between non-estrogen supplement and estrogen supplement women. Obstet Gynecol 1988;71:823–8.
10. Wilson PD, Barker G, Barnard RJ. Steroid hormone receptors in the female lower urinary tract. Urol Int 1984;39:5.
11. Bhatia NN, Bergman A, Karram MM. Effects of estrogen on urethral function in women with urinary incontinence. Am J Obstet Gynecol 1989;160:176.
12. Baden WF, Walker TR. Genesis of the vaginal profile: a correlated classification of vaginal relaxation. Clin Obstet Gynecol 1972;15:1048–54.
13. Beecham CT. Classification of vaginal relaxation. Am J Obstet Gynecol 1980;136:957–8.

14. Bump RC, Mattiasson A, Bo K, Brubaker LP, DeLancey JOL, Klarskow P, Shull BL, Smith ARB. The standardization of terminology of female pelvic organ prolapse and pelvic floor dysfunction. Am J Obstet Gynecol 1996;175:10–17.
15. Kobak WC, Rosenberger K, Walters MD. Inter observer variation in the assessment of pelvic organ prolapse. Int Urogynecol J 1996;7:121–4.
16. Richardson AC, Lyon JB, Williams NL. A new look at pelvic relaxation. Am J Obstet Gynecol 1976;126:568–73.
17. Benson JT. Vaginal approach to cystocele repair. In: Benson JT, editor. Female Pelvic Floor Disorders: Investigation and Management. New York, 1992; 289–94.
18. Schüssler B. Aims of pelvic floor evaluation. In: Schüssler B, Laycock J, Norton P, Stanton S, editors. Pelvic Floor Re-education. London: Springer-Verlag, 1994; 39–41.
19. Laycock J. Clinical evaluation of the pelvic floor. In: Schüssler B, Laycock J, Norton P, Stanton S, editors. Pelvic Floor Re-education, London: Springer-Verlag, 1994; 42–8.
20. Karram MM. Lower urinary tract infection. In: Ostergard DR, Bent AE, editors. Urogynecology and Urodynamics: Theory and Practice, 3rd edn. Baltimore, MD: Williams & Wilkins, 1991; 306–28.

9 Urodynamics of the Female Lower Urinary Tract, Resting and Stress Urethral Pressure Profiles and Leak Point Pressures

Sidney B. Radomski

Introduction

The most accurate tools that are available for the investigation of the lower female urinary tract in those with voiding dysfunction include a history, physical examination and urodynamic studies. Urodynamic studies have become more and more sophisticated over the last few years. These studies include filling cystometrogram(CMG), pressure flow studies, electromyography(EMG) studies, urethral pressure profile(UPP) studies, Valsalva leak point pressure (VLPP) and video or fluoroscopic urodynamics. All these studies can be done at one sitting to give us the most accurate assessment of a female patient's lower urinary tract function. This information, however, must be used in conjunction with the patient's clinical symptoms and treatment should not be based solely on the urodynamic findings. Lastly, not every female patient with a lower urinary tract problem not requires urodynamic investigation. These sophisticated studies should be generally reserved for patients with complex problems and those who have failed therapy. In this chapter we will discuss non-video urodynamic testing of the lower female urinary tract.

Urodynamics

Urodynamic testing can vary in complexity from a simple "eye ball" CMG [1] to video multichannel urodynamics. What is used is based on what is available for the clinician and the patient's problem. If simple bladder instability needs to be demonstrated then a simple CMG can be adequate. If a patient has had multiple incontinence procedures and is still

incontinent video multichannel urodynamics are required.

Cystometrogram (CMG)

CMG is the most simple urodynamic test available. It can be done in the office or in the cystoscopy suite by simply inserting a 14 French Foley catheter into the bladder once the patient has voided. In the past some clinicians have used a suprapubic catheter instead of a urethral catheter. There is no real advantage in using a suprapubic catheter and it is much more invasive. It has been essentially abandoned in most centers. The insertion of the catheter provides a post-void residual to start with. Once the bladder is empty a 500 ml saline intravenous bag and tubing with a drip chamber is connected to the catheter with the patient in the sitting or standing position. Fluid is run into the bladder at a slow or moderate rate (i.e. 25–50 ml/minute). The intravenous bag must be kept above the patient's pubis at a height of 15–20 cm to run in. If the patient has an unstable contraction the fluid inflow will back up as seen in the intravenous tubing drip chamber and/or it will leak around the catheter. Once the patient is filled to a comfortable capacity the catheter is removed and the patient can be stress tested (i.e. coughing, straining etc.) for urinary leakage and then asked to void. The volume voided is measured and the residual can be determined with reasonable accuracy by subtracting the volume infused by how much was voided and leaked out. Simple CMG electronic equipment is now readily available. It can provide more accurate results than an "eye ball" CMG by picking up low pressure instability and can document the actual pressure increase (i.e. cmH_2O). CMG electronic equipment uses a pressure transducer to pick up changes in bladder pressure. Numerous models are available at varying costs. A three-way stopcock is attached to the drainage port of the Foley catheter with an adapter. The second port is for infusion of saline and the third port is for the CMG pressure transducer. The tubing for the pressure transducer is fluid filled. Filling is then started and the CMG pressure transducer is zeroed. Filling should be at a constant rate. The CMG is zeroed once the infusion is started since the infusion rate affects bladder pressure readings when both infusion and pressure measurements are done through a single lumen (Foley catheter). Any increase in pressure in the bladder is picked up by the transducer and is recorded. When the infusion is stopped the pressure transducer may record a negative pressure and this may need to be zeroed once again.

An even simpler technique than using a stopcock is to use a dual lumen catheter. One port is for infusion and the other port is for pressure readings with a transducer. The dual lumen catheter prevents the infusion of fluid affecting pressure measurements. The dual lumen catheter may be costly.

The major problem with a simple CMG is that it is only a single channel. In other words, we are only measuring intravesical pressure. Intravesical pressure will include any effect from the detrusor itself (i.e. a detrusor contraction) and outside effects (i.e. coughing, talking and straining). As a result, with a simple CMG low pressure unstable contractions may not as readily be picked up and straining may be misinterpreted as an unstable detrusor contraction.

Some clinicians have advocated using gas infusion instead of saline. The use of gas such as carbon dioxide has multiple problems associated with it. There is considerable variability and poor reproducibility in results when the test is repeated in the same patient. Gas can leak around the catheter unnoticed and result in false negative results for detrusor instability [2–4]. It is more difficult to monitor the exact amount of gas infused and hence a risk of bladder perforation in the elderly. Lastly, saline, like urine, is incompressible. In contrast, gas is compressible and hence can cause artifacts during urodynamics. In the majority of urodynamic laboratories, saline or H_2O is used and is more similar physiologically to urine. Also, saline infusion allows for other tests to be performed such as a flow study and stress testing. Temperature of the infusion liquid may have an effect on bladder contractions. Saline or H_2O at room temperature is recommended. In some cases such as a neurogenic bladder ice water is used to provoke detrusor hyperreflexia ("ice water test").

Lastly, the indications for a simple CMG are as follows (these are relative): (1) history of pure urgency or urge incontinence; (2) leakage without warning (no stress incontinence).

Multichannel Urodynamics

For complex cases of voiding dysfunction multichannel urodynamics is used. Adding simultaneous fluoroscopy/video makes this test the most accurate available to assess voiding dysfunction. As the name implies, multiple channels are used. In other words with a simple CMG we measure only intravesical pressure. With multichannel testing we can measure intravesical pressure, rectal pressure (intra-abdominal pressure), true detrusor pressure and EMG. We can also measure volume infused, volume voided and flow rate. All of this information can be printed out in a coordinated chart form (Figure 9.1). This allows for simultaneous comparison of all the parameters at the exact intervals during filling.

Rectal pressure can be measured in numerous ways. It is supposed to reflect intra-abdominal pressure, which can obviously affect intravesical pressure. Rectal pressure can be measured by a simple balloon catheter inserted into the rectum. The balloon catheter is filled with fluid and attached to a pressure transducer via fluid-filled tubing. Another method is to insert a small 8 French feeding tube into the rectum and very slowly infuse saline (5 ml/minute) through the feeding tube into the rectum. The feeding tube is attached via fluid-filled tubing to a pressure transducer. A feeding tube is less costly than a balloon catheter but has some pitfalls. In using a slow infusion through a feeding tube fluid may leak out of the rectum and may be mistaken for urinary leakage. The last method to measure rectal pressure is to use a rectal pressure microtransducer tip catheter. These catheters are expensive. They can be reused but they can potentially be contaminated and transmit disease. As a result, they are not commonly used. We generally use a new rectal balloon catheter or feeding tube which does not have to be sterile.

Intravesical pressure can be measured by two methods. The first involves inserting a dual lumen catheter with one port for infusion and one port for measuring pressure with a pressure transducer via fluid-filled tubing. Drawbacks in using such a catheter is that it is generally 12 French or larger and this size of catheter may be obstructing and will affect flow rate and voiding pressure during pressure/flow studies [5]. We recommend the second method, which uses a 14 or 12 French Foley catheter with a 5 French pressure catheter inserted together.

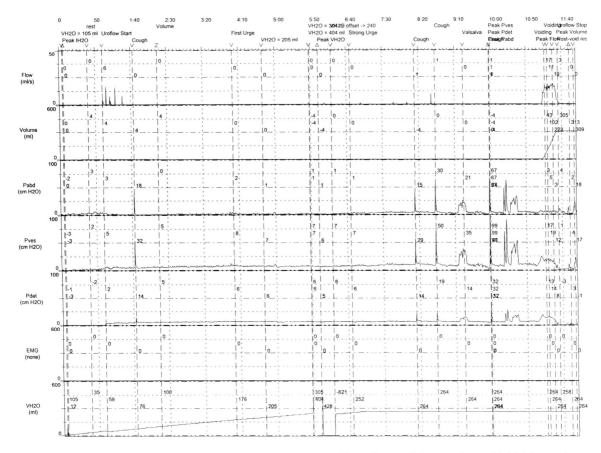

Figure 9.1   A typical multichannel urodynamic study without EMG in a woman.(Flow = flow rate, Volume = volume voided, Pabd = rectal pressure, Pves = intravesical pressure, Pdet = Pves – Pabd or true detrusor pressure, EMG = electromyography, VH2O = volume infused.)

The 5 French catheter is attached to a pressure transducer via fluid-filled tubing and can record intravesical pressure. The 5 French catheter comes with an intraluminal stylet which feeds into the Foley catheter eyelet. Once both catheters are introduced together into the bladder the stylet is removed, allowing the 5 French pressure catheter to disengage from the Foley catheter to float freely in the bladder. The Foley catheter balloon is inflated to prevent the catheter from falling out. Care must be taking to ensure the balloon of the catheter is not over-inflated as this may provoke bladder instability. With this technique infusion of saline can occur into the bladder without affecting the 5 French bladder pressure catheter. The 5 French pressure catheter measures total intravesical pressure changes. These are affected by detrusor contractions and intra-abdominal pressure changes such as coughing and straining. Once infusion is completed the Foley catheter can be removed and the patient can void easily around the small 5 French pressure catheter. This small size catheter is not obstructing and true flow and voiding pressure can be recorded simultaneously. Once all the catheters are inserted the pressure transducers (rectal and intravesical) can be zeroed. Furthermore, the transducers must be at the level of the patient's pubis at all times during the study. If the patient's position is altered (i.e. from sitting to standing) the transducers are altered or the change in pressure with the change in position must be documented and taken into account when recording values.

With the presence of a rectal pressure catheter and an intravesical pressure catheter we can determine true detrusor pressure values. By subtracting the intravesical pressure (total bladder pressure) from the rectal pressure (intra-abdominal pressure), we can determine true detrusor pressure changes such as hyperreflexia or instability or poor compliance. With these two catheters we can accurately determine bladder pressure changes by eliminating confusing artifacts such as straining, talking and coughing which will increase intra-abdominal (rectal) pressure and hence intravesical pressure.

This aspect alone makes multichannel urodynamics more accurate than a single channel simple CMG. Furthermore, subtle changes in bladder pressure increases (i.e. pressure changes less than 10 cmH$_2$O) may be picked up with multichannel testing.

With coughing and straining rectal pressure readings may not equal intravesical pressure readings at times. There may be some subtle differences which cause this. The catheters used to measure rectal and bladder pressure may be different sizes and the techniques of measurement of pressure are different. Also intra-abdominal pressures may not be transmitted evenly to the bladder and rectum. As a result, at the beginning of each study the difference between rectal and bladder pressure with coughing or straining should be made equal or noted and then the instrumentation should be zeroed. If a difference is recorded between rectal and bladder pressure catheters prior to starting the test, it must be taken into account for all later readings.

Infusion Rate and Measurement

An intravenous bag of saline is hung from an infusion weight transducer at a height of 15–25 cm. When the infusion starts the weight of the intravenous bag decreases and the transducer records this as the volume infused. With this method the rate of infusion can also be measured. Different infusion rates are used during urodynamics. A slow fill, which we consider to be <25 ml/minute, can be used in patients with severe instability to allow an adequate volume of fluid to be infused. This rate of infusion is often used in patients with neurogenic bladders. Medium fill is at approximately 25–50 ml/minute and is used in most patients to start with. Fast fill at >50 ml/minute can be used to provoke bladder instability or hyperreflexia. One potential pitfall with a fast fill infusion rate is that it may give a false positive finding of poor compliance (a significant pressure rise with filling)[6]. The cause of this is not exactly clear but may be related to the inability of the bladder to accommodate fluid so rapidly. In most individuals the average urine output is 30–100 ml/hour. In a urodynamic study the infusion rate can be 50 ml/minute or 3000 ml/hour. This clearly is not a physiological infusion rate.

Positioning

Positioning can be very important. We perform urodynamics in the sitting position in most patients. In patients who are immobile we will perform testing in the supine position. It has been shown that 58% of "unstable bladders" will remain undetected if the urodynamics is only performed in the supine position instead of being done in the sitting or upright position [7,8]. Other maneuvers such as jumping, walking on the spot or coughing or straining can also provoke an unstable bladder contraction. Placing the patient's hand in warm or cold water or the sound of running water may also provoke an unstable bladder contraction.

Uroflow

Flow rate and volume voided is measured also by collection of the fluid voided into a container sitting on a weight transducer which measures the volume voided over a time interval (cc/second). Peak flow rate appears to be the most important parameter used. Close assessment of the peak flow rate on the graph must be done to rule out artifacts such as shifting of the weight transducer. Other parameters such as voiding time and volume voided are also important. Generally speaking, a voided volume of >150 ml is needed to assess peak flow rate accurately. Lower volumes voided may not adequately stretch the detrusor muscle to allow full muscle fiber contraction and hence a lower flow rate.

Electromyography (EMG)

EMG is the study of electrical potentials produced by the depolarization of the muscle membrane. EMG studies are used to assess the activity of the pelvic floor muscles and external sphincter. There are two methods used for EMG studies. For both methods the patient must be grounded. Surface electrodes placed on the perineum are easy to do and are attached to an EMG recorder. This recorder will show a visual scale indicating pelvic floor activity. Often this scale is used with an auditory scale also (i.e. increased noise = increased pelvic floor activity). Unfortunately, surface electrodes are not accurate and have a tendency to fall off. Needle EMG electrodes are either very small needles or needles with small wires (the needles are removed and the wires are left in) which are placed in the perineum. This is far more accurate than surface electrodes. These needles need to be placed very accurately into the perineal musculature associated with the external sphincter. This may be very difficult and takes a great deal of experience. EMG studies are used to rule out a spastic external sphincter. In patients with detrusor external sphincter dyssynergia (DSD) the external sphincter fails to relax when the detrusor is contracting. In this case EMG activity of the external sphincter will be high during a bladder contraction and voiding. A spinal cord injury between the brainstem and sacral cord or other lesions that affect this area of the spinal cord (i.e. multiple sclerosis) can cause DSD. In the majority of female patients EMG studies are rarely needed and other measurements can be used to rule out excessive external sphincter activity (DSD) or urethral "spasms".

Normal Filling and Voiding

In normal individuals as the bladder fills it accommodates fluid without a rise in intraluminal pressure. As the bladder fills pelvic floor activity and urethral pressure rises to maintain continence (i.e. a slow rise in EMG activity). As the bladder reaches capacity the pressure rises slightly. When the patient voids there is a rise in intraluminal bladder pressure

(usually <40 cmH$_2$O),and the bladder neck, external sphincter and urethra relax (minimal EMG activity). When this occurs the urine is propelled through the urethra and meatus. There are a number of abnormal things that can occur during the filling and voiding phases of multichannel urodynamics that can be recorded.

Urodynamic Dysfunction

Filling Phase

Compliance is the ability of the bladder to accommodate fluid without a rise in pressure. It is defined as C = change in volume/change in pressure. Low detrusor compliance or poor compliance is a rapid increase in detrusor pressure for a small volume (Figure 9.2). Generally, an increase in pressure greater than 3.3 cmH$_2$O per 100 ml filled is considered abnormal [9]. True detrusor pressure should be

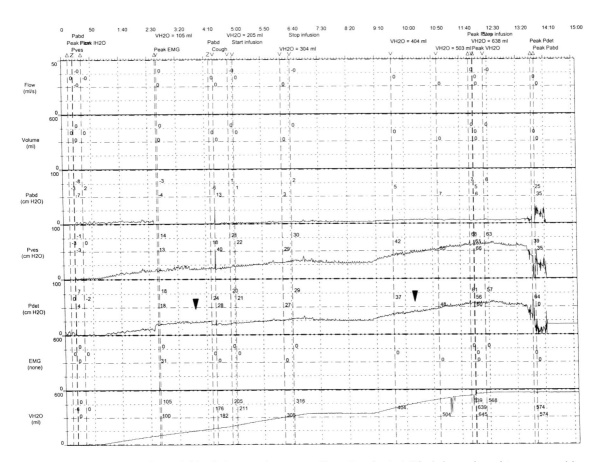

Figure 9.2 A young woman with spina bifida who has poor detrusor compliance. Note the rise in Pdet (subtracted true detrusor pressure) (see arrows) as the bladder is filled (VH2O).

Table 9.1 Causes of low or poor compliance

| Indwelling chronic catheter |
| Inflammation |
| Infection |
| Tuberculosis |
| Schistosomiasis |
| Amyloidosis |
| Obstruction |
| Neurogenic (myelodysplasia) |

lower than 15–20 cmH$_2$O [9]. We like to use the end filling pressure at a certain volume. We record the true detrusor pressure at a certain volume which is usually capacity. If there is no leakage this is termed the end filling pressure. It is important also to record the volume with which this occurs. Normally, the detrusor pressure stays below 10 cmH2O regardless of volume until the individual is ready to void. Hence an end filling pressure of 20 cmH$_2$O at a volume of 200 ml is considered poor compliance in the absence of an unstable contraction. In some cases poor compliance may be difficult to differentiate from bladder instability. In these cases we stop the infusion and wait for the pressure rise to subside. If after a period of time the pressure does not go down this is suggestive of poor compliance as opposed to bladder instability. If the pressure rise goes down with time, then this pressure rise represents bladder instability. The causes of poor or low compliance are listed in Table 9.1. Basically, any process which affects the bladder wall itself or the nerves which supply the bladder can cause poor compliance. Poor or low compliance can result in discomfort upon bladder filling, urinary frequency or incontinence and possible damage to the upper urinary tract due to high pressures within the bladder. In some cases a weak detrusor is also present resulting in poor emptying.

High compliance is the ability of the bladder to accommodate abnormally high volumes without a significant rise in bladder pressure. This may be as a result of the detrusor muscle being chronically overstretched. This can occur in individuals who delay voiding, who void infrequently or who drink large volumes of fluid per day. These individuals will carry large bladder volumes between voids or empty very poorly. In some patients who have high compliance they may be able to empty out their large volumes with normal voiding pressures. In many of these patients bladder sensation is decreased. Hence, conditions which result in polydipsia or polyuria such as diabetes mellitus or insipidus can result in this problem. Psychiatric patients who are on antipsychotic medications with anticholinergic side effects often have a dry mouth, polydipsia and

polyuria. This will result in large bladder volumes, high compliance and poor emptying. Furthermore, the anticholinergic side effect of bladder relaxation can also contribute to this problem.

The other cause of high compliance is poor sensation. Diabetes mellitus can result in a sensory neuropathy in the bladder causing chronic overstretching of the detrusor muscle. Pernicious anemia can also cause a sensory neuropathy of the bladder causing high compliance. In the acute phase of a neurological injury such as a stroke or spinal cord injury this can result in a high compliance low pressure detrusor curve. This should be dealt with aggressively by preventing the bladder wall from being overstretched; otherwise high compliance may be prolonged or a permanent finding. In patients with a peripheral nerve injury to the detrusor nerves such as a cauda equina injury, colon surgery or radical pelvic surgery in woman can also result in a high compliance low pressure bladder.

Bladder Sensation

Sensation of the bladder upon filling is relatively subjective. We like to record the patient's first sensation. Normally this occurs between 150 and 250 ml of volume infused. We then also assess sensation near capacity. A lack of sensation at 750 ml infused is clearly abnormal. The extremes of sensation, i.e. increased sensation and lack of sensation, are probably the most important findings to record [10]. Increased sensation, fullness or discomfort at a very low volume infused can be due to numerous causes. Poor or low compliance with a low capacity bladder can result in increased sensation. In some patients increased sensation alone is found with no other urodynamic abnormality. This is termed sensory urgency. This can occur in diseases such as interstitial cystitis or may occur in patients without any other significant illness. It can result in urinary frequency, nocturia, urgency and suprapubic pressure. Poor sensation may be a result of a neuropathy (i.e. diabetes mellitus), spinal cord injury or chronic bladder overdistension from other causes (i.e. obstruction). Again, since sensation is very subjective, we can only assess the extremes of this finding.

Bladder Capacity

This too is a rather subjective measure. Do we measure this to be when the patient is comfortably "full" or do we fill the patient till they are in "pain? In our urodynamic laboratory we fill the bladder till the patient is comfortably full and would normally void if they could get to a bathroom. The average capacity in females ranges from 180 to 810 ml (the mean being 366 ml) [10].

Bladder Instability or Hyperreflexia

Bladder contractions which occur without the individual's control are termed detrusor instability. If the etiology has a neurogenic basis it is then called detrusor hyperreflexia. When there is a sudden rise in detrusor pressure above 15 cmH$_2$O this is considered by definition an unstable contraction (Figure 9.3) [11]. However, low pressure instability (<15 cmH$_2$O) can also occur, which can usually only be picked up with multichannel urodynamics (Figure 9.4). These pressure increases may be subtle and must be carefully watched for and correlated with the patient's sudden urge to void. Instability may be stress induced such as an

unstable contraction brought on by coughing. The significance of this is that it may mimic stress incontinence. Careful evaluation with both history and urodynamic testing will result in the correct diagnosis. The volume with which the instability occurs, the actual pressure reading and the number of unstable contractions are not specific for the specific etiology causing the bladder dysfunction. Detrusor instability or hyperreflexia can be caused by obstruction, neurogenic causes (Parkinson's disease, stroke, multiple sclerosis, spinal cord injury etc.). As mentioned previously, in many cases we cannot find a cause for the instability. This loss of control may be due to a supersensitivity of the bladder wall receptors or possibly a loss of inhibitory pathways in the brain due to subclinical ischemia [12]. We also know that bladder instability occurs more commonly as we age.

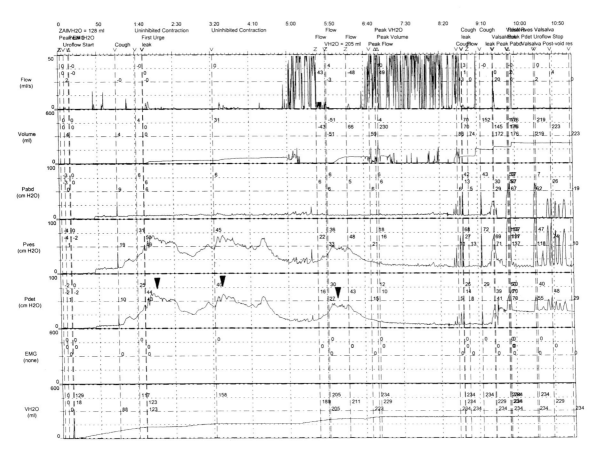

Figure 9.3   A woman with urge incontinence. Note the detrusor instability on Pdet (subtracted true detrusor pressure) (see arrows) as high as 63 cmH$_2$O.

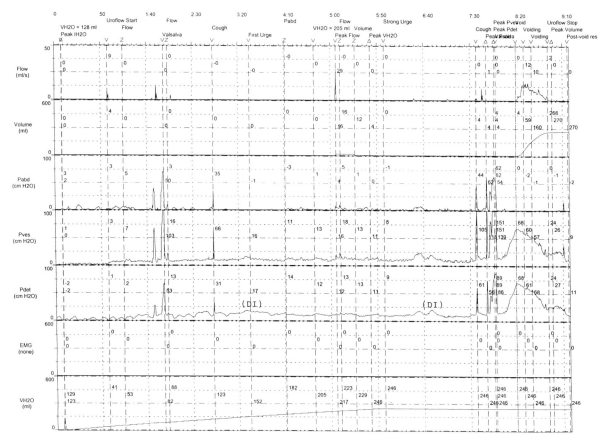

Figure 9.4   A woman with urgency and occasionally urge incontinence. Note the low pressure instability (DI) on Pdet (subtracted true detrusor pressure).

Detrusor Contractility

When a patient is asked to void we can measure the voluntary detrusor contraction. It is important that the bladder pressure catheter be small so as not to cause obstruction itself, resulting in an elevated voiding pressure. We use the voiding pressure at peak flow as our maximum voiding pressure. This must be assessed from the urodynamic graph to be accurate. We can also use the voiding pressure at the start of the flow and this is called the opening voiding pressure. In women it is not clear if maximum voiding pressure or opening voiding pressure is a more accurate assessment of detrusor contractility. The normal maximum voiding pressure in a woman is usually less than 30 cmH$_2$O (Figure 9.5). In many cases it is <20 cmH$_2$O. When the pressure is between 30 and 40 cmH$_2$O this may be elevated in some women. This region is a gray zone. When the maximum voiding pressure is >40 cmH$_2$O obstruction may be present or the

patient may be voiding with an unstable contraction. This may be difficult to differentiate but a poor flow rate will be suggestive of obstruction. A very low maximum voiding pressure (i.e. <10 cmH$_2$O) suggests minimal "urethral resistance" and may be indicative of intrinsic sphincter deficiency. However, this must be correlated with the clinical situation since this may be a normal finding in many women.

Obstruction in a woman may be due to failure of the pelvic floor to relax upon voiding, too tight of a incontinence repair or a spastic external sphincter from a neurological cause (DSD). The typical urodynamic picture in obstruction would be a low peak flow rate, a high maximum voiding pressure (> 40 cmH$_2$O) and poor emptying (Figure 9.6). EMG studies will help assess if the obstruction is due to DSD or failure of the pelvic floor or urethra to relax. In these cases EMG activity will be increased. In almost all cases of a spastic external sphincter (DSD) there is a neurological cause (i.e. spinal cord injury, multiple sclerosis etc.).

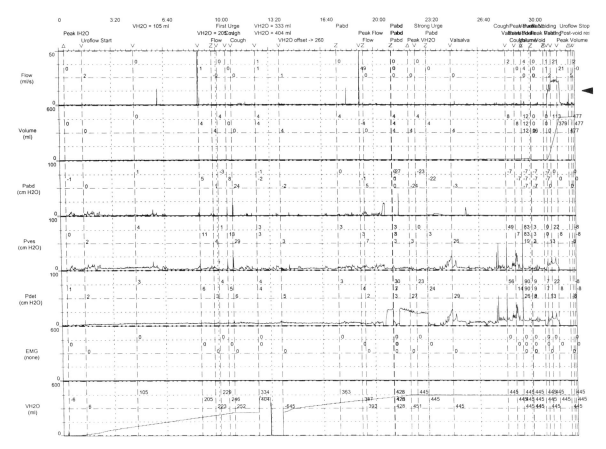

Figure 9.5   A typical flow rate in a woman. The peak flow rate (Flow) is approximately 21 ml/second (see arrow) with a voided volume (Volume) of 477 ml.

Some women cannot relax their pelvic floor or urethra when they want to void. In these women there is no neurological disorder that can be found. These women may have what has been termed as "urethral syndrome" or "urethral instability". The exact cause of this problem is unclear and is not considered to be true detrusor external sphincter dyssynergia (DSD). In many instances it may be difficult on EMG studies alone to differentiate DSD from failure of the pelvic floor to relax.

Many women during voiding often strain. In most cases this is of little importance. However, in some cases women may void entirely by straining with no detrusor contraction. Straining may be seen as an interrupted flow pattern, elevated rectal and intravesical pressure with no or minimal detrusor pressure (Figure 9.7). If it is difficult to assess we simply ask the patient to stop straining during voiding. If indeed they are straining this will result in no elevation in rectal or intravesical pressure and the flow will stop or be extremely slow. Some women will not generate a voluntary detrusor contraction and will be in retention or void a small amount with strain-

ing, leaving a large residual behind. This is termed acontractility or areflexia. An acontractile detrusor is a bladder which cannot contract. Areflexia is acontractility due to a neurological cause. Acontractility may be a result of the detrusor being chronically overstretched and unable to contract or it may be due to a neurological cause such as an injury to the nerves of the bladder (i.e. cauda equina injury or colon surgery). Often in these patients with areflexia there is no instability. Patients with a spinal cord injury between the brainstem and sacral spinal cord may have no voluntary detrusor contractions but rather hyperreflexia. Aging itself will cause bladder contractility to deteriorate [13]. In elderly women a condition termed detrusor hyperactivity with impaired contractility (DHIC) may be found [13]. These women present with a weak detrusor with low pressure instability. This results in poor emptying with urgency, frequency and/or urge incontinence. In these women care must be taken when giving anticholinergic medication to treat urge incontinence because it may put them in retention. In most woman with retention or poor empty-

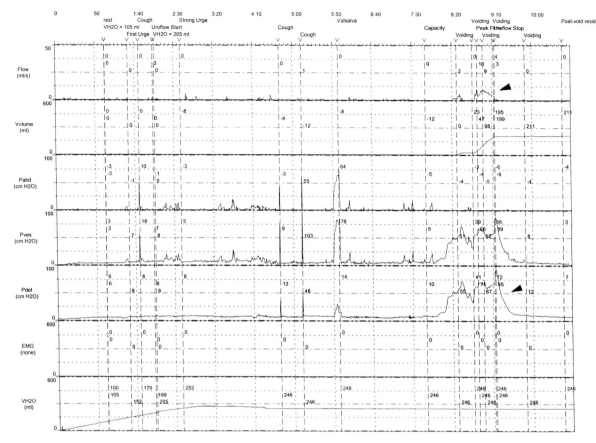

Figure 9.6 A young woman with urinary frequency and a slow stream due to the failure of the pelvic floor and urethra to relax. Note the elevated voiding pressure (Pdet = subtracted true detrusor pressure) and poor flow rate (Flow) (see arrows).

ing the cause is a hypocontractile bladder rather than obstruction [14,15].

Lastly, some patients may have trouble voiding in the presence of health care workers and with urodynamic catheters in place. This unfortunately is the nature of the testing and failure to void in the laboratory may not represent pathology in these patients. We often have these patients void in a private bathroom and record their voided volume.

Flow Rate

In most women flow rates are rarely obstructed. Poor flow rates (<15 ml/second) can occur due to obstruction from a suspension procedure, DSD or pelvic floor spasms, a very large pelvic floor prolapse that may include a cystocele, uterine or posthysterectomy vault prolapse or rectocele. A poor flow can also occur with a weak detrusor. This is the most common cause in women with a poor flow.

Post-void Residuals

Measuring post-void residual is important to assess detrusor contractility and ability to empty the bladder. Residual volume must be measured more than once to get an accurate assessment. The significance of the residual volume depends on the clinical situation. Individuals who are asymptomatic from a 100 ml residual do not need to be treated. However, females with repeated infections, urge incontinence or urinary frequency would benefit from treatment if they had a 100 ml residual. Clearly, small residuals (i.e. <75 ml) will cause fewer problems than residuals that are high (i.e. >300 ml).

Urethral Pressure Profile (UPP)

UPP is the measurement of the urethral pressure from the bladder to the tip of the urethra. Resting UPP is the pressure measurement within the urethra

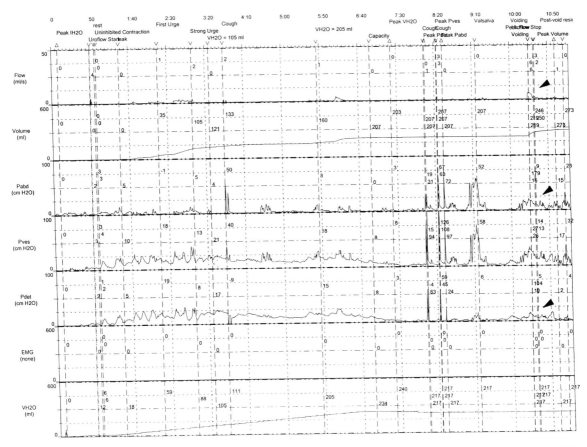

Figure 9.7   An elderly woman who voids with straining and has a weak detrusor. Note the elevated Pabd (rectal) pressure and low Pdet (subtracted true detrusor pressure) with a poor flow (Flow) (see arrows).

at a certain bladder volume at "rest". Filling UPP is the pressure measurement within the urethra with simultaneous filling. Stress UPP is the pressure measurement within the urethra with coughing or straining at a certain bladder volume. Micturational UPP is the pressure measurement within the urethra during voiding.

Today the most accurate way to perform a UPP is with a microtransducer tip catheter. Several variations in the type of catheters (i.e. size, multiple lumens, location of the sensors on the catheter) exist depending on the type of UPP performed. A considerable amount of controversy exists regarding the exact clinical value of the UPP. We believe its use is limited and more accurate and reliable tests such as video multichannel urodynamics with EMG and Valsalva leak point pressure (VLPP) have replaced its use. However, when the above tests are not available, or in centers with significant experience in using UPP, adequate data regarding the female urethra can be determined.

UPP Definitions

Functional urethral length(FUL) is the length of the urethra in which the urethral pressure exceeds the detrusor pressure(Figure 9.8). Maximum urethral pressure(MUP) is the maximum pressure rise in the urethra (Figure 9.8). Maximum urethral closure pressure is the difference between the maximum urethral pressure and the intrinsic bladder pressure [16].

Technique

"Static" or resting UPP is performed by pulling a microtransducer tip catheter at a constant rate (either by hand or by machine at a set rate) from the bladder to the tip of the urethra at a set bladder volume and measuring and recording the pressure during this pull. With a dual lumen microtransducer catheter with multiple sensors along the catheter to measure pressure along the urethra, a filling UPP

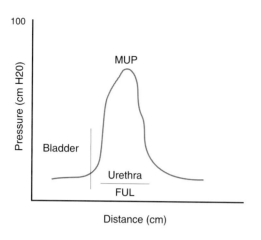

Figure 9.8 Urethral Pressure Profile Graph. MUP = Maximum urethral pressure. FUL = Functional urethral length.

without pulling can be performed. Stress UPP can also be done this way but the catheter must be small; otherwise it may be obstructive. Stress UPP can also be done with a microtransducer tip catheter being moved either antegrade or retrograde during straining. Micturational UPP can be done with a small dual lumen microtransducer catheter with multiple sensors along the catheter. During voiding the urethral pressure is recorded. Again, a large catheter may itself be obstructive and give inaccurate results.

Technical Problems

As can be imagined, a number of technical problems may occur during these tests. Manually pulling out the microtransducer catheter does not give a consistent pull rate and hence readings may be inaccurate. Mechanical pull machines are more consistent. However, the pull rate has not been clearly defined. Position of the transducer in relationship to the urethral wall will affect pressure measurements [17–19]. The exact positioning of the microtransducer tip in the urethra is very hard to tell even on fluoroscopy. Bladder volumes at which to record resting or static UPP have not been determined adequately. Bladder filling during UPP measurement may cause unpredictable results [20]. Posture will also affect UPP results [19]. Lastly, many women with a low UPP are continent and vice versa.

Indications for UPP

In our laboratory the indications are minimal in female patients. It can be used in women with stress incontinence when video multichannel urodynamics is not available, in women with intrinsic sphincter deficiency, or after intraurethral bulking agent injections (collagen, Teflon etc.) or after suspension procedures. It can also be used in neurogenic bladder dysfunction to assess urethral function. In almost all of the above indications, better and more accurate testing is available using video multichannel urodynamics with EMG and VLPP testing, which can easily assess all of the above problems.

Valsalva Leak Point Pressure (VLPP)

This is defined as the minimal pressure within the bladder to cause urinary leakage in the absence of a bladder contraction [21]. This measurement is a more accurate assessment of urethral function and resistance than the UPP. VLPP is reproducible and correlates reasonably well with the degree and type of stress incontinence (i.e. hypermobility versus intrinsic sphincter deficiency) [22]. In a normal urethra the VLPP is infinite since no leakage occurs. Severe urethral dysfunction results in a very low VLPP. VLPP is performed to assess the type and degree of stress urinary incontinence.

VLPP Pitfalls

VLPP should be determined at bladder volumes of 250–300 ml since they provide the most accurate results [23]. Any form of pelvic prolapse may cause obstruction and hence a falsely elevated VLPP. Detrusor instability occurring during testing of VLPP may give an inaccurate assessment. Some elderly females are not able to generate an adequate Valsalva pressure to leak, hence giving false negative results. Lastly, the exact interpretation of VLPP has also not been fully established. However, in general terms a VLPP of less than 60–65 cm H_2O suggests intrinsic sphincter deficiency (ISD). VLPP values greater than 90–100 cmH_2O suggest the incontinence is due to urethral hypermobility. Values between these two points (i.e. 65–90 cmH_2O) suggests some degree of hypermobility and ISD [24,25]. Although the interpretation of the VLPP values can be variable it is still far superior to UPP. VLPP should be used in conjunction with the physical examination (pelvic examination) and multichannel urodynamics. During testing it is highly recommended that multiple measurements be taken to confirm the VLPP value.

Technique

VLPP can be done using either a rectal pressure catheter or an intravesical catheter. In the absence of a detrusor contraction both methods should yield the same results. However, as mentioned earlier, rectal pressure values may not be equal to intravesical pressures and may be lower. In our laboratory we use an intravesical 5 French bladder pressure catheter and perform the testing during video and non-video multichannel urodynamics (we also record rectal pressures during VLPP testing) (Figure 9.9a, b and c). If only a VLPP is required, as in patients after incontinence surgery to assess improvement, only a rectal tube can be used to assess the VLPP rather than a full urodynamic setup. It is very important that the intravesical catheter used is small to prevent obstruction which could falsely elevate the VLPP. We test for VLPP after filling the patient to a comfortable volume of 250–400 ml. In the sitting position, the patient begins with a weak Valsalva, increasing the strength of the Valsalva to the point that the patient leaks. We will repeat this many times to confirm the value. We will also record this maneuver on video fluoroscopy. If the patient does not leak, we will have them cough or stand to provoke leakage and record the pressure. We have found, as have others, that coughing to determine VLPP may yield a higher VLPP than pure Valsalva or straining [26]. The cause of this may be that the external sphincter may fatigue more readily with Valsalva and result in a lower VLPP than with coughing. If the patient still does not leak and she has achieved an intravesical pressure of 150 cmH$_2$O or higher, she has either no stress incontinence or a very minimal degree of stress leakage.

Despite its pitfalls, VLPP is an excellent and reproducible test in assessing the degree and type of stress incontinence. Furthermore, it gives a superior

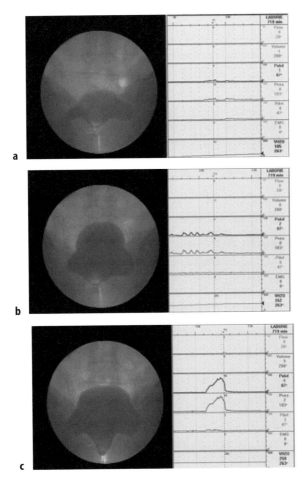

Figure 9.9 Videourodynamics of a woman with stress urinary incontinence. **a** Image at rest, note bladder neck position **b** Image at capacity. **c** Image at VLPP (Pves = 85 cmH$_2$O) with leakage. Note bladder neck position compared to images **a** and **b**.

assessment of urethral function and resistance as compared to UPP testing.

Typical Urodynamic Study

Our typical routine for urodynamic testing is to have the patient void first. We then place them in the lithotomy position and perform a pelvic examination. We then stress test the patient with coughing and straining in this position. Next, we insert a 14 French Foley catheter with a 5 French bladder pressure catheter into the bladder. We record their postvoid residual. We then insert an 8 French feeding tube into the rectum to record rectal pressure. All the catheters are secured with tape. The patient is then moved to a commode on our fluoroscopic table in the sitting position. This allows us to perform video or non-video urodynamics. The rectal and bladder pressure catheters are connected to fluid-filled tubing which is connected to the pressure transducers. The Foley is connected to our infusion of saline at room temperature. We then flush all the tubing and then start a very slow 5 ml/minute infusion through the rectal pressure tubing. We then have the patient cough to check for an increase in our pressure readings. If there is no pressure rise we again flush and readjust our catheters. Once this is corrected we then zero all our catheters and begin infusion at 25–50 ml/minute. We record compliance, first sensation, instability and urge incontinence. If necessary we will have the patient cough, strain, stand, place their hand in warm or cold water or run the water tap or increase the infusion rate to >50 ml/minute to provoke instability. We fill the patient to a comfortable capacity (>250 ml) and then remove the Foley catheter and stress test the patient many times recording the VLPP. If necessary we have the patient stand and stress test her in this position. Once this is completed we have the patient void, and peak flow, maximum voiding pressure, volume voided and residual are recorded. If the patient does not empty we ask her to void in a private bathroom and measure the volume voided.

Conclusions

A significant amount of important information can be determined with multichannel urodynamics and its associated tests. Multichannel urodynamics will be extremely helpful in complex voiding dysfunction problems. This form of testing complements the history and physical examination and can direct the clinician to an appropriate treatment plan based on all of the facts available.

References

1. Romanzi LJ, Heritz DM, Blaivas JG. Preliminary assessment of the incontinent woman. Urol Clin North Am 1995;22:513–20.
2. Gleason D, Reilly B. Gas cystometry. Urol Clin North Am 1979;6:1.
3. Hublet D, Kaechkenbeck B, Baker DE. Etude comparative entre la cystometrie a l'eau et au gaz. Acta Urol Belg 1980;48:4.
4. Wein AJ, Hanno PM, Dixon DO, Raezer D, Benson GS. The reproducibility and interpretation of carbon dioxide cystometry. J Urol 1978;120(2):205–6.
5. Tessier J, Schick E. Does urethral instrumentation affect uroflowmetry measurements. Br J Urol 1990;65:261.
6. Coolsaet BL, Van Duyl WA, Van Mastright R, van der Zwart A. Stepwise cystometry of urinary bladder. Urology 1973;2(3):255–7.
7. Arnold EP. Cystometry. Postural effects in incontinent women. Urol Int 1974;29:185–6.
8. Ramsden RD et al. The unstable bladder – fact or artifact? Br J Urol 1977;49:633–9.
9. Stephenson TP. The interpretation of conventional urodynamics. In Mundy AR, Stephenson TP, Wein AJ, editors. Urodynamics: Principles, Practice and Application. Edinburgh: Churchill Livingstone, 1994; 113.
10. Merrill DC, Bradley WE, MarklandC. Air cystometry. II. A clinical evaluation of normal adults. J Urol 1972;108:85.
11. Abrams P, Blaivas JG, Stanton SL, et al. Standardization of terminology of lower urinary tract function. Neurourol Urodyn 1988;7:403.
12. Susset, JG. Cystometry. In: Krane, RJ, Siroky, MB, editors. Clinical Neuro-urology, 2nd edn. Little, Brown and Co, 1991; 163–84.
13. Resnick NM, Yalla SV. Management of urinary incontinence in the elderly. N Engl J Med 1985;313:800–5.
14. Faerber GJ. Urinary retention and urethral obstruction. In: Kursh ED, McGuire EJ, editors. Female Urology. Philadelphia: JB Lippincott, 1994; 517.
15. Wheeler Jr JS, Culkin DJ, Walter JS et al. Female urinary retention. Urology 1990;35:428.
16. International Continence Society. First report on the standardization of terminology of lower urinary tract function. Br J Urol 1976;48:39.
17. Hilton P, Stanton SL. Urethral pressure measurement by microtransducer. Proceedings of the 11th Annual Meeting of the International Continence Society, 1981; 69–71.
18. Hilton P et al. Urethral pressure measurements before and after Burch Colposuspension: results in patients with cured and recurrent stress incontinence and with voiding difficulties. Proceedings of the 12th Annual Meeting of the International Continence Society, 1982; 130–1.
19. Van Geelen JM et al. Female urethral pressure profile; reproducibility, axial variation and effects of low dose oral contraceptives. J Urol 1984;131:394–8.
20. Raz S, Kaufman JJ. Carbon dioxide urethral pressure profile. J Urol 1976;117:765–9.
21. McGuire, EJ, Fitzpatrick, CC, Wan, J, et al. Clinical assessment of urethral sphincter function. J Urol 1993;150:1452–4.
22. Song JT, Campo R, Chai TC, Rozanski TA, Belville WD. Observer variability in stress leak point pressure measurement using fluorourodynamics. J Urol 1995; part 2, 153:492A, abstract 1056.

23. Faerber GJ, Vashi AR. Variations in Valsalva leak pressure with increasing vesical volume. J Urol 1998;159:1909–11.

24. Webster GD, Kreder KJ. The neurourologic evaluation. In: Walsh PC, Retik AB, Vaughan ED Jr, Wein AJ, editors. Campbell's Urology, 7th edn. Philadelphia: WB Saunders Company, 1998; 927–52.

25. McGuire, EJ, Cespedes, RD, O'Connell, HE. Leak-point pressures. Urol Clin North Am 1996;23:253–62.

26. Miklos JR, Sze EH, Karram MM. A critical appraisal of the methods of measuring leak point pressures in woman with stress incontinence. Obstet Gynecol 1995;86:349.

10 Videourodynamics

Sender Herschorn and Gary Peers

Introduction

The first synchronization of urodynamics with cineradiography was in the in the early 1950s through the pioneering efforts of E.R. Miller [1,2]. The initial goal was to minimize the radiation exposure to the patient during cystourethrography. At first the patient exposure was high when movies were taken, but with the advent of image intensifiers, video transduction, and later videotape recording the patient exposure was reduced. This permitted bursts of continuous activity to be recorded during critical phases of lower urinary tract activity without overexposing the patient. Today most studies can be done with less than 1 minute of fluoroscopy time [3]. These developments contributed a wealth of information to our knowledge about lower urinary tract function and dysfunction. Modern videourodynamic techniques incorporate fluoroscopy with the evolution of the urodynamic machine from a strip chart recorder to a microcomputer.

Videourodynamic studies are not necessary in every patient and simpler studies frequently provide enough information to adequately delineate and treat the dysfunction. Videourodynamic studies are beneficial when simultaneous evaluation of function and anatomy are needed to provide detailed information about the whole or parts of the storage and emptying phases. Complex incontinence where the history does not fit with the findings on preliminary investigations, incontinence that has previously been operated on, and incontinence in the face of a neurologic abnormality are well suited for videourodynamic evaluation.

The cost involved in the technique as a result of the time and effort of the personnel and the expense of the machinery, however, can be justified by its utility in solving complicated problems. It also limits it to larger centers where a large enough patient base justifies the expense. In this chapter the procedures that are carried out will be outlined. Examples of the applications will be provided and the limitations will be discussed.

Components of Videourodynamics

A typical arrangement for videourodynamic studies is shown in Figure 10.1. The fluoroscopic table is used in both the supine and upright positions. A video recorder may be used to record the studies for future review.

Tests Performed

Uroflow [4]

Although the urodynamic catheters have less effect on voiding patterns in females than males, it is still useful to obtain a uroflow on arrival that may be compared with the flow data generated during the urodynamic study. After the uroflow is done the patient's post-void residual can be determined on introduction of the urodynamic catheters.

Cystometry

The first part of the study is cystometry, the method by which the pressure-volume relationship of the bladder is measured [5]. It is used to assess detrusor activity, sensation, capacity and compliance. The detrusor pressure (Pdet) is calculated by subtraction

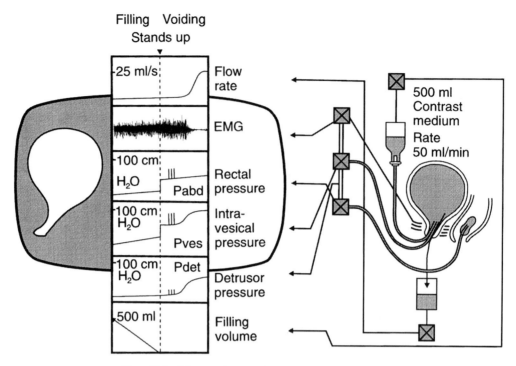

Figure 10.1   Schematic diagram of videourodynamic setup.

of the abdominal pressure (Pabd), as measured by a rectal balloon, from the total intravesical pressure (Pves). The subtracted detrusor pressure reflects the activity and pressures generated by the detrusor muscle alone. However, artifacts on the Pdet may be produced by intrinsic rectal contractions [5].

Overactive detrusor function is characterized by spontaneous or provoked involuntary contractions, which the patient cannot completely suppress [5]. Any such contraction seen while the patient is attempting to inhibit micturition is termed *detrusor instability*. Although originally defined as a minimum pressure rise of 15 cm water [6], the same diagnosis can be made if the patient's symptoms are reproduced by lesser rises of pressure [7,8]. *Motor urgency* is caused by overactive detrusor function and *sensory urgency* by a hypersensitive bladder [5]. However, it is possible that they are both conditions in the same spectrum and that patients with sensory urgency are able to inhibit the unstable contractions during cystometry but not during activities of normal living [9]. The term *detrusor hyperreflexia*, to describe the uninhibited contractions, is used when there is objective evidence of an associated neurological disorder [5].

Another type of overactive bladder dysfunction is reduced compliance. *Bladder compliance* is defined as the change in pressure for a given change in volume [3]. It is calculated by dividing the volume change by the change in detrusor pressure during that change in bladder volume, and is expressed as millimeters per cmH_2O [5]. Normal bladder compliance is high and in the laboratory the normal pressure rise is less than 6–10 cmH_2O [3]. Low bladder compliance implies a poorly distensible bladder. The actual numeric values to indicate normal, high or low compliance are not yet defined [5].

The finding of bladder overactivity on cystometry is important if it correlates with the clinical condition of the patient. Bladder instability has been reported in 30–35% of patients with stress incontinence undergoing surgery. It resolves in the majority following repairs and does not have a significant impact on outcomes [10,11]. Alternatively, if the patient's symptoms are primarily from bladder overactivity or if other factors predisposing to abnormal bladder behavior are present, the cystometric findings will influence treatment. These include a history of radiation, chronic bladder inflammation, indwelling catheter, chronic infection, chemotherapy, voiding dysfunction following pelvic surgery or other neurological conditions.

Leak Point Pressures

The Valsalva or abdominal leak point pressure (VLPP) tests the strength of the urethra and is the total abdominal pressure (Pves or Pabd) at which leakage occurs during a progressive Valsalva maneuver or cough in the absence of a bladder contraction [12]. The study is performed in the sitting or standing position with at least 150–200 ml of fluid in the bladder. A VLPP of less than 60 cmH_2O is evidence of significant intrinsic sphincter deficiency (ISD) and correlates well with severe leakage. A VLPP of between 60 and 90 cmH_2O suggests a component of ISD and a VLPP of greater than 90 cmH_2O suggests minimal ISD with leakage mainly due to hypermobility [3]. A cystocele may produce inferior pressure on an incompetent urethra that will prevent incontinence and falsely elevate the VLPP. When a cystocele is present the VLPP should be repeated with the prolapse reduced by insertion of a vaginal pack. The VLPP has been shown to be reproducible [13] but has not yet been standardized.

The detrusor or bladder leak point pressure is the detrusor pressure (Pdet) at which urethral leakage occurs during bladder filling on cystometry. This parameter is used to investigate and follow patients with neurogenic and low compliant bladders. In general, patients with a detrusor LPP of greater than approximately 25–30 cmH_2O are at risk for upper tract deterioration from reflux or obstruction [8,14]. In these patients it is necessary to assess compliance as well. A high detrusor LPP indicates poor compliance with urethral obstruction whereas a low detrusor LPP is seen in patients with incompetent urethras. In order to demonstrate poor compliance in these patients filling may be done with a Foley catheter to obstruct the outlet [15]. If both the compliance and the detrusor LPP are low, treatment has to be directed to the bladder as well as the outlet.

Pressure-Flow Studies

Pressure-flow studies are designed to provide dynamic information on the emptying phase of lower urinary tract function. Obstruction is not common in females [16] but may be found after surgical correction of stress urinary incontinence and less commonly with detrusor sphincter dyssynergia, pseudodyssynergia [17] and rarely with stricture disease. Interference with voiding may also be associated with pelvic organ prolapse. Although there are no established nomograms to depict pressure/flow in women, as there are in men, the pattern of high detrusor pressure and low urinary flow indicates obstruction (Figure 10.2). Simultaneous cystography may demonstrate the level.

Detrusor pressure during voiding is characteristically low in females. A preoperative study that demonstrates a low detrusor pressure with a low flow rate, if the free flow rate is low as well, may aid in counseling the patient about postoperative urinary retention after stress incontinence surgery.

Electromyography

Striated sphincter activity during filling and voiding can be demonstrated by sphincter electromyography (EMG) during videourodynamics. This type of kinesiologic study can be performed with surface electrodes, vaginal or anal probes, and needles. Normal sphincter EMG activity has characteristic audio quality that may be monitored simultaneously. Its most important role is the identification of abnormal sphincter activity in patients with neuro-

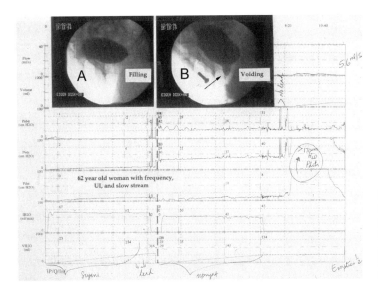

Figure 10.2 Videourodynamic study of a 62-year-old woman with urgency, frequency and slow stream following multiple urethral dilatations. The study shows a stable bladder on filling. Her voiding pressure exceeds 170 cmH_2O and her flow rate is low. There is a urethral stricture visible (arrow in B) with proximal urethral dilatation.

genic bladder dysfunction and in those with voiding dysfunction of behavioral origin [18]. EMG recordings are not necessary in routine videourodynamics for incontinence in females who have no neurologic abnormalities.

Urodynamic Equipment

Uroflow Meters

Flow meters are commonly of one of three types: weight, electronic dip-stick, or rotating disk [7]. The first measures the weight of the collected urine. The second measures the changes in electrical capacitance of a dip-stick mounted in the collecting chamber. The third measures the power required to keep a rotating disk rotating at a constant speed while the urine, which tends to slow it down, is directed towards it. All three can provide high sensitivity and reproducibility of data.

Multichannel Recorder

A multichannel recorder is required to measure simultaneous pressures during both phases of lower urinary tract function and flow during the voiding phase. There are many systems available [19] and most of them have dispensed with a strip chart output in favor of television monitor display of the procedure.

The choice of components of the study is up to the individual clinician. Figure 10.1 illustrates possible inclusions. The channels demonstrating volume of fluid instilled and volume voided are helpful but not essential as they can be measured manually. The EMG channel is not necessary for routine clinical practice but can be helpful in patients with neurologic disease, although the fluoroscopy component will demonstrate detrusor external sphincter dyssynergia in patients with suprasacral lesions and show urethral obstruction in patients with dysfunctional voiding.

Some controversy exists regarding the use of subtracted detrusor pressure versus intravesical pressure although most reports at present are with subtracted pressures. Bladder pressures are recorded via the pressure line in the bladder. This pressure is affected by intra-abdominal pressure that can be measured separately by a rectal catheter. Increases intra-abdominal can be from straining, the upright position, and other provocative activities such as coughing, jumping, and heel jouncing. In order to get an accurate recording of bladder pressure and to eliminate the effect of intra-abdominal pressure, Bates et al. [20] emphasized the value of electronically subtracting the intra-abdomi-

nal pressure from the intravesical pressure. However, even with the patient quiescent and totally cooperative, artifacts may be produced by intrinsic rectal contractions [5] since the bladder pressure is derived from the electronic subtraction. On the other hand, McGuire et al. [21] do not measure rectal or abdominal pressure with a separate catheter. They monitor urethral pressure along with bladder pressure via two lumens of the same catheter. They state that urethral pressure reflects rectal or abdominal pressure, allowing them to differentiate bladder contractions from abdominal straining. In our unit, we use subtracted detrusor pressures.

Fluoroscopy

A good quality fluoroscopy unit with high resolution image intensifier and a table that can function in both supine and erect positions are required. Fluoroscopic images are obtained selectively during the filling and voiding study and are either superimposed on the pressure-flow tracing or displayed on a separate screen. The fluoroscopic images can be stored and reproduced individually or as continuous clips during key parts of the study. A recording can be made of the procedure for subsequent review.

Since the contrast medium instilled into bladder is unlikely to be absorbed we generally use the less expensive high-osmolality contrast media. A dilute solution of one liter of Hypaque7 is prepared by the hospital pharmacy and supplied in sterile intravenous bags.

Videourodynamic Technique

The patient attends the examination with a full bladder and a flow rate is obtained. The patient is then catheterized with the urodynamics catheters and the equipment is zeroed. Two (38 cm) 8 French infant feeding tubes, one for filling which is removed prior to the voiding study and one for pressure measurements, are inserted into the bladder. Residual urine is measured. The rectal catheter is a 42 cm 14 French with a balloon over the tip.

The study is conducted by a urodynamics specialist who is present in the room, communicating with the patient throughout the procedure, and records the findings manually and electronically (Figure 10.3). A supine or semi-oblique filling study is carried out and various measurements are taken during the study and responses to actions such as Credé, cough, and Valsalva are recorded. The filling is usually at a medium rate of 50–75 ml per minute [5]. The bladder is filled, emptied and then refilled

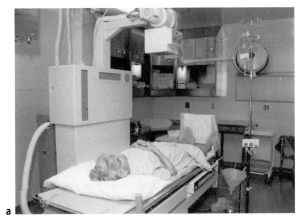

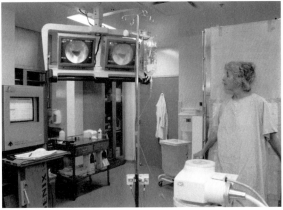

Figure 10.3 **a** The patient has been catheterized and her bladder is being filled in the supine position. **b** The patient is in the upright position after the filling catheter has been removed. She will be asked to cough and strain to demonstrate stress incontinence and then to void. The study will be stored on the multichannel recorder.

in the patient's usual voiding position (lying, sitting or standing). Two bladder fillings are usually done since decreased compliance may be a result of the medium filling [22] and a second test verifies it. The upright position of the second filling is also a provocative test for instability [5]. Additional responses to Credé, cough, and Valsalva are again

recorded. A commonly used method is to fill the bladder supine and stand the patient up for provocative maneuvers.

During the study, recordings are made of bladder images in the filling phase in the supine and/or in the upright positions. Antero-posterior (AP) and oblique views are obtained. The AP position permits documentation of reflux and its extent, and in the oblique position the course of the urethra can be seen separate from a cystocele. Note is made of the bladder outline and its position relative to the symphysis and appearance of the bladder neck at rest and with straining and coughing. Leakage of urine with instability, decreased compliance, or with various stress maneuvers is recorded. In the upright position, the presence of a cystocele and its relationship to the urethra are also noted. The voiding phase or parts of it are recorded if the patient can void in front of the camera. The patient is asked to void in front of the camera and the pressures and flow are recorded along with the fluoroscopic image. If the patient cannot void with the catheters in place they are removed and a uroflow may be done. The voided volume is measured. Total fluoroscopy time is usually less than one minute.

The recorded study provides an opportunity for the case to be reviewed and discussed. All of the events of the study are recorded and displayed on the monitor during the study. The urodynamic machine is usually equipped with the capability of compressing the study so that it can be viewed on an ordinary letter size sheet of paper.

Indications and Examples

Urinary Incontinence

Fluoroscopic imaging during the urodynamic study provides an anatomic impression of the function or dysfunction. The technique is ideally suited to evaluation of incontinence. A useful anatomic/radiologic classification of female incontinence, devised by

Table 10.1 Radiologic type of stress incontinence [23]

Type 0:	Vesical neck and proximal urethra closed at rest and situated at or above the lower end of the symphysis pubis. They descend during stress but incontinence is not seen.
Type I:	Vesical neck closed at rest and is well above the inferior margin of the symphysis. During stress the vesical neck and proximal urethra open and descend less than 2 cm. Incontinence is seen.
Type IIa:	Vesical neck closed at rest and is above the inferior margin of the symphysis. During stress the vesical neck and proximal urethra open and descend more than 2 cm. Incontinence is seen.
Type IIb:	Vesical neck closed at rest and is at or below the inferior margin of the symphysis. During stress there may or may not be further descent but as the proximal urethra opens incontinence is seen.
Type III:	Vesical neck and proximal urethra are open at rest. The proximal urethra no longer functions as a sphincter. There is obvious urinary leakage with minimal increases in intravesical pressure.

Blaivas [23], is shown in Table 10.1. We use this classification to determine the radiologic abnormality and add to it the information from the VLPP and the position of the urethra in relation to the cystocele to describe the functional problem. Each of the urodynamic tracings in the figures is shown in full with annotations made during the study. The video recordings depicting parts of the studies were obtained from a video printer connected to the fluoroscopy.

Type I abnormalities are illustrated in Figures 10.4 and 10.5. The patient in Figure 10.4 leaks with a VLPP of 62 cmH$_2$O, indicating most likely a component of ISD in her incontinence. The patient in Figure 10.5 also has a high VLPP of >120 cmH$_2$O on straining during upright filling. At the end of filling, a cough caused a large leak without much hypermobility and appears to be accompanied by a small bladder contraction. This indicates that she has stress incontinence as well as cough-induced instability.

Figures 10.6 to 10.9 demonstrate type IIa abnormalities. The patient in Figure 10.6 has a high VLPP indicating primarily a hypermobile urethra without any appreciable cystocele. In Figure 10.7, the patient has an unstable contraction with incontinence in the upright position. She also has a high VLPP. The patient shown in Figure 10.8 has a grade II cystocele that appears with straining. She probably has mainly a lateral defect [24].

The patient in Figure 10.9 complained primarily of urgency incontinence. Although she has a type IIa defect, no leakage was demonstrated (type 0). She has small contractions at the end of the upright filling showing bladder instability.

Type IIb abnormalities are shown in Figures 10.10 to 10.12. The bladder neck in Figure 10.10 is seen well below the lower margin of the symphysis and is associated with a moderate cystocele. Since the bladder neck is above the base of the cystocele, but below the lower margin of the symphysis, the patient most likely has a combined central and lateral defect. In Figure 10.11, the large cystocele is not associated with demonstrable stress incontinence, despite coughing and straining pressures of greater than 100 cmH$_2$O. It appears to be primarily a central defect. Clinical examination must include reducing the cystocele and checking for stress incontinence. The patient in Figure 10.12 has a combined central and lateral defect. She has marked bladder instability with urgency incontinence but stress incontinence is not demonstrated most likely because of the compressive effect of the cystocele.

Type III incontinence or pure ISD is demonstrated by the patient in Figure 10.13. Her bladder neck is open at rest, no appreciable descensus is seen with coughing or straining and her VLPP is low at 59 cmH$_2$O.

Neurogenic Bladder Dysfunction

Videourodynamics can be helpful in assessing bladder dysfunction patients with neurologic disorders. Since incontinence and upper tract dilatation can be prevented and treated by achieving low-pressure bladder storage and emptying [14,25], the urodynamic study provides a framework for treatment. Anatomic abnormalities can also be correlated with pressure changes.

Examples of neurogenic problems are shown in Figures 10.14 to 10.16. Since the flow rate is not measured in Figures 10.14 and 10.15, fewer channels are used during the study.

The patient in Figure 10.14 has a small capacity hyperreflexic but compliant bladder with grade 1 left vesicoureteral reflux. Her main problem was incontinence between catheterizations and treatment was anticholinergics and monitoring of her upper tracts. The patient in Figure 10.15 has a markedly trabeculated hyperreflexic bladder with filling pressures of greater than 100 cmH$_2$O. The study demonstrates detrusor external sphincter dyssynergia with an open bladder neck and tight sphincter. She also had bilateral hydronephrosis on upper tract imaging and required an augmentation cystoplasty for management. Since she was quadriplegic a continent abdominal stoma was brought from the augmentation to the umbilicus to permit self-intermittent catheterization.

The patient in Figure 10.16 developed increasing hydronephrosis and elevated creatinine after insertion of an artificial sphincter for urinary incontinence. She had previously undergone multiple bilateral ureteral reimplants for reflux. The study shows a bladder with poor compliance and gross bilateral reflux. The refluxing ureters probably dampen the bladder pressure thus improving the appearance of the compliance curve. She was also treated with an augmentation cystoplasty.

Other Urodynamic Problems

Obstruction
Although outflow obstruction is uncommon in females [17], it is occasionally seen. The patient in Figure 10.2 had an iatrogenic and functionally significant urethral obstruction that was treated with a visual internal urethrotomy and subsequent long-term self-dilation.

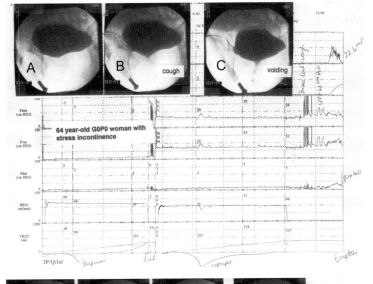

Figure 10.4 Videourodynamic study of a 64-year-old G0P0 woman with type I stress incontinence. She has a bladder capacity of more than 300 ml. The bladder neck is slightly open at rest (A). With coughing there is a small amount of descent and her VLPP is 62 cmH₂O. She has no apparent cystocele and her voiding phase is normal.

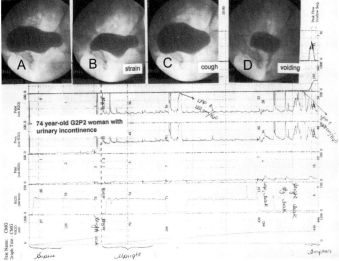

Figure 10.5 Videourodynamic study of a 74-year-old G2P2 woman with type I stress incontinence. Her bladder neck is slightly open at rest (A). In the upright position (B) she leaks with straining and a VLPP of 122 cmH₂O. She also leaks with coughing that is followed by a detrusor contraction (arrow). Her voiding is normal (D).

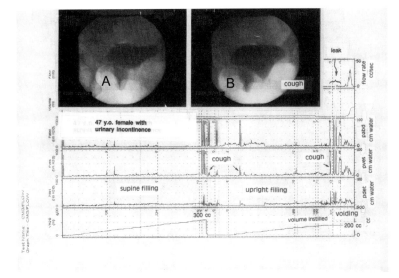

Figure 10.6 Videourodynamic study of a 47-year-old G1P1 woman with type IIa stress incontinence. Her bladder neck is open at rest (A). Leakage and hypermobility is seen with coughing (B).

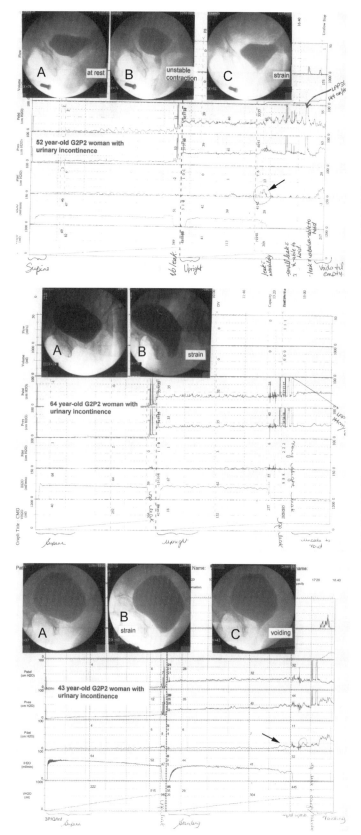

Figure 10.7 Videourodynamic study of a 52-year-old G2P2 woman with a type IIa abnormality who complains of both stress and urgency incontinence. The bladder neck is slightly open at rest (A). She has an unstable contraction (arrow) on upright filling that results in incontinence (B). With straining she leaks with a VLPP of more than 140 cmH₂O (C).

Figure 10.8 Videourodynamic study of a 64-year-old G2P2 woman with type IIa stress incontinence. Her bladder neck is well supported on upright filling (A) and with straining she leaks with a VLPP of 144 cmH₂O and a cystocele is demonstrated. She most likely has mainly a lateral defect.

Figure 10.9 Videourodynamic study of a 43-year-old G2P2 woman with urgency incontinence. Her capacity is more 500 ml and the bladder neck at rest is above the lower margin of the symphysis (A). On straining (B), she has type IIa descent but no incontinence is seen (type 0). She also has unstable contractions at the end of upright filling (arrows). Her voiding is normal (C).

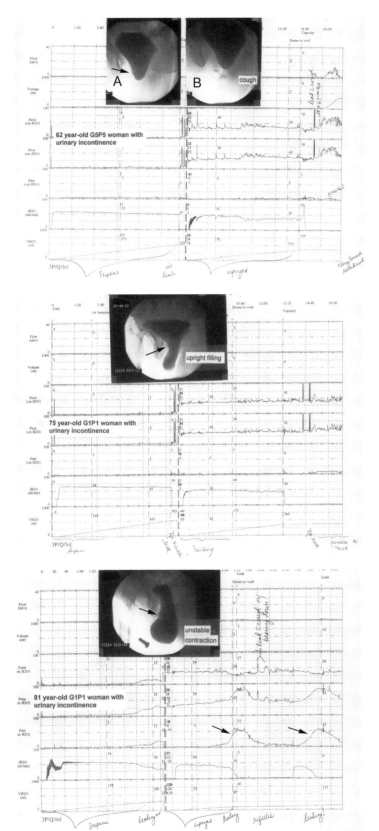

Figure 10.10 Videourodynamic study of a 62-year-old G5P5 woman with type IIb stress incontinence. Her bladder neck (arrow) on filling (A) is below the symphyseal margin and a cystocele is seen. She most likely has a combined central and lateral defect. She has leakage with coughing (B) and a VLPP of 62 cmH₂O on straining.

Figure 10.11 Videourodynamic study of a 75-year-old G1P1 woman with a large cystocele. Although she complains of stress incontinence it is not visible on this study. Her bladder neck (arrow) is at the lower margin of the symphysis. The cystocele appears primarily to be a central defect. Clinical evaluation must include reducing the cystocele and testing for stress incontinence.

Figure 10.12 Videourodynamic study of an 81-year-old G1P1 woman with a central and lateral defect. The bladder neck is below the symphysis (arrow). She has marked instability on supine and upright filling (arrows). Although she complains of stress, in addition to urge incontinence, it is not demonstrated on this study.

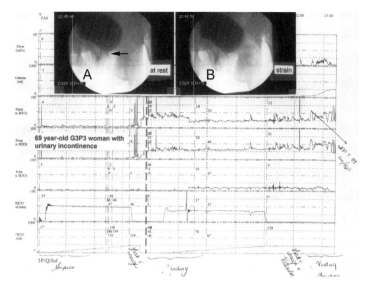

Figure 10.13 Videourodynamic study of a 69 year-old G3P3 woman with type III abnormality after 2 previous stress incontinence repairs. Her bladder neck is open at rest (arrow in A). On straining (B) there is almost no urethral movement on straining and her VLPP is 59 cmH$_2$O.

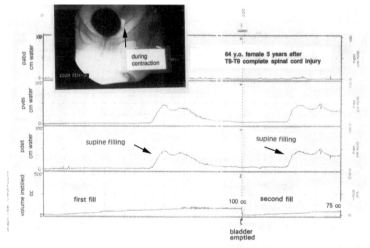

Figure 10.14 Videourodynamic study of a 64-year-old woman 5 years after a T8–9 spinal cord injury following a motor vehicle accident. She has left vesicoureteral reflux (arrow) seen during hyperreflexic contractions (arrows).

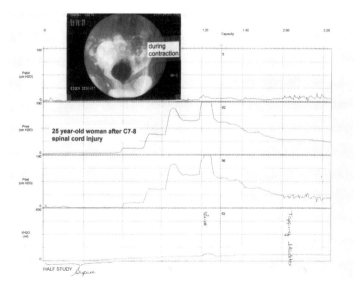

Figure 10.15 Videourodynamic study of a 25-year-old woman with C7–8 lesion 16 months after spinal cord injury following a motor vehicle accident. She needed an indwelling catheter for repeated attacks of autonomic dysreflexia and her upper tracts showed marked bilateral hydronephrosis. Her bladder is markedly trabeculated and during contractions of greater than 75–100 cmH$_2$O her external sphincter remains tight, consistent with detrusor sphincter dyssynergia. She was subsequently treated with an ileal augmentation cystoplasty and a continent abdominal stoma.

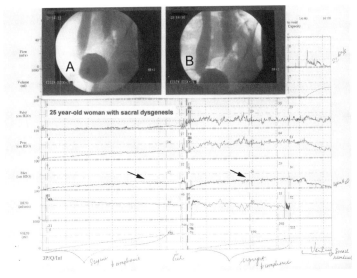

Figure 10.16 Videourodynamic study of a 25-year-old woman with sacral dysgenesis. She had an artificial sphincter inserted for urinary incontinence at age 14 and then developed bilateral vesicoureteral reflux unresponsive to multiple ureteral reimplantations. The study shows decreased bladder compliance on filling (arrows). She has gross bilateral reflux and a small capacity bladder. The reflux most likely dampens the poor compliance measurement. She subsequently underwent augmentation ileal cystoplasty and bilateral reimplants.

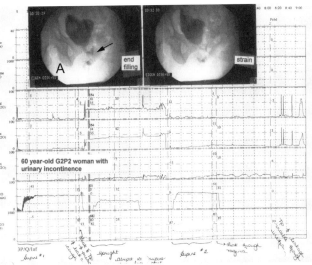

Figure 10.17 Videourodynamic study of a 60-year-old G2P2 woman who underwent an ileal neobladder to her urethra after cystectomy for muscle invasive carcinoma of the bladder. The study was done with a Foley catheter blocking the urethra to test compliance (A) which is normal. All of the leakage was demonstrated to exit the fistula at the anastomosis (arrow in A). She underwent a transvaginal fistula repair with a Martius labial fat pad flap.

Complex Problems

The patient in Figure 10.17 had a fistula at the anastomosis between an ileal neobladder and the urethra after a cystectomy for bladder cancer. The study was done with a Foley catheter obstructing the bladder neck to test the compliance. The neobladder was compliant and stable and was not contributing to the incontinence. No urethral leakage was seen with stress. All of the contrast emanated through the vagina. She was treated with a transvaginal fistula repair with a labial fat pad flap.

Pitfalls of Videourodynamics

Patient cooperation, comfort and compliance are necessary in order to obtain a meaningful and rele-

vant study. Occasionally apprehensive patients will faint when the table is moved from the supine to the upright position and the study cannot be completed. In addition, with an anxious patient stress incontinence may not be demonstrated. Of 1103 studies that we reviewed in our laboratory for neurologically normal women whose chief complaint was stress incontinence, we were unable to demonstrate stress incontinence on fluoroscopy in 239 (21.6%). It is also difficult for many patients to void in front of the camera with catheters in the bladder and rectum and observers watching them. In our series, only 585 patients (53%) were able to void and some of these did so with abdominal straining. The others were unable to void during the procedure and the voiding data was obtained from the uroflow.

To optimize visibility of the lower urinary tract on fluoroscopy patient position has to be correct.

However, visibility may be poor or absent with very obese patients. The clinician also has to maintain a dialogue with the patient to image crucial events as the patient must relay changes in sensation during filling and may be the first to sense incontinence.

The radiation equipment must be well maintained and undergo regular maintenance and safety inspections. Since fluoroscopy time is short, radiation exposure to the patient should not be a problem. However, the clinician should use radiation protection such as aprons and thyroid shields.

The other pitfalls relate to the urodynamic aspects and are similar to those previously outlined by O'Donnell [26]. Standardized terminology to communicate results and concepts should always be used. The testing procedures and equipment should be compatible with commonly accepted methodologies. The value and limitations of each measurement must be realized; for example, the VLPP may not be useful in the presence of a large prolapsing cystocele. To confirm reliability within a particular laboratory it is necessary to have a high test–retest correlation of studies. The validity of a test refers to its ability to measure what it is supposed to measure. The clinician must always be aware of how it compares to a "gold standard" test, which in urodynamics may be difficult to establish. The urodynamic studies should correlate with other clinical data. The voiding history, the physical examination, the endoscopic examination, and the urodynamic evaluation, and in this case the radiologic studies, should serve to validate one another and strengthen the clinical assessment. Finally, the failure to maintain equipment may lead to inaccurate results.

Conclusion

Videourodynamic techniques have evolved over the years with improvements in technology and refinements in the concepts of lower urinary tract structure, function, treatment. There are exciting developments in other newer imaging technologies. Ultrasound can be used during urodynamic studies but the vaginal probe may alter bladder neck position and perineal probes are undergoing investigation [27]. Magnetic resonance (MR) imaging has provided significant advances in knowledge about the pelvic floor [28] but it is carried out in the supine position and interventional MR has not yet been adapted to the technique. The tests are still applicable today, for the appropriate indications, as when they were first developed almost 50 years ago.

References

1. Miller E. The beginnings. Urol Clin North Am 1979;6:7–9.
2. Enhörning G, Miller ER, Hinman Jr F. Urethral closure studied cine-roentgenography and simultaneous bladder-urethra pressure recording. Surg Gynecol Obstet 1964;118:507–16.
3. Webster GD, Kreder KJ. The neurourologic evaluation. In: Walsh PC, Retik AB, Vaughan Jr. ED, Wein AJ, editors. Campbell's Urology, 7th edn. Philadelphia: WB Saunders, 1998; 927–52.
4. Abrams P, Torrens M. Urine flow studies. Urol Clin North Am 1979;6:71–9.
5. Abrams P, Blaivas JG, Stanton SL, Andersen JT. Standardisation of terminology of lower urinary tract function. Neurourol Urodyn 1988;7:403–27.
6. Bates P, Bradley WE, Glen E et al. First report on the standardization of terminology of lower urinary tract function. Br J Urol 1976;48:39–42.
7. Massey A, Abrams P. Urodynamics of the female lower urinary tract. Studies Urol Clin North Am 1985;12:231–246.
8. Baivas JG. Cystometry. In: Blaivas JG, editor. Atlas of Urodynamics. Baltimore: Williams & Wilkins, 1996; 31–47.
9. Creighton SM, Pearce JM, Robson I et al. Sensory urgency: How full is your bladder? Br J Obstet Gynaecol 1991;98:1287–9.
10. Awad SA, Flood HD, Acker KL. The significance of prior anti-incontinence surgery n women who present with urinary incontinence. J Urol 1988;140:514–17.
11. McGuire EJ. Bladder instability in stress incontinence. Neurourol Urodyn 1988;7:563.
12. McGuire EJ, Fitzpatrick CC, Wan J et al. Clinical assessment of urethral sphincter function. J Urol 1993;150:1452–4.
13. Heritz DM, Blaivas JG. Reliability and specificity of the leak point pressure. J Urol 1995;153:492A.
14. McGuire EJ, Woodside JR, Borden TA, Weiss RM. Prognostic value of urodynamic studies in myelodysplastic children. J Urol 1981;126:205–9.
15. Woodside JR, McGuire EJ. Technique for detection of detrusor hypertonia in the presence of urethral sphincteric incompetence. J Urol 1982; 127:740–3.
16. Farrar D, Turner-Warwick R. Outflow obstruction in the female studies. Urol Clin North Am 1979; 6:217–25.
17. Wein AJ, Barrett DM. Other voiding dysfunctions and related topics. In: Wein, AJ, Barrett, DM, editors. Voiding Function and Dysfunction. Chicago: Year Book, 1988;274–301.
18. Fowler C. Electromyography. In: Blaivas JG, editor. Atlas of Urodynamics. Baltimore: Williams & Wilkins, 1996; 60–76.
19. Blaivas JG. Deciding on the right urodynamic equipment. In: Blaivas JG, editor. Atlas of Urodynamics. Baltimore: Williams & Wilkins, 1996; 19–28.
20. Bates CP, Whiteside G, Turner-Warwick R. Synchronous cine/pressure/flow cysto-urethrography with special reference to stress and urge incontinence. Br J Urol 1970;42:714–23.
21. McGuire EJ, Cespedes RD, Cross CA, O'Connell HE. Videourodynamic studies. Urol Clini North Am 1996;23:309–21.
22. Webb RJ, Styles RA, Griffiths CJ, Ramsden PD, Neal DE. Ambulatory monitoring of patients with low compliance as a result of neurogenic bladder dysfunction. Br J Urol 1989;64:150–4.
23. Blaivas JG, Olsson CA. Stress incontinence: Classification and surgical approach. J Urol 1988;139:727–31.
24. Raz S, Stothers L, Chopra A. Vaginal reconstructive surgery for incontinence and prolapse. In: Walsh PC, Retik AB,

Vaughan Jr. ED, Wein AJ, editors. Campbell's Urology, 7th edn. Philadelphia: WB Saunders, 1998; 1059–94.

25. Barkin M, Dolfin D, Herschorn S. The urologic care of the spinal cord injured patient. J Urol 1983;129:335–9.

26. O'Donnell PD. Pitfalls of urodynamic testing. Urol Clin North Am 1991;18:257–68.

27. Virtanen HS, Kiilhoma PJA. Ultrasound urodynamics. In: Blaivas JG, editor. Atlas of Urodynamics. Baltimore: Williams & Wilkins, 1996; 117–25.

28. Yang A, Mostwin JL, Rosenshein N, Zerhouni EA. Pelvic floor descent in women: dynamic evaluation with fast MR imaging and cinematic display. Radiology 1991;179:25–33.

11 Role of Ultrasound in the Investigation of Urinary and Fecal Incontinence

Heinz Koelbl

Introduction

Ultrasound was first introduced into medicine in 1942 by the Viennese neurologist Dussik for locating brain tumors. In 1958 Donald used this diagnostic method for intrauterine measurements of the fetus. Since then, ultrasonic investigation has become an indispensable part of the diagnostic repertoire in obstetrics and gynecology [1]. Attempts to determine the functional interactions within the pelvis, including the bladder, the urethra and the pelvic floor, have prompted the study of urethrovesical relationships by numerous methods, mostly radiographic techniques of urethrocystography [2,3]. Ultrasound has many advantages over other imaging systems in that it is possible to visualize fluid-filled structures without the use of contrast medium. Ultrasound allows soft tissues to be seen, including the kidney, the bladder and its wall, the urethra and the urethral sphincter. The main advantage with ultrasound is that there is no ionizing radiation used and this means that tests may be repeated as frequently as required. There is no risk to the patient or ultrasonographer from ionizing radiation, and urine within the bladder and urethra is clearly visualized. The installation and operating costs of ultrasound are significantly less than those of similar radiological equipment.

While sonographic urethrocystography by perineal, introital or vaginal ultrasound is replacing radiography in routine clinical use, more detailed information about the urethra and periurethral tissues has been obtained by three-dimensional sonography and intraluminal high frequency ultrasound. However, the latter techniques are still the subject of research.

Ultrasonographic evaluation of the upper urinary tract belongs to routine assessment in the pre- and post-therapeutic concept of urogynecology. Measurement of the kidneys and the calices complements detection of hydronephrosis, hydroureters and parenchymal cysts of the kidneys in the diagnostic program of upper urinary tract alterations. Ultrasound has also been suggested as an alternative source for imaging the urethrovesical anatomy [3]. Although the clinical significance of various radiological parameters in patients with pelvic floor relaxation, especially associated with genuine stress incontinence (GSI), is controversial, basic evaluation of its use was sufficient to justify introduction of sonography as an alternative to commonly used radiological procedures. Ultrasound has been used to detect anatomic alterations associated with GSI, to select the appropriate type of surgery, to assess surgical results, and postoperative complications. Moreover, ultrasound imaging is regarded as an investigation complementing the evaluation of pelvic floor muscle function. Movement of intrapelvic structures (e.g. urethrovesical junction, bladder base) can be evaluated as a consequence of pelvic floor muscle contraction.

Instrumentation

Ultrasound refers to sound energy with a frequency above 20 MHz. The sound waves are produced and received by piezoelectric crystals. The sound beam itself is propagated as a longitudinal wave through human soft tissue at a speed of 1.54 km/second. Penetration of tissue depends on the frequency of the sound waves. The higher the frequency, the shorter the wavelength and deeper the tissue penetration. Since frequency selection involves a compromise between better image resolution (high frequency) and deeper tissue penetration (low frequency), the decision must be based on the position of the organs to be examined.

There are various types of ultrasound transducers currently being used, each with an advantage in certain applications. The advantages of sector scanners include easy handling of the transducer head and a very small contact site. Linear-array scanners have a large number of crystals arranged in a linear fashion. Curved linear-array scanners offer the improved handling of sector scanners without the limitations of narrow proximal field widths encountered with vaginal or rectal endoprobes.

Real-time imaging is particularly suitable for examination of the bladder and the urethra. In these areas it provides a mode of dynamic echography in which two-dimensional images are continuously updated. It allows the sonographer to scan the bladder and the urethra with speed and precision. Among the various real-time scanners available, the linear-array and sector scanners have been recommended and most widely used in patients with stress incontinence and pelvic floor disorders.

Vaginal and transrectal probes and sector scanners have overcome some of the difficulties associated with conventional linear-array machines; they provide a sharper, better focused picture with good resolution. The endoprobe may be straight or flexible; however, it is commonly angulated up to 45∞ to facilitate visualization of the pelvic organs. This angulation also allows for less external movement of the probe and better patient comfort. A permanent record of the scan can be obtained by attaching a camera to the cathode ray tube. A videotape recorder is also useful for obtaining records for teaching the patient and for future comparisons of results after treatment. The advanced technology of urodynamic instruments allows direct sonographic and tonometric registration on single- or double-screens with a high reproducibility. Most of them are on-line with computers provided with improving software and picture-archiving systems. Thus, data storage of both tonometric and sonographic results, essential for patient care and follow-up, for scientific work, and for forensic reasons, can be easily obtained.

With advanced technology the size of the scanners has become smaller and meets most of the requirements for an acceptable investigation with high resolution. The ongoing development of microprobes will increase knowledge about the physiology and pathophysiology of the relevant morphology. Small endoprobes have been used for demonstration of the sphincteric function of the urethra and intravesical ultrasound. For urogynecological investigation commonly employed frequencies for the transducers range from 2.4 to 5 MHz for transabdominal ultrasound, 5 to 7 MHz for endosonography, introital and perineal techniques, and 20 MHz for three-dimensional ultrasound.

Abdominal Sonography

Upper Urinary Tract

Meanwhile, ultrasonographic evaluation of the upper urinary tract belongs to routine assessment in the pre- and post-therapeutic concept of urogynecology [2]. The use of ultrasound for evaluation of the upper urinary tract has evolved from merely using the bladder as a transparent window to scan pelvic structures. Ultrasound is used to evaluate the upper urinary tract, particularly for the detection of hydronephrosis, renal stones, and to assess renal parenchyma. Besides measurement of the kidneys and the renal pelvis with its calices, and detection of hydroureters, ultrasound is the relevant diagnostic modality in the detection of upper urinary tract lesions [4]. It is quick and easy to perform and thus useful not only in the pre- and post-therapeutic assessment, but also for the staging of gynecological malignancies. Difficulties exist in the differentiation between obstructive and non-obstructive patterns of hydroureters [5]. Doppler ultrasound studies are capable of differentiating between these two entities. As yet, ultrasound studies may detect hydronephrosis, which is suggestive of ureteral damage, but it will not detect a ureter that has been injured and is leaking into the peritoneal cavity, nor one that is obstructed but has not yet produced genitourinary anomalies, such as aplasia, hypoplasia and horseshoe kidney; ultrasound diagnosis must be confirmed by radiological procedures.

Ultrasound of the Bladder

Bladder and post-void residual volumes can be determined transabdominally, although accuracy is not reliable for volumes less than 50 ml [6]. With transabdominal ultrasound the bladder is scanned in two perpendicular planes (transverse and sagittal) and three diameters (height, width, and depth) are measured. Height corresponds to the greatest superoinferior measurement; depth corresponds to the greatest antero-posterior (AP) measurement (Figure 11.1). Both are obtained in sagittal plane scan. The simplest formula used to estimate volume by abdominal ultrasound is bladder volume (ml) = (H × W × D) × (0.7). The correction factor 0.7 is needed because the shape of the bladder is not circular until it is almost completely full. The same formula can be used for pre-micturition and post-

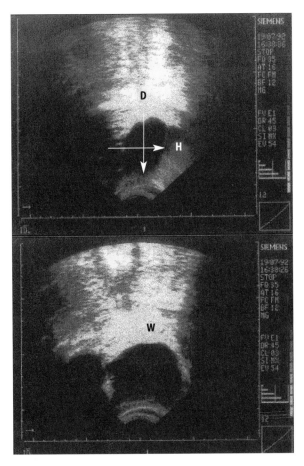

Figure 11.1 Sonographic assessment of bladder (residual) volume using transabdominal ultrasound. Measurement of depth (D) and height (H) in sagittal plane (top) and width (W) in transversal plane (bottom) – bladder volume (ml) = (H × W × D) × (0.7.)

micturition volume assessments. The error rate of this formula is approximately 21%.

Recently, small portable ultrasound units have been developed. These portable units are easy to use and serve solely for the measurement of residual urine volumes, including special software to calculate bladder volume, automatically. Meanwhile, a variety of successive models are available. These ultrasound systems demonstrate excellent test–retest and interrater reliability [7–9].

Transabdominal ultrasound has also proven valuable in the evaluation of the urinary tract in neuromuscular bladder dysfunction and detrusor instability. Brandt and others found that ultrasound of the bladder yielded significantly more diagnostic information than radiography in 27% of their study group. Brandt also demonstrated bladder trabeculation as well as dilated ureters in neuromuscular dysfunction using abdominal sonography [10].

Sonogaphic Urethrocystography

Numerous studies have demonstrated real-time ultrasonography to be useful in evaluating the anatomic relationship of the bladder, the urethrovesical junction (UVJ), and the proximal urethra. With careful observation, the changes in the shape and position of the vesical neck and the proximal urethra can be determined while the patient is performing a Valsalva maneuver or coughing. However, although the bladder neck can be seen on transabdominal ultrasound, it is occasionally hidden behind the symphysis pubis. The bladder neck is especially difficult to locate in obese patients and in women with severe genitourinary prolapse. This is the result of significant intervening tissue affecting sound wave penetration (attenuation) and acoustic shading from the symphysis. A transurethral catheter may be needed to demonstrate the urethral axis. As a consequence, transabdominal ultrasound may be used to determine the extent of mobility of the bladder and urethra and to detect detrusor instability in some patients. However, the pitfalls of this technique in evaluating the urethrovesical anatomy have to be considered.

Perineal Ultrasound

Newer applications of sonography place the transducer on the perineum. Avoiding excessive pressure to the perineal region this scanning technique does not alter anatomic relationships. However, its application in patients with severe genitourinary prolapse is limited.

Ultrasonic urethrocystography by perineal scanning for evaluation of female stress urinary incontinence was suggested by Kohorn and others [11]. The procedure is carried out with the patient in various positions (upright, supine) with legs slightly abducted to allow access of the transducer to the perineum. A linear-array or curved-array transducer scanner is positioned in a sagittal orientation to visualize the bladder, bladder base, urethrovesical junction, and the pubic symphysis (Figure 11.2). Comparative results between radiologic and perineal sonographic urethrocystography have been reported, and give comparable and reproducible results [12–16]. Perineal ultrasound for pelvic floor exercises as a biofeedback instrument is recommended by Martan et al. [17] and demonstrated in Figure 11.3. Moreover, changes in bladder neck mobility in nulliparous continent women, during pelvic floor muscle contraction, before and after tension-free vaginal tape (TVT) surgery and Burch

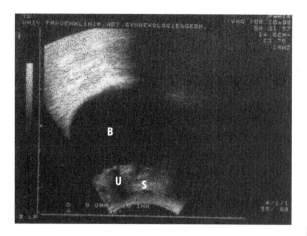

Figure 11.2 Sonographic urethrocystography with perineal ultrasound (B, bladder; U, urethra; S, pubic symphysis).

colposuspension have been published recently [18–21].

A standardization of functional sonography has been published by the German Association of Urogynecology in 1996 aiming at a common understanding and interpretation of pictures with high quality and reproducibility [22]. Of the various sonographic techniques used to perform urethrocystography, perineal and introital ultrasound have been widely used and recommended as the most reliable. Measurement methods for the two techniques have now been standardized as shown in Figure 11.4. Moreover, picture orientation, comparison between radiology, and principles of the respective investigation, including examination position, bladder filling, provocation tests and variations caused by the ultrasound probes, have been pointed out.

Introital Ultrasound

Regional distortion using vaginal or rectal endosonography, even with small endoprobes, was the reason for development of introital sonography [23]. The technique involves placing a vaginal sector scanner to the vulva just underneath the external urethral orifice, visualizing the bladder, urethrovesical junction, urethra and symphysis (Figure 11.5). Modern vaginal probes are thin and give good visualization of the lower urinary tract when placed only a short distance into the vagina. Thus, this technique is devoid of any potential morphological artifact as a result of urethral or bladder neck distortion. Using introital sonography, Hanzal et al. prospectively determined the influence of transurethral catheters used for cystometry on bladder neck anatomy [24].

This study revealed similar results for the assessment of bladder neck location and the posterior urethrovesical angle at rest and during straining, with and without a catheter in place. Urethral width was significantly greater with a catheter in situ. From these data it appears that catheters used for urodynamic assessment increase urethral width but do not affect bladder neck location and urethral mobility. The exact location of microtip pressure transducers can easily be determined while visualizing the bladder neck and the urethra during filling [25]. The voiding phase can also be evaluated even

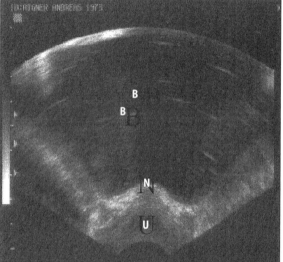

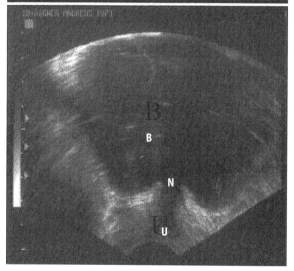

Figure 11.3 Sonographic demonstration of the bladder using perineal sonography. The bladder is visualized in sagittal plane at rest (top) and during contraction of the pelvic floor with marked elevation of the bladder neck (bottom) (B, bladder; U, urethra; N, bladder neck).

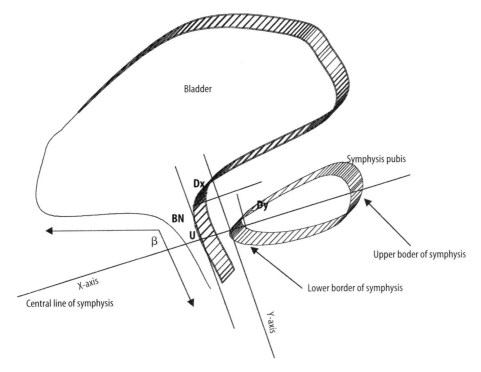

Figure 11.4 Sonographic urethrocystography – assessment of the relevant parameters – a line is drawn through the pubic symphysis between the upper and the lower edge of the pubic bone. (BN, bladder neck, U, urethra, Dy, distance from bladder neck to central line of symphysis, Dx, distance bladder neck to lower border of symphysis; β, retrovesical angle.) Recommendations of the German Association of Urogynecology on functional sonography of the lower urinary tract [22].

without the use of catheters. Micturition, and the patient's ability to stop voiding, which demonstrates the voluntary musculature and the urethral "milk-back" mechanism, can be visualized and evaluated. Wavelike detrusor contractions accompanied by bladder neck opening may be seen in patients with an unstable bladder. Inadequate emptying associated with urethral obstruction may be seen in patients following an overzealous urethropexy. Uncoordinated emptying may be seen in patients with detrusor-sphincter dyssynergia and can be verified by simultaneous electromyographic study. The location of the urethrovesical junction can be readily determined. Successful colposuspension is found to be associated with a urethrovesical location which is more anterior, although not necessarily more elevated. In addition, overcorrection in anti-incontinence surgery causing postoperative micturition disorders can be visualized by ultrasound as shown in Figure 11.6, as a hypermobile urethra is easily seen on ultrasound and according to this study may help to distinguish different causes of GSI. Movement of the bladder and the urethra during real-time sonography indirectly reflects pelvic floor action during both contraction and relaxation. Pelvic floor defects can be indirectly visualized with both perineal and introital sonography as demonstrated in Figure 11.7. However, owing to the prolapse, the probes may alter lower urinary tract anatomy and give erroneous results. First attempts to identify lesions of the attachments of the lateral vagina to the tendineal arc of the levator ani, termed paravaginal defects, are promising.

Vaginal and Rectal Endosonography

Vaginal or rectal ultrasound techniques involve probes of higher frequencies than transabdominal linear-array scanners and, therefore, afford sharper better focused pictures with high resolution [26]. The endosonographic probes avoid interference from the symphysis pubis and subcutaneous fat. Transrectal sonography produces a good view of the bladder, urethra and the bladder neck, although the rectal probe can occasionally alter the alignment of the bladder neck movement during Valsalva maneu-

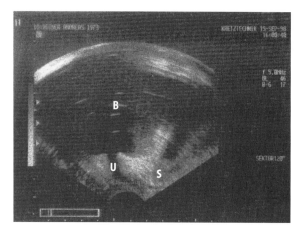

Figure 11.5 Sonographic urethrocystography with introital sonography (B, bladder; U, urethra; S, pubic symphysis).

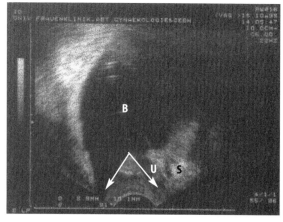

Figure 11.6 Introital sonography of a patient after Burch colposuspension with voiding disorders at 4 weeks after surgery. The patient revealed bladder residual volumes up to 150 ml. Sonographic urethrocystography shows an elevated bladder neck due to overcorrection. The retrovesical angle (between arrows) is small (B, bladder; U, urethra).

vers or coughing [27]. They cannot be used in patients with significant pelvic relaxation.

Vaginal Sonography

Vaginal ultrasound has been proposed as a suitable alternative to conventional radiological urethrocystography. In order to quantify displacement of the urethrovesical junction, Hol et al. introduced a simple, well-standardized vaginal ultrasound technique and compared the position and mobility of the bladder neck in 160 continent women and patients with GSI [28]. Examinations were carried out with a Foley catheter introduced into the bladder, where the balloon half-filled with soapy water and half with air to give a recognizable fluid level, paralleled the horizontal axis of the patients.

Compared to continent women, the position of the bladder neck in patients with GSI was significantly lower and more posterior at rest, during straining and squeezing. However, the authors observed a considerable overlap between the two groups for all parameters. This study clearly demonstrates the necessity of indicating patient position and a point of reference (inferior edge of the pubic symphysis) for reliable and standardized evaluation of bladder neck position. Moreover, assessment of bladder wall thickness of > 5 mm was found to be associated with detrusor instability with a positive predictive value of 94% [29].

Some concern exists that the use of a transvaginal probe which lies in direct contact with the bladder neck may alter lower urinary tract anatomy

and give erroneous results. Mouritsen et al. evaluated the effect of a vaginal ultrasound probe on bladder neck anatomy and mobility in 20 women [30]. Colpo-cysto-urethrography (CCU) during rest, Valsalva and withholding maneuvers were carried out with and without simultaneous vaginal sonography. CCU findings and measurements of bladder neck position and mobility were reported to be unaffected by insertion of the probe. In another investigation Mouritsen et al. studied patients after bladder neck suspension using CCU and vaginal sonography [31]. The measurements of bladder-to-

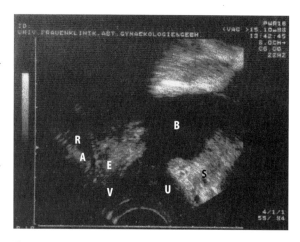

Figure 11.7 Sonographic visualization (introital ultrasound) of a pelvic floor defect in the anterior and middle compartment assessed during Valsalva maneuver (B, bladder; U, urethra; E, enterocele; V, vagina; R, rectum; A, anorectal angle).

symphysis distance and rotation angle in relation to the symphysis pubis were almost identical for the two procedures. From these studies it appears that vaginal ultrasound is a reliable and convenient technique for pre- and postoperative evaluation of bladder neck anatomy and mobility.

Quinn et al. (1988) described vaginal sonography in a series of 100 women with a range of urinary symptoms [26]. The inferior border of the pubic symphysis was used as a "key landmark". A level mounted on the endoprobe ensured the maintenance of a horizontal position during scanning, thus avoiding any distortion of urethrovesical anatomy caused by the probe. In 19/23 patients with genuine stress incontinence the UVJ was inferior to the level of the mid-symphysis at rest, and in 18 there was opening and descent of the bladder neck during coughing. Meanwhile most of the studies report that vaginal ultrasound is an accurate method for recording anatomical changes, especially the mobility of the bladder neck. Beside its easy feasibility and reproducibility, Bergman and co-workers reported that descent of the urethrovesical junction of more than 1 cm on straining correlated with stress urinary incontinence [6]. On the other hand, a considerable overlap in the position of the bladder neck at rest as well as during straining and sneezing was observed by Carey and Dwyer [33]. Hol and co-workers (1994) used a Foley catheter and introduced it into the bladder, with the balloon half-filled with soapy water [28]. Thus, a recognizable fluid level which is parallel to the horizontal axis of the patient is produced and serves as a reference to assess mobility of the bladder neck during a standardized Valsalva force. Compared with a healthy control group, patients with genuine stress incontinence revealed a significantly lower and more posterior position of the bladder at rest, during straining and squeezing. However, there was a considerable interindividual overlap between the two groups for all parameters. Alterations due to pelvic floor muscle contraction and straining can be evaluated by "still" pictures comparing the situation at rest with the extent of displacement at maximal effort. However, rapid movement of the urethrovesical unit, e.g. during coughing, can be measured only when a video recorder is attached to the ultrasound machine.

Vaginal ultrasonography has been proposed as a suitable alternative to videocystourethrography. However, in a study of 44 women with urinary incontinence, Wise and co-workers [27] found an increase of the maximum urethral pressure and the functional urethral length, and an improvement of the pressure transmission caused by the endoprobe inserted 2 cm into the vagina. The authors conclude that the use of a vaginal probe results in compression of the urethra and therefore may reduce the likelihood of detecting incontinence in women with genuine stress incontinence or underestimate the severity of GSI diagnosed [27].

Assessment of Bladder (Residual) Volume

Beside visualization of the bladder and urethra, vaginal scanning is also valuable in the assessment of urethral diverticula. However, the diagnosis of this entity should be confirmed by cystoscopy and radiological procedures. Until recently, residual urines have been measured by transabdominal ultrasound only. However, it can be difficult to visualize low bladder volumes from the abdominal wall because of distortion and diffraction of the long ultrasonic beam. Haylen et al. (1989) have used a transvaginal linear-array ultrasound scanner to measure bladder volumes in the range 2–300 ml [34]. The method is simple, atraumatic and acceptable to patients, and a clear picture of the bladder is obtained (in the sagittal plane) even at low bladder volumes. From the maximum dimensions of the bladder in this plane (horizontal = H, vertical depth = D) an unknown bladder volume can be calculated from the formula: bladder volume (ml) = $5.9 \times H \times D - 14.6$.

Assessment of Bladder Wall Displacement and Infiltration

Determination of bladder wall displacement and/or infiltration caused by cervical cancer is an important part of the staging procedure. In a comparative study of computed tomography (CT), cystoscopy, and magnetic resonance imaging (MRI), 21 women with stage Ib–IIIb cervical cancer were evaluated with vaginal ultrasound to diagnose invasion of the bladder wall. Mobility of the bladder wall against the vaginal ultrasound probe in the region of the anterior vaginal fornix was considered to exclude infiltration. This test showed an accuracy of 95%, while it was 76%, 86% and 80% for CT, cystoscopy, and MRI, respectively [35]. From these data it appears that transvaginal ultrasonographic examination is a useful adjunct in detecting invasion of the bladder wall in patients with advanced cervical cancer.

Rectal Sonography

Placing a linear-array transducer within the rectum to improve imaging of the bladder base and neck was described by Nishizawa and co-workers [36]. The authors described how the technique may be used to replace X-ray cystography during urodynamic imaging. Shapeero et al. used the same technique to visualize the bladder base and proximal urethra in males suspected of having neuromuscular dysfunction of the bladder [37]. They performed sonographic and radiologic voiding cystourethrography on all patients, and concluded that the sonographic examination is as good, and occasionally better than the radiographic method. The technique of using a transrectal probe for the investigation of women with urinary incontinence was introduced by Brown and co-workers [38]. However, questions arose regarding endoprobe movement during straining maneuvers, thereby creating artifacts, attendant discomfort, and possible inhibition of bladder neck movement. Bergman and colleagues established that insertion of the rectal probe did not alter urethral junction mobility as evaluated by the Q-tip angle change [10]. Using the UVJ drop as a comparative parameter they reported a sensitivity of 86% and specificity of 92% in the evaluation of women with genuine stress urinary incontinence. However, the potential problems of endoprobe movement during straining were also noted by these authors. On the basis of findings on rectal ultrasound combined with urodynamic observations, Kuo et al. observed the occurrence of various patterns in patients with GSI [39]. Funneling of the bladder neck, urethral hypermobility, an incompetent urethral sphincter and a cystocele were found to occur alone or in conjunction with any other of these findings. These data highlight the importance of urodynamic and sonographic assessment to identify various combinations of defects responsible for GSI, which may have implications for the choice of treatment.

Cystosonography

Similar to vaginal ultrasound, cystosonography is a helpful diagnostic intravesical procedure to scan the bladder wall, its wall displacement and/or invasion from gynecological malignancies [40]. This endosonographic method is performed with a rotation scanner which has a range of 360° and a frequency of 6 MHz. The scanner is introduced via a 24-Charrière resectoscope shaft. Cystosonography should be preceded by cystoscopy to avoid inadvertent bleeding (urethral strictures, bladder tumors). This type of endosonography is able to detect edema and/or tumor invasion of the bladder mucosa. Whereas cystoscopy is capable of demon-

strating superficial changes of the bladder mucosa, cystosonography permits visualization of deeper layers of the bladder wall. Moreover, it is possible to obtain biopsy specimens under direct ultrasound control that cannot be detected by cystoscopy alone. Compared with transcutaneous sonography, the endosonographic evaluation of tumor spread is more precise, because of the short distance to the transducer head and the higher frequencies being applied.

Intraurethral Ultrasound

Intraurethral ultrasound (IUUS) is a new endosonographic technique providing high resolution imaging (20 MHz) of the urethra and the surrounding tissues. This technique is recommended for the diagnosis of diverticula and urinary incontinence, since other imaging methods do not provide much information on the urethra and its sphincter. In a pilot study Kirschner-Hermanns et al. investigated the sphincteric region in women using IUUS. Examination of 44 stress incontinent and healthy women revealed a negative correlation between the external urethral sphincter (area and circumference) and the grade of stress incontinence (p < 0.01). In no patient with normal urinary continence was the sphincter reduced in size [41]. The meaning of these findings in relation to urethral pressure measurements merits further evaluation, since it could be helpful in the choice of treatment. Endoluminal ultrasound has also been applied during surgical treatment of urethral diverticula [42]. Intraoperatively, the diverticula were well visualized by endoluminal ultrasound, which demonstrated improved identification of the size and orientation of urethral diverticula, sludge within the diverticula, the extent of periurethral inflammation, diverticular wall thickness, and the distance between the diverticular wall and urethral lumen, compared to traditional imaging techniques.

Three-dimensional Ultrasound

The three-dimensional (3D) reconstruction of ultrasound images has become a widespread option in ultrasound equipment since the early 1990s [43]. Some catheters with an ultrasound transducer in the tip have been tested for studies of bladder volume. In a prospective study 249 adult outpatients were tested for accuracy, by comparing scan versus catheter volumes [44]. The device exhibited a sensitivity of 97%, a specificity of 91% and an overall accuracy of 94%. Three-dimensional ultrasound of the urethra has also has attracted scientific interest. Khullar et al. scanned women with urinary symptoms with a 5 MHz three-dimensional perineal ultrasound [45]. All women with urethral sphincter incompetence had a continuous hypoechoic area from the bladder neck to the urethral meatus. Some of the women with severe GSI had breaks in the continuous circle of the "rhabdosphincter" and it was replaced by hyperechoic areas. The authors believe that these observations may indicate damage to the urethral sphincter. Further studies are needed to confirm these observations and to elucidate the clinical implications of three-dimensional ultrasound findings. Moreover, similar results have been obtained with three-dimensional ultrasound of the female urethra comparing transvaginal and transrectal scanning [46].

Ultrasound and Fecal Incontinence

Before the introduction of ultrasound, defects of the external anal sphincter had traditionally been diagnosed by palpation, anal manometry and electromyography. Now endo- and exoanal techniques provide information on normal anatomy and on defects of the anal sphincter [47].

Ultrasound with an endoanal probe has added significantly to our ability to determine accurately the occurrence and extent of anatomical anal sphincter mechanism damage. Comparing clinical and histological findings with endoanal ultrasound observations, Sultan et al. showed that the sonographic technique is capable of identifying such defects resulting in a more precise evaluation of such lesions shown in Figure 11.8 [48,49]. The sonographic findings showed external sphincter defects as hypoechoic, or amorphous and of mixed echogenicity. Anal endosonography was performed using a 7 MHz rotating endoprobe with a focal range 2–5 cm. To identify external sphincter defects, anal endosonography was ascribed more sensitivity (100%) than clinical (56%) and conventional physiological methods (89% EMG, 67% manometry) [49]. Occult sphincter defects after vaginal delivery were found by Sultan et al. in 35% diagnosed by anal endosonography, most of them caused by forceps delivery [50,51]. Internal sphincter defects were associated with a significantly lower mean resting anal pressure and external sphincter defects were associated with a significantly lower squeeze pressure.

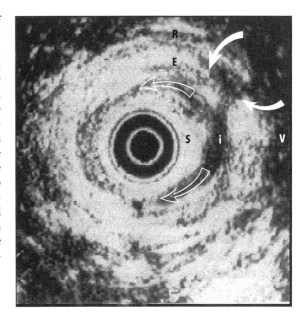

Figure 11.8 Anal endosonographic image of a 64-year-old woman with fecal incontinence. Anterior is to the right of the image. An amorphous external sphincter defect of mixed echogenicity is delineated by arrows (V, vagina; E, external anal sphincter; I, internal anal sphincter). (From Sultan et al., Br J Surg 1994; 81:465 [40], with permission.)

Peschers et al. described an exoanal ultrasound technique using a conventional 5 MHz convex transducer placed on the perineum [52]. The axial images of a normal and a damaged anal sphincter complex are shown in Figure 11.9. Twenty-five women with fecal incontinence were investigated and compared to 43 asymptomatic women. Sphincter defects were detected in 20 women. The internal anal sphincter has been shown to be visible as a hypoechoic circle, the external anal sphincter showed a hyperechoic pattern. Whether the exoanal probe provides as much information as the endoanal one remains to be seen.

Conclusion

Recent observations confirm that ultrasound is gaining more importance in the assessment of both lower urinary tract function and fecal incontinence. Data comparing ultrasound with radiologic techniques justify the use of ultrasound for various diagnostic procedures. Compared with radiology, sonographic investigation is simple to perform, can be performed using one hand, lacks side effects, is minimally invasive and therefore highly acceptable for most patients. As yet, and similar to conventional radiology ultrasound, it is not able to provide con-

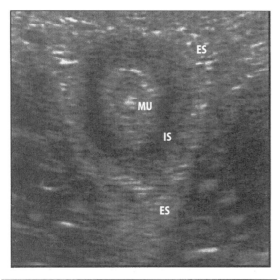

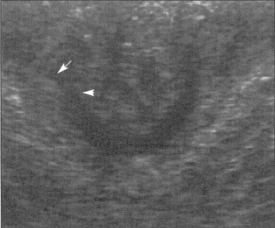

Figure 11.9   Top: Axial images of a normal anal sphincter complex (above). The internal anal sphincter (IS) appears as a hypoechoic circle surrounded by the hyperechoic external anal sphincter (ES; MU, mucosa and submucosa). The top of the image indicates the anterior part of the sphincter.
Bottom: Axial images of internal and external anal sphincter defects. The defect appears as an anterior gap in the continuity of the dark circle (internal sphincter, arrowhead) and the hyperechoic circle (external anal sphincter, arrow). (From Peschers et al., Br J Obstet Gynaecol 1997;104:1000–1 [52], with permission.)

clusive and discriminatory diagnostic information, but rather to supply complementary data to be used in conjunction with other diagnostic tools.

Ultrasound has become an essential procedure in modern urogynecology to assess upper urinary tract lesions, morphologic changes associated with female urinary incontinence, pelvic floor disorders including external and internal anal sphincter defects. Its simplicity, cost effectiveness, and availability in gynecology favor its use as a basic urogy-

necologic screening procedure, especially before and after conservative or surgical treatment. Meanwhile, ultrasound has become a potential alternative to conventional radiological procedures and improvements are continuing. As a consequence a diagnostic regimen for the sequential use of ultrasound in urogynecology can be recommended as the result of scientific work.

Exclusion of upper urinary tract lesions is carried out with the use of ultrasound, especially in patients undergoing gynecologic surgery. However, there are difficulties in the recognition of congenital anomalies and therefore radiology still has its place for selected indications. Surgical complications causing upper urinary tract lesions should be screened by ultrasound and completed by radiological procedures when indicated.

Many radiographic studies have been published evaluating the mobility of the bladder base, the urethrovesical junction, urethra, and support of the surrounding soft tissues in women thought to have an anatomic defect as the basis for stress urinary incontinence. Cinefluoroscopy is still in routine use, although urinary incontinence cannot be visualized adequately using static methods such as the lateral urethrocystogram. Therefore, ultrasound is particularly suitable for dynamic examination of the bladder and the urethra without time limits, especially because of the lack of side effects. Perineal scanning and introital sonography are less invasive than transvaginal and transrectal endosonographic methods. Moreover, demonstration of the urethra does not necessarily require catheterization.

Ultrasound evaluation of the bladder neck and urethra provides a wide range of information for the urogynecologist. Moreover, neighboring structures can be visualized at the same time giving more complex information. The position of the bladder neck in the relaxed state and the degree of displacement with reference to the symphysis pubis can be measured. This information can be helpful in determining the type of surgical procedure. Surgical correction of the anatomic defect can be assessed. Application of visualization techniques to demonstrate the urethrovesical anatomy in patients with genuine stress incontinence relates to one of the aims of anti-incontinence bladder surgery: to elevate the bladder neck to a position within the abdominal cavity. Conversely, failure of adequate bladder neck elevation is a factor leading to recurrent genuine stress incontinence after surgery. Thus, the ability to measure objectively the descent of the bladder neck pre- and postoperatively is important. Although intraoperative use of ultrasound to assess these changes has been attempted by some urogynecologists, its clinical value and feasibility during anti-incontinence surgery has not yet been proven. Detrusor contractions with concomitant funneling of the bladder neck are occasionally detected during scanning. Finally, postoperative voiding difficulties can be evaluated sonographically to determine the location of obstruction and the volume of residual volume.

Rapid development, especially the application of higher frequencies with small transducers, the availability of ultrasound instruments in gynecology, its cost-effectiveness, and the lack of radiation without the need for lead shielding make ultrasound a valuable diagnostic procedure which remains in one hand and can be used in conjunction with other urogynecologic investigational techniques. Moreover, there is no limit to investigation time and no contrast media reaction, which favors its clinical application. Compared with radiology, the increasing number of comparable results and the technical developments of smaller endoprobes and three-dimensional scanners will increase the diagnostic field in urogynecology, resulting in a better understanding of function and dysfunction.

Ultrasound in urogynecology is on its way to replacing conventional radiological procedures. Moreover ultrasound has contributed to a better understanding of physiology and pathophysiology of both the lower urinary tract and the pelvic floor. However, as with conventional radiology, it does not yet appear to provide conclusive and discriminatory diagnostic information, but supplies complementary data to be used in conjunction with other diagnostic tools.

References

1. Donald I, MacVican J, Brown T. Examination of abdominal masses by pulsed ultrasound. Lancet 1958;i:1188–91.
2. Nargund VH, Lomas K, Sapherson DA, Flannigan GM, Stewart PA. Radiographer-performed abdominal and pelvic ultrasound: its value in a urology out-patient clinic. Br J Urol 1994;73:366–9.
3. White RD, McQuown D, McCarthy TA, Ostergard DR. Real time ultrasonography in evaluation of urinary stress incontinence. Am J Obstet Gynecol 1980;138:235–7.
4. Spencer J, Lindsell D, Mastorakou I. Ultrasonography compared with intravenous urography in the investigation of adults with haematuria. BMJ 1990;301:1074–6.
5. Ellenbogen PH, Scheible FW, Talner LB. Sensitivity of Gray scale ultrasound in detecting upper urinary tract obstruction. Am J Roentgenol 1978;130:731–6.
6. Orgaz RE, Gomez AZ, Ramirez CT. Application of bladder ultrasonography I. Bladder content and residue. J Urol 1981;125:174–6.
7. Henriksson L, Marsal K. Bedside ultrasound diagnosis of residual urine volume. Arch Gynecol Obstet 1982;231:129–33.
8. Ouslander JG, Simmons S, Tuico E, Nigam JG, Fingold S, Bates Jensen B, Schnelle JF. Use of a portable ultrasound device to measure post-void residual volume among incontinent nursing home residents. J Am Geriatr Soc 1994, 42:1189–92.
9. Coombes GM, Millard RJ. The accuracy of portable ultrasound scanning in the measurement of residual urine volume. J Urol 1994,152:2083–5.
10. Brandt TD, Harrey N, Calenoff L, Greenberg M, Kaplan P, Nanninga J. Ultrasound evaluation of the urinary system in spinal chord injury patients. Radioliology 1981;141:473–8.
11. Kohorn EI, Scioscia AL, Jeanty P. Ultrasound cystourethrography by perineal scanning for the assessment of female stress urinary incontinence. Obstet Gynecol 1986;68:269–72.
12. Koelbl H, Bernaschek G, Wolf G. A comparative study of perineal ultrasound scanning and urethrocystography in patients with genuine stress incontinence. Arch Obstet Gynecol 1988;244:39–45.
13. Gordon D, Pearce M, Norton P, Stanton S. Comparison of ultrasound and lateral chain urethrocystography in the determination of bladder neck descent. Am J Obstet Gynecol 1989;160:182–5.
14. Schaer GN, Koechli OR, Schuessler B, Haller U. Perineal ultrasound for evaluating the bladder neck in urinary stress incontinence. Obstet Gynecol 1995;85:220.
15. Schaer GN, Koechli OR, Schuessler B, Haller U. Usefulness of ultrasound contrast medium in perineal sonography for visualization of bladder neck funneling-first observations. Urology 1996; 47:452.
16. Schaer GN, Koechli OR, Schuessler B, Haller U. Can simultaneous perineal sonography and urethrocystometry help explain urethral pressure variations? Neurourol Urodyn 1997;16:31.
17. Martan A, Halaska M, Voigt R, Drbohlav B. Sonographie des Blasenhals-Urethra-Uberganges vor und nach Beckenbodentraining mit Kolpexin. Zentralbl Gynakol 1994,116:416–18.
18. Peschers UM, Fanger G; Schaer GN, Vodusek DB, DeLancey JO, Schuessler B. Bladder neck mobility in continent nulliparous women. Br J Obstet Gynaecol 2001;108(3):320–4.
19. Miller JM, Perucchini D, Carchidi LT, DeLancey JO, Ashton-Miller J. Pelvic floor muscle contraction during a cough and decreased vesical neck mobility. Obstet Gynecol 2001;97(2):255–60.
20. Atherton MJ, Stanton SL. A comparison of bladder neck movement and elevation after tension-free vaginal tape and colposuspension. Br J Obstet Gynaecol 2000;107(11):1366–70.
21. Martan A, Masata, Halaska M, Voigt R. Ultrasound imaging of the lower urinary system in women after Burch colposuspension. Ultrasound Obstet Gynecol 2001 17(1):58–64.
22. Schaer G, Koelbl H, Voigt R, Merz E, Anthuber Ch, Niemayer R, Ralph G, Bader W, Fink D, Grischke E, Hanzal E, Koechli OR, Koehler K, Munz E, Perucchini D, Peschers U, Sam C, Schwenke A. Recommendations of the German Association of Urogynecology on functional sonography of the lower female urinary tract. Int Urogynecol J 1996;7:105–8.
23. Koelbl H, Bernaschek G. A new method for sonographic urethrocystography and simultaneous pressure-flow measurements. Obstet Gynecol 1989;74:417–22.
24. Hanzal E, Joura EM, Haeusler G, Koelbl H. Influence of catheterisation on the results of sonographic urethrocystography in patients with genuine stress incontinence. Arch Gynecol Obstet 1994, 255:189–93.
25. Koelbl H, Bernaschek G, Deutinger J. Assessment of female urinary incontinence by introital sonography. J Clin Ultrasound 1990;18:370–4.
26. Quinn MJ, Beynon J, McMortensen NUJ, Smith PJB. Transvaginal endosonography: a new method to study the anatomy of the lower urinary tract in urinary stress incontinence. Br J Urol 1988;62:414–17.

27. Wise BG, Burton G, Cutner A, Cardozo L. Effect of vaginal ultrasound probe on lower urinary tract function. Br J Urol 1992;70:12–16.

28. Hol M, Van Bolhuis C, Vierhout ME. Vaginal ultrasound studies of bladder neck mobility. Br J Obstet Gynaecol 1995,102:47–53.

29. Khullar V, Cardozo LD, Salvatore S, Hill S. Ultrasound: a noninvasive screening test for detrusor instability. Br J Obstet Gynaecol 1996;103:904–8.

30. Mouritsen L, Strandberg C, Frimodt-Moller C. Bladder neck anatomy and mobility: effect of vaginal ultrasound probe. Br J Urol 1994,74:749–52.

31. Mouritsen L, Strandberg C. Vaginal ultrasonography versus colpo-cysto-urethrography in the evaluation of female urinary incontinence. Acta Obstet Scand 1994;73:338–42.

32. Bergman A, Vermesh M, Ballard AC, Platt LD. Role of ultrasound in urinary incontinence. Urology 1989;33:443–4.

33. Carey M, Dwyer PL. Position and mobility of the urethrovesical junction in continent and stress incontinent women before and after successful surgery. Aust NZ J Obstet Gynaecol 1991;31:279–84.

34. Haylen BT, Frazer MI, Sutherst JR, West CR. Transvaginal ultrasound in the measurement of bladder volumes in women: preliminary report. Br J Urol 1989;63:152–4.

35. Iwamoto K, Kigawa J, Minagawa Y, Miura H, Terakawa N. Transvaginal ultrasonographic diagnosis of bladder-wall invasion in patients with cervical cancer. Obstet Gynecol 1994;83:217–19.

36. Nishizawa O, Takada H, Sakamoto F. Combined urodynamic and ultrasonic techniques: a new diagnostic method for the lower urinary tract. Tohoku J Exp Med 1982;136:231–2.

37. Shapeero LG, Friedland GW, Perkash I. Transrectal sonographic voiding cystourethrography: studies in neuromuscular bladder dysfunction. Am J Radiol 1983;141:83–90.

38. Brown MC, Sutherst J, Murray A. Potential use of ultrasound in place of X-ray fluoroscopy in urodynamics. Br J Urol 1985;57:88–90.

39. Kuo HC, Chang SC, Hsu T. Application of transrectal ultrasound in the diagnosis and treatment of female stress urinary incontinence. Eur Urol 1994, 26:77–84.

40. Koelbl H, Bernaschek G. Cystosonography: a diagnostic adjunct for the staging of advanced gynecologic malignancies. Obstet Gynecol 1988;72:951–4.

41. Kirschner-Hermanns R, Klein HM, Muller U, Schaefer W, Jakse G. Intra-urethral ultrasound in women with stress incontinence. Br J Urol 1994;74:315–18.

42. Chancellor MB, Liu JB, Rivas DA, Karasick S, Bagley DH, Goldberg BB. Intraoperative endo-luminal ultrasound evaluation of urethral diverticula. J Urol 1995;153:72–5.

43. Campani R, Bottinelli O, Calliada F, Coscia D. The latest in ultrasound: three-dimensional imaging. Part II. Eur J Radiol 1998; 27:183–7.

44. Marks LS, Dorey FJ, Macairan ML, Park C, deKernion JB. Three-dimensional ultrasound device for rapid determination of bladder volume. Urology 1997;50:341–8.

45. Khullar V, Salvatore S, Cardozo LD, Hill S, Kelleher CJ: Three dimensional ultrasound of the urethra and urethral sphincter – a new diagnostic technique. Neurourol Urodyn 1994;13:352–3.

46. Umek WH, Obermair A, Stutterecker D, Hausler G, Leodolter S, Hanzal E. Three-dimensional ultrasound of the female urethra: comparing transvaginal and transrectal scanning. Ultrasound Obstet Gynecol 2001;17(5):425–30.

47. Sentovich SM, Blatchford GJ, Rivela LJ, Lin K, Thorson AG, Christensen MA. Diagnosing anal sphincter injury with transanal ultrasound and manometry. Dis Colon Rectum 1997;40:1430–4.

48. Sultan AH, Nicholls RJ, Kamm MA, Hudson CN, Beynon J, Bartram CI. Anal endosonography and correlation with in vitro and in vivo anatomy. Br J Surg 1993;80:508–11.

49. Sultan AH, Kamm MA, Talbot IC, Nicholls RJ, Bartram CI. Anal endosonography for identifying external sphincter defects confirmed histologically. Br J Surg 1994;81:463–5.

50. Sultan AH, Kamm MA, Hudson CN, Thomas JM, Bartram CI. Anal sphincter disruption during vaginal delivery. N Engl J Med 1993;329:1905–11.

51. Campbell DM, Behan M, Donnelly VS, O'Herlihy C, O'Connell PR. Endosonographic assessment of postpartum anal sphincter injury using a 120 degree sector scanner. Clin Radiol 1996;51:559–61.

52. Peschers U, DeLancey JOL, Schaer G, Schuessler B. Exoanal ultrasound of the anal sphincter: normal anatomy and sphincter defects. Br J Obstet Gynaecol 1997;104:999–1003.

12 Anorectal Testing: Defecography and Anorectal Manometry

N.E. Diamant

There are many tests of anorectal function and a recent review identifies the capabilities of these various tests and techniques, and provides some direction for their use in patients with the common conditions of fecal incontinence, constipation and anorectal pain [1]. The present discussion will deal with two tests of the anorectal area that are frequently used in the assessment of pelvic floor disorders, defecography (evacuation proctography) and anorectal manometry.

Defecography (Evacuation Proctography)

Defecography involves imaging the rectum with contrast material and using fluoroscopic techniques to observe the defecation process and the accompanying changes in anorectal structure [2–7]. The procedure has the potential to provide information about anorectal, puborectalis and levator muscle, and rectal function as well as anatomical defects of the anorectal area. Various contrast materials have been used, including esophageal contrast barium, and barium mixed with potato starch, or other viscous materials. After filling the rectum with the contrast material, the external anal opening is usually outlined by smearing it with barium-impregnated gel and a contrast-soaked tampon is inserted by women to define the anterior vaginal wall. With the subject positioned sitting on a commode-like chair, video fluoroscopic images are obtained during a number of maneuvers: resting state, voluntary and maximum contraction of the sphincter and pelvic floor muscles ("squeeze"), and during defecation.

The radiographic images are analyzed to assess a number of static and movement derived parameters, and other radiographic features. Static measurements can include: anal canal length; anorectal angle; position of anorectal junction; and rectosacral gap (Figures 12.1 and 12.2). The derived measurements can include: change in anorectal length; change in anorectal angle; anal canal angulation; perineal elevation, descent, and total movement; horizontal movement of the anorectal junction; and rectal evacuation. Other features that may be noted are: mucosal prolapse and intussusception; rectocele; suspected enterocele; posterior wall squeeze impression; rectoanal junction appearances; and anal canal closure 7 (Figures 12.3 and 12.4).

Defecography is not a study of normal defecation in response to a desire to defecate. Therefore study subjects are often embarrassed by the nature and the setting of the test, which may inhibit or alter the defecation process and emptying of the contrast

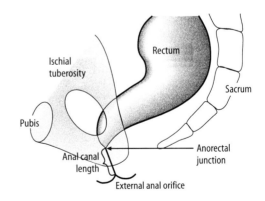

Figure 12.1 Anorectal landmarks. The anorectal junction can be measured with reference to the inferior margin of the ischial tuberosity, the anal canal length as the distance from the external anal orifice to where the parallel sides of the anal canal diverge to form the rectal walls, and the rectosacral gap as the space taken at the S3 level.

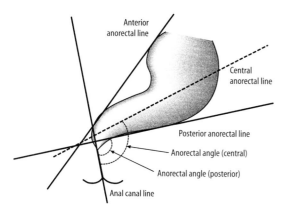

Figure 12.2 The anorectal angle. The posterior anorectal angle is formed by the intersection of the posterior anorectal line with the anal canal line; the central anorectal angle by the intersection of the anal canal line with the line that bisects the angle between the anterior and posterior anorectal lines.

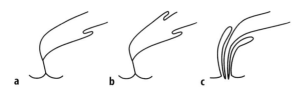

Figure 12.3 Mucosal prolapse and intussusception. Mucosal prolapse can occur unilaterally (**a**), circumferentially (**b**), and form an intussusception even to the extent of external prolapse (**c**).

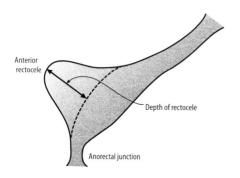

Figure 12.4 Anterior rectocele. This common rectocele is seen as an anterior wall protrusion beyond the expected line of the rectum.

material. Furthermore, there are a number of aspects that signal caution in the use of the technique, in interpretation of the findings, and in subsequent clinical decision-making [1]: (1) There is disagreement over the measurement of the anorectal angle, a parameter thought to be critical to the interpretation of defecography results [8,9]. It is uncertain whether to use the central axis of the rectum [4,7], the entire posterior wall of the rectum

[10] or the most distal portion of the posterior wall [2,3,6,7,11]. (2) Some of the often reported findings, especially rectocele, descent of the pelvic floor, and internal intussusception, are seen in a high proportion of asymptomatic individuals [6,7,11,12], and the presence of these entities does not correlate with impaired rectal emptying [12]. (3) Normal values of rectal emptying vary widely [13,14]. (4) Rectal evacuation does not correlate with symptoms (or distinguish between symptoms such as infrequent defecation versus impaired defecation), colonic transit, or anal manometry [12,13]. (5) Arguments are made that defecography adds little additional data to anorectal manometry [15,16] and/or does not differentiate patients with impaired defecation from those with fecal incontinence or from normal controls [17]. (6) There are significant differences between men and women, and age-related differences. (7) Finally, the method of performance of the technique varies considerably from center to center [3,4,7–9,17–20], and factors such as the consistency of the barium can affect the findings [7]. Nevertheless, when used in conjunction with a good history and physical examination, and with other tests of anorectal function, there are some potential uses of this technique.

Because of the limitations of the technique noted above, there are no generally accepted normal values and findings that are universally applicable. Some indication of values for the anorectal angle, position of the anorectal junction, perineal movement, and anal canal length are shown in Tables 12.1–12.4. Some generalizations can be made but the wide variation in normal values makes application of these questionable. Men tend to have a longer anal canal, while women tend to have a greater anorectal angle. Voluntary "squeeze" decreases the anorectal angle, while "strain" and defecation increase the angle.

Rectocele

There is some merit to the objective demonstration of a large rectocele in patients with incomplete evacuation, and who are helped by rectal or vaginal digitation during defecation. However, rectoceles less than 2 cm diameter are normal in women [7]. Even large rectoceles can be asymptomtomatic, and the correlation between the presence of such a finding, symptoms, and improvement with surgery is not predictable [21].

Intussusception

Internal rectal intussusception has been suggested as a cause of symptoms and of solitary rectal ulcer.

Table 12.1 Anorectal angle

	Rest	Squeeze	Strain	Reference
Posterior anorectal angle (°)[a]				
Men	96 ± 17 (64–125) {25}[b]	80 ± 16 (45–116) {25}	98 ± 19 (67–123) {17}	Shorvon et al. [7]
Women	95 ± 16 (70–134) {22}	71 ± 12 (54–95) {22}	103 ± 15 (75–128) {15}	Shorvon et al. [7]
Men {4} + Women {6}	93.7 ± 2.3	—	123 ± 6.7	Mantzikopoulos et al. [80]
Men {22} + Women {34}	92.0 ± 1.5	—	136.6 ± 1.5	Mahieu et al. [3]
[c] Men {2} + Women {14}	92 (88–100)	—	130 (120–150)	Womack et al. [81]
Central anorectal angle (°)[a]				
Men	118 ± 12 (91–140) {25}	113 ± 17 (90–160) {25}	118 ± 12 (97–136) {17}	Shorvon et al. [7]
Men {7} + Women {14}	98.6 (74–121)	—	121.6 (90–156)	Freimanis et al. [20]
Women {25}	108 (94–119)	—	—	Skomorowska et al. [82]
Men {40}	127 (101–155)	—	—	Skomorowska and Hegedus [19]
Women {40}	108 (90–120)	—	—	Skomorowska and Hegedus [19]

[a] Mean ± SD (Range).
[b] {} = n.
[c] Central or posterior angle – not stated.

Table 12.2 Position of anorectal junction

	Rest	Squeeze	Strain	Reference
[c]*Position (mm)[a]*				
Men	16 ± 9 (0–31) {25}[b]	28 ± 9 (9–41) {25}	-4 ± 9 (–22 to +31) {17}	Shorvon et al. [7]
Women	4 ± 13 (–32 to +21) {22}	14 ± 12 (–20 to +25) {22}	16 ± 15 (–48 to +12) {15}	Shorvon et al. [7]

[a] Mean ± SD (Range).
[b] {} = n.
[c] Distance between upper anal canal and inferior margins of the ischial tuberosities.

Table 12.3 Perineal movement (mm)[a]

	Elevation (squeeze)	Descent (defecation)	Reference
Men {17}[b]	13 ± 7	19 ± 10 (2–39)	Shorvon et al. [7]
Women {15}	10 ± 7	20 ± 15 (0–54)	Shorvon et al. [7]
Men {40}	—	45 (20–80)	Skomorowska and Hegedus [19]
Women {40}	—	45 (20–70)	Skomorowska and Hegedus [19]
Women {25}	—	45 (25–70)	Skomorowska et al. [82]
Men {22} + women {34}	—	<20	Mahieu et al. [3]
Men {4} + women {6}	—	35 ± 9	Mantzikopoulos et al. [80]

[a] Mean ± SD (Range).
[b] {} = n.

Table 12.4   Anal canal length (mm)[a]

	Rest	Squeeze	Strain	Reference
Men	22 ± 7 (10–37)	28 ± 9 (12–45)	17 ± 6 (9–27)	Shorvon et al. [7]
	{25}[b]	{25}	{17}	
Women	16 ± 5 (6–26)	19 ± 6 (6–26)	14 ± 5 (6–20)	Shorvon et al. [7]
	{22}	{22}	{15}	

[a] Mean ± SD (Range).
[b] {} = n.

However, its correction correlates poorly with symptomatic benefit, and mucosal prolapse and rectal intussusception have been reported in normal subjects [7, 20].

Rectal Prolapse

Defecography can demonstrate external rectal prolapse [22–27], a finding readily demonstrated on the commode without radiology.

Enterocele

Defecography combined with filling of the small bowel with barium from above may be useful in demonstrating an enterocele [4], and therefore may aid in the evaluation of patients with impaired defecation and proctalgia.

Rectal Evacuation

In theory, the quantification of rectal evacuation could be helpful in patients with constipation attributed to pelvic floor dysfunction or dyssynergia [2–5,28]. For example, some patients with constipation have poor rectal emptying on proctography [12,29]. However, the finding is nonspecific and no differences were observed in patterns of rectal emptying of barium contrast among four study groups: patients with infrequent defecation and normal colonic transit, those with infrequent defecation with proximal slowing of colonic transit, patients with defecatory difficulty only and control subjects [12]. Further, rectal emptying is subject to many variables including backflow into the sigmoid, barium consistency, and rectal size. Finally, information about evacuation has not been proven to alter management or to predict the outcome of treatments such as colectomy in younger patients [30]. Therefore, the degree of overlap renders defecography of limited importance in management decisions in patients with constipation. However, if the results of defecography (e.g. inappropriate contraction of

the puborectalis muscle) corroborate other studies of anorectal function, they may serve to reinforce the validity of such testing, and provide direction for therapy such as biofeedback training [31].

Fecal Incontinence

There is no evidence that evacuation proctography is of established value in patients with fecal incontinence.

Constipation

Proctography is of potential value in patients with constipation where the following problems are suspected as the cause of impaired defecation, and physical examination and other tests support the findings: (a) inappropriate contraction of the puborectalis muscle; (b) enterocele (e.g. after hysterectomy); and (c) anterior rectocele (e.g. history of manipulation of the rectal wall per vaginam).

Anorectal Manometry

Anorectal manometry provides information about the nature and behavior of the anorectal area by measuring pressures in the anal canal and rectum. Figure 12.5 shows the major anorectal structures. Measurements are made at rest, with voluntary contraction of the external anal sphincter and pelvic floor, and with straining as if to have a bowel movement. The measurement technique usually includes balloon distension of the rectum to assess reflex anal sphincter responses, and to obtain some measure of rectal sensation. Anorectal manometry can also be used to perform biofeedback therapy for anorectal disorders. The technique has been applied to the assessment of conditions such as constipation, fecal incontinence and anorectal pain.

Anal canal pressures and anal sphincter responses can be measured with open-tipped or side-opening water-perfused catheters, solid state microtransducers, or air- or water-filled balloons of various sizes

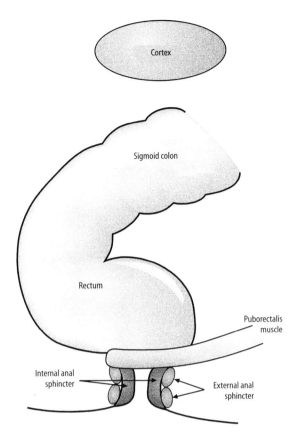

Figure 12.5 Maintenance of continence. In addition to voluntary control of the defecation process and the external anal sphincter, and the influence of colonic function and stool consistency, anorectal structures and function are important and include: rectal compliance and sensation of urgency; internal and external anal sphincter integrity; contraction of the puborectalis muscle; and the anorectal angle.

and configurations. However, although balloon probes can assess sphincter responses to rectal distension and other stimuli, they cannot adequately measure resting pressures of the anal canal. To eval-uate the measurements properly, normal values must be established for each technique.

By manometry, the anal canal is seen as a region of higher resting pressure that separates the rectum from the exterior. Males have longer anal canals than do women [32–36] with considerable overlap (Table 12.5, see also Table 12.4). Normal anal canal pressures vary according to gender, age and tech-niques employed (Tables 12.6 and 12.7). In general, pressures are higher in males and in younger persons but there is a considerable overlap in values. The pressure decrease with age is particularly marked in women over the age of 50–55.

Resting Anal Canal Pressures (RAP)

These may be assessed by station pull-through or rapid pull-through techniques [32,34, 36–41], and tend to be higher with the rapid pull-through (Table 12.6). Tonic activities of both the internal (IAS) and external anal sphincters (EAS) contribute to the resting pressure with approximately 75–85% of this pressure derived from the IAS. However, if the patient is not completely relaxed, a larger contribu-tion from the EAS (and therefore higher pressures) will be recorded.

Squeeze Pressures

These are obtained by asking the patient to maximally contract (MSP) the EAS, and considerable variation in normal values exists (Table 12.7). The duration of maximal squeeze can also be obtained, and normal subjects can maintain an increase of 10 mmHg for 49 ± 1 s and of 5 mmHg for 122 ± 37 s. [37,42].

Reflex Anal Sphincter Responses

The IAS and EAS are normally inhibited either in response to rectal distension or during attempted

Table 12.5 Normal values of length (cm) of anal canal

Women	n	Men	n	Reference
4.0 ± 1.0^c	18	4.0 ± 1.0^c	18	[32]
$3.1 (2.0–4.2)^b$	20	$3.6 (2.4–4.4)^b$	20	[33]
$2.2 (2.2–3.8)^c$	35	$2.8 (2.1–3.7)^c$	23^a	[34]
3.7 ± 0.2	10	4.0 ± 0.6^b	12	[36]

Values expressed as mean ± SEM or mean (range).
[a] Expressed as median (range).
[b] Significantly different.
[c] Not significantly different.
From Diamant et al. [1], with permission.

Table 12.6   Representative normal values of maximal resting anal canal pressures determined manometrically

	Women	n	Men	n	Reference
Station pull-through	58 ± 3	22	66 ± 6	15	[37]
	54 ± 5	12	Not studied		[38]
	50 ± 13	18[a]	63 ± 12	18	[39]
	49 ± 3	12	49 ± 3	7	[40]
Slow pull-through					
	46 (range 40–58)	35	60 (range 51–98) 23		[34]
Rapid pull-through	100 ± 22	10[a]	Not studied		[32]
	106 ± 18	10[a]	Not studied		[32]
	102 ± 19	35[b]	100 ± 21	27[b]	[41]
	76 ± 24	40[c]	97 ± 20	31[c]	[41]
	53 ± 22	17[d]	72 ± 23	3[d]	[41]

Values expressed as mmHg (mean ± SEM) unless indicated.
[a] Significant difference between sexes but not age.
[b] Ages 20–39 years.
[c] Ages 40–69 years.
[d] Ages 70+ years.
From Diamant et al. [1], with permission.

Table 12.7   Representative normal values of maximal squeeze anal canal pressures determined manometrically

	Women	n	Men	n	Reference
Station pull-through	135 ± 15	22	218 ± 18	15	[37]
	90 ± 9	12	Not studied		[38]
	159 ± 45	18[a]	238 ± 38	18	[32]
Slow pull-through					
	103 (range 78–190)	35	163 (range 76–234)	23	[34]
Rapid pull-through					
	179 ± 55	10[a]	Not studied		[39]
	159 ± 35	10	Not studied		[39]
	171 ± 40	35[b]	240 ± 65	27[b]	[41]
	132 ± 169	40[c]	203 ± 45	30[c]	[41]
	116 ± 40	17[d]	219 ± 32	3[d]	[41]

Values expressed as mmHg (mean ± SEM) unless otherwise indicated.
[a] Significant difference between sexes but not age.
[b] Ages 20–39 years.
[c] Ages 40–69 years.
[d] Ages 70 + years.
From Diamant et al. [1], with permission.

defecation (Figure 12.6). This reflex inhibition can be elicited by distending a rectal balloon or by asking the subject to expel the manometer (pseudo defecation) [32,38,42–44] (Table 12.8). If the rectum is enlarged (megarectum), greater volumes of rectal distension are required to elicit the inhibitory reflex. The decrease in pressure is largely that of the IAS which makes up the majority of the resting pressure. This balloon distension reflex of the IAS remains intact in patients with extrinsic denervation but disappears with neuropathy and loss of ganglion cells of the myenteric plexus (e.g. Hirschsprung's disease) and/or with atrophy and fibrosis of the IAS [45,46]. Although EAS inhibition can be assessed with all types of anorectal manometers, simultaneous EMG recordings ensure that inhibition of EAS activity contributes to the decreased pressures. A transient reflex EAS contraction is often seen prior to the reflex inhibition, and this contraction can be enhanced by biofeedback training for the treatment of fecal incontinence.

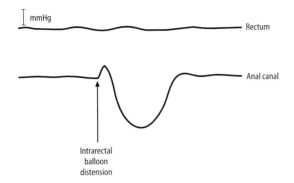

Figure 12.6 Reflex activity of the anal sphincter. Transient intrarectal balloon distension normally produces a relaxation of the internal anal sphincter and cessation of external sphincter contraction, which is recorded as a decrease in resting sphincter pressure. A transient external sphincter contraction may also be seen as an increase in pressure prior to the relaxation.

Prolonged Anorectal Manometry

Methods are available to monitor anorectal motor events over prolonged periods of time and in fully ambulant subjects [40,47–49]. The clinical applicability of these techniques has not as yet been established.

Vector Manometry (Vectometry)

The radial pressure profile along the anal sphincter is measured by circumferentially placed recording ports, and it is likely that up to eight radially-oriented recording ports are necessary for adequate resolution [50–53]. The technique is used to try and localize weakness of the IAS and/or EAS due to damage or disruption of the sphincters; this is recognized by a decrease in pressure in a particular radial orientation (Figure 12.7). This information is of value in patients with fecal incontinence, particularly women who may have suffered sphincter damage at the time of delivery. However, the technique has limitations which make it less satisfactory than other methods such as anal ultrasound. Agreement with ultrasound and needle electromyography has been variable [50–54]. The sensitivity and specificity of vector manometry are too low to determine which patients should have surgical management [53]. The technique cannot readily distinguish IAS from EAS damage.

Therefore, although some of the data can be interpreted as indicating that vectometry is of clinical value in identifying patients with traumatic sphincter injury, anal canal ultrasound if available is a preferable test for identifying such patients [55–59].

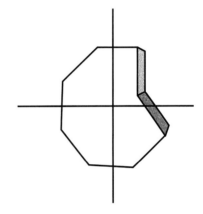

Figure 12.7 Vector manometry of the anal canal. Multiple recording ports circumferentially placed can help detect local areas of the anal sphincter which are weak or damaged. These are seen as a decrease in pressure in a specific radial location.

Table 12.8 Thresholds of IAS relaxation (ml)

Thresholds[d]	n	Characteristics of distending balloon	Reference
14 ± 1	16	5 cm long, 5 cm from anal verge	[42]
20 (10–30)	11	5 cm long, 5 cm from anal verge	[43]
22 ± 3 (10–40)	12	5 cm long, 5 cm from anal verge	[38]
25 ± 2	17[a]	5 cm long, 5 cm from anal verge	[44]
19 ± 6	18[b]	2.5 × 3 cm, 5 cm from anal verge	[32]
23 ± 11	18[c]	2.5 × 3 cm, 5 cm from anal verge	[32]

[a] Elderly >age 60 years.
[b] Elderly >age 66 years.
[c] Young; ages 21–40 years.
[d] Expressed as mean ± SEM and or (range).
From Diamant et al. [1], with permission.

Table 12.9   Representative normal values for thresholds of conscious perception of rectal distension

Rectal sensation (ml)[a]	n	Technique	Reference
12 ± 1	16	Balloon 5.5 × 4 cm, 5 cm from anal verge	[42]
13 ± 2 (10–30)	11	Balloon 5 cm long, 5 cm from anal verge	[43]
13 ± 3 (5–30)	12	Balloon 5 cm long, 5 cm from anal verge	[38]
14 ± 3	17[b]	Balloon 5 cm long, 5 cm from anal verge	[44]
17 ± 9	36	Balloon 2.5 × 3 cm, 5 cm from anal verge	[39]

[a] Mean ± SEM (range).
[b] Ages 60–79 years; no differences between gender or age.
From Diamant et al. [1], with permission.

Rectal Sensation

Balloon distension is used to detect the threshold (smallest volume of rectal distension) for three common sensations, the first detectable sensation (rectal sensory threshold), the sensation of urgency to defecate, and the sensation of pain (often defined as maximum tolerable volume). The clinical significance of the latter two thresholds is less well established than that of the first. The type of inflation (phasic versus continuous) and the speed of continuous inflation affect the threshold volume required for healthy controls to perceive rectal distensions [60]. Also, the size and shape of the balloon will affect the threshold volume, and thresholds appear to vary with the distance of the balloon from the anal verge. Therefore, within groups, sensory thresholds vary widely, with an upper range of normal of 30 ml for a latex balloon 5 × 4 cm situated 5 cm above the anal verge (Table 12.9).

The maximum tolerable volume or pain threshold may be reduced in patients who have a non-compliant rectum (e.g., abdomino-perineal pull-through, proctitis, rectal ischemia) [61], and the pain threshold may also be reduced in patients with functional bowel disorders [61–65]. On the other hand, the thresholds for first detectable sensation and the urge to defecate are often elevated in patients with constipation. Significant loss of or delay in the ability to sense rectal distension (rectal sensory threshold) is a sufficient but not a necessary condition for fecal incontinence [15, 66, 67].

Fecal Incontinence

Anal canal pressures are often low in patients with fecal incontinence, which has led to studies for discriminating fecally incontinent patients from continent patients and controls [67, 68]. However, it is not logical to expect anal canal pressure to be perfectly correlated with continence because of the wide range of normal pressures, and there are other factors which may cause fecal incontinence in the absence of decreased anal canal pressures.

A decrease in MSP has the greatest sensitivity and specificity for discrimination of fecal incontinence, the efficiency of this measurement depending on the cut-off pressure considered as normal and the sex of the patient. For example, taking the mean minus 2 SD for controls as the cut-off, the sensitivity is 92% and specificity is 97% [67]. RAP is decreased but the sensitivity of this decrease is poor in discriminating the incontinent patients from normal subjects [67, 68]. The duration of maximum squeeze (e.g. >5 mmHg in lower anal canal) is about 2 minutes, and is decreased in patients with incontinence [39,41]. Incontinence to liquids is associated primarily with low internal anal sphincter pressures; patients incontinent to both liquids and solids have abnormally low squeeze pressures (external anal sphincter) in addition [69].

Other manometric features may be seen in patients with incontinence. These include an increase in spontaneous internal sphincter relaxations which are not associated with compensatory increases in external sphincter activity. These last about 45 seconds and are more frequently associated with increases in rectal pressure in the incontinent patients [67,70]. In addition to increased spontaneous transient relaxations, these incontinent patients have low thresholds for balloon-induced relaxations and show post-squeeze or post-strain relaxations, the latter not usually seen in normal subjects [70]. Therefore, especially if there is some loss of rectal sensation, internal sphincter relaxation can occur before a rectal stimulus is sensed and before compensatory external sphincter contraction can be initiated, resulting in fecal incontinence. On the other hand, the finding of a low threshold to induce a pain or a desire to defecate may have value by indicating the presence of visceral hypersensitivity, poor rectal compliance, or rectal irritability in patients with fecal incontinence.

Constipation

Manometry may be utilized to assess anorectal function in patients with chronic constipation. The absence of internal anal sphincter relaxation in response to rectal distension strongly suggests Hirschsprung's disease in the appropriate clinical setting [71], while the presence of internal sphincter relaxation excludes Hirschsprung's disease from consideration. Therefore, manometry is a relatively noninvasive screening technique for this uncommon disorder.

Manometry may be used to assess anorectal patterns during attempted defecation such as with expulsion of a rectal balloon (pseudodefecation). Intrarectal pressure is recorded as an indication of intra-abdominal pressures generated, while at the same time, pressure recordings from the anal canal indicate the normal presence of relaxation or inappropriate contraction of the external anal sphincter [5]. The latter pattern suggests the presence of pelvic floor dyssynergia, also known as anismus or the puborectalis syndrome [72]. However, it is uncertain whether a manometric pattern suggesting dyssynergia alone is a sufficient diagnostic criterion [12].

Therefore, anorectal manometry is clinically useful in relatively few patients with chronic constipation. The technique has potential value to exclude Hirschsprung's disease, and in the assessment and management of constipated adults who exhibit pelvic floor dyssynergia, especially if this is corroborated by anal sphincter EMG and by impaired expulsion of contrast with defecography.

Anorectal Pain Syndromes

Two main syndromes occur, the levator ani syndrome and proctalgia fugax. The irritable bowel syndrome may also be associated with rectal pain and patients with the syndrome report pain at a lower volume of rectal distension than do healthy controls [62]. However, there are no specific manometric features of the syndrome.

Levator ani syndrome is defined as a chronic or intermittent dull, aching pain or discomfort in the rectum [73, 74] and the symptoms may also include a chronic sensation of rectal fullness and urge to defecate. Although the physiological mechanism for the syndrome is not firmly established, the syndrome has been attributed to chronic tension in the striated pelvic floor muscles [74]. The diagnosis is based on clinical symptoms and physical examination; anorectal manometry is not required although it may be helpful in confirming the association of the symptoms with elevated pelvic floor or anal canal muscle tension.

Proctalgia fugax refers to sharp, fleeting pains from the anal canal or rectum [73, 74]. The physiological basis for these symptoms is also unknown and the diagnosis is based solely on symptom criteria and exclusion of other diseases. A small group of patients with severe proctalgia may have a myopathy of the internal anal sphincter [75], and in some patients paroxysms of contraction of the anal canal may be involved [76]. However, at present anorectal manometry plays no role in the diagnosis or treatment of proctalgia fugax.

Biofeedback Therapy

Anorectal manometry can be used to perform this therapy for both fecal incontinence and constipation [31]. There is as yet no evidence that anorectal manometry has predictive value for the use of this therapy.

For fecal incontinence the biofeedback training is designed to teach the patient (a) how to recognize small volumes of rectal distension, and (b) how to contract the external anal sphincter while simultaneously keeping intra-abdominal pressure low [77,78]. To accomplish these goals, one needs to be able to display to the patient a measure of sphincter contraction, which can be based on anal canal pressures or pelvic floor EMG; and a measure of abdominal wall contraction, which can be based on pressures in a rectal balloon or a skin surface measure of rectus abdominis EMG. One also needs to be able to distend the rectum with graded volumes of air in a balloon. Therefore objective monitoring of outcome requires the use of anorectal study techniques.

Biofeedback techniques have value in patients with constipation with associated pelvic floor dyssynergia [79]. To perform these studies, anorectal testing techniques are required: (a) pelvic floor dyssynergia should be corroborated by at least two different tests from among the following: manometry, defecography and sphincter EMG, and (b) sphincter EMG or manometric techniques are utilized for the biofeedback training sessions where the patients are taught to relax the anal sphincter and pelvic floor muscles.

References

1. Diamant NE, Kamm MA, Wald A, Whitehead WE. AGA Technical Review on Anorectal Testing Techniques. Gastroenterology 1999;116:735–60.

2. Mahieu P, Pringot J, Bodart P. Defecography: II. Contribution to the diagnosis of defecation disorders. Gastrointest Radiol 1984;9:253–61.

3. Mahieu P, Pringot J, Bodart P. Defecography: I. Description of a new procedure and results in normal patients. Gastrointest Radiol 1984;9:247–51.

4. Ekberg O, Nylander G, Fork F-T. Defecography. Radiology 1985;155:45–8.

5. Loening-Baucke V, Cruikshank BM. Abnormal defecation dynamics in chronically constipated children with encopresis. J Pediatr 1986;108:562–6.

6. Bartram CI, Turnbull GK, Lennard-Jones JE. Evacuation proctography: An investigation of rectal expulsion in 20 subjects without defecatory disturbance. Gastrointest Radiol 1988;13:72–80.

7. Shorvon PJ, McHugh S, Diamant NE, Somers S, Stevenson GW. Defecography in normal volunteers: results and implications. Gut 1989;30:1737–49.

8. Penninckx F, Debruyne C, Lestar B, Kerremans R. Observer variation in the radiological measurement of the anorectal angle. Int J Colorectal Dis 1990;5:94–7.

9. Ferrante SL, Perry RE, Schreiman JS, Cheng S-C, Frick MP. The reproducibility of measuring the anorectal angle in defecography. Dis Colon Rectum 1991;34:51–5.

10. Papachrysostomou M, Stevenson AJM, Ferrington C, Merrick MV, Smith AN. Evaluation of isotope proctography in constipated subjects. Int J Colorectal Dis 1993;8:18–23.

11. Turnbull GK, Bartram CI, Lennard-Jones JE. Radiologic studies of rectal evacuation in adults with idiopathic constipation. Dis Colon Rectum 1988;31:190–7.

12. Wald A, Caruana BJ, Freimanis MG, Bauman DH, Hinds JP. Contributions of evacuation proctography and anorectal manometry to evaluation of adults with constipation and defecatory difficulty. Dig Dis Sci 1990;35:481–7.

13. Wald A, Jafri F, Rehder J, Holeva K. Scintigraphic studies of rectal emptying in patients with constipation and defecatory difficulty. Dig Dis Sci 1993;38:353–8.

14. Hutchinson R, Mostafa AB, Grant EA. Scintigraphic defecography: Quantitative and dynamic assessment of anorectal function. Dis Colon Rectum 1993;36:1132–8.

15. Rex DK, Lappas JC. Combined anorectal manometry and defecography in 50 consecutive adults with fecal incontinence. Dis Colon Rectum 1992;35:1040–5.

16. Berkelmans I, Heresbach D, Leroi A-M et al. Perineal descent at defecography in women with straining at stool: a lack of specificity or predictive value for future anal incontinence? Eur J Gastroenterol Hepatol 1995;7:75–9.

17. Hiltunen K-M, Kolehmainen H, Matikainen M. Does defecography help in diagnosis and clinical decision-making in defecation disorders? Abdom Imaging 1994;19:355–8.

18. Halligan S, McGee S, Bartram CI. Quantification of evacuation proctography. Dis Colon Rectum 1994;37:1151–4.

19. Skomorowska E, Hegedus V. Sex differences in anorectal angle and perineal descent. Gastrointest Radiol 1987;12:353–5.

20. Freimanis MG, Wald A, Caruana B, Bauman DH. Evacuation proctolography in normal volunteers. Invest Radiol 1991;26:581–5.

21. Siproudhis L, Ropert A, Lucas J et al. Defecatory disorders, anorectal and pelvic floor dysfunction: a polygamy? Int J Colorectal Dis 1992;7:102–7.

22. Broden B, Snellman B. Procidentia of the rectum studied with cineradiography: A contribution to the discussion of causative mechanism. Dis Colon Rectum 1968;11:330–47.

23. Bacon HE. Anus, rectum, sigmoid colon: diagnosis and treatment. In: Anonymous. Prolapse and Procidentia. New York: Lippincott, 1941; 400–41.

24. Fry IK, Griffiths JD, Smart PJG. Some observations on the movement of the pelvic floor and rectum with special reference to rectal prolapse. Br J Surg 1966;53:784–7.

25. Goei R, Baeten C, Arends JW. Solitary rectal ulcer syndrome: Findings at barium enema study and defecography. Radiology 1988;168:303–6.

26. Kuijpers JH, DeMorree H. Toward a selection of the most appropriate procedure in the treatment of complete rectal prolapse. Dis Colon Rectum 1988;31:355–7.

27. Kuijpers HC, Strijk SP. Diagnosis of disturbances of continence and defecation. Dis Colon Rectum 1984;27:658–62.

28. Whitehead WE, Chaussade S, Corazziari E, Kumar D. Report of an international workshop on management of constipation. Gastroenterol Int 1991;4:99–113.

29. Turnbull GK, Lennard-Jones JE, Bartram CI. Failure of rectal expulsion as a cause of constipation: Why fiber and laxatives sometimes fail. Lancet 1986;767–9.

30. van der Sijp JRM, Kamm MA, Lennard-Jones JE. Age of onset and rectal emptying: predicting outcome of colectomy for severe idiopathic constipation. Int J Colorectal Dis 1992;7:35–7.

31. Rao SSC, Enck P, Loening-Baucke V. Biofeedback therapy for defecation disorders. Dig Dis 1997;15:78–92.

32. Loening-Baucke V, Anuras S. Anorectal manometry in healthy elderly subjects. Am J Geriatr Soc 1984;32:636–9.

33. Rasmussen H. Dynamic anal manometry: Physiological variations and pathophysiological findings in fecal incontinence. Gastroenterology 1992;103:103–13.

34. Pedersen IK, Christiansen J. A study of the physiological variation in anal manometry. Br J Surg 1989;76:69–71.

35. Taylor BM, Beart RW, Jr., Phillips SF. Longitudinal and radial variations of pressure in the human anal sphincter. Gastroenterology 1984;86:693–7.

36. McHugh SM, Diamant NE. Anal canal pressure profile: a reappraisal as determined by rapid pullthrough technique. Gut 1987;28:1234–41.

37. Read NW, Harford WV, Schmulen AC, Read MG, Santa Ana C, Fordtran JS. A clinical study of patients with fecal incontinence and diarrhea. Gastroenterology 1979;76:747–56.

38. Caruana BJ, Wald A, Hinds JP, Eidelman BH. Anorectal sensory and motor function in neurogenic fecal incontinence. Comparison between multiple sclerosis and diabetes mellitus. Gastroenterology 1991;100:465–70.

39. Loening-Baucke V, Anuras S. Effects of age and sex on anorectal manometry. Am J Gastroenterol 1985;80:50–3.

40. Orkin BA, Hanson RB, Kelly KA, Phillips SF, Dent J. Human anal motility while fasting, after feeding, and during sleep. Gastroenterology 1991;100:1016–23.

41. McHugh SM, Diamant NE. Effect of age, gender, and parity on anal canal pressures. Contribution of impaired anal sphincter function to fecal incontinence. Dig Dis Sci 1987;32:726–36.

42. Chiarioni G. Liquid stool incontinence with severe urgency: anorectal function and effective biofeedback treatment. Gut 1993;34:1576–80.

43. Wald A, Tunuguntla AK. Anorectal sensorimotor dysfunction in fecal incontinence and diabetes mellitus. Modification with biofeedback therapy. N Engl J Med 1984;310:1282–7.

44. Merkel IS, Locher J, Burgio K, Towers A, Wald A. Physiologic and psychologic characteristics of an elderly population with chronic constipation. Am J Gastroenterol 1993;88:1854–9.

45. Chiou AWH, Lin J-K, Wang F-M. Anorectal abnormalities in progressive systemic sclerosis. Dis Colon Rectum 1989;32:417–21.

46. Engel AF, Kamm MA, Talbot IC. Progressive systemic sclerosis of the internal anal sphincter leading to passive faecal incontinence. Gut 1991;35:857–9.

47. Kumar D, Waldron D, Williams NS, Browning C, Hutton MRE, Wingate DL. Prolonged anorectal manometry and external anal sphincter electromyography in ambulant human subjects. Dig Dis Sci 1990;35:641–8.

48. Ferrara A, Pemberton JH, Grotz RL, Hanson RB. Prolonged ambulatory recording of anorectal motility in patients with slow-transit constipation. Am J Surg 1994;167:73–9.

49. Ferrara A, Pemberton JH, Levin KE, Hanson RB. Relationship between anal canal tone and rectal motor activity. Dis Colon Rectum 1993;36:337–42.

50. Tjandra JJ, Sharma BRK, McKirdy HC, Lowndes RH, Mansel RE. Anorectal physiological testing in defecatory disorders: A prospective study. Aust NZ J Surg 1994;64:322–6.

51. Braun JC, Treutner KH, Dreuw B, Klimaszewski M, Schumpelick V. Vectormanometry for differential diagnosis of fecal incontinence. Dis Colon Rectum 1994;37:989–96.

52. Yang Y-K, Wexner SD. Anal pressure vectography is of no apparent benefit for sphincter evaluation. Int J Colorectal Dis 1994;9:92–5.

53. Perry RE, Blatchford GJ, Christensen MA, Thorson AG, Attwood SEA. Manometric diagnosis of anal sphincter injuries. Am J Surg 1990;159:112–17.

54. Eberi T, Zeller C, Barnert J, Wienbeck M. Anal pressure vectography and transanal ultrasonography: which method is best in anal sphincter assessment? Gastroenterology 1996;110:A659(Abstract).

55. Law PJ, Kamm MA, Bartram CI. A comparison between electromyography and anal endosonography in mapping external anal sphincter defects. Dis Colon Rectum 1990;33:370–3.

56. Burnett SJD, Speakman CTM, Kamm MA, Bartram CI. Confirmation of endosonographic detection of external anal sphincter defects by simultaneous electromyographic mapping. Br J Surg 1991;78:448–50.

57. Felt-Bersma RJF, Cuesta MA, Koorevaar M et al. Anal endosonography: Relationship with anal manometry and neurophysiologic tests. Dis Colon Rectum 1992;35:944–9.

58. Sultan AH, Kamm MA, Talbot IC, Nicholls RJ, Bartram CI. Anal endosonography for identifying external sphincter defects confirmed histologically. Br J Surg 1994;81:463–5.

59. Felt-Bersma RJF, vanBaren R, Koorevaar M, Strijers RLM, Cuesta MA. Unsuspected sphincter defects shown by anal endosonography after anorectal surgery. A prospective study. Dis Colon Rectum 1995;38:249–53.

60. Sun WM, Read NW, Prior A, Daly J-A, Chea SK, Grundy D. Sensory and motor responses to rectal distension vary according to rate and pattern of balloon inflation. Gastroenterology 1990;99:1008–15.

61. Whitehead WE, Schuster MM. Gastrointestinal Disorders: Behavioral and Physiological Basis for Treatment. Orlando, FL: Academic Press, 1985.

62. Mayer EA, Gebhart GF. Basic and clinical aspects of visceral hyperalgesia. Gastroenterology 1994;107:271–93.

63. Prior A, Maxton DG, Whorwell PJ. Anorectal manometry in irritable bowel syndrome: differences between diarrhoea and constipation predominant subjects. Gut 1990;31:458–62.

64. Whitehead WE, Engel BT, Schuster MM. Irritable bowel syndrome. Physiological and psychological differences between diarrhea-predominant and constipation-predominant patients. Dig Dis Sci 1980;25:404–13.

65. Whitehead WE, Holtkotter B, Enck P et al. Tolerance for rectosigmoid distention in irritable bowel syndrome. Gastroenterology 1990;98:1187–92.

66. Buser WD, Miner PBJ. Delayed rectal sensation with fecal incontinence. Gastroenterology 1986;91:1186–91.

67. Sun WM, Donnelly TC, Read NW. Utility of a combined test of anorectal manometry, electromyography, and sensation in determining the mechanism of "idiopathic" faecal incontinence. Gut 1992;33:807–13.

68. Felt-Bersma RJF, Klinkenberg-Knol EC, Meuwissen SGM. Anorectal function investigations in incontinent and continent patients. Dis Colon Rectum 1990;33:479–86.

69. Read NW, Bartolo DCC, Read MG. Differences in anal function in patients with incontinence to solids and in patients with incontinence to liquids. Br J Surg 1984;71:39–42.

70. Sun WM, Read NW, Milner PB, Kerrigan DD, Donnelly TC. The role of transient internal sphincter relaxation in faecal incontinence? Int J Colorectal Dis 1990;5:31–6.

71. Tobon F, Reid NCRW, Talbert JL, Schuster MM. Nonsurgical test for the diagnosis of Hirschsprung's disease. N Engl J Med 1968;278:188–94.

72. Preston DM, Lennard-Jones JE. Anismus in chronic constipation. Dig Dis Sci 1985;30:413–18.

73. Drossman DA, Funch-Jensen P, Janssens J, Talley NJ, Thompson WG, Whitehead WE. Identification of sub-groups of functional gastrointestinal disorders. Gastroenterol Int 1990;3:159–72.

74. Whitehead WE. Functional disorders of the anus and rectum. In: Drossman DA, Richter JE, Talley NJ, Thompson WG, Corazziari E, Whitehead WE, editors. The Functional Gastrointestinal Disorders. Boston: Brown, 1994; 217–63.

75. Kamm MA, Hoyle CHV, Burleigh D et al. Hereditary internal anal sphincter myopathy causing proctalgia fugax and constipation. A newly identified condition. Gastroenterology 1991;100:805–10.

76. Rao SSC, Hatfield RA. Paroxysmal anal hyperkinesis: a characteristic feature of proctalgia fugax. Gut 1996;39:609–12.

77. Whitehead WE, Thompson WG. Motility as a therapeutic modality. In: Schuster MM, editor. Atlas of Gastrointestinal Motility in Health and Disease. Baltimore: Williams & Wilkins, 1994; 300–16.

78. Enck P, Daublin G, Lubke HJ, Strohmeyer G. Long-term efficacy of biofeedback training for fecal incontinence. Dis Colon Rectum 1994;37:997–1001.

79. Enck P. Biofeedback training in disordered defecation: A critical review. Dig Dis Sci 1993;38:1953–60.

80. Mantzikopoulos G, Spiliadis C, Alexacos J et al. Chronic distal constipation evaluated with defecography. Hellenic J Gastroenterol 1991;4:117–24.

81. Womack NR, Williams NS, Holmfield JH, Morrison JF, Simpkins KC. New method for the dynamic assessment of anorectal function in constipation. Br J Surg 1985;72:994–8.

82. Skomorowska E, Henrichsen S, Christiansen J, Hegedus V. Videodefaecography combined with measurement of the anorectal angle and of perineal descent. Acta Radiol Suppl 1987;28:559–62.

13 MRI Studies in the Evaluation of Pelvic Floor Disorders

Marie-Andrée Harvey and Eboo Versi

Introduction

Traditional knowledge of pelvic floor anatomy has been obtained by anatomists working on cadavers and consequently all our information is based on this mode of investigation. However, as a result of the embalming process, anatomic artifacts have been described and consequently our understanding of living anatomy is distorted. Furthermore, because ante-mortem clinical information is often lacking, such studies are limited in their ability to correlate anatomy with functional status.

Recently, with the advent of magnetic resonance imaging (MRI), evaluation of functional anatomy has become possible in the live subject. This tool has become invaluable in the description of live and dynamic anatomy of the pelvic floor. In contrast to radiology and fluoroscopy, this form of investigation permits the evaluation of soft tissue without the risk of radiation exposure and is non-invasive and preferable for the patient. Regrettably, it is very costly. Nonetheless, MRI, when available, has now become the instrument of choice in structural research of pelvic floor disorders. Its actual role in the clinical setting remains limited not only for reasons of cost but also because there is little data supporting its usefulness in clinical decision making.

This chapter will attempt to briefly explain MRI technology. The anatomical information accessed by this technology will be compared with that obtained by histology and other types of imaging studies. Finally, the pathophysiology of pelvic floor support and continence mechanisms will be discussed in the context of this new imaging facility.

MRI Technology at a Glance

MRI uses the natural electromagnetic fields produced by the spinning protons of the atoms present in different tissues of the body [1]. The electric charge of the proton produces an electrical current as the proton rotates within the nucleus of the atom. This electric current in turn induces a magnetic field. This magnetic field assumes random direction (vector) as the atoms themselves may be positioned randomly in space. When a patient is placed in a strong external magnetic field (such as in an MRI machine), the electromagnetic fields (vectors) of the individual atoms align with the external magnetic field.

MRI utilizes a pulse of electromagnetic wave (radio frequency) that disturbs this alignment, changing the magnetic vectors (direction) of the patient's electromagnetic fields (which were aligned parallel to the magnetic field). The pulse is of a brief duration and after this, the magnetic vectors again change towards the initial alignment. The same way an electrical current produces a magnetic field, a shifting magnetic field produces a current. Therefore, as the magnetic field resumes its original alignment, a current is produced (also called the MRI signal) and this is "received" in an "antenna" (the coil).

How does this translate into an image? The rotational speed of the protons within a magnetic field is dependent on the strength of the magnet (given in teslas). The stronger the magnet (greater number of teslas), the faster the rotation (the higher the frequency). By placing the patient in a magnetic field that has different (graded) strength at different

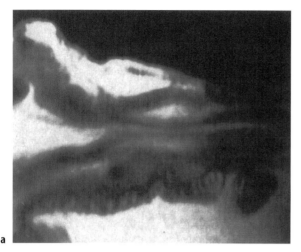

a

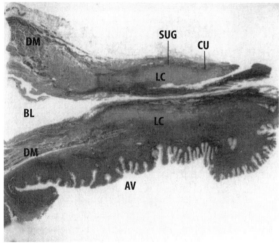

b

Figure 13.1   Midline sagittal T2-weighted MRI image (**a**) and corresponding histologic section (**b**). BL, bladder; DM, detrusor muscle; AV, anterior vaginal wall; LC longitudinal and circular muscles, SUG, striated urogenital muscle; CU compressor urethrae. (From Strohnbehn K et al., Obstet Gynecol 1996;87:752, with permission.)

pendicular) vectors. Each vector is independent. The time it takes the longitudinal vector to resume its original value is named T1 (longitudinal relaxation time). Similarly, the time it takes the transversal vector to vanish as the field resumes its parallel position to the external magnetic field is named T2 (transversal relaxation time). Liquids have a long T1 and T2 time, whereas fat has a short T1 and T2. By varying the time to repeat (TR) of the radio pulses' frequency and direction, we can "T1- or T2-weight" the image, i.e. manipulate the time it takes the two vectors to resume their original positions. Such manipulation results in differences in the intensity of the MR signal received by the coil. This results in the enhancement of the contrast between different tissues, as each tissue contain different atoms, whose protons spin at different frequencies. In a T1-weighted image, fluids tend to be darker than solids, and in T2-weighted images, fluids appear rather white. In this way, tissue contrast is obtained and images are developed with excellent resolution.

Anatomical Studies

A full description of anatomical structures of the pelvic floor can be found in Chapter 3. We will limit our review to the MRI contribution to the fund of current knowledge.

Multiple studies have evaluated the anatomy of the pelvic floor, comparing it to cadaver sections [2–6], confirming previously described structures [3,7,8] or describing new ones [5,7,9,10].

The four layers of the urethra, namely the mucosa, submucosa, smooth muscle and striated muscles, have been visualized with MRI. Strohbhen et al. [4] correlated side by side the MRI images and the histological appearance of a cadaver specimen. T2-weighted images were found to produce the best multilayered urethral soft tissues. The mucosa was bright, circled by submucosa that appeared dark, bright smooth muscle and finally dark striated muscle (Figure 13.1). Others [5,7] have obtained similar results. In addition, Strohbhen et al. [4] compared the MRI appearance of cadavers (pre- and post-fixation), as well as cadavers versus live subjects. The signal characteristics and ring appearance remained constant on subjective evaluation pre- and post-fixation. Findings were also comparable between living subjects and cadavers except for the mucosa, which was darker in the living on T2-weighted images; and the submucosa, which was brighter in the living than the already bright appearance in the cadaver. The urethral volume measured by endorectal coil showed an inverse correlation with advancing age [11].

points, the frequency of rotation of each proton will be different, resulting in an MR signal of different frequency sent to the receiver coil. A location can therefore be assigned for a certain frequency. The computer, by the means of a mathematical process (the Fourier transformation), analyzes how much signal of a specific frequency is received. As each frequency represents a location, the image can be reconstructed.

As the magnetic field vector (originally aligned parallel to the external magnetic field of the MRI) is disturbed by the radio frequency pulses (therefore becoming perpendicular to the MRI magnetic field), its final vector (direction) is the addition of longitudinal (parallel to the MRI field) and transverse (per-

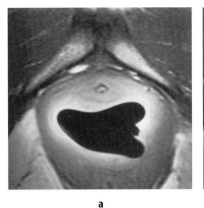 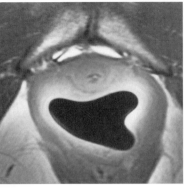 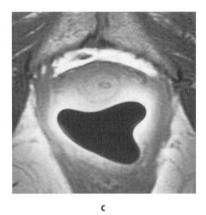

Figure 13.2 Serial T1-weighted axial images from a continent nulliparous woman, from proximal to the urogenital diaphragm (**a**) through the mid-urethra (**c**). (From Aronson MP et al., AM J Obstet Gynecol 1995;173:1707, with permission.)

Furthermore, histologic studies and MRI imaging demonstrated that the urethra and bladder neck were in close apposition with the vaginal mucosa [2,6,7]. This substantiates the hypothesis that the endopelvic fascia, located ventral to the vagina, provides the primary urethral support. This endopelvic fascia is the fused layer between the urethra and vagina and is responsible for the hammock-type of support of the former. That "fascia", composed of connective tissue and smooth muscle, is attached to the arcus tendineus fasciae pelvis, which runs from the posterior aspect of the pubis to the ischial spine on each side. The distal portion of this structure is often referred to as the "posterior pubourethral ligament". Attachment of the endopelvic fascia to the arcus is visible on MRI on T1-weighted axial images [7] (Figure 13.2).

In a study comparing endovaginal (Figure 13.3a) to body coil (Figures 13.3b) imaging, Tan et al. [8] noted that with the endovaginal coil, a sling-like structure ventral to the urethra, connecting it to the levator ani muscle, was shown (Figure 13.3), with a signal intensity suggestive of ligamentous tissue. This structure was named the "urethropelvic sling" by the authors. This could correspond to the compressor urethrae described by DeLancey [12] and identified by us on both supine and erect MRI [13]. Other authors found a similar structure on MRI using endovaginal and endorectal coils [11].

Whether or not there is a connection between the urethra and the levator ani is controversial as some authors have identified it [9] with a 0.3 T magnet and others [14] not even when a 1.5 T magnet and endovaginal coil were used [14]. Histological studies [15] suggest that only the connections between the levator ani and the vagina on one hand, and between the urethra and vagina on the other, control the urethral support, rather than there being a direct con-

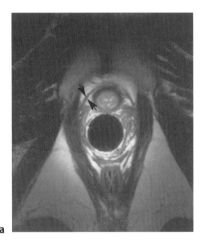

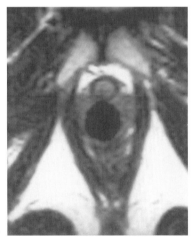

Figure 13.3 Axial T2-weighted slice through the level of the mid-urethra showing an elliptic ligamentous loop running ventral to the urethra (star), the urethropelvic sling (arrows). Note the connection of the sling with the levator ani muscle. **a** Endovaginal coil. **b** Body coil. (From Tan IL et al., MAGMA 1997;5:61, with permission.)

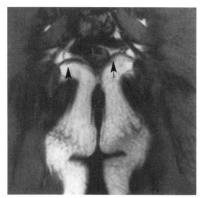

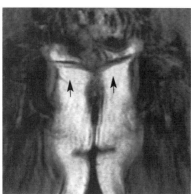

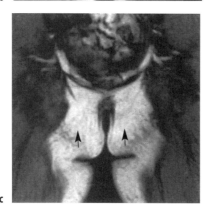

Figure 13.4 MRI coronal image of a female nulliparous pelvic floor at rest (**a**), during a pelvic floor contraction (**b**) and during straining (**c**). (From Hjartardóttir S et al., Acta Obstet Gynecol Scand 1997;76:569, with permission.)

between the urethra/rectum and the vagina is formed by a conglomerate consisting of vascular and connective tissue.

The cardinal and uterosacral ligaments provide support of the uterus and colpos. The cardinal ligaments are not visible on MRI. Histologic studies in fact reveal that the paracervical area is filled with adipose tissue, vessels and nerves and MRI confirms this [2]. The uterosacral ligaments, in contrast, are visible on MRI scanning and on histologic sections [2]. They commence at the lateral margin of the cervix and vault. They run dorsally to connect with the parietal pelvic fascia that covers the sacrospinous ligaments, coccygeus muscle and the presacral space.

The levator ani can also be assessed using MRI scanning [3,9,17]. Although initially described as a basin by anatomists, the actual shape is rather like two contiguous domes at rest (Figure 13.4a) [17]. Axial imaging demonstrates the pubovisceralis muscle, a thick U-shaped muscle, which runs from the posterior aspect of the pubic bone and circles the rectum as a sling. The pubovisceralis muscle is attached to the distal vagina by smooth muscle, collagen and elastin fibers [15], which are visible on MRI [10]. The iliococcygeus muscle, thin and flat, arises from a fibrous band, the arcus tendineus levator ani, which overlies the obturator internus muscle and stretches from the pubic bone to the ischial spine.

Most MRI studies of the pelvic floor have been performed in the supine position. The disadvantage of this is that the effect of gravity on the pelvic floor distorts the tissues posteriorly and the supporting table further compounds this, resulting in their artificial imaging. In recent years, General Electric Medical Systems (Schenectady, NY), in conjunction with researchers at Brigham & Women's Hospital (Boston, MA) have designed a 0.5 T interventional magnet, which allows surgeons to operate under direct MRI guidance. We have proved that such a magnet can permit imaging of the pelvic floor, and have assessed the differences between supine and erect imaging. In a pilot study [13], we have demonstrated that this magnet system can be used to identify pelvic floor structures and that most of these were stable in both positions, with the exception of the posterior urethrovesical angle, which increased significantly in the erect position.

MRI in the Dynamic Evaluation of the Pelvic Floor

Evaluation of the pelvic floor during a pelvic floor muscle contraction and a Valsalva maneuver can provide invaluable information on the dynamics of

nection between the urethra and the levator ani. This has recently been substantiated by DeLancey's team [16]. They reported evidence of urethral support being through a hammock-like structure provided by the attachment of the vaginal sidewalls to the fascia of the levator ani. No proper endopelvic or rectovaginal fascia have been demonstrated on MRI or histological studies. Instead the space support and continence mechanisms. Quantification of normal descent of the pelvic organs associated with a Valsalva was defined by Yang et al. [18]. The bladder base and vaginal cuff/cervix should not descend more that 1 cm below the pubococcygeal line (PCL – line extending from the most inferior portion of the symphysis pubis to the tangent of the coccygeal curve at the last coccygeal joint). The rectum did not descend to more than 2.5 cm below the same reference line. Other authors [19], using the same pubococcygeal line, documented in nulliparous continent women the following maximal descent: the bladder base was located at a distance of 1.1 ± 0.9 cm (mean $\pm$ SD) above the PCL, the cervix, at 2.2 ± 0.5 cm. Finally, these measurements were repeated more recently, with some variability by Law et al. [20]. The mean distance between the bladder base and the PCL at maximal strain was 0 cm, between the cervix and the PCL 0.6 cm, and between the rectum (anorectal angle) and PCL 1.3 cm (i.e. below the PCL).

In studies involving normal volunteers performing a contraction (Kegel), pelvic structures moved anteriorly and cephalad with a narrowing of the retropubic space [17,20,21]. The levator plate reached a position closer to the horizontal. On coronal views, the levator ani lost its double dome appearance, with the muscle reaching a more horizontal position (Figure 13.4b) [17]. The bladder base and upper vagina followed in the same direction. The anorectal angle decreased [22].

During Valsalva, sagittal views of the levator plate revealed an increased inclination towards the vertical, away from the PCL. This inclination, however, was very slight (only 15 degree) [23]. The width of the levator hiatus increased by a mean of 8 mm in nulliparas and the bladder base descended by a mean of 14 mm in these women [17]. The levator assumed a basin shape (Figure 13.4c) and the anorectal angle increased [22]. The uterus was noted to initially move posteriorly, towards the sacrum, then inferiorly onto the levator plate with increasing degree of strain [23]. This further supports the theory that the levator is the main means of support. With maximal Valsalva, the pelvic organs rest on the levator plate [24].

Correlation of MRI with Clinical Findings

Prolapse

Studies correlating physical examination with MRI detection of prolapse are scant, and the quality varies.

Yang et al. [18] reviewed retrospectively the charts of the women who participated in their study on dynamic evaluation of pelvic floor, for evidence of prolapse on physical examination. The prolapse was assessed by compartment (anterior – cystocele, apical – vault/uterine descent, posterior – rectocele) and the authors assumed that a compartment not mentioned in the chart note was devoid of prolapse. The specialty of the examining physician was not systematically recorded but has included internists who may not be used to routinely quantifying prolapse. Out of 26 subjects, they found corroboration with MRI in 20 patients with a clinical cystocele, 24 with an apical descent and 18 with a rectocele. Lienemann et al. [25] reported the presence of prolapse on MRI, compared to clinical evaluation. Out of 46 patients, 33 had on physical examination a cystocele and an equal number a vault prolapse. MRI detected 31 of these 33 cases (94% $\pm$ 4%) for each type of prolapse. Physical examination demonstrated uterine prolapse in 7 patients, all of which were detected on MRI. Including findings at time or surgery (in 8 of the patients), 19 women had a clinical enterocele, of which MRI documented 18 (95% $\pm$ 5%). Finally, 17 subjects presented a rectocele on examination. MRI detected 13 of them (77% $\pm$ 10%). In another study, Goodrich et al. [23] noted that 6 out of 10 women (60% $\pm$ 15%) had a cystocele on physical examination; MRI disclosed them all, plus an additional one. Five women (50% $\pm$ 16%) had a rectocele and three (30% $\pm$ 15%) an enterocele on clinical evaluation. MRI detected all 5 rectoceles plus an additional one, and all 3 enteroceles. Finally four women presented with vault or uterine descent on physical examination and all four were detected on MRI. The degree of prolapse as evaluated by MRI was similar to that of examination in 6 out of 10 for cystocele and rectocele, 9 out of 10 for enterocele and 7 out of 10 for uterine/vault descent. When the grade of prolapse was different from physical examination, MRI showed a greater degree of prolapse in all patients for all four types of prolapse, except for one patient with a cystocele that was downgraded with MRI from grade 2 to grade 1. Notwithstanding the flaws in the methodology employed, these studies suggest that a very good correlation exists between clinical and MRI diagnoses.

More recently, Gousse et al. [26] reported on a study aimed at developing a fast cost-effective MRI assessment for staging prolapse. They studied 100 women (of whom, 65 had symptoms of prolapse and 35 not). They performed a physical examination using the halfway system. Of the women with prolapse, 45 underwent surgical correction. Intraoperative findings were considered the gold standard against which physical examination and

MR were compared. Physical examination was highly sensitive in detecting urethrocele, cystocele, cuff prolapse and rectocele (100, 97, 100, 97%, respectively). Good sensitivity was noted for the detection of uterine prolapse (87%), but physical examination was less sensitive for detecting enterocele (73%). In comparison, MRI had greater sensitivity than physical examination only for enteroceles (87%). It had otherwise equal (urethrocele, cystocele, cuff prolapse) or inferior (uterine prolapse: 83%, rectocele: 76%) sensitivity. The specificity of physical examination was greater for the detection of urethrocele, cystocele, cuff prolapse and enterocele than that of MRI (83 versus 75%, 100 versus 83%, 83 versus 54% and 83 versus 80%, respectively) or equal. In a qualitative comparison pilot study, Tunn et al. [27] evaluated 13 patients (who subsequently underwent surgical repair) by physical examination using the Pelvic Organ Prolapse Quantification (POP-Q) system (International Continence Society, 1996) [28] and with MRI. Physical examination disclosed all pelvic floor defects with the exception of one enterocele, which was picked up on MRI. MRI staging was not performed. Singh et al. [29] sought to establish an MRI grading system which would best correlate with the physical examination (using the POP-Q). They used the mid-pubic line as a proxy of the hymen (which is used as reference line in the POP-Q) and a composite outcome measure made up of the absolute descent measured and of the distance from the mid-pelvic line during maximal strain. Data to establish normality were obtained through MRI from 10 asymptomatic nulliparous patients presumed to be devoid of prolapse. Twenty patients were recruited in this study. Eleven had mild prolapse (POP-Q stage I–II), and 9 had severe prolapse (stage III–IV). MRI correlated with the clinical staging in 15 cases (kappa = 0.61). In 5 cases, the MRI upgraded by one stage the clinical staging. They did not, however, report on the site-specific prolapse findings. In a study aimed specifically at enterocele detection, Lienemann et al. [30] compared MR colpocystorectography (where contrast material in placed in the bladder, vagina and rectum) to physical examination. Physical examination (supine, during maximal strain using a speculum) revealed 43 cases of enteroceles out of 55 patients, compared to 49 cases detected by MRI.

All of these studies provided data supporting the accuracy and sometimes the superiority of physical examination, except for the detection of enterocele. One should note that in none of the studies were patients examined standing, using a bi-digital technique, with one digit in the vagina and the other in the rectum during maximal Valsalva, which is the method of choice for the clinical diagnosis of an enterocele [31]. MRI tended to upgrade the degree of prolapse; however, this could be artifactual since MRI grading uses different landmarks as reference points. Nevertheless, only MRI will provide additional information (over physical examination) such as detailed utero-ovarian anatomy, ureteric dilatation, diverticulum etc. Also, while physical examination may be accurate at detecting a defect in the pelvic floor, MRI can definitely determine which organ occupies the prolapsed bulge.

Studies have looked at comparing different radiological imaging techniques in patients with prolapse. In particular, cystocolpoproctography (also referred to as cystocolpodefecography by certain authors) has been compared. In all studies where the small bowel was opacified by oral barium ingestion, cystocolpoproctography was superior in detecting all the "celes" [32,41] although only marginally in one study [33]. One study, performed specifically to assess the presence of enterocele [30], showed divergent results. The small bowel was not opacified, but the rectum, vagina and bladder were for both examinations. Fluoroscopy was performed in the standing position, rather than sitting as in other publications. The authors reported on the superiority of MR in detecting enterocele over fluoroscopy, as the latter missed 15/34 enteroceles.

Comparison between (bead-chain) cystourethrography and MRI [34] in a study on 27 women with symptoms of stress incontinence, has found very high significant correlation between the two tests for the bladder neck position (r = 0.95) and presence of a cystocele (r = 0.92) during strain. The posterior vesicourethral angle did not significantly correlate with MRI, the latter showing higher angulation.

Anatomical differences between women with and without prolapse have also been the subject of MRI studies. Aronson et al. [7] noted that patients with prolapse tended to have an attenuation or loss of the pubourethral ligaments (also referred to as the most anterior part of the arcus tendineus fasciae pelvis). In addition, paravaginal defects found on physical examination were confirmed on MRI. Furthermore, the levator plate was more vertical (greater angle with PCL), the hiatus wider, and the bladder base and apex showed greater descent than in patients without prolapse [23]. Ozasa et al. [35] documented a change in the levator plate in patients with uterine prolapse compared to normal controls. The former had a levator plate assuming a more vertical orientation.

Stress Incontinence

As in the case of studies of prolapse and its symptomatology, very few articles are published correlating the symptoms of stress incontinence with MRI imaging. Some studies compared anatomical differences between stress incontinent and continent women.

Detailed anatomical differences were noted by Aronson et al. [7], who documented that, compared to continent women (n = 4), stress incontinent subjects (n = 4) presented an attenuation of the pubourethral ligament (distal portion of the arcus tendineus fasciae pelvis that inserts behind the pubis). However, all incontinent women also had prolapse and all continent women did not. Thus, this finding cannot be attributed specifically to either the incontinence or the prolapse. In addition, funneling of the urethra was present in two incontinent subjects.

Kirschner-Hermans et al. [14], comparing 24 women with stress incontinence to 6 healthy volunteers, noted that 66% of the former group showed a loss of the dorsal angle of the levator sling. In addition, 66% of the incontinent women revealed changes thought to be due to muscle degeneration (increased hypodensity on T1-weighted imaging). A study comparing 20 women without symptoms of prolapse or of urinary incontinence to a group of 49 women with such symptoms [36] revealed an increased signal intensity in the levator muscle compared to the internus muscle amongst women with prolapse or incontinence (protons density-weighted images). This was suggestive of a reduction in striated muscle in favor of an increased content of fat and water, according to the authors. However, such findings should be interpreted with caution, as chemical-shift artifacts (artifact arising at the interface of tissues of which one contains predominantly water and fat protons) could influence signal intensity.

Klutke et al. [9] noted in incontinent women the change in the "urethropelvic ligament" (extension originating at the levator muscle from the arcuate line – arcus tendineus fasciae pelvis – to the bladder neck and proximal urethra): they seemed to have lost their attachment to the levator ani. In none of these studies were symptoms correlated with findings.

Various authors reported gross anatomical dissimilarities. Unterweger et al. [19] compared 30 continent (10 nulliparous, 10 previous cesarean delivery, 10 previous vaginal delivery) to 10 stress incontinent women. None were examined for detection of prolapse. Significantly greater bladder and cervical descent on straining was noted in the incontinent group compared to the continent group. The symptom of urinary incontinence, as graded on a visual analogue scale scaled from 0 to 10, did not correlate with the amplitude of either bladder floor

or cervical descent. The authors concluded that the pelvic floor laxity was greater in the stress incontinent group than in continent groups, including the continent women group who had experienced a prior vaginal delivery. No detailed anatomical differences were studied. Other authors reported similar results [21], in addition to describing an increased pelvic floor descent in multiparous compared to nulliparous women. They were also unable to demonstrate a difference between multiparous women before and after the menopause.

Differences between patients with prolapse and those with urinary incontinence were sought by Tunn et al. [27]. No differences between the two groups were detected. Both groups showed a loss of the hammock-like shape of the vagina. Therefore, no MRI criteria to date can differentiate stress incontinent women from women with prolapse.

Only one study correlated different MRI and urodynamic parameters [27]. The authors found no correlation between any of the MRI criteria and urethral closure pressure at rest or pressure transmission.

MRI in Intervention Studies

A few studies looked specifically at pre- versus postoperative changes on MRI. Goodrich et al. [23] studied five women with clinical pelvic floor relaxation preoperatively. Surgical procedures were not described. On physical examination, all postoperative patients no longer showed signs of prolapse. On MRI, the pelvic organs returned to a more anatomically normal position postoperatively, both at rest and with Valsalva. Nonetheless, the levator plate became more inclined towards the vertical than preoperatively, the hiatus was wider, and the urethrovesical angle at strain was decreased (Figure 13.5).

Huddleston et al. [37] studied 12 patients with anatomic stress incontinence (hypermobility) on urodynamic studies. All 12 patients had a cystocele. Clinical evaluation of paravaginal defect was not reported. Preoperative MRI was performed and revealed bilateral paravaginal defects on all 12 subjects. At time of surgery, the presence of the paravaginal defects was noted. The operative finding of a paravaginal defect was found in all patients with such defects noted on MRI. It is unknown whether the surgeon was blinded to the results of the MRI study. Postoperatively (surgical procedure unreported), MRI demonstrated a disappearance of the defects in three women, with a cure of their stress incontinence and reduction of cystocele on clinical examination. In two patients postoperatively, MRI

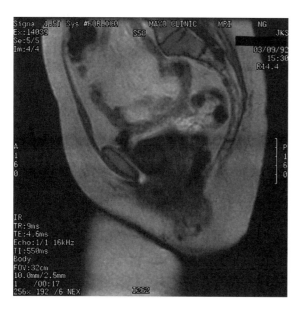

Figure 13.5 Postoperative scan of patient at maximal strain. Although the plane of the levator plate is vertical, there was no sign of pelvic floor dysfunction after surgical repair, based on either physical examination of MRI. (From Goodrich MA et al., Obstet Gynecol 1993;82:883--91, with permission.)

detected persistence of defects and this correlated with a clinically persistent cystocele.

The effect of periurethral collagen injection at the bladder neck in women with stress incontinence was evaluated using MRI [38]. Thirty-two women were studied at a median of 12 months post-injection. MRI easily imaged collagen. Neither volume nor position of retained collagen was predictive of clinical outcome. The mean retained volume of collagen (2.4 ml) was 25% of the mean injected volume (9.7 ml).

Magnetic resonance imaging was also used to depict postoperative anatomy and function following sacrocolpopexy [39]. No preoperative physical or MRI examinations are reported. Sacrocolpopexy was the sole surgery performed on the 25 women although attachment of the mesh differed if an anterior wall (ventral attachment) or posterior wall (dorsal attachment) were present. The mesh attachment site could be identified on the vagina and on the sacrum. Half the women had the mesh fixed at the level of S2, others at S1 and S3. The vaginal axis was on average at an angle of 142° (presumably from the pubococcygeal line). The mesh could be visualized entirely in most patients. On physical examination, recurrent prolapse (site unspecified) was found in 15 women (most with stage I, but 3 women had stage III vaginal vault prolapse). MRI found a mean apex position at rest of +3.8 cm from the pubococcygeal line, and of +2.2 cm with strain (range +4.7

to −3.2 cm – a negative value indicates a prolapse below the pubococcygeal line). Direct comparison of mean descent or staging between physical examination and MRI was not performed.

A French group evaluated the anatomical modifications induced by an intravaginal continence device (IVD – Temporella, Biogyne Groupe Poli, France) in a pilot study on 10 women with symptom of stress incontinence [40]. This device oval-shaped, devised as a space-occupying apparatus to relieve stress incontinence. Self inserted, all IVDs were located underneath the bladder base, above the levator plate. The IVD resulted in a statistically significant elevation of the bladder neck (using the pubococcygeal line as reference) both at rest and during strain. It brought the urethra and bladder neck upward and forward, towards the pubic bone. The IVD produced a 0.7 cm elevation at rest and 1.5 cm during strain.

Kaufman et al. evaluated whether or not MRI testing affected surgical management [41]. Detection of levator ani hernias, for which the clinical significance is unknown but appears to be associated with obstructed defecation, was the one defect that was specifically picked up by MRI. Consequently, the authors modified the surgery to include correction of this defect.

MRI in Postpartum Studies

Few published reports evaluated the changes in pelvic floor immediately after vaginal delivery. In the first reported study [42], 14 women (6 primigravidas, 8 multigravidas) were recruited for the prospective evaluation of the involuting uterus following vaginal delivery. Supine MRI was done at rest within 30 hours of delivery, at 1, 2 and 6 weeks as well as at 6 months after delivery. Measurements between several anatomical landmarks (urethra, vaginal, anus) and the symphysis pubis, urethrovesical angle and vaginal, urethral and anal length were taken in sagittal and axial views. Only the distance between the symphysis and the distal vagina showed a statistical change over time, but no clear trend in any direction (decreased or increase) was noted. No comparison was made between primi- and multigravidas or with nulliparas.

In a pilot study (data not published), we have shown the differences between a group of nulliparas (n = 9) and a group of primiparas (n = 5), at rest and with Valsalva, using a 0.5T interventional MRI. Such MRI allows positioning in the sitting position, thus allowing the normal gravity effect on the pelvic floor. All primiparas had a vaginal delivery. In brief, we noted a significant increased distance between the pubis and the bladder neck in primigravidas compared to nulligravidas at rest. The distance between the bladder neck and the pubococcygeal line was smaller is primigravidas (i.e. the bladder neck was lower in absolute terms) than in nulliparas. Of interest, the contour of the left levator ani was more commonly found to be irregular in postpartum subjects, possibly suggesting a detachment of the levator ani from its insertion site.

More recently, DeLancey's group [43] reviewed images obtained during studies aimed at assessing the uterine involution in the postpartum period [42,44]. They found chemical changes within the levator ani, which could be related to muscular structure damage (such as edema, change in fat content, infarction, and denervation), 1 day postpartum with only partial recovery by 6 months. The delay in recovery of the chemical changes may help in future studies to deduce what type of injury is responsible for each type of damage (denervation, direct muscular damage). Furthermore, they noted an increase in the urogenital hiatus, which correlated with midline episiotomy use and birthweight (only at 1 day postpartum for the latter), but not with parity. The size of the urogenital and levator ani hiatus decreased significantly in the 2 weeks following childbirth, which implies a return to levator ani geometry (provided by the resting tone of the striated muscles) as early as 2 weeks postpartum. However, the posterior displacement of the sagging perineal body during the postpartum period persisted for up to 6 months, suggesting a delayed recovery of connective tissue remodeling.

MRI Use in Anorectal Diseases

Magnetic resonance imaging techniques have been more extensively used in the study of anorectal anatomy [45–49], its diseases such as fecal incontinence or constipation [50,51], and in comparative study with other testing [46] and imaging techniques [25,52].

A controversy surrounds the anatomy of the anal sphincters, with the external sphincter being divided into one [53], two [54] or three parts [55] or not at all [56] on histological studies. MR imaging using body coil [48] documented two distinct muscle masses that were noted on histological sections: the first one, dorsal and cranial, corresponded to the puborectalis muscle. The second, more caudal, represented the combination of the subcutaneous and deep part of the external anal canal, which could not be distinguished. The authors

reported difficulties in identifying the internal sphincter due to lack of contrast in signal intensity, a difficulty encountered by other authors [49]. Gross anatomy was described from MRI done in continent nulliparous women [45,46] and in continent healthy volunteers (men and women) [49]. The mean anterior sphincter length was 28 mm in the first study and 22.6 mm in the second. The mean posterior sphincter length was 31.5 mm and 27.3 mm, respectively. In both, the internal sphincter was noted to represent approximately 50% of the total thickness. More detailed anatomical description was not reported. The mean thickness of the internal sphincter was 1.72 mm and that of the external sphincter, 3.99 mm. Inter-observer agreement was high for the external sphincter but low for the internal one.

Anal anatomy has been further evaluated by means of endoanal MR studies. Hussain et al. [47], in an MRI study using an endoanal receive coil, noted the length of the anterior anal canal to be 36 mm, and that of the posterior canal, 42 mm. The internal anal sphincter was visible as the continuation of the circular smooth muscle of the rectum. Average thickness was 2.5 mm. A longitudinal muscle layer was then visualized, with an average thickness of 1.3 mm, as a continuation of the outer longitudinal smooth muscle of the rectum. The external anal sphincter was noted only in the lower part of the anal canal, with an average anterior length of 18 mm and a posterior length of 19 mm. It appeared to have a varying degree of septation. Cranial to the external sphincter, the puborectalis muscle was noted to complete the anal canal, with a length of 23 mm. These findings were corroborated in another study using an endoanal coil [57]. In addition, the latter study described the external sphincter as consisting of a subcutaneous, a superficial and a deep part. This is consistent with a study evaluating the sphincter anatomy on cadaveric sections of anal sphincters [48] compared with MRI of anal canal in the living; a clear subcutaneous and deep portions of the external anal sphincter were identified on anatomical sections. Furthermore, no age-related differences in the lengths of the anal canal, external sphincter and puborectal muscle were found. However, women had a significant increase in thickness of the internal but a decrease of the longitudinal muscles with advancing age. Non-significant decreases in external sphincter thickness were noted.

Morphological studies of the anal sphincters have yielded inconsistent results (Table 13.1). Part of the difference encountered in morphometry was the imaging technique, where Aronson et al. [45] and Fenner et al. [46] used external receive coils and Hussain et al. [47] used an endoanal receive coil

Table 13.1 Anal canal morphometric measurements in different studies [45–47]

	Length (mm)		Width (thickness; mm)		Proportion of thickness attributed to internal sphincter (%)	
	Anterior	Posterior	Anterior	Posterior	Anterior	Posterior
Aronson et al. [45]	28	31.5	18.3	25.8	45	49
Fenner et al. [46]	22.6	27.3	15.6	34.3	56–58	28–39
Hussain et al. [47]	36	42	6.3	19.8	60	20

which could have resulted in a thinning effect. In addition, the first two studies included only female subjects, whereas the third pooled results from male and female volunteers. All the studies were small, with 10 or fewer subjects. However, recently a relationship between atrophic findings on MR and histologically demonstrated atrophy was documented [58]. Such atrophy on MR has been associated with impaired continence following sphincteroplasty, with patient's outcome being significantly better in patients without atrophy (92% versus 26%) [59]. Atrophy of the external sphincter was described as extreme thinning of its fibers or generalized fatty infiltration.

Two studies looked at anorectal symptoms and MRI findings [50,51]. Healy et al. [50] compared the incidence of prolapse and anorectal descent evaluated on MRI to anorectal symptomatology in three groups: constipation and straining (group 1, n = 10), women with fecal incontinence (group 2, n = 10) and asymptomatic women (group 3, n = 10). Constipated women had a greater incidence of prolapse on MRI than fecally incontinent women or asymptomatic women, but there was no difference between fecally incontinent women and asymptomatic women. Anorectal junction descent was greater in women with constipation than in asymptomatic women, but the same as in women with fecal incontinence. Women with fecal incontinence also had a greater degree of anorectal junction descent when compared to asymptomatic women.

In another study, Healy et al. [51] compared women with obstructed defecation (straining, incomplete emptying and perineal digital manipulation) to asymptomatic women using MRI and normal evacuation proctography and anorectal physiology tests. They found no difference at rest. However, with straining, symptomatic women had a greater descent of the bladder base, uterocervical and anorectal junction than asymptomatic women, a wider pelvic floor hiatus, a more acute anorectal angle and an increased levator plate angle with the pubococcygeal line.

Correlation of MRI findings with anal manometry [46] showed a positive correlation between the mean posterior sphincter length measured on MRI and the mean high-pressure zone length with squeeze recorded on manometry. This high-pressure zone represents the continence zone. The sphincter thickness did not correlate with manometric pressures. In a more recent study [60], cross-sectional external anal sphincter area, measured on MRI, was found to correlate with maximal squeeze pressure. This study also evaluated correlation with pudendal nerve terminal motor latencies, and the latter was not found to correlate with squeeze pressure, percentage fat content in the external sphincter or mean external sphincter area. Other authors did not find a similar correlation [61].

MRI has been compared to fluoroscopic defecography [22] and standard evacuation proctography [52] in patients with constipation. Schoenenberger et al. [22] evaluated 15 patients with chronic constipation using fluoroscopic defecography and MRI defecography in a 0.5 T open-configuration magnet which allows imaging in the sitting position. The standard of reference for the diagnosis was the combined result of the history, physical examination, laboratory studies and imaging (fluoroscopy and MRI) data. The anorectal angle correlated very well ($R^2 = 0.984$) between the fluoroscopic and MRI measurement. Pathologies could be multiple in any given patients, with 19 pathologies present in total (rectocele, spastic pelvic floor syndrome, intussusception, descending perineum syndrome, prostatitis, rectal prolapse and stenosis, and hypertrophic puborectalis muscle). Fluoroscopic defecography missed 4 pathologic conditions out of the 19, thus detecting 79% of the pathologies present. MRI, on the other hand, showed all but one (95%) of the pathologies.

Healy et al. [52] compared parameters of anorectal configuration by standard proctography and by MRI in 10 women experiencing difficulty with defecation. They found no correlation of any parameters at rest. During straining, the measurement on MRI of the rectal axis (angle formed by the longitudinal axis of the anal canal and the longitudinal axis of the rectum), the anorectal junction descent and the anorectal angle change correlated significantly

($r = 0.62$, 0.7 and 0.78, respectively) with standard proctography.

Finally, in a comparative study of normal anatomy between MRI and anal endosonography imaging on 8 normal volunteers, Schäfer et al. [49] demonstrated a significant correlation ($r = 0.818$) between the muscle thickness (MRI) and the muscle diameter (sonography). However, as with prior anatomic studies of the anal canal using a body coil [45,46], MRI could not differentiate between mucosa, submucosa and internal anal canal, whereas this was possible with high-resolution sonography. Malouf and co-workers performed a comparison of anal sonogram with endoanal MRI in 52 patients with fecal incontinence, using clinical consensus as the gold standard (based on symptoms, trauma, clinical examination and anorectal physiologic testing) [60]. Complete agreement was found in only 62% of the patients. They concluded that MRI was equivalent in the diagnosis of external anal sphincter injury, but MR imaging was inferior in diagnosing internal anal sphincter injury. This is in slight contrast to findings reported by another group [62]. Using surgical finding as the gold standard, these authors reported that MR and ultrasound detected 10/12 defects of the internal sphincter and respectively 12 and 11 out of 13 external defects. However, MRI was superior in detecting sphincter thinning (suggestive of atrophy).

MRI and Three-dimensional Reconstruction Studies

The original study reporting on the use of computer-generated three-dimensional (3D) reconstruction was applied to a cadaver specimen [3]. Topography of the muscles was reconstructed to demonstrate the topography of the levator ani.

The first study of the application of pelvic floor 3D modeling in the live subject was performed by Lennox Hoyte's group [63]. This group studied 10 young nulliparous women using a 1.5 T magnet and external coil. Two-dimensional images were recorded, then the information was segmented into anatomical components using manual editing. Then integrated software produced the 3D reconstructed image. Levator ani volume was then measured. The combined volume of the coccygeus, puborectalis and iliococcygeus was 46.6 ± 5.9 ml, with a range between 39 and 57 ml, and this was not associated with body mass index.

More recently, the same group [64] found in a pilot study that there seemed to be a relationship between levator volume and pelvic floor dysfunction diagnosis. Volume was lowest in the woman with prolapse and highest in the continent female. In a follow-up study [65], the authors compared three groups of 10 women. The first groups were controls – no symptoms of incontinence or prolapse; the second group was incontinent– symptomatic of stress incontinence and with documented genuine stress incontinence on urodynamic studies, with no prolapse on examination; the third group had prolapse – anterior wall prolapse protruding beyond introitus, with symptoms of prolapse. Their results were similar to that found in their pilot study. Controls had a mean levator volume of 32.2 (± 7.0) cm³, subjects with genuine stress incontinence had a mean volume of 23.2 (± 5.8) cm³ and subjects with prolapse had a mean volume of 18.4 (± 7.7) cm³. Although the mean volumes were significantly different, there was overlapping in the range of levator ani volume found between the three groups. The study suggested that levator ani mass either plays a role in female pelvic floor dysfunction or it is impacted by dysfunction of the latter.

Conclusion

MRI opens up tremendous research opportunities in imaging of the pelvic floor. Elucidation of the mechanisms of diseases such as pelvic floor dysfunction and stress incontinence are still in their infancy and correlation with symptoms, physical finding and urodynamic testing almost non-existent. For these reasons, MRI remains, for now, part of the investigational armamentarium and should be used in well-designed research protocols and not for clinical evaluation.

References

1. Schild HH. MRI made easy (… well almost). Berlex Laboratories: Wayne, NJ. 1994.
2. Fritsch J, Hötzinger H. Tomographical anatomy of the pelvis, visceral pelvic connective tissue, and its compartments. Clin Anat 1995;8:17–24.
3. Strohbhen K, Ellis JH, Strohbhen JA, DeLancey JOL. Magnetic resonance imaging of the levator ani with anatomic correlation. Obstet Gynecol 1996;87:277–85.
4. Strohbhen K, Quint LE, Prince MR, Wojno KJ, DeLancey JOL. Magnetic resonance imaging anatomy of the female urethra: A direct histologic comparison. Obstet Gynecol 1996;88:8750–6.
5. Tan IL, Stoker J, Zwamborn AW, Entius KAC, Calame JJ, Laméris JS. Female pelvic floor: Endovaginal MR imaging of normal anatomy. Radiology 1998;206:777–83.
6. Fauconnier A, Delmas V, Lassau JP, Boccon-Gibod L. Ventral tethering of the vagina and its role in the kinetics of urethra and bladder-neck straining. Surg Radiol Anat 1996;18:81–7.

7. Aronson MP, Bates SM, Jacoby AF, Chelmow D, Sant GR. Periurethral and paravaginal anatomy: An endovaginal magnetic resonance imaging study. Am J Obstet Gynecol 1995;173:1702–10.

8. Tan IL, Stoker J, Laméris JS. Magnetic resonance imaging of the female pelvic floor and urethra: body coil versus endovaginal coil. MAGMA 1997;5:59–63.

9. Klutke C, Golomb J, Barbaric Z, Raz S. The anatomy of stress incontinence: magnetic resonance imaging of the female bladder neck and urethra. J Urol 1990;143:563–6.

10. Tunn R, Fischer W, Paris ST. MR imaging study of birth-related changes in the attachment between the vagina and the pubococcygeus muscle. Urogyneecol Int J 1998;12:57–61.

11. Nurenberg P, Forte TB, Zimmern PE. Etude de l'anatomie urétrale et du plancher pelvien pr IRM avec antenne de surface et antenne endorectale. Progrès en Urologie 2000;10:224–30.

12. DeLancey JOL. Anatomy and physiology of urinary incontinence. Clin Obstet Gynecol 1990;33:298–307.

13. Fielding JR, Versi E, Mulkern RV, Lerner MH, Griffiths DJ, Jolesz FA. MR imaging of the female pelvic floor in the supine and upright positions. JMRI 1996;6:961–3.

14. Kirschner-Hermans R, Wein B, Niehaus S, Schaefer W, Jakse G. The contribution of magnetic resonance imaging of the pelvic floor to the understanding of urinary incontinence. Br J Urol 1993;72:715–18.

15. DeLancey JOL, Starr RA. Histology of the connection between the vagina and levator ani muscle. J Reprod Med 1990;35:765–71.

16. Tunn R, DeLancey JOL, Quint EE. Visibility of pelvic organ support system structures in magnetic resonance images without an endovaginal coil. Am J Obstet Gynecol 2001;184:1156–63.

17. Hjartardottir S, Nilsson J, Petersen C, Lingman G. The female pelvic floor: A dome – not a basin. Acta Obstet Gynecol Scand 1997;76:567–71.

18. Yang A, Mostwin JL, Rosenshein NB, Zerhouni EA. Pelvic floor descent in women: Dynamic evaluation with fast MR imaging and cinematic display. Radiology 1991;179:25-33.

19. Unterweger M, Marincek B, Gottstein-Aalame N et al. Ultrafast MR imaging of the pelvic floor. AJR Am J Roentgenol 2001;176:959–63.

20. Law PQ, Danin JC, Lamb GM, Regan L, Darzi A, Gedroyc WM. Dynamic imaging of the pelvic floor using an open-configuration magnetic resonance scanner. J Magn Reson Imaging 2001;13:923–9.

21. Christensen LL, Djurhuus JC, Constantinou CE. Imaging of pelvic floor contractions using MRI. Neurourol Urodyn 1995;14:209–16.

22. Schoenenberger AW, Debatin JF, Guldenschuh I, Hany TF, Steiner P, Krestin GP. Dynamic MR defecography with a superconducting, open-configuration MR system. Radiology 1998;206:641–6.

23. Goodrich MA, Webb MJ, King BF, Bampton AEH, Campeau NG, Riederer SJ. Magnetic resonance imaging of pelvic floor relaxation: Dynamic analysis and evaluation of patients before and after surgical repair. Obstet Gynecol 1993;82:883–91.

24. DeLancey JOL. Anatomy and biomechanics of genital prolapse. Clin Obstet Gynecol 1993;36:897–909.

25. Lienemann A, Anthuber C, Baron A, Kohz P, Reiser M. Dynamic MR colpocystorectography assessing pelvic floor descent. Eur Radiol 1997;7:1309–17.

26. Gousse AE, Barbaric ZL, Safir MH, Madjar S, Marumoto AK, Raz S. Dynamic half Fourier acquisition, single shot turbo spin-echo magnetic resonance imaging for evaluating the female pelvis. J Urol 2000;164:1606–13.

27. Tunn R, Paris ST, Taupitz M, Hamm B, Fisher W. MR imaging in post-hysterectomy vaginal prolapse. Int Urogynecol J 2000;11:87–92.

28. Bump RC, Mattiasson A, Bo K Brubaker LP, DeLancey JOL, Klarskov P. The standardization of terminology of female pelvic organ prolapse and pelvic floor dysfunction. Am J Obstet Gynecol 1996;175:10–17.

29. Singh K, Reid WMN, Berger LA. Assessment and grading of pelvic organ prolapse by use of dynamic magnetic resonance imaging. Am J Obstet Gynecol 2001;185:71–7.

30. Lienemann A, Anthuber C, Baron A, Reiser M. Diagnosing enteroceles using dynamic magnetic resonance imaging. Dis Colon Rectum 2000;43:205–13.

31. Nichols DH. Enterocele and massive eversion of the vagina. In: Thompson JD, Rock JA, editors. Te Linde's Operative Gynecology, 7th edn. Philadelphia: JB Lippincott, 1992; 862.

32. Vanbeckvoort D, Van Hoe L, Oyen R, Ponette E, De Ridder D, Deprest J. Pelvic floor descent in females: Comparative study of colpocystodefecography and dynamic fast MR imaging. J Magn Reson Imaging 1999;9:373–7.

33. Kelvin FM, Maglinte DDT, Hale DS, Benson JT. Female pelvic organ prolapse: A comparison of triphasic dynamic MR imaging and triphasic fluoroscopic cystocolpoproctography. AJR Am J Roentgenol 2000;174:81–8.

34. Gufler H, DeGregorio G, Allmann K-H, Kundt G, Dohnicht S. Comparison of cystourethrography and dynamic MRI in bladder neck descent. J Comput Assist Tomogr 2000;24:382–8.

35. Ozasa H, Mori T, Togashi K. Study of uterine prolapse by magnetic resonance imaging: Topographical changes involving the levator ani muscle and the vagina. Gynecol Obstet Invest 1992;34:43–8.

36. Tunn R, Paris S, Fisher W, Hamm B, Kuchinke J. Static magnetic resonance imaging of the pelvic floor muscle morphology in women with stress incontinence and pelvic prolapse. Neurourol Urodyn 1998;17:579–89.

37. Huddleston HT, Dunnihoo DR, Huddleston III PM, Meyers PC. Magnetic resonance imaging of defects in DeLancey's vaginal support levels I, II and III. Am J Obstet Gynecol 1995;172:1778–84.

38. Carr LK, Herschorn S, Leonhardt C. Magnetic resonance imaging after intraurethral collagen injected for stress urinary incontinence. J Urol 1996;155:1253–5.

39. Lienemann A, Sprencer D, Anthuber C, Baron A, Reiser M. Functional cine magnetic resonance imaging in women after abdominal sacrocolpopexy. Obstet Gynecol 2001;97:81–5.

40. Maubon AJ, Boncoeur-Martel MP, Juhan V et al. Static and dynamic MRI of a urinary control intra-vaginal device. Eur Radiol 2000;10:879–84.

41. Kaufman HS, Buller JL, Thompson JR et al. Dynamic pelvic magnetic resonance imaging and cystocolpoproctography alter surgical management of pelvic floor disorders. Dis Colon Rectum 2001;44:1575-84.

42. Hayat SK, Thorp JM, Kuller JA, Brown BD, Semelka RC. Magnetic resonance of the pelvic floor in the post-partum patient. Int Urogynecol J 1996;7:321–4.

43. Tunn R, DeLancey JOL, Howard D, Thorp JM, Ashton-Miller JA, Quint LE. MR imaging of levator ani muscle recovery following vaginal delivery. Int Urogynecol J 1999;10:300–7.

44. Willms AB, Brown ED, Kettritz UI, Kuller JA, Semelka RC. Anatomic changes in the pelvis after uncomplicated vaginal delivery: evaluation with serial MR imaging. Radiology 1995;195:91–4.

45. Aronson MP, Lee RA, Berquist TH. Anatomy of anal sphincters and related structures in continent women studied with magnetic resonance imaging. Obstet Gynecol 1990;76:846–51.

46. Fenner DE, Kriegshauser JS, Lee HH, Beart RW, Weaver A, Cornella JL. Anatomic and physiologic measurements of the internal and external anal sphincters in normal females. Obstet Gynecol 1998;91:369–74.

47. Hussain SM, Stoker J, Laméris JS. Anal sphincter complex: Endoanal MR imaging of normal anatomy. Radiology 1995;197:671–7.

48. Peschers UM, DeLancey JOL, Fritsch H, Quint LE, Prince MR. Cross-sectional imaging anatomy of the anal sphincters. Obstet Gynecol 1997;90:839–44.

49. Schäfer A, Enck P, Fürst G, Kahn T, Frieling T, Lübke HJ. Anatomy of the anal sphincter. Comparison of anal endosonography to magnetic resonance imaging. Dis Colon Rectum 1994;37:777–81.

50. Healy JC, Halligan S, Reznek RH, Watson S, Phillips RKS, Armstrong P. Patterns of prolapse in women with symptoms of pelvic floor weakness: Assessment with MR imaging. Radiology 1997;203:77–81.

51. Healy JC, Halligan S, Reznek RH, Watson S, Bartram CI, Kamm MA, Phillips RKS, Armstrong P. Magnetic resonance imaging of the pelvic floor in patients with obstructed defecation. Br J Surg 1997;84:1555–8.

52. Healy JC, Halligan S, Reznek RH, Watson S, Bartram CI, Phillips R, Armstrong P. Dynamic MR imaging compared with evacuation proctography when evaluating anorectal configuration and pelvic floor movement. AJR Am J Roentgenol 1997;169:775–9.

53. Ayoub SF. Anatomy of the external anal sphincter in men. Acta Anat 1979;105:25–36.

54. Oh C, Kark AE. Anatomy of the external anal sphincter. Br J Surg 1972;59:717–23.

55. Milligan ETC, Morgan CN. Surgical anatomy of the anal canal with special reference to anorectal fistula (I). Lancet 1934;ii:1150–6.

56. Golingher J. Surgery of the Anus, Rectum and Colon, 2nd edn. London: Baillière Tindall, 1967.

57. Rociu E, Stoker J, Eijkemans MJC, Laméris JS. Normal anal sphincter anatomy and age- and sex-related variations at high-spatial-resolution endoanal MR imaging. Radiology 2000;217:395–401.

58. Briel JW, Zimmerman DDE, Stoker J et al. Relationship between sphincter morphology on endoanal MRI and histopathological aspects of the external anal sphincter. Int J Colorectal Dis 2000;15:87–90.

59. Briel JW, Stoker J, Rociu E, Laméris JS, Hop WC, Schouten WR. External anal sphincter atrophy on endoanal magnetic resonance imaging adversely affects continence after sphincteroplasty. Br J Surg 1999;86:1322–7.

60. Williams AB, Malouf AJ, Bartram CI, Hallign S, Kamm MA, Kmiot WA. Assessment of external anal sphincter morphology in idiopathic fecal incontinence with endocoil magnetic resonance imaging. Dig Dis Sci 2001;46:1466–71.

61. Zbar AP, Kmiot WA, Aslam M et al. Use of vector manometry and endoanal magnetic resonance imaging in the adult female for assessment of anal sphincter dysfunction. Dis Colon Rectum 1999;42:1411–18.

62. Rociu E, Stoker J, Eijkemans MJC, Schouten WR, Laméris JS. Fecal incontinence: Endoanal US versus endoanal MR imaging. Radiology 1999;212:453–8.

63. Fielding JR, Dumanli H, Schreyer G et al. MR-based three-dimensional modeling of the normal pelvic floor in women: Quantification of muscle mass. AJR Am J Roentgenol 2000;174:657–60.

64. Hoyte L, Fielding JR, Versi E et al. MR-based three-dimensional modeling of levator ani: First studies of muscle volume and geometry in living women with normal GU function, prolapse and genuine stress incontinence. Arch Esp Urol 2001;54(6):532-539.

65. Hoyte L, Schierlitz L, Zou K, Flesh G, Fielding JR. Two- and 3-dimensional MRI comparison of levator ani structure, volume and integrity in women with stress incontinence and prolapse. Am J Obstet Gynecol 2001; 185:11–19.

14 Pelvic Floor Neurophysiologic Testing

Dana Soroka and Harold P. Drutz

Bladder Function

The two functions of the bladder are urine storage at low pressure without leaking and periodic evacuation; these are under the control of the peripheral, autonomic and central nervous systems.

Urine Storage

The storage of urine is under the control of the sympathetic nervous system. There is a continuous tonic stimulation to the urethra (smooth muscle) via α-adrenergic receptors of the sympathetic nervous system. In addition, there is an added voluntary tone exerted by the external urethra (striated muscle) and the levator ani muscles for short bursts via the pudendal nerve and the sacral reflex. The final urethra continence mechanism is coaptation of the urethra due to the urethral vascular plexus (Figures 14.1 and 14.2).

These mechanisms are further enhanced by progesterone stimulation of β-receptors of the bladder and estrogen stimulates the α-receptors of the urethra.

The detrusor muscle is inhibited via β-adrenergic receptors stimulation to allow the bladder to fill without increasing intravesical pressure (i.e. accommodation) (Figures 14.1 and 14.2).

Bladder Emptying

Once bladder volume reaches maximum capacity and the intravesical pressure <15–20 mmH$_2$O, the receptors within the detrusor muscles signal higher cortical centers to initiate bladder emptying (Figures 14.1 and 14.2).

In order for the bladder to empty intravesical pressure must exceed intraurethral pressure. This requires the parasympathetic coordination of ure-

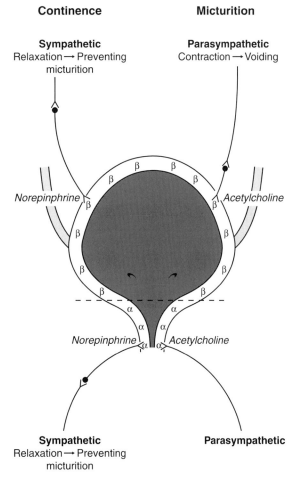

Figure 14.1 Voiding loops. (Reproduced with permission from Herst AL et al., editors. Comprehensive Gynecology. Mosby Year Book, 1992.)

159

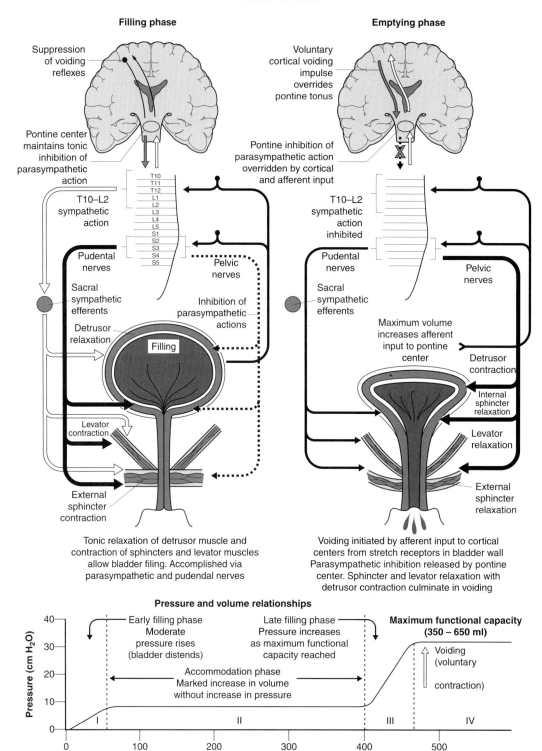

Figure 14.2   Micturition and urine storage. (Reproduced with permission from Retzky SS and Rogers RM. Clinical Symposia. Ciba 1996 November 2.)

Table 14.1 The four basic loops controlling bladder function

Loop I originates in the frontal lobe and terminates in the brainstem where it modifies input from loop II. Lesions in this loop leads to detrusor hyperreflexia with urinary frequency, urgency and diurnal urge incontinence [2]. Diseases associated with lesions of this pathway include cerebrovascular disease, brain tumors, Parkinson's disease, multiple system atrophy and multiple sclerosis.

Loop II originates in the bladder wall (detrusor muscle) and the sacral micturition center (spinal cord) and terminates in the brainstem detrusor nucleus (brainstem). The signal from this loop is inhibited by loop I or stimulates loop III. Loop II facilitates the emptying of the bladder by maintenance and amplification of the detrusor contraction. Complete interruption to this loop leads to urinary retention, partial lesions lead to incomplete emptying [3]. Disorders associated with interruption of this pathway include spinal cord trauma and multiple sclerosis.

Loop III: sensory afferents in the bladder wall (detrusor muscle) go to the sacral micturition center (spinal cord) then to the spinal pudendal motor nucleus with motor fibers which terminate in the striated urethral sphincter to allow relaxation of urethra at time of detrusor contraction (i.e. coordinates urethral contraction immediately prior to detrusor contraction). Lesions affecting this loop lead to detrusor sphincter dyssynergia, incomplete emptying and intermittent voiding [4]. Defects associated with interference of the neuronal pathway include spinal trauma, tethered cord syndrome, multiple sclerosis, diabetic neuropathy, tabes dorsalis and pernicious anemia.

Loop IV originates in the frontal lobe (cerebral cortex) to the pudendal nucleus (spinal sacral micturition center) and terminates in the urethral striated muscle and allows volitional control of the striated urethral sphincter during the storage phase of urine and voiding. Lesions affecting this loop will lead to maintenance of urethral tone with loss of voluntary control [2]. Diseases associated with lesions include cerebrovascular disease, brain tumors, multiple system atrophy, spinal cord trauma and multiple sclerosis.

thral relaxation followed closely by detrusor contraction (Figures 14.1 and 14.2).

There are four basic loops which coordinate bladder function [1] (Table 1; Figure 14.3).

Neurophysiologic Focused Lower Urinary Tract Assessment

When assessing the bladder it is important to start with a history and physical examination.

History

A full history of the present illness should be obtained, with emphasis on the onset and evolution of the symptoms, as well as a full medical and medication history. It is also important to take a full bowel and sexual function history.

Physical Examination [4]

Physical examination should include the following:

- Mental status
- Cranial nerves
- Cerebellum
- Muscle strength
- Deep tendon reflexes
- Sensory function

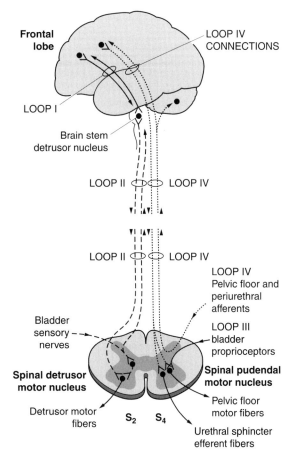

Figure 14.3 Sympathetic and parasympathetic innervation of the bladder loops. (Reproduced with permission from Herst AL et al., editors. Comprehensive Gynecology. Mosby Year Book, 1992.)

Diseases Affecting the Lower Urinary Tract

Diseases of the Central Nervous System Affecting the Lower Urinary Tract

Diseases that affect the central nervous system include dementia, cerebral vascular accidents, tumor, trauma and hydrocephalus. These diseases should be picked up on history, mental status examinations, loss of muscle strength or asymmetrical deep tendon reflexes.

Cerebrovascular Disease

Acute cerebral vascular disease can be associated with urinary retention. Long-term problems are associated with abnormalities in loops I and IV. Detrusor dyssynergia can result from loss of loop one leading to urinary urgency with maintenance of voluntary urethral control [5,6].

Brain Tumor

Frontal lobe tumors will lead to detrusor hyperreflexia with loss of loops I and IV. When a midline paracentral gyrus lesion is present there is loss of voluntary relaxation of the striated urethral sphincter (loop IV) with urinary retention [7,8].

Parkinson's Disease

This is a disease of dopamine deficiency leading to predominance of the cholinergic system in the corpus striatum (loop I). Twenty-five to 75% of patients will have symptoms of urgency, frequency, nocturia and urge incontinence. The most common findings are detrusor hyperreflexia with or without sphincter contraction [6,9].

Shy–Drager Syndrome (Multiple System Atrophy)

This is a rare degenerative disease which has Parkinsonian features but involves degeneration of the cerebellum, brainstem peripheral autonomic ganglia and thoracolumbar preganglionic sympathetic neurons. The most common voiding dysfunction in this group is detrusor hyperreflexia (loss of loop I inhibition of loop II), with denervation of the striated sphincter leading to an open bladder neck (loop IV) [9].

Spinal Cord Injuries

The sacral spinal cord starts at T12 to L1 and terminates in the cauda equina.

Suprasacral Injury. Initial spinal trauma associated with spinal shock will lead to hypotonic bladder with sphincter spasticity leading to urinary retention.

Lesions above T6 will lead to detrusor hyperreflexia, smooth and striated muscle sphincter dyssynergia. If the lesion is between T6 and the sacral spinal cord there will be detrusor hyperreflexia with striated sphincter dyssynergia but smooth sphincter synergia [9].

Sacral Spinal Cord. Lesions of the spinal cord lead to detrusor areflexia with failure of smooth muscle relaxation; striated sphincter tone remains but voluntary control is lost [7].

Tethered Cord Syndrome. Tethered cord syndrome is a congenital neurogenic bladder syndrome that is the result of traction of the lower spinal cord segment.

Incomplete detrusor contraction increases urethral resistance leading to detrusor sphincter dyssynergia. There is decreased detrusor contraction due to sacral micturition center damage (loop III) [10].

Spinal Dysraphism. Incontinence involves stress incontinence due to intrinsic sphincter deficiency and detrusor hyperactivity [11].

Myelomeningocele. Varying degrees of lesions can be present [12,13]: (a) contractile bladder with 52% bladder neck competence, and 48% incompetence and 95% detrusor sphincter dyssynergia; (b) intermediate or acontractile bladder with static urethra that does not respond to bladder pressure or volume; (c) 6% of patients will have incomplete cord lesions and have competent sphincter mechanisms and detrusor hyperreflexia.

Multiple Sclerosis (MS)

MS is a disease in which symptoms wax and wane and is associated with multiple lesions of the central nervous system. As it has multiple lesions it can affect all the loops associated with bladder function. Voiding dysfunction is the presenting symptom in about 10% of women with MS, and 50–90% of women with MS will have voiding dysfunction. The most common voiding dysfunction is detrusor dyssynergia, often associated with striated dyssynergia. Some women will also have symptoms of urinary retention [14–16].

Detrusor instability and hyperreflexia

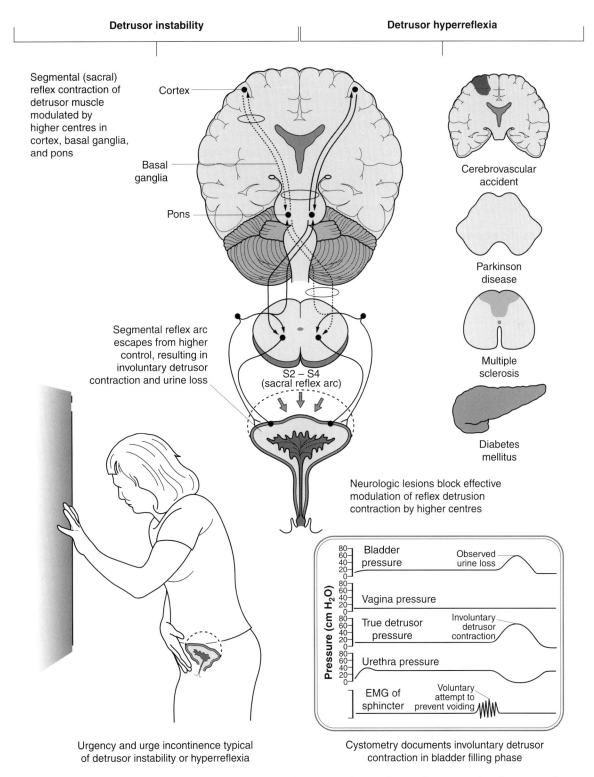

Detrusor instability

Segmental (sacral) reflex contraction of detrusor muscle modulated by higher centres in cortex, basal ganglia, and pons

Cortex

Basal ganglia

Pons

Segmental reflex arc escapes from higher control, resulting in involuntary detrusor contraction and urine loss

S2 – S4 (sacral reflex arc)

Detrusor hyperreflexia

Cerebrovascular accident

Parkinson disease

Multiple sclerosis

Diabetes mellitus

Neurologic lesions block effective modulation of reflex detrusion contraction by higher centres

Bladder pressure — Observed urine loss

Vagina pressure

True detrusor pressure — Involuntary detrusor contraction

Urethra pressure

Pressure (cm H$_2$O)

EMG of sphincter — Voluntary attempt to prevent voiding

Urgency and urge incontinence typical of detrusor instability or hyperreflexia

Cystometry documents involuntary detrusor contraction in bladder filling phase

Figure 14.4 Detrusor instability and hyperreflexia. (Reproduced with permission from Retzky SS and Rogers RM. Clinical Symposia. Ciba 1996 November 2.)

Diseases of the Peripheral Nervous System Affecting the Lower Urinary Tract

Diabetes Mellitus (DM)

The Schwann cell demyelination that occurs as a result of the metabolic abnormalities associated with DM leads to gradual loss of bladder sensation. This leads to recurrent prolonged detrusor stretching and over time there is loss of detrusor contractility. In addition, a variety of pathologic findings are present: detrusor hyperreflexia, impaired detrusor contractility, detrusor areflexia, intermediate and normal [8,17–19].

Tabes Dorsalis and Pernicious Anemia

These two diseases have the same effect on the bladder as diabetes mellitus [20].

Guillain–Barré Syndrome

Guillain-Barré syndrome most commonly affects large myelinated fibers but there may also be involvement of small myelinated fibers and inflammatory infiltration of the lumbosacral spinal roots and thoracolumbar sympathetic chain. This leads to micturitional disturbances in about 25% of people with this syndrome. Abnormalities seen include evacuation, storage abnormalities, bladder areflexia, disturbance of bladder sensation, decreased maximum cystometric capacity and detrusor overactivity or non-relaxing sphincter with neurogenic changes [21].

The symptoms seen in these patients include nocturnal or diurnal urinary frequency, sensation of urgency, urinary incontinence and enuresis, difficulty voiding and urinary retention. Symptoms follow onset of weakness, and resolve with other symptoms [22,23].

Herpes Zoster

This virus invades the sacral spinal ganglia and when it erupts, women may experience urinary urgency, frequency and retention. These symptoms resolve spontaneously [20].

Spinal Disk Disease

When lumbar disk disease of the L4–5 or L5–S1 leads to compression of the spinal cord, voiding dysfunction results. This may include detrusor areflexia with or without loss of striated sphincter function. The status of the sphincter determines if there is urinary incontinence or retention [24].

Radical Pelvic Surgery

Acute voiding dysfunction is most commonly associated with abdominal perineal resection and radical hysterectomy. Some of these women will go on to have permanent voiding dysfunction. The most common abnormalities in these women are loss of bladder sensation followed by decreased detrusor contractility and loss of voluntary control of the striated sphincter which leads to outlet obstruction [25].

In any disease that leads to obstruction of bladder emptying, treatment is vital to avoid upper tract injury, which occurs if intravesical pressure exceeds 40 mmH$_2$O [26].

Clinical Neurophysiological Testing

If a neurologic deficit is elicited on simple screening, neurophysiological testing may be considered.

Electrophysiologic testing examines striated muscle motor and sensory function, smooth muscle function and autonomic nerve pathways. The somatic motor sensory system is evaluated by electromyography (EMG), terminal motor latency measurements, and motor evoked potential (MEP). Sensory evoked potentials assess the sensory system. Autonomic nervous system tests relate to function of the sympathetic or parasympathetic fibers [27].

Neurophysiological Tests

Neurophysiologic testing is the assessment of nerve function by stimulation at one site by various means (electrical, mechanical, thermal or magnetic). Unfortunately, its role in the assessment of the pelvis and patients with incontinence is still in its experimental stages. The following are tests that are available at present [27].

Electromyography (EMG)

Recording of bioelectrical activity of striated muscle during the tested time period usually correlates with other urodynamic parameters (kinesiological EMG).

Motor unit EMG helps differentiate between normal, denervated/reinnervated and myopathic muscle.

EMG is used to assess pelvic floor muscle behavior during bladder filling and voiding. This demonstrates voluntary and reflex activation of pelvic floor muscles. Concentric needle EMG is used to diagnose lower motor neuron units abnormalities [27].

Concentric Needle EMG

This is used to distinguish diseased from normal striated muscle. However, it is difficult to assess the urethral sphincter and it is not standardized.

The test can help differentiate between multiple system atrophy (Shy–Drager syndrome) and idiopathic Parkinson's disease [28].

Concentric needle EMG changes have been detected in women who are incontinent 8 weeks postpartum and they are associated with prolonged second stage and heavier babies [29].

Single Fiber EMG

Once a muscle has undergone denervation there will be reinnervation with reorganization of motor units and these abnormalities can be detected using single fiber EMG. This is an important test for women with unexplained urinary retention without obvious cause. It has been standardized; it does involve some pain.

EMG can detect changes associated with cauda equina lesion and lumbosacral myelomeningocele. It can also help distinguish multiple system atrophy (Shy–Drager syndrome) from Parkinson's disease and progressive supranuclear palsy [30].

Pudendal Nerve Conduction Test

Pudendal nerve latency is used to assess nerve function. Perineal latency is abnormally prolonged in patients with urinary stress incontinence [31,32]. It has been found that there is an increase in the mean pudendal nerve terminal motor latency 48–72 hours after vaginal delivery but in 60% of women this had returned to normal 2 months later [33].

Long-term postpartum changes in pudendal nerve latency are controversial [34,35]. Pudendal nerve latency is prolonged in women with prolapse and further prolonged after a vaginal repair [36,37]. The validity of this test is unclear as different laboratories and different techniques have different normal values.

Electrical stimulation may disturb cardiac pacemaker activity.

Anterior Sacral Root (Cauda Equina) Stimulation

This test is used to identify and to assess pathology of sacral roots. Invasive stimulation of individual roots in sacral foramina has been advocated as a

diagnostic procedure before the implantation of electrodes which are to be used with implanted electrical stimulators for treatment of selected types of lower urinary tract dysfunction [38]. It may be used to differentiate between motor and sensory involvement of the sacral reflex arc [27].

There is a question regarding its validity because latencies differ from laboratory to laboratory and with different electrodes [27]. There is limited normative data.

Motor Evoked Potentials

Motor evoked potentials are used to demonstrate the patency of the pyramidal tracts and to reveal pathological conduction of pyramidal tracts.

Sensory System Tests

Initial screening includes testing of skin sensation of the pelvic floor with touch and pin prick as well as testing of sensation during cystometry.

Peripheral sensory pathways are tested by sensory neurography and the central nervous system by somatosensory evoked potentials [27].

Quantitative Sensory Testing

The aim of this form of testing is to provide quantifiable, reproducible and sensitive data on sensory deficits in response to specific stimuli.

During cystometry, first sensation of bladder filling, first desire to void and strong desire to void are recorded.

The International Continence Society's sixth report on standardization of the terminology of the lower urinary tract function suggests the following details be included when reporting sensory testing: patient's position, bladder volume, site of applied stimulus, number of times the stimulus was applied, number of responses recorded, sensation that was recorded, and type of stimulus applied. Normal values from the laboratory doing the testing should be included in the reporting [39].

Mechanical stimulation, by measuring the force applied to a Foley bulb needed to initiate sensation in the trigone, is neither specific nor reliable [40].

Vibration has not been established to assess lower urinary tract function.

Temperature can be used as a stimulation tool in the assessment of the bladder. There is some evidence that filling the bladder with cold water facilitates the diagnosis of detrusor instability as a test of thin autonomic fibers, but its usefulness is still questioned [41].

Electrical current can be used for urethral assessment as urethral electrosensitivity has been found to correlate with first desire to void and maximum cystometric capacity on urodynamics in normal subjects. Its role in clinical practice has yet to be determined [42].

Benefits
Urodynamics give reproducible sensory data that may be enhanced by the temperature testing as they test two different sensory mechanisms.

Limitations
There have been no standard sets of tests established for the urogenital area.

Risks are those associated with catheter insertion.

Sensory neurography can only be used in males.

Electroneurography of Dorsal Sacral Root

Electroneurography has been used to identify posterior roots, and to reveal pathological conduction of roots. Its application is for intraoperative identification of nerve roots in order to preserve perineal sensation and avoid voiding dysfunction of spastic children undergoing dorsal rhizotomy [43].

The clinical usefulness of this test is still undetermined.

Somatosensory Evoked Potential (SEP)

SEP is used to demonstrate patency of the somatosensory pathways and to reveal pathological conduction of somatosensory pathways to the parietal cortex.

- Spinal SEP – technically difficult in women; therefore not used.
- Cerebral SEP – a stimulating electrode is placed in the periphery and the impulse is recorded centrally.
- Pudendal SEP [27] – its role is to differentiate between motor and sensory fibers, and normal values have been established. However, physical examination of lower limb abnormalities (hyperreflexia) is more sensitive then recording evoked potential from the pudendal nerve in patients with MS.
- Evoked potential mapping–not currently applicable to incontinent patients.

Sacral Reflexes

Sacral reflex responses on stimulation of the dorsal clitoris nerve have been proposed to be of value in patients with lower motor neuron lesions and have been found to be absent or delayed in incontinent patients with conus/cauda involvement.

The sacral reflex can be elicited mechanically, electrically and magnetically. The simplest method is by mechanical stimulation and there are reported normative data in the literature. To date there is no data on the sensitivity or specificity of this test [44,45].

Autonomic Nervous System Tests

Sympathetic skin response testing is the standard test used to assess autonomic function but has not been established clinically for testing incontinent patients.

Conclusion

It is important to have a basic understanding of the neuroanatomy of the bladder and pelvic floor before going on to assess it.

Clinical neurophysiologic testing is for the most part only for clinical research at this time. It should be considered only in a select group of patients suspected or known to have abnormalities of the neuromuscular system and should be carried out by a trained professional.

To date there are no generally accepted guidelines for performing neurophysiologic tests.

The future of clinical neurophysiology testing [27]:

- Correlation of test results with both the underlying lesion and disturbed function.
- Pathophysiology of different types of incontinence.
- Usefulness of tests in clinical practice for better diagnosis and evaluation of some physiologically based treatment modalities such as pelvic floor muscle exercises, biofeedback and electrical stimulation.
- Usefulness of tests for intraoperative monitoring.
- Such research will generally further insight into pathophysiology of lower urinary tract dysfunction.

References

1. Bradley WE, Rockswold GL, Timm GW et al. Neurourology of micturition. J Urol 1976;115:481–6.

2. Sand P. The evaluation of the incontinent female. Curr Probl Obstet Gynecol Fertil 1992;109–51.

3. Bradley WE, Timm GW, Scott FB. Innervation of the detrusor muscle and urethra. Urol Clin North Am 1974;1:3–27.

4. Karram MM, Bhatia NN. Importance of neurologic evaluation in women with lower urinary tract dysfunction. J Reprod Med 1990;35(8):799–804.

5. Wein AJ, Barrett DM. Etiologic possibilities for increased pelvic floor electromyography activity during bladder filling. J Urol 1982;127:949–52.

6. Barrett DM, Wein AJ. Voiding dysfunction: diagnosis, classification, and management. In: Gillenwater JY, Grayhack JT, Howards SS, Duckett JW, editors. Adult and Pediatric Urology, 2nd edn. St Louis: Mosby Year Book, 1991; 1001–99.

7. Soler D, Boreyskowski M. et al. Lower urinary tract dysfunction in children with central nervous system tumors. Arch Dis Child 1998;79(4):344–7.

8. Lang EW, Chestnut RM et al. Urinary retention with supratentorial cortical lesions. Eur Neurol 1996;36(1):43–7.

9. Blaivais JG. Non-traumatic neurogenic voiding dysfunction in the adult. I. Physiology and approach to therapy. AUA Update Series; 1985, lesson 11, vol. 4.

10. 10. Fukui J, Kakizaki T. Urodynamic evaluation of tethered cord syndrome including tight filum terminale: prolonged follow-up observations after intraspinal operation. Urology 1980;16(5):539–52.

11. Perez LM, Smith EA et al. Outcome of sling cystourothropexy in the pediatric population: A critical review. J Urol 1996;156:642–6.

12. Mundy AR, Shab PJR et al. Sphincter behavior in myelomeningocele. Br J Urol 1985;57:647–51.

13. Keshtgar AS, Rickwood AMK. Urologic consequences of incomplete cord lesions in patients with myelomeningocele. Br J Urol 1988;82:258–60.

14. Miller H, Simpson CA et al. Bladder dysfunction in multiple sclerosis. Br Med J 1965;i:1265–9.

15. McGuire EJ, Savastana JA. Urodynamic functioning and long term outcome management of patients with multiple sclerosis induced lower urinary tract dysfunction. J Urol 1984;132:713–15.

16. Awad SA, Gajewski JB et al. Relationship between neurological and urological status in patients with multiple sclerosis. J Urol 1984;132:499–502.

17. Mundy AR, Blaivas JG. Non-traumatic neurologic disorders. In: Mundy AR, Stevenson TP, Wein AJ, editors. Urodynamics: Principles, Practice and Application. New York: Churchill Livingstone, 1984; 278–87.

18. Kaplan SA, Blavais JG. Diabetic cystopathy. J Diabet Complications 1988;2(3):133–9.

19. Kaplan SA, Te AE. Urodynamic findings in patients with diabetic cystopathology. J Urol 1995;153(2):352–3.

20. Hald T, Bradley WE. The urinary bladder – neurology and dynamics. Baltimore: Williams & Wilkins, 1982; 160–5.

21. Kanda T, Hayashi H et al. A fulminate case of Guillain–Barré Syndrome; topographic and fiber size related analysis of demyelinating changes. J Neurol Neurosurg Psychiatry 1989;52:857–64.

22. Honavar M, Tharakan JKL et al. A clinicopathological study of Guillain–Barré syndrome: 9 cases and literature review. Brain 1991;114:1245–69.

23. Sakakibara R, Hattori T et al. Micturitional disturbance in patients with Guillain-Barré Syndrome. J Neurol Neurosurg Psychiatry 1997;63:649–53.

24. Goldman HB, Appell RA. Symposium: Neurogenic bladder dysfunction: Voiding dysfunction in women with lumbar disc prolapse. Int Urogynecol J 1999;10:134–8.

25. Havengak, Ender WE et al. Male and female sexual and urinary function after total mesorectal excision with autonomic nerve preservation for carcinoma of the rectum. J Am Coll Surg 1996;182:495–502.

26. McGuire EJ, Woodside JR et al. The prognostic significance of urodynamic testing in myelodysplastic patients. J Urol 1981;126:205–9.

27. Vodusek DB, Belmelmans B, Chanellor M, Coates K, van Kerrebroeck P, Opsomer RJ, Schmidt R, Swash M, Fowler CJ. Clinical neurophysiology. In: Abrams P., Khoury S, Wein A, editors. Incontinence. Plymouth, 1999; 156–95.

28. Schwarz J, Kornhuber M. Electromyography of the external anal sphincter in patients with Parkinson's disease and multiple system atrophy: Frequency of abnormal spontaneous activity and polyphasic motor unit potentials. Muscle Nerve 1997;20:1167–72.

29. Beck RO, Betts CD et al. Genitourinary dysfunction in multiple system atrophy: Clinical features and treatment in 62 cases. J Urol 1994;151:1336–41.

30. Allen R, Hosker G et al. Pelvic floor damage and childbirth: a neurophyiological study. Br J Obstet Gynecol 1990;97:770–9.

31. Snooks SJ, Badenoch DE et al. Perineal nerve damage in genuine stress incontinence. Br J Urol 1985;57:422–6.

32. Smith A., Hoskner G. et al. The role of pudendal nerve damage in the etiology of genuine stress incontinence in women. Br J Obstet Gynaecol 1989;96:29–32.

33. Snooks SJ, Swash M et al. Injury of the pelvic floor sphincter musculature in childbirth. Lancet 1984;ii(8402):546–50.

34. Jameson JS, Chia YW et al. Effect of age, sex, parity on anorectal function. Br J Surg 1994;81:1689.

35. Snooks SJ, Swash M et al. Effect of vaginal delivery on the pelvic floor, a 5 year follow-up. Br J Surg 1990;77:1358–60.

36. Smith ARB, Hosker GL et al. The role of partial denervation of the pelvic floor in etiology of genitourinary prolapse and stress incontinence A neurophysiological study. Br J Obstet Gynaecol 1989(b);96(1):24–8.

37. Benson T, McClellan E. The effect of vaginal dissection on the pudendal nerve. Obstet Gynecol 1993;82(3):387–9.

38. Madersbacher H, Fischer J. Sacral anterior root stimulation: prerequisite test indications. Neurol Urodyn 1993;12(5):489–94.

39. Abrams P, Blaivas JG et al. The standardization of terminology of lower urinary tract function. Scand J Urol Nephrol 1988(S114):5–19.

40. Frazer MI, Haylen BT. Trigone sensitivity testing in women. J Urol 1989;141(2):356–8.

41. Hellstrom PA, Tamela TLJ et al. The bladder cooling test for urodynamic assessment analysis of 400 examinations. Br J Urol 1991;67(3):275–9.

42. Powell PH, Feneley RCL. The role of urethral sensation in clinical urology. Br J Urol 1980;52(6):539–41.

43. Deletis V, Vodusek DB et al. Intraoperative monitoring of dorsal sacral roots: minimizing the risk of iatrogenic micturition disorders. Neurosurgery 1992;30(1):72–5.

44. Ertekin C, Reel F. Bulbocavernosus reflex in normal men and patients with neurogenic bladder and/or impotence. J Neurol Sci 1976;28(1):1–15.

45. Ertekin C, Hansen M et al. Examination of the descending pathway to the external anal sphincter and pelvic floor muscles by transcranial cortical stimulation. Electro encephalogr Clin Neurophysiol 1990;75:500–10.

15 Cystoscopy, Urethroscopy and Dynamic Cystourethroscopy

Patrick J. Culligan and Peter K. Sand

Background and History

Urethroscopy, cystoscopy and dynamic cystourethroscopy are valuable diagnostic and therapeutic tools which are essential to the practice of urogynecology.

Bozzini [1], who designed a scope that used a candle for illumination, published the first description of endoscopic visualization of the female bladder nearly 200 years ago. The technique and equipment used for cystoscopy were refined during the nineteenth century by Desmormeaux [2], Nitze [3] and Grunfeld [4]. However, it was not until Kelly [5] introduced his scope and method of air distension of the bladder, with the patient in the knee–chest position, that cystoscopy became widely used (Figure 15.1).

The development of the fiberoptic telescope in 1954 marked the beginning of modern endoscopy [6]. This innovation allowed the examiner to view the bladder through angled lenses, greatly improving the extent of visualization. While ideal for cystoscopy, these angled lenses made visualization of the urethra quite difficult prompting Robertson [7] to develop a 0∞ angle, or "straight ahead", scope specifically for urethroscopy. Robertson's technique of dynamic cystourethroscopy greatly improved diagnostic evaluation of the lower urinary tract. In 1964, cystoscopy using flexible fiberoptic technology was described [8]. Today, the techniques of rigid and flexible cystourethroscopy are used for an ever-expanding array of diagnostic and therapeutic procedures in the office and operating room.

Equipment

Three basic components are necessary for endoscopic visualization of the bladder and urethra: the scope, the light source, and the distending medium.

Rigid Scopes

There are three parts that make up the rigid cystoscope: the telescope, the bridge and the sheath (Figure 15.2). The telescope contains an eyepiece, which can be used with or without a camera; fiberoptic bundles that carry high-intensity light; and a lens. Telescopes vary with respect to the lens angle relative to the long axis of the instrument. Common viewing angles are 0° (straight-ahead), 25–30° (forward oblique), 70–75° (lateral) and 120° (retrograde). These different angles facilitate visualization of all areas of the urethra and bladder. The 0∞ scope is used for urethroscopy but should not be considered adequate for cystoscopy. The 25–30° scopes are most widely used for diagnostic cystoscopy, while the 70–75° scopes are useful for both surgical and diagnostic techniques. The 120° scope is less widely used than the others, but can be useful for visualizing irregular contours within the bladder.

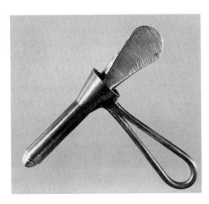

Figure 15.1 The Kelly cystoscope.

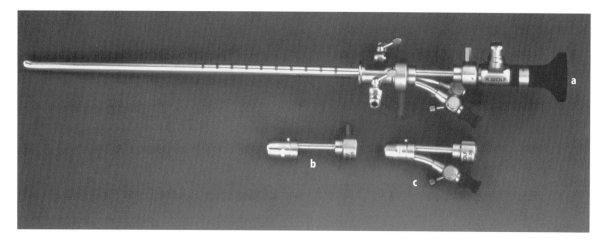

Figure 15.2 Modern rigid cystoscope. **a** Fully assembled; **b** simple bridge; **c** bridge with operative port.

The telescopes are interchangeable within the sheath, which can be left in place throughout a given procedure. Sheaths, which are available in various shapes and diameters, provide a lumen for the introduction of distending media and surgical instruments. Sheath diameters range from 7F for pediatrics to 28F for operative cystoscopy, and the shape of the sheath may be either oval or round. The smallest adequate sheath should be used in any given case, but most women can tolerate examinations in the office with up to a 21F sheath even without the use of local anesthesia. The telescope is held in place with a locking mechanism called a bridge, which may have one or two angled sidearms allowing the introduction of instruments. A special bridge (called an Albaran bridge) can be used for manipulation of instruments within the operator's field of view. The Albaran bridge (Figure 15.3) has a deflecting mechanism, which is especially useful during biopsy, removal of foreign bodies, cauterization, and ureteral catheterization.

Flexible Scopes

Despite the refinements in rigid cystourethroscopy, some drawbacks remain. In order to view the entire urethra and bladder, at least two lenses (the 0° and either the 70° or 30°) are needed. Furthermore, rigid scopes can cause significant pain and trauma, espe-

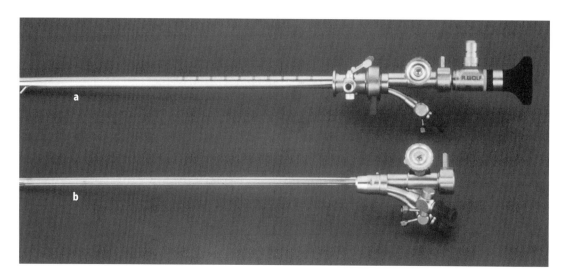

Figure 15.3 **a** Rigid cystoscope assembled with Albaran bridge; **b** Albaran bridge alone.

cially in male patients, if they are not handled properly. These and other factors have prompted many practitioners to use flexible scopes for office cysto-urethroscopy.

As mentioned previously, Marshall first described the the use of flexible fiberoptic technology for exploration of the bladder in 1964. Since then, several comparative studies have found that the diagnostic capabilities of flexible scopes are similar to those of rigid scopes [9,10].

Unlike rigid scopes, flexible scopes combine the optics, irrigation channel and instrument channel in a self-contained unit. The optical fibers are individually coated, which allows them to transmit light and images when bent. Separate bundles of fibers are used for light and image transmission. A central channel serves as both an irrigation and instrument port, and the distal tip of the scope has a deflecting mechanism (15–18F in diameter) that is capable of turning greater than 290° in a single plane.

Drawbacks of the flexible scope include a somewhat granular image quality, decreased flow rates through the irrigation channel, and their relatively fragile nature.

Light Sources

Modern scopes use a fiberoptic cable that transmits light from a high intensity light source through a connector on the telescope and down the fiberoptic bundles. Like flexible fiberoptic scopes, these light cables are somewhat fragile. A camera can be attached to the eyepiece of the telescope to allow for video monitoring.

Distending Media

As previously mentioned, air was the first distending media used for cystoscopy. Modern cystourethroscopy is usually performed using water or saline solution, but many practitioners still use carbon dioxide. Some authors report excellent results using carbon dioxide as their distending media [11,12]. The use of carbon dioxide for bladder distension may result in irritation caused by the formation of carbonic acid [13]. Because of the potential for false positive cystoscopic findings and the more physiologic properties of fluid distending media, carbon dioxide is less commonly used today.

The fluid distending media is typically delivered via gravity from a 1–3 liter bag connected by tubing to the scope. Although generally a benign process, bladder filling has been associated with sudden death due to intravascular hemolysis in the presence of a pre-existing vesical ulceration [14].

Indications and Contraindications

The most common indications for cystoscopy and urethroscopy include the work-up of hematuria, sterile pyuria or other potentially cancer-related findings as well as suspected foreign bodies, diverticula and fistulas. The precise role of cystoscopy in the evaluation of the incontinent woman is controversial.

In the past, cystourethroscopy was popularized for the complete evaluation of lower urinary tract dysfunction [7,15]. Later, retrospective studies found the technique to be a relatively insensitive screening tool when compared to urodynamic studies [16,17]. When used as an adjuvant to urodynamic studies, however, the anatomical assessment provided by cystourethroscopy is an important tool. Following a retrospective analysis of a referral population, Cundiff found that urodynamics without cystourethroscopy would have missed important diagnoses in 19% of women [18].

Most experts agree that cystourethroscopy is indicated for the evaluation of incontinent patients who have irritative voiding symptoms such as frequency, urgency and dysuria. Most urogynecologists also use the technique to evaluate persistent incontinence or voiding dysfunction following an anti-incontinence procedure. Unexplained bladder pain and failure of urodynamics to explain urogenital symptoms are other relative indications for endoscopic evaluation. Further studies are needed before cystourethroscopy can be recommended as a part of the routine evaluation of all incontinent patients.

The only true contraindication to cysto-urethroscopy is a known, active urinary tract infection.

Technique and Description of Normal Findings

Diagnostic Cystourethroscopy

The technique described below is performed in an office setting using sterile saline or water as the distending media. The patient's bladder is empty at the start of the examination. The fluid is infused via gravity as previously described. With the patient in the dorsal lithotomy position, the urethral meatus and distal anterior vaginal wall is cleansed with an antiseptic solution. While sterile technique should be observed, sterile gloves and drapes are not necessary. Even with strict adherence to sterile technique, organisms from the distal urethra can be forced into the bladder causing acute cystitis. For this reason, a prophylactic dose of an antibiotic is administered either just prior to or immediately following the examination.

The 0° urethroscope is inserted under direct visualization without the use of local anesthesia, since these agents can alter the color of the urethral mucosa. As long as the operator takes care to maintain adequate flow through the scope and inserts the scope slowly, urethral visualization is usually very well tolerated without the use of anesthesia. In order to avoid urethral trauma, the distending media should be flowing prior to insertion of the scope. Only the 0° scope is appropriate for visualization of the urethra. Scopes with angled lenses do not allow the examiner to completely visualize the circumference of the urethra. The urethra is inspected in a retrograde fashion allowing the operator to evaluate the color and topography throughout its length. As the scope is advanced, the center of the urethral lumen should be kept in the center of the visual field. The normal urethra will appear slightly pink, with numerous mucosal folds overlying a healthy vascular submucosa. In a normal urethra, when the fluid flow is interrupted, coaptation of the mucosal surfaces occurs rapidly owing to the abundance of elastic and contractile fibers present. A normal urethrovesical junction will automatically close more tightly as the bladder fills [7].

Following initial inspection, *dynamic urethroscopy* is performed during which the examiner evaluates dynamic function of the urethra and bladder during filling and various maneuvers. Dynamic urethroscopy was first described by Robertson [7]. For this technique, the urethroscope is used to observe the bladder neck during filling to diagnose detrusor overactivity, and during provocative maneuvers such as Valsalva, cough and pubococcygeus contraction to identify passive opening of the bladder neck indicating genuine stress incontinence. A normal urethrovesical junction will close during such maneuvers [15]. Cystometry is also performed during this portion of the examination. While the bladder is filling, the patient is asked to identify her first sensation of having a volume of fluid in the bladder, fullness or desire to urinate, and maximum capacity. The urethrovesical junction is kept in view during cystometry. The patient is asked to do her best to retain the fluid. During a spontaneous detrusor contraction, the urethrovesical junction and proximal urethra will open involuntarily. Although this method of detecting detrusor instability has poor sensitivity

[16], it is worthwhile based on the fact that it is easily incorporated into a standard examination during bladder filling.

When urethroscopy is complete, the examiner uses either a 30° or 70° scope for the systematic inspection of the bladder. Frequently, 0° scopes require different sheaths than the angled-lens scopes requiring removal and reinsertion of the scope. Since urethral appearance has already been assessed at this point, it is appropriate to provide local anesthesia in the form of xylocaine jelly for insertion of the angled-lens cystoscope. Removing some fluid from the bladder through the cystoscope at this time is another way to make the patient more comfortable. Flexible cystoscopes do not require removal and re-insertion, because the single unit can be used for both urethroscopy and cystoscopy.

When performing cystoscopy, the first landmark is the air bubble that invariably gets trapped against the dome of the bladder in the midline. Using the air bubble as a starting point, the entire surface of the bladder is inspected including the ureteral orifices and trigone. It is important to remember to move the air bubbles out of the way with an abdominal hand, as pathology can sometimes be found underneath them. The entire mucosal surface is examined for lesions, discoloration, diverticula, foreign bodies, trabeculations, stones, and other abnormalities. A progressive clockwise sweeping motion is used to insure that the entire surface is visualized. The examiner should maintain proper orientation throughout the procedure, and keep the bladder mucosa under direct visualization at all times to avoid bladder perforation with the scope. When distended, the bladder wall should appear smooth, pale pink to whitish in color and roughly spherical in shape. An abundance of blood vessels are usually apparent just beneath the mucosal surface. When present, the uterus and cervix can usually be seen indenting the posterior surface of the bladder. The ureteral orifices usually can be seen during this examination approximately 1.5–2 cm from midline in either side of the trigone. One should be able to see efflux of urine from each orifice. Failure to see such efflux should be followed up by an intravenous pyelogram to rule out the possibility of congenitally absent kidney or previous iatrogenic ureteral damage. Rarely, duplicated ureters are seen, usually entering the bladder slightly superior to the trigone in proximity to the ipsilateral orifice. Manual pressure over the dome of the bladder towards the symphysis allows easy visualization of the anterior portion of the bladder. When pelvic organ prolapse is prominent, it is usually helpful to place a finger inside the vagina to elevate hidden parts of the bladder. As the scope is withdrawn, the examiner's finger is placed into the vagina to palpate the urethral wall against the scope. When the full length of the scope cannot be palpated distinctly, occult urethral diverticulum must be suspected [19].

Operative Cystoscopy

Apart from some minor procedures that are easily performed in either an office or operating room setting, urogynecologists typically refer patients to urologists for operative cystoscopy. Examples of these minor procedures include removal of foreign bodies including intravesical sutures; biopsy of small lesions; and the placement or removal of ureteral stents. Of course, periurethral injections for the treatment of stress incontinence are also performed under direct endoscopic visualization. A complete discussion of periurethral bulking agents for the treatment of stress incontinence can be found in Chapter 36. A full discussion of operative cystoscopic techniques is beyond the scope of this chapter.

Intraoperative Diagnostic Cystoscopy

Cystoscopy is an integral part of virtually all urogynecologic procedures. In a retrospective analysis, Harris [20] reported a 4% incidence of ureteral or bladder injury during complex urogynecologic procedures. Since none of these injuries were appreciated until intraoperative cystoscopy was performed, these authors concluded that cystoscopic confirmation of bladder integrity and ureteral function should be considered a part of all such procedures. More recently, Jabs and Drutz [21] recommended that cystoscopy be used liberally to reduce the frequency of serious sequelae from urinary tract injury during incontinence and prolapse surgery. Intraoperative cystoscopy can be also useful for guidance in suprapubic catheter placement and for distinguishing between the bladder and an anterior enterocele sac at the outset of a vaginal procedure to correct prolapse. Urogynecologists and urologists have traditionally used intraoperative visualization of the bladder neck to assess the tension of an anti-incontinence procedure. However, this practice has recently been shown to be neither reproducible nor predictive of postoperative success [22].

The technique of assessing bladder integrity and ureteral function is similar to the technique for office cystoscopy described above. Intravenous injection of 5 ml of indigo carmine dye approximately 5–10 minutes prior to cystoscopy is very helpful when looking for ureteral function. A blue jet of dye should efflux from each ureteral orifice. If after an appropriate interval no dye is seen coming from a ureteral orifice, three possibilities should be considered: the ureter in question has been ligated during the operation; an undiagnosed preoperative condition exists such as ligation with prior surgery or congenital absence; or the bladder is so distended that back pressure on the ureteral orifices is too great to allow efflux of dye. It is also important to note the quality of the stream of dye-stained urine coming from each ureter. A slow trickle of blue dye coming from one or both ureters could be indicative of partial ureteral obstruction and should not be considered reassuring.

Unrecognized ureteral or bladder injuries can lead to postoperative complications of unexplained fever, ileus, flank pain, hematuria, urinoma, urinary ascites, and fistula. Loss of renal function and death from infectious complications can also occur. Therefore, it is reasonable to include cystoscopic confirmation of ureteral and bladder integrity into all major gynecologic operations performed as part of a resident training program [23]. In fact, with the increasing popularity of minimally invasive suburethral sling procedures that incorporate cystoscopy (e.g. the tension-free vaginal tape (Johnson and Johnson, Sommerville, NJ), such credentialing is more important than ever.

At times, the surgical approach to incontinence or prolapse does not lend itself well to transurethral cystoscopy. When this is the case, the technique of suprapubic teloscopy may be employed. For this approach, cystoscopy is performed through the bladder dome by means of a stab wound that will later serve as the site for suprapubic catheter placement. Excellent descriptions of both an open and laparoscopic approach to suprapubic teloscopy have been published [24,25]. Briefly, after completion of the surgical procedure, the bladder is filled with 300–400 ml of sterile saline in a retrograde fashion through a three-way transurethral Foley catheter. A purse-string of absorbable suture is placed in the dome of the bladder, and a small stab wound is then made through the center of the purse-string. The 30° telescope is inserted into the wound, and the ends of the suture are held tightly to make the defect water-tight. Systematic inspection of the entire bladder mucosa is then performed. The same defect can then be used for suprapubic catheter placement.

Interpretation of Findings

Urethroscopy

Normal urethroscopic findings are described above. Some of the most common abnormal urethral findings are discussed here.

Diverticula are discussed in detail in Chapter 41 of this text. They occur in up to 5% of women [26]. While the diagnosis is typically made by clinical history and physical examination, some diverticula are only appreciated with radiologic, urodynamic or urethroscopic investigation. For direct urethroscopic visualization of the diverticular orifice, the examiner places a finger inside the patient's vagina, massaging the urethra against the scope. Pus and/or urine can then frequently be seen exuding from the opening of a diverticulum. As mentioned above, another clue to the presence of a urethral diverticulum is the inability of the examiner to distinctly palpate the entire length of the scope inside of the urethra. It is important to remember that between 20% and 50% of patients have multiple diverticula [27,28].

Atrophic changes are seen secondary to estrogen deficiency. Estrogen receptors are found virtually throughout the female urogenital tract [29]. The decreased periurethral blood supply associated with estrogen deficiency can adversely affect urethral coaptation and cause patients to experience dysuria, urgency, dyspareunia, and incontinence. Physical examination will frequently reveal a urethral caruncle, and urethroscopy will reveal a pale epithelium and loss of the coapting urethral folds. These findings can be seen even in women who are faithful in taking their standard estrogen replacement dose, since these dosing schedules were determined with osteoporosis and not urogenital symptoms in mind. Virtually all of the atrophic changes associated with estrogen deficiency are reversible with local estrogen replacement.

Urethritis is a nonspecific term that encompasses both chronic and acute conditions that cause various changes in the endoscopic appearance of the urethra, the most common of which are redness and exudate.

Pseudo-polyps or "fronds" are frequently seen at the urethrovesical junction and can even be considered normal. These fronds are typically transparent and are of no clinical significance. They are sometimes are attributed to chronic inflammation, but when this is the case, other inflammatory findings should be present as well. Any urethral polypoid lesion seen proximal to the urethrovesical junction should be biopsied to rule out malignancy.

Condylomata of the urethra are commonly found in its distal third. Urethral involvement has been reported in 5–35% of female patients with genital condyloma acuminatum, with most lesions occurring within or near the meatus [30].

Carcinoma of the urethra is an extremely rare condition accounting for less than 0.02% of all cancers in women. The most common type is squamous cell cancer which typically involves the entire urethra. However, adenocarcinoma, transitional cell cancer, malignant melanoma, and undifferentiated primary cancers of the urethra have been reported as well [31].

Fistulas are discussed in Section 8 of this text.

Intrinsic sphincter deficiency (ISD) is generally thought to be a diagnosis that should be based on a combination of historical, urodynamic and urethroscopic parameters most of which are not strictly defined. Typical endoscopic findings in a patient with ISD include an open patulous proximal urethra at rest that may or may not be hypermobile with increased intra-abdominal pressure. In severe cases, submucosal scarring and fibrosis can lead to a rigid, "pipe-stem" appearance.

Cystoscopy

Normal cystoscopic findings are discussed above. Some of the most common abnormal findings are discussed here.

Cystitis is a nonspecific term that means inflammation of the bladder. The various causes of cystitis are discussed in detail in Section 4 of this text. Below are descriptions of the cystoscopic findings associated with various forms of cystitis.

Bacterial cystitis is a contraindication for cystoscopy, but when it is encountered inadvertently it can have a wide range of appearances based on clinical severity. These can range from the presence of a few papules all the way to the finding of hemorrhagic cystitis.

Chronic trigonitis is another name for the common finding of *squamous metaplasia* overlying the trigone. The finding, characterized by granular, pearly gray-white epithelium with irregular borders, is most common in patients who are middle-aged or older but can be seen at any age [32]. The etiology of squamous metaplasia is not known. One theory is that is it an anatomic epithelial variant that develops under the influence of hormonal stimulation or lack thereof [33]. Another theory holds that the finding is a result of irritation from chronic urinary tract infections. Biopsies of these lesions consistently show squamous replacement of the urothelial transitional epithelium without hyperplasia or abnormal maturation [32].

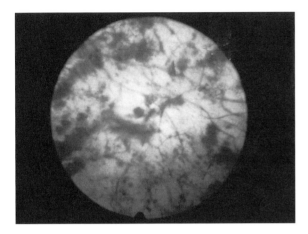

Figure 15.4 Glomerulations associated with interstitial cystitis.

Cystitis cystica and cystitis glandularis are also common findings associated with chronic urothelial inflammation. Cystitis cystica is characterized by multiple uniform clear mucosal cysts usually found along the posterior bladder mucosa. Cystitis glandularis looks like cystitis cystica, except the cysts are not clear and do not have a uniform appearance. Both types of cysts arise from glandular metaplasia. While cystitis cystica is a uniformly benign finding, cystitis glandularis is thought to occasionally transform into adenocarcinoma [34,35] and should be followed with serial cystoscopy and biopsy as appropriate.

Interstitial cystitis is a chronic, non-infectious, inflammatory condition of the bladder. A complete discussion of this debilitating condition is found in Chapter 18 of this text. Hunner's ulcers are considered the pathognomonic cystoscopic finding for interstitial cystitis, but they are seen in only about 10% of cases [36]. A more common finding in these patients is the presence of glomerulations (Figure 15.4), or diffuse submucosal hemorrhagic spots, seen with overdistension of the bladder. These spots often appear only on refilling of the bladder to supraphysiologic volumes. The patient may require general anesthesia in order to tolerate this examination.

Radiation cystitis results from injury to the bladder associated with radiation therapy for uterine, cervical or colonic malignancies. The clinical presentation of an acute cystitis typically begins 4–6 weeks after treatment, but late reactions can occur months to years following cessation of treatment [37]. The cystoscopic appearance of radiation cystitis is dependent on time interval from treatment, but most commonly extensive vascular dilatation is seen.

Atrophic changes within the bladder associated with estrogen deficiency are similar to those of the urethra described above. Urothelial paleness is the most common cystoscopic appearance of this condition.

Diverticula of the bladder are relatively common clinical disorders that rarely require treatment, although progressive enlargement to enormous proportions has been reported [38]. Some studies indicate that they result from increased intravesical pressure secondary to some form of outlet obstruction [39]. Endoscopic visualization of the entire diverticulum can be difficult, when the neck of the structure is relatively small. However, either direct visualization or cytologic evaluation of the space is necessary, since malignancies arising from diverticula have been reported [40].

Bladder stones (Figure 15.5) can result from urinary retention or the presence of a foreign body such as a non-absorbable suture from a previous operation. Urinary retention presumably causes calculi by allowing inflammatory exudate to come together forming a nidus. Bladder stones may vary quite a bit in appearance, but they all tend to have a rather smooth surface.

Trabeculations appear as interlaced cords or muscular ridges beneath the mucosal lining of a distended bladder. In men, trabeculations are thought to result from chronic outlet obstruction. However, this etiology does not necessarily apply to women, since outlet obstruction is a rare phenomenon in females. Detrusor instability with chronic voluntary suppression seems to be a more likely cause for this invariably benign finding [41].

Fistulas are discussed in a comprehensive fashion in Section 8 of this text.

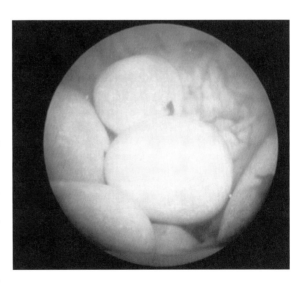

Figure 15.5 Bladder stones.

Endometriosis is a common gynecologic disorder characterized by abnormal growth of endometrial glands and stroma outside of the uterine cavity. The classic presenting symptom of intravesical endometriosis is cyclic pain and irritative voiding symptoms. Less than 30% of these women report cyclic hematuria [42]. Cystoscopy will reveal a hemorrhagic lesion within the bladder mucosa. Histologic confirmation is required for the diagnosis. There are rare reports of malignant transformation of vesical endometriosis, so long-term follow-up is necessary [43].

Ureteral ectopy is the name given to a ureteral orifice that lies outside the boundary of the trigone. Most commonly, this condition is associated with a duplicated collecting system draining the upper of two kidney pelves [44]. If the ectopic ureter opens into the urethra, severe urinary incontinence can result.

A *ureterocele* is a cystic dilation of the terminal intravesical portion of the ureter. Ureteroceles are thought to result from chronic pressure such as the type that would be exerted against a stenotic ureteral orifice [45]. Ureteroceles are also commonly seen when there is a duplicated kidney and collecting system. Most commonly, ureteroceles are not a clinically significant finding, but surgery can be necessary when the patient experiences ureterovesical obstruction, ascending infection, secondary urethrolithiasis, flank pain, and recurrent hematuria.

Bladder cancer is the most common urinary tract cancer in women. Approximately 14 900 new cases of bladder cancer are diagnosed in the United States annually, making it essentially as common as cervical cancer [46]. Transitional cell carcinoma (Figure 15.6) is the most common cell type followed by adenocarcinoma and squamous cell carcinoma. Cystoscopic appearance varies with histologic type and extent of disease. Although these lesions will generally appear as obvious raised papillary or villous lesions, carcinoma in situ can be difficult to identify. The lesions may be multicentric, requiring multiple biopsies. In a recent prospective study including comprehensive evaluations of 1930 patients (736 females) with hematuria, Khadra et al. recommended cystoscopic evaluation of all such patients after finding 230 cases of bladder cancer – 7 of which were found in women younger than 40 [47].

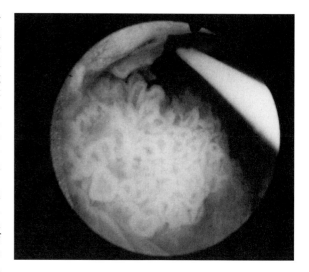

Figure 15.6   Transitional cell bladder cancer.

tract. The techniques of cystoscopy, urethroscopy and dynamic cystourethroscopy are invaluable to the pelvic surgeon in both the operating room and office setting. The diagnostic and therapeutic advantages of these techniques should not be underestimated.

References

1. Bozzini P. Lichtieter, eine erfindung zur anschung innerer thiele, und krukheiten nebst abbilding. J Pract Arzeykunde 1805;24:107.
2. Desmormeaux AJ. Transactions of the Societe Chirurgie, Paris: Gazette des Hop, 1865.
3. Nitze M. Eine neue balbachtungs-und untersuchunigsmethods fur harnrohre, harnbiase und rectum. Wein Med Wochenschr 1879;24:649.
4. Grunfeld I. Der harnrohrenspiegel (das endoscope), seine diagnostische und therapeutische anwendung. Vienna: Deutsch Chirugie, 1881.
5. Kelly HA. The direct examination of the female bladder with elevated pelvis-the catheterization of the ureters under direct inspection, with and without elevation of the pelvis. Am J Obstet Dis Wom Child 1894;25:1–19.
6. Hopkins HH, Kopany NS. A flexible fiberscope using static scanning. Nature 1954;179:39–41.
7. Robertson JR. Air cystoscopy. Obstet Gynecol 1968;32:328–30.
8. Marshall VF. Fiberoptics in urology. J Urol 1964;91:110–12.
9. Figueroa TE, Thomas R, Moon TD. Taking the pain out of cystoscopy: a comparison of rigid with flexible instruments. J Louisiana St Med Soc 1987;139:26–8.
10. Clayman RV, Reddy P, Lange PH. Flexible fiberoptic and rigid-rod lens endoscopy of the lower urinary tract: a prospective controlled comparison. J Urol 1984;131:715–16.
11. Matthews PN, Skewes DG, Kothari JJ, Woodhouse CRJ, Hendry WF. Carbon dioxide versus water for cystoscopy: a comparative study. Br J Urol 1983;55:364–6.

Summary

Technological advances have vastly improved the utility of endoscopic evaluation of the lower urinary

12. Matthews PN, Bagood KA, Woodhouse CRJ. CO_2 cystoscopy using a flexible fiberoptic endoscope. Br J Urol 1984;56:188–90.
13. Wein AJ, Hanno PM, Dixon DO. The reproducibility and interpretation of carbon dioxide cystometry. J Urol 1978;120:205–7.
14. Bell MD, Sudden death due to intravascular hemolysis after bladder irrigation with distilled water. J Forensic Sci 1992;37(5):1401–6.
15. Robertson JR. Gynecologic urethroscopy. Am J Obstet Gynecol 1972;115:986–9.
16. Sand PK, Hill RC, Ostergard DR. Supine urethroscopic and standing cystometery as screening methods for the detection of detrusor instability. Obstet Gynecol 1987;70:57–60.
17. Scotti RJ, Ostergard DR, Guillaume AA, Kohatsu KE. Predictive value of urethroscopy as compared to urodynamics in the diagnosis of genuine stress incontinence. J Reprod Med 1990;35:772–6.
18. Cundiff GW, Bent AE. The contribution of urethrocystoscopy to evaluation of lower urinary tract dysfunction in women. Int Urogynecol J 1996;7:307–11.
19. Julian TM. Simple examination techniques to aid in the diagnosis of urethral diverticulum. Obstet Gynecol 1990;76:910–12.
20. Harris RL, Cundiff GW, Theofrastus JP et al. The value of intraoperative cystoscopy in urogynecologic and reconstructive pelvic surgery. Am J Obstet Gynecol 1997;177(6):1367–71.
21. Jabs CF, Drutz HP. The role of intraoperative cystoscopy in prolapse and incontinence surgery. Am J Obstet Gynecol 2001;185(6):1368–73.
22. Bump RC, Hurt WG, Addison WA, Fantl JA, McClish DK. Reliability and correlation of measurements during and after bladder neck surgery. The Continence Program for Women Research Group. Br J Urol 1998;82(5):628–33.
23. Hibbert ML, Salminen ER, Dainty LA, Davis GD, Perez RP. Credentialing residents for intraoperative cystoscopy. Obstet Gynecol 2000;96(6):1014–17.
24. Timmons CM, Addison WA. Obstet Gynecol 1990;75(1):137–9.
25. Miklos JR, Kohli N, Sze EH, Saye WB. Obstet Gynecol 1997;89(3):476–8.
26. Roehrborn CG. Long term follow-up study of the marsupialization technique for urethral diverticula in women. Surg Gynecol Obstet 1988;167:191–6.
27. Lee RA. Diverticulum of the urethra: clinical presentation, diagnosis, and management. Obstet Gynecol. 1984;27:490–8.
28. Robertson JR. Urethral Diverticula. In: Ostergard DR, Bent AE, editors. Urogynecology and Urodynamics: Theory and Practice, 4th edn. Baltimore: Williams & Wilkins, 1996; 361–70.
29. Iosif CS, Batra S, Ed A et al. Estrogen receptors in the human female lower urinary tract. Am J Obstet Gynecol 1981;141:817–22.
30. Sand PK, Shen W, Bowen LW, Ostergard DR. Cryotherapy for the treatment of proximal urethral condyloma accuminatum. J Urol 1987;137:874–6.
31. Johnson DE, O'Connell JR. Primary carcinoma of the urethra. Urology 1983;21:42–5.
32. Benson RC, Swanson SK, Farrow GM. Relationship of leukoplakia to urethral malignancy. J Urol 1987;137:979–82.
33. Packham DA. The epithelial lining of the female trigone and urethra. Br J Urol 1971;43:201–3.
34. Edwards PD, Hurm RA, Jaeschke WH. Conversion of cystitis glandularis to adenocarcinoma. J Urol 1972;108:568–70.
35. Susmano D, Rubenstein AB, Dakin AR et al. Cystitis glandularis and adenocarcinoma of the bladder. J Urol 1991;105:671–4.
36. Messing EM, Stamey TA. Interstitial cystitis: early diagnosis, pathology, and treatment. Urology 1978;12:381–92.
37. Fajardo LF, Berthrong M. Radiation injury in surgical pathology. Am J Surg Pathol 1978;2:159–63.
38. Miller A. The aetiology and treatment of diverticulum of the bladder. Br J Urol 1958;30:87–91.
39. Barrett DM, Malek RS, Kelalis PP. Observations on vesical diverticulum in childhood. J Urol 1976;116:284–8.
40. McCormick SR, Dodds PR, Kraus PA et al. Non-epithelial neoplasms arising within vesical diverticula. Urology 1985;25:405–8.
41. Bassi P, Artibani W, Pegovavo V et al. Obstruction or no obstruction. Int J Urol Nephrol 1988;20:489–93.
42. Shook TE, Nyberg LM. Endometriosis of the urinary tract. Urology 1988;31:1–6.
43. Price DT, Maloney KE, Ibrahim GK, Cundiff GW, Leder RA, Anderson EE. Vesical endometriosis: Report of two cases and review of the literature. Urology 1996;48(4):639–43.
44. Young DW, Lebowitz RL. Congenital abnormalities of the ureter. Semin Roentgenol 1986;21:172–8.
45. Tanagho EA. Anatomy and management of ureteroceles. J Urol 1972;107:729–32.
46. Droller MJ. Bladder cancer: State of the art. CA Cancer J Clin 1998;48:269–84.
47. Khadra MH, Pickard RS, Charlton M, Powell PH, Neal DE. A prospective analysis of 1,930 patients with hematuria to evaluate current diagnostic practice. J Urol 2000;163:524–7.

4 Inflammatory Conditions, Painful Bladder and Pelvic Syndromes, Common Bowel Problems

16 Urinary Tract Infections in the Non-pregnant Woman

Abheha Satkunaratnam and Harold P. Drutz

Introduction

Infections of the urinary tract are common problems encountered in primary care and specialty care practice. There are an estimated seven to eight million physician visits for acute uncomplicated urinary tract infections and more than one million hospitalizations annually in the United States [1]. They account for over US$1 billion in health care costs annually in the United States [2]. This figure would be much higher if other costs were included such as laboratory tests, outpatient-therapy, and missed days from work or school. Women are more afflicted by urinary tract infections compared to men except at the extremes of age. Indeed, urinary tract infections are the most frequent bacterial infection in women. Approximately half of adult women report an experience with urinary tract infection at some point in their lives [3]. Of women who experience an initial infection, 25–30% will have recurrent episodes [4]. Women with recurrent urinary tract infections account for a significant portion of referrals to gynecologists, urologists, and urogynecologists.

The entire spectrum of urinary tract infection (UTI) including uncomplicated cystitis is associated with significant morbidity. The impact of UTI-related morbidity on society is significant due to its high prevalence. One study of the effects of UTI infection in university women reported the following per annum rates: inability to attend school or work 1.2 days, restricted activity 2.4 days, and time in bed 0.4 days [5]. Similar findings have been reported in other groups of women. Among older women, UTI is a leading cause of Gram-negative bacteremia and potential life-threatening septicemia. In Canada, 526 patients died of UTI in 1997 [6]. Postmenopausal status is recognized as an independent risk factor for new onset and recurrent urinary tract infections [7]. With the worldwide aging population, this disease will continue to increase in both incidence and prevalence among postmenopausal woman. With emerging antimicrobial resistance to urinary tract pathogens, safe and effective management strategies are necessary for improving patient morbidity, while minimizing antimicrobial resistance.

Epidemiology

Approximately 50–70% of women will experience a urinary tract infection (UTI) in their lifetime and 25–30% will have recurrent episodes [4]. The prevalence of acute UTI increases with age, reaching approximately 7% in women aged 50 or older [8]. In the elderly population, the incidence of UTI rises dramatically. Bacteriuria, or colonization of urine by bacteria, is a prerequisite for the development of urinary tract infection or symptomatic bacteriuria. At least 20% of elderly, non-institutionalized women have bacteriuria [9]. In the institutionalized population this figure is thought to be higher [10]. Women aged 80 years or more have a reported bacteriuria rate of 25–50% [11]. Despite these figures, the factors predisposing postmenopausal women to UTIs are yet to be elicited when compared to those in pre- and perimenopausal women.

In the premenopausal group, several predisposing factors have been suggested, but very few scientifically verified. Those factors that are recognized include coitus, the use of a diaphragm or spermicidal lubricant for contraception, catheterization, urinary tract calculi, impaired host defenses, and previous cystitis [12]. Low socioeconomic status, recent upper respiratory tract infection, and recent use of antibiotics have also been identified as risk factors for UTI [13]. Other risk factors such as poor menstrual and toilet hygiene, use of tampons or douching, and infrequent voiding lack qualified scientific support [14,15]. Among postmenopausal women, cystocele, post-void residual volume and urinary incontinence are strongly associated with recurrent UTI [16]. Urogenital or gynecologic surgery is a risk factor for new onset and recurrent UTI. Estrogen deficiency is also recognized as an independent risk factor for the development of urinary tract infection, recurrent urinary tract infection, and urinary incontinence [17].

Classification

The classification of urinary tract infections has little scientific basis. The terms uncomplicated and complicated have simplified the approach to urinary tract infections for the practicing clinician but continue to categorically group a wide variety of patients and pathogens at the expense of the individual patient at hand. However, the distinction of complicated UTI from uncomplicated UTI is impor-

tant owing to the increased risk and incidence of acquiring new infections, the potential for adverse systemic or local complications, the likelihood of therapeutic failure, and the emergence of antimicrobial resistance. For the patient, these adverse complications may include urosepsis, abscess formation, renal scarring, or potentially renal failure and end-stage renal disease.

Historically, the term complicated urinary tract infection described a subset of patients who did not adequately respond to conservative short-term treatment with antibiotics. Today, this term is applied to UTI occurring in the presence of structural urinary tract abnormalities (including catheterization), metabolic and hormonal abnormalities, impaired host defenses, or unusual pathogens (Table 16.1). The epidemiology, natural history and burden of illness of complicated UTI are poorly understood [18]. The literature pertaining to complicated UTI is scientifically poor, primarily employing retrospective reviews, and we remain in the process of eliciting its pathogenesis. This diagnostic conundrum is the product of inadequate knowledge and insufficient scientific evidence [18]. To simplify, these are factors that increase the risk of

Table 16.1 Classification of women at risk of complicated urinary tract infections

Structural abnormalities	(a)	Increased post-void residual – pelvic floor prolapse
	(b)	Obstruction – bladder outlet obstruction
	(c)	Foreign bodies – catheterization, nephrostomy tubes, ureteral stents
	(d)	Congenital abnormalities – vesicoureteral reflux, ureteral duplication
	(e)	Urinary calculi
	(f)	Neurogenic bladder
	(g)	Urinary diversion procedures
	(h)	Infected cysts
	(i)	Bladder or renal abscess
	(j)	Fistulas
Metabolic and hormonal abnormalities	(a)	Diabetes mellitus
	(b)	Pregnancy
	(c)	Renal impairment and renal disorders – azotemia, polycystic kidney disease, papillary necrosis, nephropathies
	(d)	Xanthogranulomatous pyelonephritis
	(e)	Malakoplakia
	(f)	Primary biliary cirrhosis
Impaired host defenses	(a)	Elderly patients
	(b)	Transplant recipients
	(c)	Neutropenia, immunosuppressive therapy
	(d)	Congenital or acquired immunodeficiency syndromes
Unusual pathogens	(a)	Nosocomial infections and resistant organisms
	(b)	Long-term institution
	(c)	Yeasts and fungi
	(d)	*Mycoplasma* spp.
	(e)	Resistant bacteria including *Pseudomonas aeruginosa*
	(f)	Metastatic bacterial infections (*Staphylococcus* spp.)
	(g)	Calculi – predisposing bacteria (*Proteus* spp. and *Corynebacterium urealyticum*)

acquiring bacteriuria, promote an infection, and/or contribute to the persistence of an infection that may lead to adverse consequences. The labeling of a patient with complicated UTI can lead to a lifelong experience of extended, and occasionally more sophisticated yet unyielding investigations, alternative treatment modalities, prolonged courses of antibiotics, and protracted follow-up. It must be remembered that conventional treatment with antimicrobial therapy will predictably cure 75–80% of patients with supposed complicated UTI. Thus, the term complicated UTI should be employed carefully and reserved for patients within those groups who fail therapy because of relapse or persistence of infection.

Etiology

In uncomplicated UTIs, *Escherichia coli* is the predominant causative pathogen, accounting for 70–90% of infections. *Staphylococcus saprophyticus* accounts for approximately 5–15%, and enterococci and non-*E. coli* aerobic Gram-negatives including *Klebsiella* spp. and *Proteus mirabilis* the remaining 5–10% [19,20].

In complicated UTIs, which include nosocomial-acquired infections, drug-resistant *E. coli* and Gram-negative aerobic bacilli other than *E. coli* are responsible. These include *Enterobacter* spp., *Klebsiella* spp., *Serratia* spp., *Citrobacter* spp., *Providencia* spp., *Acinetobacter* spp., *Pseudomonas* spp., as well as Gram-positive cocci, such as Enterococci and Staphylococci [18,20,21].

Diagnosis

Urinary tract infection is often, but not always, accompanied by the symptoms of dysuria, frequency, urgency, and possibly nocturia. Fever is rare in cystitis, but has been reported. Acute pyelonephritis is a syndrome of localized flank or back pain accompanied by systemic symptoms of fever, chills, and prostration.

Diagnostic testing includes urinary dipstick screening and urinary culture. Urinary dipstick has been used as a screen for pyuria and hematuria which are thought to occur in women with UTI. Urinary dipsticks which detect leukocyte esterase activity (LE) as an indicator of pyuria and urinary nitrite production (NIT) as an indicator of bacteriuria have been shown to improve detection of

*FDA – Food and Drug Administration, United States

significant bacteriuria (colony counts $\geq 10^5$ colony-forming units (CFU)/ml) [22]. However, many women have urinary tract symptoms with colony counts as low as 10^3 CFU/ml [21–23]. Semeniuk and Church [23] have demonstrated poor positive predictive value of urinary dipstick with LE and NIT ranging from 0% with a bacterial colony count of 10^3 CFU/ml to 84% with 10^5 CFU/ml. However, the negative predictive value of a negative result with both LE and NIT ranges from 99.1% with 10^3 CFU/ml to 98.3% with 10^5 CFU/ml. Thus, owing to the high specificity of the test, a negative urinalysis could be used as a screen to eliminate UTI, as well as avoid unnecessary urinary culture [23].

Urinary culture and sensitivity remains the gold standard of diagnostic testing for UTI. Midstream or "clean-catch", and catheterized specimens should be collected for testing to avoid contamination from external genitalia and skin.

Management of Urinary Tract Infections

Acute Uncomplicated Lower Urinary Tract Infection

Currently used antimicrobial agents to treat uncomplicated, community-acquired UTI include trimethoprim-sulfamethoxazole (TMP-SMX), nitrofurantoin, ß-lactams, fluoroquinolones, and fosfomycin, all of which achieve high concentrations in the urine. As a rule, currently available single-dose therapy is less effective than the same antimicrobials used for longer duration [24]. Currently, TMP-SMX for 3 days should be considered first-line standard therapy [25]. Three-day treatment with TMP-SMX and fluoroquinolones are equivalent to regimens of longer duration but with fewer side effects [25–28]. It should be noted that ciprofloxacin and ofloxacin are the only FDA*-approved short-course (3-day) regimens for cystitis except for fosfomycin tromethamine, which is the first FDA-approved single-dose therapy for UTI [26]. Trimethoprim alone, and ofloxacin are equivalent to TMP-SMX [27,28]. *β*-Lactams, as a group, are less effective than TMP-SMX when given for 3 days and thus should be avoided.

Resistance of *E. coli* and other uropathogens to *β*-lactams continues to increase and now approaches 23–67% in most studies [26,27,29,30]. Nitrofurantoin and fluoroquinolones have generally maintained their effectiveness against *E. coli* isolates

Table 16.2 In vitro susceptibility of *E. coli* from North American studies of women with urinary tract infection. Reproduced with permission from Gupta et al. Increasing antimicrobial resistance and the management of uncomplicated community-acquired urinary tract infections. *Ann Intern Med* 2001; 135: 41–50.

Study site	Year	Study sample	TMP-SMX resistance (%)	Nitrofurantoin resistance (%)	Fluoroquinolone resistance (%)	Reference
United States	1990s	Outpatient women age 18–93	7	N/A	0	[32]
Washington state	1995	Outpatient university women	11	0.6	0.2	[19]
Washington state	1996	Outpatient women aged 18–50	18	0.2	0.2	[33]
California	1997	Outpatient university women	15	0	0	[34]
United States	1998	Outpatient women aged 15–50	18	1	1	[35]
Canada	1998	Outpatients	19	0.1	1	[36]
Ontario province	1998	Outpatients	8.4	4.6	0	[30ᵃ]

ᵃ All isolates included, of which *E. coli* accounted for 91.8%.
Adapted from Gupta et al. [29].

Table 16.3 In vitro susceptibility of *E. coli* from non-North American studies of women with urinary tract infection. Reproduced with permission from Gupta et al. Increasing antimicrobial resistance and the management of uncomplicated community-acquired urinary tract infections. *Ann Intern Med* 2001; 135: 41–50.

Study site	Year	Study sample	TMP-SMX resistance (%)	Nitrofurantoin resistance (%)	Fluoroquinolone resistance (%)	Reference
Netherlands	1991	Outpatients	12	7	0	[37]
United Kingdom	1992	Outpatients	19	6	1	[38]
France	1995	Outpatients	13	N/A	0	[39]
Israel	1995	Outpatients	31	N/A	4	[40]
Belgium	1995/6	Outpatients	17	1	1	[41]
Trinidad	1995	Outpatients	17	11	1	[42]
Bangladesh	1996/7	Outpatients	60	N/A	18	[43]
Spain	Unspecified	Outpatients	32ᵃ	N/A	13	[44]

ᵃ All isolates included of which 84% *E. coli*.
Adapted from Gupta et al. [29]

that cause community-acquired UTI (>95–99%) [31]. However, nitrofurantoin is less effective against non-*E. coli* Gram-negative rods and *Proteus* and *Pseudomonas* species [29,31]. Nitrofurantoin is equally effective in a 5–7-day course as TMP-SMX in bacterial eradication of *E. coli* [28]. With 7-day courses of nitrofurantoin, more gastrointestinal side effects were noted than equal duration of treatment with either TMP-SMX or fluoroquinolones [28].

Current TMP-SMX-resistant *E. coli* varies greatly from region to region. In southern Ontario, Canada, the resistance rate of *E. coli* is 8.4% to TMP-SMX, and 4.6% to nitrofurantoin [30]. In the United States there is a reported range of TMP-SMX-resistant *E. coli* from 7 to 18% [19,29,30,32–36] (Table 16.2). Table 16.3 summarizes the reported resistance of *E. coli* to TMP-SMX from 12 to 60% in the world literature [29,37–44].

Current recommendations are that TMP-SMX remain the first-line antimicrobial of choice in areas that demonstrate <10–20% resistant *E. coli* rate [29]. In endemic areas where *E. coli* resistance is >20%, fluoroquinolones should be the first-line manage-

ment. Nitrofurantoin is especially useful in these microbial-resistant times and should be considered for first-line therapy in endemic areas. β-Lactams should be employed sparingly and only in cases of documented culture demonstrating Gram-positive cocci or other sensitive uropathogens.

Acute Uncomplicated Upper Urinary Tract Infection

Traditionally, acute uncomplicated pyelonephritis was managed by hospitalization and treatment with intravenous antibiotics for up to 6 weeks. Current evidence suggests that most young healthy women with uncomplicated upper urinary tract infection will have a satisfactory outcome with 2 weeks of antimicrobial therapy [45,46]. Patients treated for a 2-week duration for uncomplicated upper urinary tract infection had similar outcomes as those treated for the traditional 3–6 weeks [47,48]. It has also been suggested that the route of treatment need not be parenteral [49,50]. Mild cases of uncomplicated

Table 16.4 Management of uncomplicated upper urinary tract infection

Mild acute pyelonephritis:	Outpatient treatment
Uncomplicated urinary tract and patient profile Low-grade fever Mild to moderate costovertebral angle tenderness Absence of nausea or vomiting Normal or slightly elevated leukocyte count	First line: PO fluoroquinolones × 2 weeks (i.e. ciprofloxacin 500 mg twice daily) Second line: PO TMP-SMX × 2 weeks (i.e. Septra DS twice daily) Third line (or Gram-positive cocci culture positive): PO amoxicillin or amoxicillin/clavulanic acid × 10–14 days (i.e. Clavulin 500 mg four times daily) Inpatient treatment First line: IV fluoroquinolones, aminoglycoside, or third-generation cephalosporin × 1 dose – 24 hours Followed by PO fluoroquinolones, TMP-SMX based on culture × 2 week total Second line: IV aminoglycoside ± ampicillin × 24 h then PO amoxicillin/clavulanic acid × 2 week total
Severe acute pyelonephritis	Inpatient management Appropriate imaging IV fluoroquinolones, aminoglycoside ± ampicillin, or third-generation cephalosporin × 48–72 hours or resolution of fever Followed by PO fluroquinolones, amoxicilin/clavulanic acid, TMP–SMX, nitrofurantoin based on culture × 2 week total

PO, by mouth; IV, intravenous.
Warren et al. [27].

pyelonephritis (uncomplicated urinary tract and patient profile, low-grade fever, moderate costovertebral angle tenderness, absence of nausea or vomiting, and normal or slightly elevated leukocyte count) in the compliant woman may be managed with oral antimicrobials for 7–14 days as an outpatient [51,52]. A reasonable treatment option is admission for observation for 12–24 hours with either intravenous or oral antimicrobial therapy. Fluoroquinolones should be employed as first-line empirical therapy, or if the organism is known to be susceptible, oral TMP-SMX may be employed. If Gram-positive cocci are responsible, amoxicillin or amoxicillin/clavulanic acid may be used [25–27].

Criteria for acute uncomplicated upper UTI requiring admission to hospital has not been well studied in the literature. If the patient profile is complicated, clinical presentation is severe (with high fever, markedly elevated leukocyte count, vomiting, dehydration, sepsis, acute complication such as perinephric abscess), or if the patient fails to improve during an initial outpatient treatment period, she should be admitted to hospital. Appropriate investigations include complete blood count, serum electrolytes and creatinine if renal compromise is suspected, and urine culture; blood cultures should also be performed if the patient is febrile (defined as temperature ≥38.5°C). Management should commence with intravenous antimicrobials after blood and urine cultures have been taken (Table 16.4). Current recommendations include parenteral fluoroquinolone, an aminoglycoside with or without ampicillin, or an extended third-generation cephalosporin with or without an aminoglycoside. If the patient improves clinically in 48–72 hours, she may be managed by oral antimicrobials directed at the cultured organism or, if unknown, empirically with fluoroquinolones, TMP-SMX, or nitrofurantoin. If Gram-positive cocci are isolated, ampicillin with or without an aminoglycoside should be used and the patient continued on amoxicillin or amoxicillin/clavulanic acid orally after clinical improvement [27]. Medical imaging as clinically indicated should be performed early in the course of management.

The Infectious Diseases Society of America (IDSA) has developed evidence-based, peer-reviewed practice guidelines for treatment of acute uncomplicated lower and upper urinary tract infection in women which have been endorsed by both the American Urologic Association and European Society of Clinical Microbiology and Infectious Diseases [25]. It will continue to be updated every 2 years on the IDSA homepage (*http://www.idsociety.org*).

Acute Complicated Lower and Upper Urinary Tract Infection

If patients with factors mentioned earlier (see Table 16.1) present with symptoms and signs of acute lower or upper urinary tract infection, adequate medical evaluation prior to embarking on empirical therapy is vital. Again, all patients with the underlying factors mentioned earlier should not automatically be labeled as having a "complicated UTI". Untreated infection does not always lead to serious morbidity or mortality in the "complicated UTI" [53–55]. Treatment of asymptomatic bacteriuria should be considered carefully as not all patients with a complicating risk factor should be empirically treated. Empirical treatment of these patients leads to the potential for increased resistant microbial pathogens, side effects, allergic reactions, and health care expenditures. Its use would be considered appropriate in asymptomatic patients where the potential exists for serious morbidity. These may include, but are not limited to, the diabetic, the leukopenic or immunocompromised patient, immunosuppressed transplant patient, and pregnancy [54]. Treatment of asymptomatic bacteriuria has been demonstrated to be beneficial in pregnancy (see Chapter 7). Treatment is clearly indicated in the symptomatic bacteriuric patient.

The medical literature is sparse in well-designed treatment trials for complicated UTIs and thus no definitive guidelines are available to aid in managing these patients. We continue to have unproven empiric therapy for most patients with such infections [51–52]. Urine dipstick screening in the diagnosis of UTI is a test with poor positive predictive value. The importance of proper urinary culture, be it by midstream, clean-catch specimen or catheterized sample, cannot be sufficiently emphasized for this group of patients. The decision to embark on empiric treatment versus awaiting urinary culture results should be individualized based on the severity of the patient's illness. Of the multiple organisms that may cause UTI in the complicated patient, resistant *E. coli* and *Klebsiella* spp. are more common in women [56].

The choice of antimicrobials should take into account the wide array of potential uropathogens that may affect this group of patients. For patients with systemic illness, septicemia, or urosepsis, admission to hospital and empiric treatment with broad-spectrum antibiotics should be initiated prior to identification of the affecting organism. However, urine, and if indicated blood cultures, should be drawn immediately prior to initiating therapy. First-line empirical therapy should provide coverage for *Enterobacteriaceae* spp., *Klebsiella* spp., *Enterococcus* spp., and *Pseudomonas* spp. Acceptable choices would include broad-spectrum penicillin with β-lactamase inhibitor combined with an aminoglycoside. A third-generation cephalosporin with pseudomonal coverage would also be acceptable first-line therapy. Alternatives include parenteral fluoroquinolones. Therapy should be targeted with narrower-spectrum antibiotics when organisms and their susceptibility are discerned. Duration of treatment is dependent on the severity of illness and the individual clinical setting. Generally a treatment consisting of parenteral antibiotics for a period of 48–72 hours until clinical resolution followed by targeted antimicrobial therapy based on susceptibility data for a minimum of 2 weeks is acceptable.

Medical imaging is used predominantly in patients with complicated *upper* UTI. However, its use in complicated and uncomplicated *lower* UTI cannot be ruled out entirely and, again, should be individualized. Ultrasonography is generally accepted as the most sensitive technique for ruling out urinary tract obstruction [57,58]. This technique is also the quickest and most sensitive technique in identification of abscess formation [59]. An early baseline ultrasound in the clinically well patient with a febrile UTI is valuable for future management [60,61]. In selected cases, where there is persistence of clinical disease (fever, elevated leukocyte count), computed tomography (CT) may be used to exclude abscess formation [59]. The excretory urogram has become less useful with the advancement of imaging modalities and should be used in conjunction with urologic and radiologic consultation owing to the potential nephrotoxic effects. The role of renal cortical scintigraphy with technetium 99m-dimercaptosuccinic acid (^{99m}Tc-DMSA) in the management of acute complicated UTI has not been fully evaluated but may be of use in the future [62].

Patients with urinary obstruction should have ultrasonography to visualize the renal tract for identification and localization of the obstruction, for identification of hydroureter, hydronephrosis, possible pyonephrosis, and identifying potential complications such as renal abscess [62]. Proper management of the obstruction with elimination of the calculi will aid in achieving cure for the patient and minimize potential complications including recurrence. If perinephric or renal abscess is identified, urologic consultation should be obtained for potential surgical drainage. These patients may require prolonged courses of antibiotics for complete recovery.

If the patient is found to have atrophic kidneys with severe pyelonephritic scarring, they are at risk of relapse and persistence of UTI, which may necessitate nephrectomy [63]. Another complicating factor of pyelonephritis which may lead to end-stage renal disease is renal papillary necrosis [64]. Persistence of bacteria in the necrotic papillae can be cured with extraction, or by partial or total nephrectomy [18]. Identification of polycystic renal disease may identify women at risk of recurrent pyelonephritis. Aerobic Gram-negative bacilli are the most common cause of infected cysts and approximately one-quarter of patients experience perinephric abscess and substantial mortality [3]. Aminoglycosides and ß-lactams penetrate the cyst wall poorly; thus lipophilic antibiotics that can transfer across the epithelial barrier (i.e. TMP-SMX or fluoroquinolones) should be employed [65].

Special Focus Patients

The Postmenopausal Woman

The postmenopausal woman is at increased risk for urinary tract infections. Microbiologic observations in the elderly suggest a wide spectrum of infecting organisms with a tendency toward pathogens with increased antimicrobial resistance [66]. *E. coli* is isolated in 50–60% of infections, with *P. mirabilis* and *Klebsiella pneumoniae* also being frequent. Urinary incontinence, increased post-void residual volume, pelvic floor prolapse and in particular cystocele are risk factors for UTI in the elderly. Estrogen deficiency has an important role in the development of bacteriuria and subsequent UTI. Estrogen maintains the acidic pH of the vagina through the stimulation of *Lactobacillus* proliferation in the vaginal epithelium. The acidic pH of the vagina prevents vaginal colonization by *Enterobacteriaceae* spp., one of the main urinary tract pathogens from the rectum. In addition, host susceptibility plays an important role in the development of UTI. Vaginal mucosal susceptibility to bacterial adherence has been demonstrated to be increased in epithelial cells at higher vaginal pH [67]. Vaginal fluid contains various antibodies that are thought to provide immune defenses against mucosal pathogens through inhibition of bacterial adherence to host cells [68]. These immune defenses may be negatively affected by increasing age and estrogen deficiency.

Treatment of UTI in the postmenopausal woman should include evaluation of the lower genital tract for estrogen deficiency, and the initiation of local or systemic estrogen. Local estrogen treatment has been demonstrated to reduce the incidence of UTI in elderly women [69]. It may be in the form of vaginal estriol or estrogen cream, or an estradiol-releasing vaginal ring. It has also been demonstrated to reduce the incidence of recurrent UTI [70]. In addition, means to reduce post-void residual secondary to incomplete emptying or pelvic-floor prolapse should be addressed. Estrogen also has beneficial effects on pelvic floor prolapse and incontinence, which may secondarily impact on the incidence of UTI and recurrent UTI.

The Catheterized Patient

Indications for urethral catheterization are many but can be grouped into the categories of surgery, urine output measurement, urinary retention, and urinary incontinence. Virtually all complications of urinary catheterization are the results of subsequent bacteriuria [71]. The risk of catheter-associated infection increases by 5–8% per day, so that by the end of one month, well over 90% of patients with indwelling catheters are bacteriuric [72]. The risk of intermittent catheterization is far less at <1% [71]. Endogenous bacteria are the most common pathogen in the catheterized patient. Its entry is facilitated by the indwelling catheter, which acts as a conduit for entry along both internal and external surfaces of the catheter. A biofilm which covers and secures bacteria, while potentially facilitating its transport, has been identified and demonstrated on both urethral and ureteric catheters [73]. Mechanical damage to the urinary epithelium may occur, leading to decreased epithelial host defenses. As a foreign object, the catheter may decrease antibacterial polymorphonuclear leukocyte formation [74].

Most catheter infections are from single organisms but up to 15% may be polymicrobial [75]. *E. coli* remains the most frequent organism isolated. However, *Enterococcus*, *Pseudomonas aeruginosa*, *Klebsiella pneumoniae*, *Proteus mirabilis*, *Enterobacter* spp., *Staphylococcus epidermis*, and *Staphylococcus aureus* are more common than in the non-catheterized patient. Less familiar species include *Providencia stuartii* and *Morganella morganii* [76]. Long-term catheterization for more than 30 days can lead to complications such as urinary obstruction, urinary tract stones, chronic pyelonephritis, and potentially bladder cancer [77]. Bacteriuria caused by *P. mirabilis* is associated with catheter obstruction through its hydrolysis of urea to ammonia leading to increased urinary pH and crystallization of struvite and apatite within the catheter lumen [78].

Minimizing the frequency and duration of catheterization, as well as keeping a closed catheter system, seem to be the most effective steps in the prevention of bacteriuria [77]. Prophylactic antibiotics appear to decrease the initial incidence of bacteriuria but long-term studies suggest no difference in infection rate. With emerging antimicrobial resistance, their use should be avoided. Patients with catheters should be judiciously cultured and treatment individualized based on the results. Empirical treatment should be reserved for the clinically ill patient. Treating UTI in catheterized patients include removal or replacement of the catheter due to the presence of bacteria on the biofilm, and a search for urinary stones and urinary obstruction with ultrasonography. Fungal infections with *Candida* species may develop in the catheterized patient but are generally asymptomatic. Removal of the catheter results in disappearance of candiduria in up to 40% of patients [77]. Oral fluconazole or bladder irrigation with amphotericin B results in similar eradication rates [79].

The Diabetic Patient

Bacteriuria and urinary tract infections are four times as common in diabetic women as in non-diabetic women [80]. Diabetes mellitus causes several changes in the genitourinary system including impaired host defense mechanisms, diabetic nephropathy, renal artery stenosis, and cystopathy or impaired bladder tone and function. Complications of UTI in the diabetic woman include renal and perirenal abscess, gas-forming infections such as emphysematous pyelonephritis and emphysematous cystitis, fungal infections, xanthogranulomatous pyelonephritis, and renal papillary necrosis. Lower and upper urinary tract infection may be asymptomatic in the diabetic patient. *E. coli* remains the most common uropathogen, with *Klebsiella pneumoniae* in particular being more common in the diabetic patient [80].

Urinary culture is mandatory in the diabetic patient because of the higher incidence of microbial resistance [81]. When clinically indicated, ultrasonography or plain abdominal X-ray should be performed to rule out diabetic-related complications as listed above. Treatment for the asymptomatic diabetic with bacteriuria is controversial, because of the possibility of progression to upper urinary tract infection. Some experts do recommend treating the asymptomatic bacteriuric, diabetic patient. However, if the patient's glycemic control is optimized, therapy should be reserved for the symptomatic patient due to difficulty in bacterial eradication and emerging antimicrobial resistance.

Recurrent UTI and Preventive Measures

Recurrent UTI is defined as a symptomatic UTI that follows clinical resolution of an earlier treated or untreated UTI. The vast majority of recurrent UTI is due to reinfection as opposed to persistent infec-

tion. Relapse is clinically defined as a UTI that is caused by the same species as the original UTI occurring within 2 weeks after completion of treatment. Underlying susceptibility to vaginal colonization with uropathogens is more common in women with recurrent UTI [82]. The underlying mechanism by which this occurs has yet to be established but appears to be based on the greater ability for uropathogenic coliforms to adhere to uroepithelial cells in patients with recurrent UTI [83]. The discovery of these mechanisms may hold the answer to the prevention of UTI and recurrent UTI.

In premenopausal women, the frequency of sexual intercourse appears to be the greatest risk factor for recurrent UTI [84]. In addition, spermicide use, having a new partner within the last year, having a first UTI before the age of 15 years, and having a mother with a history of UTIs appear to be risk factors for recurrent UTI [84]. Behavioral factors have not been evaluated in a prospective fashion. Pelvic anatomy, such as distance from urethra to anus, may play a role in some women with recurrent UTI [85]. Hypoestrogenemia in the postmenopausal woman contributes to the occurrence of recurrent UTI. The use of vaginal estrogens has been demonstrated in prospective studies to decrease the incidence of recurrent UTI [69,70].

Urinary culture is mandatory in the patient with recurrent UTI who has been treated. Antimicrobial therapy must be directed at the offending agent for sufficient duration as outlined by the Infectious Disease Society of America. Prevention strategies such as elimination of spermicide-containing products in the premenopausal woman, and use of vaginal estrogen in the postmenopausal woman are recommended. Addressing the occurrence of UTI symptoms in relation to sexual intercourse will help in identifying those women who may benefit from post-coital antibiotic prophylaxis. Prophylactic antibiotics should be reserved for patients who experience significant distress from their symptoms. Prophylaxis has been advocated for women experiencing two or more symptomatic UTIs in a 6-month period to three or more symptomatic UTIs in a 12-month period [86,87]. The infections should be verified and documented to be culture positive.

Continuous prophylaxis, post-coital prophylaxis, and intermittent self-treatment have been demonstrated to be effective in the management of recurrent uncomplicated UTI [88]. Several regimens have been attempted, including daily or post-coital TMP-SMX, nitrofurantoin, fluoroquinolones, and first-generation cephalosporins. Continuous prophylaxis has been demonstrated to be effective in reducing recurrent UTI [89–91]. There are varying recommendations as to the duration of treatment from an initial 6-month trial period to a 2-year trial period [88,89]. Treatment regimens include TMP-SMX 40/200 mg daily or thrice weekly, daily nitrofurantoin 50–100 mg, daily norfloxacin 200 mg or ciprofloxacin 125 mg, and daily ceflacor 250 mg or cefalexin 125–250 mg [89]. Post-coital prophylaxis has also been demonstrated to be effective in prevention of recurrent UTI [88,92]. In the only placebo-controlled trial performed to date, post-coital TMP-SMX 40/200 mg single-dose therapy was effective in reducing the rate of recurrent UTI [92]. Other treatment regimens have included single-day therapy with TMP-SMX 80/400 mg, nitrofurantoin 50–100 mg, ciprofloxacin 125 mg, norfloxacin 200 mg, ofloxacin 100 mg, cinoxacin 250 mg, and cefalexin 250 mg [88,92]. Prophylactic or self-initiated treatment should be reserved for the reliable patient who is motivated and compliant with medical instructions. They should be instructed to notify their physician or seek medical attention if their symptoms are not completely resolved within 48 hours [88–92].

Fruit juices, and in particular cranberry juice, have been suggested as effective in UTI prevention. Recent studies suggest that there may be a protective effect against UTI in the premenopausal age group [93]. It was initially thought to be effective in UTI prevention by lowering urinary pH but scientific evaluation has not confirmed this hypothesis [94]. It is thought that cranberry juice inhibits *E. coli* and other Gram-negative uropathogen adherence to uroepithelial cells [95,96]. Only cranberry and blueberry juices are known to possess these anti-adherence compounds [97]. In the postmenopausal age group, a prospective, placebo-controlled, randomized study demonstrated a statistically significant difference in the incidence of asymptomatic bacteriuria and antibiotic use, with a trend towards decreased incidence of symptomatic UTI in women randomized to prophylactic cranberry juice ingestion [94]. There are insufficient studies with significant power to state that cranberry juice is effective in preventing or treating symptomatic UTI. Probiotic agents such as *Lactobacillus* also have a potential role in UTI prevention. They function in this role through their competitive colonization of the vagina with uropathogens through various mechanisms. *Lactobacillus* species has been shown to block potential sites of bacterial attachment, inhibit bacterial growth, maintain a low vaginal pH, and produce hydrogen peroxide (H_2O_2), a harmful chemical to some uropathogens such as *Enterococcus* [98–102]. Well-designed treatment trials for the prevention of UTI or recurrent UTI with probiotic agents have yet to be performed.

Future Directions

As clinicians and researchers in women's health, we must better understand the epidemiology and pathogenesis of urinary tract infections. The prevalence of this disease demands further research and development of diagnostic, therapeutic, and preventive strategies. We are still dependent on traditional urine culture for diagnosis of urinary tract infection. Patient care would benefit greatly from the development of a rapid, accurate, inexpensive bedside test that would allow the practitioner to decide whom to treat at the time of examination [103]. In development is a rapid, automated urine analyzer which measures the number and size of all urine particles including bacteria, red blood cells, and white blood cells by electrical flow impedance [104]. These urine-screening tests are being evaluated for identification of samples that will likely result in negative urine cultures. These rapid analyzers would enable clinical decision-making at the time of presentation, as well as potentially eliminating costly, time-consuming, and resource-intensive urine cultures in patients with negative screening tests.

Management strategies need to be re-evaluated on an ongoing basis to reduce laboratory testing, patient visits and hospital admissions, while improving clinical and bacterial eradication rates and minimizing antimicrobial resistance. Strategies in patient-initiated home therapy have been successful in clinical outcome studies but have the potential for unnecessary treatment and further development of antimicrobial resistance [105]. Hospitals and regional microbiology divisions should collect data regarding endemic antibiotic resistance on an ongoing basis to decrease patient morbidity and improve bacterial eradication rates.

Evolving knowledge of the biofilm will direct pharmacological research while allowing further understanding of the pathophysiology behind urinary tract infections. In the future, biofilm-directed antimicrobials may emerge as first-line agents for urinary tract infections. Development of probiotic *Lactobacillus* strains that adhere to vaginal cells and have antimicrobial mechanisms, such as surfactant and H_2O_2 production, will help prevent bacterial colonization and subsequent urinary tract infection [103]. Vaccination would be an effective means of decreasing the incidence and prevalence of urinary tract infection. One of many promising strategies for the prevention of urinary tract infection is the development of vaccines that target the mechanisms by which uropathogens adhere to urogenital epithelium. FimH adhesin molecule is located on the filamentous type 1-pilus protein appendages on the surface of *E. coli* [106]. Antibody production against these adherence molecules may decrease urogenital colonization and subsequent development of bacteriuria. Vaginal mucosal immunization with whole-cell vaccine containing heat-killed bacteria has been suggested to stimulate local cervicovaginal antibodies [107]. These techniques, aimed at increasing local mucosal immunity to various uropathogens, are presently in phase II of its clinical trials [108]. These immunologic approaches to the prevention of urinary tract infection offer therapeutic alternatives to the use of frequent or long-term antibiotics and the threat of antimicrobial resistance.

References

1. Gorbach SL, Bartlett JG, FalagasM, Damer DH. Guidelines for Infectious Diseases in Primary Care. Baltimore, MD: Williams & Wilkins, 1999.
2. Kunin CM. Urinary tract infections in females. Clin Infect Dis 1994;18:1–12.
3. Kunin CM. Urinary Tract Infections, 5th edn. Baltimore, MD: Williams & Wilkins, 1997.
4. Hooton TM. Recurrent urinary tract infections in women. Int J Antimicrob Agents 2001;17:259–68.
5. Foxman B, Frerichs RR. Epidemiology of urinary tract infections: I Diaphragm use and sexual intercourse. Am J Public Health 1985;75:1308.
6. Health Indicators 1999 CD-ROM, Statistics Canada.
7. Romano JM, Jaye D. UTI in the elderly: common yet atypical. Geriatrics 1981;36:113–15.
8. Shortliffe LMD, Stamey TA. Urinary tract infections in adult women. In: Walsh PC, Gittes RE, Permufter AF et al., editors. Campbell's Urology. Philadelphia: WS Saunders, 1986; 797–830.
9. Abrutyn E, Biscia JA, Kaye D. The treatment of asymptomatic bacteriuria in the elderly. J Am Geriatr Soc 1988;36:473–5.
10. McCue JD. Effective treatment in the long-term care setting. Geriatrics 2000;55(Sept):48–61.
11. Sourander LB. Urinary tract infection in the aged – an epidemiological study. Am Med Intern Fenn 1966;55(45):7–55.
12. Thiede HA. The prevalence of urogynecologic disorders. Obstet Gynecol Clin North Am 1989;16(4):709–16.
13. Foxman B, Somsel P, Sobel JD et al. Urinary tract infection among women aged 40–65:behavioral and sexual risk factors. J Clin Epidemiol 2001;54(7):710–18.
14. Maybeck CE. Treatment of uncomplicated urinary tract infection in nonpregnant women. Postgrad Med J 1972;48:69.
15. Kunin CM, McCormack RC. An epidemiologic study of bacteriuria and blood pressure among nuns and working women. N Engl J Med 1968;278:635.
16. Raz R, Gennesin Y, Wasser J et al. Recurrent urinary tract infections in post-menopausal women. Clin Infect Dis 2000;30:152–6.
17. Raz R. Postmenopausal women with recurrent UTI. Int J Antimicrob Agents 2001;17:269–71.
18. Ronald AR, Harding GKM. Complicated urinary tract infections. Infect Dis Clin North Am 1997;11(3):583–593.
19. Hooton TM, Stamm WE. Diagnosis and treatment of uncomplicated urinary tract infection. Infect Dis Clin North Am 1997;11:551–81.
20. McCarty JM, Richard G, Huck W et al. A randomized trial of short-course ciprofloxacin, ofloxacin, or trimethoprim/sulfamethoxazole for the treatment of acute urinary tract infection in women. Ciprofloxacin Urinary Tract Infection Group. Am J Med 1999;106:292–9.
21. Stamm WE, Counts GW, Running KR et al. Diagnosis of coliform infection in acutely dysuric women. N Engl J Med 1982;307:463–8.
22. Bartlett RC, O'Neill D, McLaughlin JC. Detection of bacteriuria by leukocyte esterase, nitrite, and the Automicrobic System. Am J Clin Pathol 1984;82:683–7.
23. Semeniuk H, Church D. Evaluation of the leukocyte esterase and nitrite urine dipstick screening tests for detection of bacteriuria in women with suspected uncomplicated urinary tract infections. J Clin Microb 1999;37(9):3051–2.
24. Leibovici L, Wysenbeek AJ. Single-dose antibiotic treatment for symptomatic urinary tract infections in women: a meta-analysis of randomized trials. Q J Med 1991;285:43.
25. Norrby SR. Short-term treatment of uncomplicated lower urinary tract infections in women. Rev Infect Dis 1990;12:458.
26. Hooton TM. Practice guidelines for urinary tract infection in the era of managed care. Int J Antimicrob Agents 1999;11:241–5.
27. Warren JW, Abrutyn E, Stamm WE et al. Guidelines for antimicrobial treatment of uncomplicated acute bacterial cystitis and acute pyelonephritis in women. Clin Infect Dis 1999;29:745–58.
28. Iravani A, Klimberg I, Echold RM et al. A trial comparing low-dose, short-course ciprofloxacin and standard 7 day therapy with co-trimoxazole or nitrofurantoin in the treatment of uncomplicated urinary tract infection. J Antimicrob Chemother 1999;43(Suppl A):67–75.
29. Gupta K, Hooton TM, Stamm WE. Increasing antimicrobial resistance under the management of uncomplicated community-acquired urinary tract infections. Ann Intern Med 2001;135:41–50.
30. Mazulli T, Skulnick M, Low DE et al. Susceptibility of community Gram negative urinary tract isolates to mecillinam and other oral agents. Presented 38th Interscience Conference on Antimicrobial Agents and Chemotherapy, San Diego, CA, 24–27 September 1998. Abstract E-038.
31. Reckendorf HK, Castringius RG, Spingler HK. Comparative pharmacodynamics, urinary excretion, and half-life determinations of nitrofurantoin sodium. Antimicrob Agents Chemother 1962;2:531–7.
32. McCarty JM, Rishard G, Huck W et al. A randomized trial of short-course ciprofloxacin, ofloxacin, or trimethoprim/sulfamethoxazole for the treatment of acute urinary tract infection in women. Ciprofloxacin Urinary Tract Infection Group. Am J Med 1999;106:292–9.
33. Gupta K, Scholes D, Stamm WE. Increasing prevalence of antimicrobial resistance among uropathogens causing acute uncomplicated cystitis in women. JAMA 1999;281:736–8.
34. Dyer IE, Sankary TM, Dawson JA. Antibiotic resistance in bacterial urinary tract infections, 199–1997. West J Med 1988;169:265–8.
35. Gupta K, Sahm DF, Mayfield D, Stamm WE. Antimicrobial resistance among uropathogens causing community acquired UTI in women: a nationwide analysis. Clin Infect Dis. 2001;33(1):89–94.
36. Zhanel GG, Karlowsky JA, Harding GK et al. A Canadian national surveillance study of urinary tract isolates from outpatients: a comparison of the activities of trimethoprim-sulfamethoxazole, ampicillin, mecillinam, nitrofurantoin,

and ciprofloxacin. The Canadian Urinary Isolate Study Group. Antimicrob Agents Chemother 2000;44:1089–92.

37. Trienekens T, Stobberingh E, Beckers F, Knottnerus A. The antibiotic susceptibility patterns of uropathogens isolated from general practice patients in southern Netherlands. J Antimicrob Chemother 1994;33:1064–6.

38. Gruneberg RN. Changes in urinary pathogens and their antibiotic sensitivities, 1971–1992. J Antimicrob Chemother 1994;33(Suppl A):1–8.

39. Perrin M, Donnio PY, Heurtin-Lecorre C et al. Comparative antimicrobial resistance and genomic diversity of *Escherichia coli* isolated from urinary tract infections in the community and in hospitals. J Hosp Infect 1999;41:273–9.

40. Weber G, Risenberg K, Schlaeffer F et al. Changing trends in frequency and antimicrobial resistance of urinary pathogens in outpatient clinics and a hospital in Southern Israel, 1991–1995. Eur J Clin Microbiol Infect Dis 1997;16:834–8.

41. Christaens TH, Heytens S, Verschraegen G et al. Which bacteria are found in women with uncomplicated urinary tract infections in primary health care, and what is their susceptibility pattern anno 95–96? Acta Clin Belg 1998;53:184–8.

42. Orrett FA, Shurland SM. The changing patterns of antimicrobial susceptibility of urinary pathogens in Trinidad. Singapore Med J 1998;39:256–9.

43. Iqbal J, Rahman M, Kabir MS, Rahman M. Increasing ciprofloxacin resistance among prevalent urinary tract bacterial isolated in Bangladesh. Jpn J Med Sci Biol 1997;50:241–50.

44. Garcia-Rodriguez JA. Bacteriological comparison of cefixime in patients with noncomplicated urinary tract infection in Spain. Preliminary results. Chemotherapy 1998;44(Suppl 1):28–30.

45. Safrin S, Siegel D, Black D. Pyelonephritis in adult women: inpatient versus outpatient therapy. Am J Med 1988;85:793–8.

46. Pinson AG, Philbrick JT, Lindbeck, Schorling JB. ED management of acute pyelonephritis in women: a cohort study. Am J Emerg Med 1994;12:271–8.

47. Stamm WE, McKevitt M, Counts GW. Acute renal infection in women: treatment with trimethoprim-sulfamethoxazole or ampicillin for two or six weeks. Ann Intern Med 1987;106:341–5.

48. Jernelius H, Zbornik J, Bauer CA. One or three weeks' treatment of acute pyelonephritis? A double blind comparison, using a fixed combination of pivampicillin plus pivmecillinam,. Acta Med Scand 1988;223:469–77.

49. Bergeron MG. Treatment of pyelonephritis in adults. Med Clin North Am 1995;79:619–49.

50. Bach D, van den Berg-Segers A, Hubner A et al. Rufloxacin once daily versus ciprofloxacin twice daily in the treatment of patients with acute uncomplicated pyelonephritis. J Urol 1995;154:19–24.

51. Bailey RR, Peddie BA. Treatment of acute urinary tract infection in women. Ann Intern Med 1987;107:430.

52. Talen D, Stamm WE, Reuning-Scherer J, Church D. Ciprofloxacin (CIP) 7 day vs. TMP/SMX 14 day +/– ceftriaxone (CRO) for acute uncomplicated pyelonephritis: a randomized, double-blind trial. Boston: International Congress of Infectious Diseases, 1988.

53. Ronald AR, Nicolle LE, Harding GKM. Standard of therapy for urinary tract infections in adults. Infection 1992;20(Suppl 3):S164–70.

54. Melekos MD, Naber KG. Complicated urinary tract infections. Int J Antimicrob Agents 2000;15:247–56.

55. Stamm WE. Catheter-associated urinary tract infections: epidemiology, pathogenesis, and prevention. Am J Med 1991;91(Suppl 3B):S65–71.

56. Kawada Y. Comparison of complicated urinary tract infections in men and women. Infection 1994;22 (Suppl 1):S55–7.

57. Bailey RR, Lynn KL, Robson RA et al. DMSA renal scans in adults with acute pyelonephritis. Clin Nephrol 1996;46:99–104.

58. Johnson JR, Vincent LM, Wanf K et al. Renal ultrasonography correlates of acute pyelonephritis. Clin Infect Dis 1992;14:15–22.

59. Talner LB, Davidson AJ, Lebowitz RL et al. Acute pyelonephritis: can we agree on terminology? Radiology 1994;192:297–305.

60. Gillenwater JY. The pathophysiology of urinary tract obstruction. In: Walsh PC, Retik AB, Stamey TA, Vaughan ED, editors. Campbell's Urology. Philadelphia: Saunders, 1992; 299–332.

61. Schaeffer JA. Infections of the urinary tract. In: Walsh PC, Retik AB, Stamey TA, Vaughan ED, editors. Campbell's Urology. Philadelphia: Saunders, 1992; 731–806.

62. Weidner W, Ludwig M, Weimar B et al. Rational diagnostic steps in acute pyelonephritis with special reference to ultrasonography and computed tomography scan. Int J Antmicrob Agents 1999;11:257–9.

63. Stamey TA. Pathogenesis and Treatment of Urinary Tract Infections. Baltimore, MD: Williams & Wilkins, 1980.

64. Huland H, Busch R. Chronic pyelonephritis as a cause of end-stage renal disease. J Urol 1982;127:642–3.

65. Sklar AH, Caruana RJ, Lammers JE, Strauser GD. Renal infections in autosomal dominant polycystic kidney disease. Am J Kidney Dis 1987;10:81–8.

66. Nicolle LE. Asymptomatic bacteriuria in the elderly. Infect Dis Clin North Am 1997;11:647–67.

67. Schaeffer AJ, Rajan N, Cao Q et al. Host pathogenesis in urinaryntract infections. Int J Antimicrob Agents 2001;17:245–51.

68. Brandtzaeg P. Mucosal immunity in the female genital tract. J Reprod Immunol 1997;36:23–50.

69. Raz R, Stamm WE. A controlled trial of intravaginal estriol in postmenopausal women with recurrent urinary tract infections. N Engl J Med 1993;329:753–6.

70. Eriksen BC. A randomized, open, parallel-group study on the preventive effect of an estradiol-releasing vaginal ring (Estring) on recurrent urinary tract infections in postmenopausal women. Am J Obstet Gynecol 1999;180:1072–9.

71. Warren JW. Catheter-associated urinary tract infections. Infect Dis Clin North Am 1997;11(3):609–22.

72. Mulhall AB, Chapman RG, Crow RA. Bacteriuria during indwelling urethral catheterisation. J Hosp Infect 1988;11:253–62.

73. Ramsay JWA, Garnham AJ, Mulhall AB et al. Biofilms, bacteria and bladder catheters. A clinical study. Br J Urol 1989;64:395–8.

74. Zimmerli W, Lew PD, Waldvogel FA. Pathogenesis of foreign body infection. Evidence for local granulocyte defect. J Clin Invest 1984;73:1191–200.

75. Rahav G, Pinco E, Silbaq F et al. Molecular epidemiology of catheter-associated bacteriuria in nursing home patients. J Clin Microbiol 1994;32:1031–4.

76. Warren JW, Tenney JH, Hoopes JM et al. A prospective microbiologic study of bacteriuria in patients with chronic indwelling urethral catheters. J Infect Dis 1982;146:719–23.

77. Warren JW. Catheter-associated urinary tract infections. Int J Antimicrob Agents 2001;17:299–303.

78. Mobley HLT, Warren JW. Urease-positive bacteriuria and obstruction of long-term urinary catheters. J Clin Microbiol 1987;25:2216–17.

79. Jacobs L, Skidmore E, Freeman K et al. Oral fluconazole compared with bladder irrigation with amphotericin B for

treatment of fungal urinary tract infections in elderly patients. Clin Infect Dis 1996;22:30–5.

80. Patterson JE, Andriole VT. Bacterial urinary tract infections in diabetes. Infect Dis Clin N Am 1997;11(3):735–49.

81. Botalla MA, Baladimos MC, Bradley RF. Bacteriuria in diabetes mellitus. Diabetologia 1971;7:297–301.

82. Stamey TA, Kaufman MF. Studies of introital colonization in women with recurrent urinary infections. II. A comparison of growth in normal vaginal fluid of common versus uncommon serogroups of *Escherichia coli*. J Urol 1975;114:264–7.

83. Schaeffer AJ, Jones JM, Dunn JK. Association of in vitro *Escherichia coli* adherence to vaginal and buccal epithelial cells with susceptibility of women to recurrent urinary-tract infections. N Engl J Med 1981;304:1062–6.

84. Scholes D, Hooton TM, Roberts PL et al. Risk factors for recurrent UTI in young women. J Infect Dis 2000;182:1177–82.

85. Hooton TM, Stapleton AE, Roberts PL et al. Perineal anatomy and urine-voiding characteristics of young women with and without recurrent urinary tract infections. N Engl J Med 1993;329:753–6.

86. Nicolle LE, Ronald AR. Recurrent urinary tract infection in adult women: diagnosis and treatment. Infect Dis Clin North Am 1987;1:793–806.

87. Ronald AR, Conway B. An approach to urinary tract infections in ambulatory women. Curr Clin Top Infect Dis 1988;9:76–125.

88. Hooton TM. Recurrent urinary tract infection in women. Int J Antimicrob Agents 2001;17:259–68.

89. Nicolle LE, Ronald AR. Recurrent urinary tract infection in adult women: diagnosis and treatment. Infect Dis Clin North Am 1987;1:793–806.

90. Nicolle LE. Prophylaxis: recurrent urinary tract infection in women. Infection 1992;20:5203–5.

91. Chew LD, Fihn SD. Recurrent cystitis in nonpregnant women. West J Med 1999;170:274–7.

92. Stapleton A, Latham RH, Johnson C, Stamm WE. Postcoital antimicrobial prophylaxis for recurrent urinary tract infection. J Infect Dis 1988;157:1239–41.

93. Foxman B, Geiger AM, Palm K et al. First-time urinary tract infection and sexual behaviour. Epidemiology 1995;6:162–8.

94. Avorn J, Monane M, Gurwitz, Gurwitz JH et al. Reduction of bacteriuria and pyuria after ingestion of cranberry juice. JAMA 1994;271:751–4.

95. Sobota AE. Inhibition of bacterial adherence by cranberry juice: potential use for the treatment of urinary tract infections. J Urol 1984:131;1013–16.

96. Schmidt DR, Sobota AW. An examination of the anti-adherence activity of cranberry juice on urinary and nonurinary bacterial isolates. Microbios 1988;55:173–81.

97. Ofek I, Goldhar J, Zafriri D et al. Anti-*Escherichia* adhesin activity of cranberry and blueberry juices. N Engl J Med 1991;324:1599.

98. Chan RCY, Bruce AW, Reid G. Adherence of cervical, vaginal and distal urethral normal microbial flora to human uroepithelial cells and the inhibition of adherence of gram-negative uropathogens by competitive exclusion. J Urol 1984;131:596–601.

99. Chan RCY, Reid G, Irwin RT et al. Competitive exclusion of uropathogens from human uroepithelial cells by *Lactobacillus* whole cells and cell wall fragments. Infect Immun 1985;47:84–9.

100. Klebanoff SJ, Hillier SL, Eschenbach DA et al. Control of microbial flora of the vagina by H_2O_2-generating lactobacilli. J Infect Dis 1991;164:94–100.

101. McGroarty JA, Reid G. Detection of a lactobacillus substance that inhibits *Escherichia coli*. Can J Microbiol 1988;34:974–8.

102. McGroarty JA, Reid G. Inhibition of enterococci by *Lactobacillus* species in vitro. Microb Ecol Health Dis 1988;1:215–19.

103. Stamm WE, Norrby SR. Urinary tract infections: disease panorama and challenges. J Infect Dis 2001;183(Suppl 1):S1–4.

104. Gentelet H, Carrricajo A, Rusch P et al. Evaluation of a new rapid urine screening analyzer: cellFacts. Pathol Biol 2001;49:262–4.

105. Gupta K, Hooton TM, Roberts PL, Stamm WE. Patient-initiated treatment of uncomplicated urinary tract infections in young women. Ann Intern Med 2001;135:9–16.

106. Langermann S, Ballou WR Jr. Vaccination utilizing the FimCH complex as a strategy to prevent *Escherichia coli* urinary tract infections. J Infect Dis 2001;183(Suppl 1):S84–6.

107. Kozlowski PA, Cu-Uvin S, Neutra MR et al. Mucosal vaccination strategies for women. J Infect Dis 1999;179(Suppl 3):S493–8.

108. Uehling DT, Hopkins WJ, Beierle LM et al. Vaginal mucosal immunization for recurrent urinary tract infection: extended phase II clinical trial. J Infect Dis 2001;183(Suppl 1):S81–3.

17 Urethral Syndrome

Sender Herschorn and Martine Jolivet-Tremblay

Introduction and Definitions

The urethral syndrome was first described in 1949 by Powell and Powell [1] in a clinicopathological study. The term was popularized in the 1960s with the work of Gallagher and co-workers [2] who wrote that 50% of female patients with lower urinary tract symptoms had no laboratory evidence of urinary infection. The traditional definition, therefore, referred to any irritative symptoms suggesting a urinary tract infection (UTI) but with a negative urine culture. The term was widely used in the past but now has evolved into a much more restrictive condition and most cases will be labeled with another entity, as will be discussed below.

The pure urethral syndrome refers to irritative and painful lower urinary tract symptoms without infection or objective urological abnormality. It can be acute or chronic.

Acute urethral syndrome is a self-limited condition that is very rare. If the midstream culture is negative but the urine analysis revealed an elevated white cell count, other causes of inflammation, such as sexually transmitted diseases, fungal infections, stone, cancer, urethral diverticula, caruncle, or condylomata, must be ruled out. If the investigations are negative, it is probably better to call the acute episode a frequency/urgency episode rather than acute urethral syndrome because of the possible future connotations. In the past twenty years, with advances in the diagnosis of uncommon or subacute infections, the term 'pure acute urethral syndrome' is rarely employed in favor of a more specific diagnosis [3].

Chronic urethral syndrome refers to irritative symptoms, without any obvious cause occurring over a long period of time. The patient can have exacerbations and remissions during this time. It is still a diagnosis of exclusion and should be used with caution only after negative investigation. Interstitial cystitis (IC) must be considered as its symptomatic manifestations may be indistinguishable from the urethral syndrome [4]. The actual diagnosis of IC may also be problematic and the reader is referred to the chapter on interstitial cystitis (Chapter 18).

The symptoms were thought to occur mainly in women as initially in the literature on the urethral syndrome it was exclusively a female diagnosis. However, male patients may actually have similar clinical presentations with non-bacterial syndromes such as chronic prostatitis or chronic pelvic pain syndrome [4–6].

Symptomatology

The urethral syndrome has a wide spectrum of non-specific symptoms: frequency, urgency, nocturia, pain or burning on urination (dysuria), suprapubic pain, and other symptoms such as dyspareunia and postcoital urethral discomfort. Since these symptoms can be caused by a large number of different etiologies (Table 17.1) there are no specific pathognomonic characteristics.

Etiology

The proposed etiologies of the urethral syndrome have been as varied as the therapeutic interventions. Table 17.2 shows some of the etiologies proposed over the years.

Table 17.1 Possible causes of irritative symptoms

Urinary tract infection
Bladder cancer
Bladder calculus
Radiation cystitis
Detrusor instability
Hyperreflexic bladder
Large post-void residual volume
Urethritis
Urethral caruncle
Urethral diverticulum
Periurethral gland infection
Condylomata
Cervicitis
Carcinoma of the vulva
Pelvic mass
Atrophic genitalia
Diabetes mellitus
Diabetes insipidus
Diuretic medication
Renal impairment
Pregnancy
Chemical irritation (BCG, contraceptive foam)
Chemotherapy

Table 17.2 Proposed etiologies

Acute urethral syndrome
Bacterial infection
Herpes
Sexually transmitted diseases
Urethral spasm
Chemical agents
Chronic urethral syndrome
Urethral stenosis
Interstitial cystitis
Psychological disorder
Hormonal imbalance
Hypospadias
Chemical agents
Allergy

Acute Urethral Syndrome

An infectious etiology has been suspected for a long time. The original definition of significant bacteriuria of 10^5 or greater bacteria per milliliter stemmed from the classic studies of Kass [7–9]. The number of bacteria was proposed to distinguish contamination from true bacteriuria. Latham and Stamm in 1984 [10], in their Urologic Clinics of North America review, lowered the number of bacteria required to

attribute the cause of symptoms to infection based on the work of Stamm and colleagues [11]. In this paper 59 women with acute urethral syndrome were compared with 35 patients with classically defined cystitis and 66 asymptomatic women. Of the 59 women with acute urethral syndrome, 42 had pyuria and 37 of these had positive cultures obtained only by catheterization or suprapubic aspiration with coliforms (24), *Staphylococcus saprophyticus* (3), and *Chlamydia trachomatis* (10). Almost no women without pyuria had positive cultures. Thus 63% of the women who were initially diagnosed as having urethral syndrome actually had bacterial infection, which was not proved on voided cultures. Latham and Stamm [10] established a new criterion for acute cystitis with concomitant findings of pyuria and hematuria in that bacteriuria of greater than 10^2 per ml, rather than 10^5 per ml, was sufficient to make the diagnosis. Hamilton-Miller [12] also found that in a population of women with recurrent urinary tract symptoms, only about 50% of the episodes were due to infections with greater than 10^5 bacteria/ml. Lowering the threshold for the definition of significant bacteriuria increased the frequency with which the symptoms were thought to be from urinary infection. Overall 30–50% of patients with symptoms of acute urethral syndrome have been found to have positive cultures with less than 10^5 bacteria/ml [13].

Sexually transmitted organisms such as *Neisseria gonorrhoeae* and *Chlamydia trachomatis* can also cause dysuria and frequency in 20–30% of women [10,14]. Primary genital herpes and vaginitis can also cause dysuria and frequency [15]. In their population of 150 women, Horner and co-workers [16] found that *C. trachomatis* of the urethra was frequent but not usually associated with frequency/dysuria symptoms. Hamilton-Miller also reported that although candidiasis and trichomoniasis are common causes of acute dysuria and frequency the presence of sexually transmitted organisms could not account for the majority of these symptoms [12].

The clinical significance of other organisms is under dispute. Stamm and colleagues [11] found *Mycoplasma hominis* and *Ureaplasma urealyticum* in both symptomatic and control groups and these organisms were not felt to be associated with urethral syndrome. Wilkins and colleagues [17] isolated fastidious organisms, *Gardnerella vaginalis* and *Lactobacillus* sp, from bladder biopsies or urine culture from patients who met the criteria for urethral syndrome or interstitial cystitis. However, they did not have a control group. Maskell [18] suggested that urethral syndrome resulted from excessive multiplication of lactobacilli in the urethra, but Cooper and colleagues [19] showed that antibiotics with *Lactobacillus* activity were no more effective in treating symptoms than those without such activity. Gillespie and colleagues [20] also found no differences in positive cultures of fastidious organisms in disease and control groups. Although Haarala and co-workers [21] in a small study demonstrated streptococci anaerobes in five patients with urethral syndrome, the significance of the finding was unclear.

Chronic Urethral Syndrome

Following the description of the urethral syndrome, urethral stenosis was regarded as a common etiology and urethral dilatation was a commonly performed treatment for many years [22,23]. Urethral cryosurgery has even been proposed to treat recurrent urethral syndrome [24]. Although many patients have been reported to benefit from dilatation, the diagnostic criteria in the reported studies have been inconsistent, histologic studies documenting periurethral fibrosis have not been shown to be reproducible, and documentation of a stenosis by objective means, such as radiography or urodynamics, has been lacking [25,26]. At this point in time urethral stenosis should be considered rare and other causes sought.

Latham and Stamm [10] evaluated women with chronic urethral syndrome for infectious causes but found inconsistent results.

Chronic urethral syndrome and interstitial cystitis share many features and in many instances are thought to be one and the same [14]. The reader is referred to the chapter on interstitial cystitis (Chapter 18) for a complete discussion.

Other theories about cause include hormonal imbalances, reactions to ingested or environmental chemicals, and allergic conditions, but little supporting evidence is available [27]. Fibromyalgia has also been associated with urethral syndrome. Paira [28] found that 18% of patients with fibromyalgia met the criteria for urethral syndrome by questionnaire compared with none in a control group. Irritative lower urinary tract symptoms have also been reported in patients with Sjogren's syndrome and systemic lupus erythematosus [29]. It is possible that the urethral syndrome is an occasional manifestation of systemic disease.

More recently, urethral instability has been proposed as a possible etiology of chronic urethral syndrome. Urethral instability is a pressure fall of more than 15 cmH$_2$O measured on urethral profilometry [30]. Clarke [31] found urethral instability in 6.4%

of 608 patients and noted that it appeared to be a cause of frequency and urgency of micturition. Weil and co-workers [32] in their study of 427 female patients found urethral instability in 16.4% of patients and showed that the instability was related to frequency, nocturia, urgency, and a history of urethral syndrome. Bernstein and colleagues [33] found evidence of a muscular abnormality, characterized by poor control and increased activity of the pelvic floor associated with pain, in a small subgroup of women with urethral syndrome These may be various types of dysfunctional voiding and can be related to chronic symptoms.

Psychological factors in urethral syndrome have also been studied but the data are conflicting. Baldoni and colleagues [34] described a relationship between micturition, stressful events, and psychological symptoms in 58 female patients evaluated by questionnaire. O'Dowd and co-workers [35] also reported a prevalence of psychosomatic complaints in patients with urethral syndrome. Carson and associates [36] proposed that the disorder was a conversion reaction or psychophysiologic abnormality. Others, however, like Sumners [37], Maskell [18] and Nazareth and King [38] could find no role for psychiatric or psychological factors in the causation. In clinical practice these patients may be very distressed by their symptoms so the cause or effect relationship may be difficult to ascertain.

Van Bogaert [39] described a very rare cause of urethral syndrome, in six female patients with hypospadias. He successfully treated their symptoms by urethral meatal transposition.

Since an actual cause of symptoms, such as IC or dysfunctional voiding, can frequently be found, the term chronic urethral syndrome is no longer used very much [40]. The diagnostic approach should focus on finding an underlying condition.

Evaluation

Because of the many possible causes of irritative and painful lower urinary tract symptoms these patients should be evaluated carefully. They should all undergo a history and physical examination. One should attempt to differentiate between acute and chronic symptoms as the management differs. The physical examination should include a careful genital and pelvic examination to rule out genital condylomata, atrophic vulvar and vaginal changes, cervicitis, periurethral gland infection, local chemical irritation, pelvic masses, and rarely vulvar carcinoma.

In patients with acute symptoms vesical, urethral and vaginal infection must be ruled out. Urinalysis and urine culture and sensitivity are done to look for Gram-negative organisms and *Staphylococcus saprophyticus*. Other organisms in the acutely symptomatic patient with pyuria such as *Chlamydia trachomatis* and sexually transmitted organisms should occasionally be looked for. Urine microscopy may miss a low-count infection and indeed low colony counts in an acutely symptomatic patient may still indicate true urethritis or cystitis rather than acute urethral syndrome [40]. Antibiotic therapy is then indicated when infection is demonstrated or strongly suspected.

Primary genital herpes (HPVII) can also causes the symptoms of urgency and frequency associated with urethral pain. Urinary tract or genital fungus infections such as candidiasis or trichomoniasis are not uncommon etiologies of nonspecific symptoms in the genito-pelvic area.

Since the acute urethral syndrome is by definition a self-limited condition, in the absence of any treatable infection or microhematuria, further diagnostic studies are not routinely indicated [40].

In patients with chronic symptoms the same work-up that essentially searches for infection should be done. If the symptoms persist for more than 6–9 months, and the infection work-up is negative, additional testing can be done primarily to look for interstitial cystitis. It is important to try to make an accurate diagnosis rather than label the patient chronic urethral syndrome.

A urinary diary or voiding log is a very helpful and simple tool that can give an indication of the daily fluid intake and voiding pattern [41].

Urine cytology and if necessary appropriate urinary tract imaging studies may be done to eliminate cancer or urethral abnormalities such as a diverticulum.

Gynecologic consultation may be worthwhile in a patient with unexplained symptoms [40]. Occasionally a psychiatric or psychological consultation may be helpful [36–38].

Cystoscopy can help evaluate the urinary tract for bladder and urethral carcinoma, urethral caruncle or diverticulum, inflammatory bladder conditions, radiation cystitis, tuberculosis, or changes associated with interstitial cystitis such as glomerulations on second fill or ulcers. Since the patients may feel extreme discomfort with this test, general or regional anesthesia may be required. Bladder biopsies and/or hydrodistension may also be done.

The value of urodynamic studies is controversial. However, it can identify patients with findings suggestive of neurologic disease such as hyperreflexia with detrusor-sphincter dyssynergia. Other conditions such as bladder instability and dysfunctional voiding may also be diagnosed.

Management

Patients with acute symptoms from a urinary tract infection should be treated with a short course of an appropriate antibiotic. In the absence of a positive culture, most patients will be treated with empiric antibiotics. Doxycycline, erythromycin, and metronidazole have been recommended to treat fastidious and anaerobic organisms potentially missed on routine culture [27]. Stamm and co-workers [42] carried out a randomized trial of doxycycline versus placebo for treatment of acute urethral syndrome. They found it to be beneficial in women with pyuria and infection due to coliforms, staphylococci, or *C. trachomatis*. Other effective choices are trimethoprim-sulfamethoxazole or tetracycline [43].

The effect of estrogen deficiency on the urethra and bladder may be associated with the urethral syndrome [44]. Estrogen may improve some of the symptoms and may protect against recurrent lower urinary tract infections [45].

Patients with dysfunctional voiding may respond to alpha-blockers or diazepam but long-term studies with these agents are lacking [46].

Management of patients with chronic symptoms is much more difficult. If an alternative cause cannot be found on clinical examination, laboratory testing, cystoscopy, and urodynamic studies, the diagnosis of IC should be suspected and the patients treated for this entity. The reader is referred to the chapter on interstitial cystitis (Chapter 18) for a complete discussion. The occasional patient may also present with fibromyalgia and may respond to antihistamines, non-steroidal anti-inflammatories, and diazepam [28]. The patient with established dysfunctional voiding may be amenable to modalities such as biofeedback, pelvic floor muscle training, or sacral neuromodulation. The reader is referred to the chapters on behavior modification techniques, biofeedback and functional electrical stimulation, and sacral nerve stimulation (Chapters 24, 25, 27) for a complete discussion.

Urethral dilatation was an option for many years but objective data proving a beneficial outcome are lacking. The original idea was that distal urethral constriction was a cause of symptoms. However, female urethral strictures are rare and Rutherford and co-workers showed a similar response in two patient groups one undergoing urethral dilatation and the other cystoscopy [26]. Sand and colleagues [24] reported a randomized trial of a cryoprobe versus urethral dilatation and massage for recurrent urethral syndrome. They reported a 91% success with cryotherapy versus 33% for dilatation. However, complications of retention, bleeding, incontinence and recurrence were seen with the technique. In a recent survey of urologists from Texas, Lemack and colleagues [47] found that 21% of urologists trained more than 10 years ago considered dilation very or extremely successful in treating urethral syndrome but 0 of 42 urologists trained more recently considered it to be successful (p = 0.014). Urethral dilatation has been relegated to a rarely used treatment for the urethral syndrome.

As with other chronic diseases, patient education, realistic expectations of treatment outcome, and a supportive approach on the part of the health care provider are very important. Additional resources may include self-help groups such as the Interstitial Cystitis Association, if appropriate. The management of these problems may be frustrating for both the physician and patient, underscoring the need for a careful and systematic approach to investigation and treatment. Since the condition is benign and may be self-limited or have remissions and exacerbations, the treatment should also do no harm.

References

1. Powell NB, Powell EB. The female urethra: a clinicopathological study. J Urol 1949;61:557–70.
2. Gallagher DJA, Montgomery JZ, North JDK. Acute infections of the urinary tract and the urethral syndrome in general practice. Br Med J 1965;i:622–6.
3. Messing EM. Interstitial cystitis and related syndromes. In: Campbell's Urology, 5th edn. Philadelphia: WB Saunders Company, 1986; 1070–92.
4. Hanno PM. Interstitial cystitis and female urethral syndrome. In: Stein BS, editor. Clinical Urological Practice. New York: WW Norton, 1995; 611–22.
5. Bodner DR. The urethral syndrome. Urol Clin North Am 1988;15:699–704.
6. Sant GR, Nickel JC. Interstitial cystitis and chronic prostatitis: the same syndrome? In: Nickel JC, editor. Textbook of Prostatitis. Oxford: Isis Medical Media, 2000; 169–76.
7. Kass EH. Chemotherapeuthic and antibiotic drugs in the management of infections of the urinary tract. Am J Med 1955;18:764–81.
8. Kass EH. Asymptomatic infection of the urinary tract. Trans Assoc Am Physicians 1956;69:56–63.
9. Kass EH. Bacteriuria and the diagnosis of infections of the urinary tract: With observation on the use of methionine as a urinary antiseptic. Arch Intern Med 1957;100:707–14.
10. Latham RH, Stamm WE. Urethral syndrome in women. Urol Clin North Am 1984;11:95–101.
11. Stamm WE, Wagner KF, Amsel R et al. Causes of the acute urethral syndrome in women. N Engl J Med 1980;303:409–15.
12. Hamilton-Miller JM. The urethral syndrome and its management. J Antimicrob Chemother 1994;33(suppl A):6–73.
13. Papapetropoulou M, Pappas A. The acute urethral syndrome in routine practice. J Infection 1987;14: 113–18.
14. Curran JW, Rendtorff RC, Chandler RW et al. Female gonorrhea: its relation to abnormal uterine bleeding, urinary tract symptoms, and cervicitis. Obstet Gynecol 1975;45:195–8.
15. Corey L, Benedetti J, Critchlow C et al. Treatment of primary first-episode genital herpes simplex virus infections with acyclovir. Results of topical, intravenous and oral therapy. J Antimicrob Chemother 1983;12(suppl B):79.
16. Horner PJ, Hay PE, Thomas BJ, Renton AM, Taylor-Robinson D. The role of Chlamydia trachomatis in urethritis and urethral symptoms in women. Int J STD AIDS 1995;6:31–4.
17. Wilkins EGL, Payne SR, Pead PJ, Moss S, Maskell RM. Interstitial cystitis and urethral syndrome: A possible answer. Br J Urol 1989;64:39–44.
18. Maskell R. Urinary tract infection. In: Clinical and laboratory Practice. London: Edward Arnold, 1988.
19. Cooper J, Raeburn A, Brumfitt W, Hamilton-Miller JMT. Single-dose and conventional treatment for acute bacterial and non-bacterial dysuria and frequency in general practice. Infection 1990;18:65–9.
20. Gillespie WA, Henderson EP, Linton KB, Smith PJ. Microbiology of the urethral (frequency and dysuria) syndrome. A controlled study with 5-year review. Br J Urol 1989;64:270–4.
21. Haarala M, Kiilholma P, Lehtonen OP. Urinary bacterial flora of women with urethral syndrome and interstitial cystitis. Gynecol Obstet Invest 1999;47:42–4.
22. Davis DM. Vesical orifice obstruction in women and its treatment by resection. J Urol 1955;73:112–16.
23. McCannel DA, Haile RW. Urethral narrowing and its treatment. Int Urol Nephrol 1982;14:407–14.
24. Sand PK, Bowen LVV, Ostergard DR, Beni A, Panganiban R. Cryosurgery versus dilatation and massage for the treatment of recurrent urethral syndrome. J Reprod Med 1989;34:499–504.
25. Zufall R. Ineffectiveness of treatment of urethral syndrome in women. Urology 1978;12:337–9.
26. Rutherford AJ, Hinshaw K, Essenhigh DM, Neal DE. Urethral dilatation compared with cystoscopy alone in the treatment of women with recurrent frequency and dysuria. Br J Urol 1988;61:500–4.
27. Messing EM. Interstitial cystitis and related syndromes. In: Walsh PC, Retik AB, Stamey TA, Vaughn ED, editors. Campbell's Urology, 6th edn. Philadelphia: WB Saunders, 1992; 997–1005.
28. Paira SO. Fibromyalgia associated with female urethral syndrome. Clin Rheumatol 1994;13:88–9.
29. Haarala M, Alanen A, Hietarinta M, Kiilholma P. Lower urinary tract symptoms in patients with Sjögren's syndrome and systemic lupus erythematosus. Int Urogynecol J 2000;11:84–6.
30. McGuire EJ. Reflex urethral instability. Br J Urol 1978;50:200–4.
31. Clarke B. Urethral instability. Austral NZ J Obstet Gynaecol 1992;32:270–5.
32. Weil A. Miege B. Rottenberg R. Krauer F. Clinical significance of urethral instability. Obstet Gynecol 1986;68:106–10.
33. Bernstein AM, Philips HC, Linden W, Fenster H. A psychophysiological evaluation of female urethral syndrome: evidence for a muscular abnormality. J Behav Med 1992;15:299–312.
34. Baldoni F, Ercolani M, Baldaro B, Ttrombini G. Stressful events and psychological symptoms in patients with functional urinary disorders. Percept Motor Skills 1995;80:605–6.
35. O'Dowd TC, Pill R, Small JE, Davis RH. Irritable urethral syndrome: follow up study in general practice. B M J Clin Res Ed 1986;292:30–2.

36. Carson CC, Segura JW, Osborne DM. Evaluation and treatment of the urethral syndrome. J Urol 1980:124:609–10.

37. Sumners D, Kelsey M, Chait I. Psychological aspects of lower urinary tract infections in women. BMJ 1992;304:17–19.

38. Nazareth I, King MB. The urethral syndrome: A controlled evaluation. J Psychosom Res 1993;37:737–43.

39. Van Bogaert LJ. Surgical repair of hypospadias in women with symptoms of urethral syndrome. J Urol 1992;147:1263–4.

40. Hanno P. Interstitial cystitis and related diseases. In: Walsh PC, Retik AB, Vaughan Jr ED, Wein AJ, editors. Campbell's Urology, 7th edn. Philadelphia: WB Saunders Company, 1998; 631–62.

41. Cardozo L. Urinary urgency and frequency. In: Stanton SL, editor. Clinical Gynecologic Urology. St Louis: CV Mosby Company, 1984; 300–4.

42. Stamm WE, Running K, McKevitt M et al. Treatment of the acute urethral syndrome. N Engl J Med 1981;304:956–8.

43. Kunin CM. Management of urinary tract infections. In: Detection, Prevention, and Management of Urinary Tract Infections. Philadelphia: Lea & Febiger, 1987; 341–2.

44. Belchetz PE. Hormonal treatment of postmenopausal women. N Engl J Med 1994;330:1062–71.

45. Walters S, Wolf H, Barlebo H, Jensen HK. Urinary incontinence in postmenopausal women treated with estrogens: a double-blind clinical trial. Urol Int 1978;33:135–43.

46. Barbalias GA, Meares EM. Female urethral syndrome: Clinical and urodynamic perspectives. Urology 1984;23:208–12.

47. Lemack GE, Foster B, Zimmern PE. Urethral dilation in women: a questionnaire-based analysis of practice patterns. Urology 1999;54:37–43.

18 Interstitial Cystitis: New Concepts in Pathogenesis, Diagnosis, and Management

C. Lowell Parsons

Introduction

Interstitial cystitis (IC) is a disorder of the lower urinary tract that causes symptoms of pelvic pain and/or urinary frequency. Often mistaken for other urologic or gynecologic disorders, it is a gradually progressive disease that may affect as many as 1 in 4.5 women, as well as a significant number of men. IC has been considered difficult to detect because of its variable presentation and the lack of a generally accepted set of criteria for diagnosis. In recent years, however, significant advances have been made in the understanding of this complex and surprisingly common disorder.

In this chapter, we will make an attempt to present a clear and up-to-date definition of IC. We will review new concepts of its pathogenesis and discuss diagnostic tools and techniques as well as recent developments in treatment. We will present IC as a disease process whose clinical presentation changes with development of the disease and with fluctuations in other health factors that may provoke symptom flares, such as allergies and hormonal fluctuations. By recognizing IC in its various stages, the physician can offer effective treatments to patients whose disease might otherwise go unrecognized.

Definition

Although IC was first reported in the literature in 1915, little progress was made in defining the IC patient population until 1987, when a group of interested researchers met at the National Institutes of Health (NIH) to establish clinical criteria for characterizing the IC syndrome patient for research studies [1]. Never intended to define IC, these criteria were designed to describe advanced and persistent disease that had perhaps caused recognizable pathologic changes. Not surprisingly, subsequent studies have confirmed that the early NIH criteria represent only a small part of the IC population. The results of two 1999 studies indicate that strictly-applied NIH criteria miss approximately two-thirds of IC cases [2,3].

In fact, IC is a clinical syndrome with, as yet, no distinct pathologic tissue or serum changes to indicate its presence. Its symptoms vary depending on whether a patient has an early-phase, milder version of the syndrome, or a later, more advanced stage as is seen in older patients. It is best to think of IC as a gradually progressive disease process, intermittent in the beginning and more persistent as the IC advances and secondary bladder changes become more apparent in advanced stages (Figure 18.1).

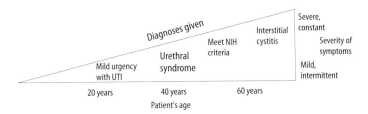

Figure 18.1 IC is a disease in a continuum. The traditional view of the IC is a syndrome of fixed severity has resulted in the misdiagnosis of the various phases of IC over the lifetime of the disease.

In general, IC is best defined by the clinical symptoms of urinary urgency, frequency and/or pelvic pain in a patient who has no other definable pathology such as urinary infection, carcinoma, or cystitis induced by radiation or medication.

Epidemiology

IC traditionally was considered quite rare, but recent data suggest that it may be much more common than early epidemiologic studies suggested.

Although IC was first identified in 1907 by Nitze, few epidemiologic studies have been reported [4]. In early reports of the incidence of IC, the numbers are low. In a Finnish study of 103 individuals with IC, for example, Oravisto estimated an annual incidence of 1.2 cases per 100 000 and a prevalence of approximately 10–11 per 100 000 [5]. Held and co-workers estimated 44 000 cases in the United States [6] with a worst-case prevalence of 450 000 [7]. In 1997, Jones and Nyberg [8] reported an incidence of 500 000 to 1 000 000 people in the US with IC.

These reports may reflect a definition of IC that encompassed only advanced-phase disease. In a large study of 1000 successive patients presenting to outpatient centers in England for a clinical trial, 50% of the patients with signs and symptoms of urinary tract infection (urgency/frequency) had negative cultures [9]. In reporting their results, the authors concluded that these patients had "the urethral syndrome", which the authors defined as the presence of signs and symptoms of infection but negative urine cultures.

It is likely, in fact, that urethral syndrome is the early or mild form of IC. In 2001, Parsons and co-workers found a positive potassium sensitivity test, indicative of an abnormal bladder epithelium, in 78% of 466 patients with clinical IC, 55% of 116 patients with urethral syndrome, and in none of 42 controls. They concluded that the finding of lower but still significant potassium sensitivity in urethral syndrome patients is supportive of the concept that IC is a continuum that begins with the mild and intermittent symptom profile that traditionally has been labeled "urethral syndrome" [10]. In addition, the results of studies in gynecologic pelvic pain patients and in men with lower urinary tract symptoms (LUTS) [11,12] indicate that there may be significant numbers of previously unrecognized cases of IC in these patient populations.

Pathogenesis

In recent years, substantial progress has been made in understanding the development of IC. It may well be that IC encompasses a number of different etiologies, culminating in a bladder insult that ultimately results in the symptoms of pain and/or urinary urgency.

Lymphatic, infectious, neurologic, psychologic, autoimmune, and vasculitic etiologies have been proposed for IC [13–20], but most of these are hypothetical, with little data to confirm or refute their role in the disease.

A number of discoveries have helped to put some of the IC puzzle pieces in place. One of the more widely accepted theories is that there is a defective bladder epithelium with loss of the "blood–urine barrier" resulting in a leaky membrane [21,22]. The permeability of the epithelium to small molecules could explain the induction of symptoms, especially if the diffusing substances stimulate the depolarization of sensory nerves [23,24]. In particular, it has been shown that diffusion of potassium across the bladder epithelium could trigger the sensory nerve endings, resulting not only in symptoms, but even in disease progression due to tissue injury from toxic levels of this cation [25]. Mast cells and their degranulation, vascular problems such as reflex sympathetic dystrophy, and probably neuro-inflammation from upregulation of the sensory nerves also play a role in IC.

Vascular Insufficiency

Reduction of vascular perfusion may negatively affect mucosal, muscle and nerve nutrition and initiate a cascade of events that causes symptoms. Radiation is known to impair blood supply by injuring the microvasculature of organs and certainly, in the case of the urinary bladder, leads to a syndrome that is basically IC with urgency, frequency, and altered epithelial permeability [26]. Other perfusion abnormalities such as reflex sympathetic dystrophy [27] may result in a secondary decrease in blood flow that also triggers events leading to symptoms in the IC syndrome. Vascular injury could even be accelerated in IC because of reduced epithelial permeability regulation resulting in a potassium leak into the bladder interstitial space. This potassium would be directly toxic to the small blood supply of the subepithelial tissues, leading to further bladder destruction.

Epithelial Leak

A widely held theory concerning the pathogenesis of IC is that of an epithelial leak. The hypothesis is that the permeability regulatory mechanism of the superficial epithelial cells is impaired, resulting in the migration of solutes across the epithelium. There had been little data to support the concept that such a leak existed [21] and a subsequent study was unable to confirm the initial observation that both normal subjects and IC patients had abnormal findings in their tight junctions relative to ruthenium red penetration. The initial report involved only three patients and no controls, however, and was primarily an anatomic study.

A well-controlled study in 56 patients provided data to support the hypothesis that the bladder surface in many IC patients may indeed leak solute [22]. This data has been supported by subsequent investigations which employed an even more sensitive "leak assay" to screen individual patients for potential aberrations in permeability. From these studies, it was estimated that at least 70–75% of the patients could be determined to have a leaky epithelium [26,28]. The caveat here is that there are false negatives to the test (probably not false positives) and epithelial problems may be present in even more patients. In addition, this was a slightly skewed population, with the patients who have a non-leaky epithelium being more difficult to treat and more likely to present to the tertiary care center.

This latter concept is supported by the fact that other investigators have found similar responses to the potassium test. To date, the results of over 1300 potassium sensitivity tests (PSTs) in IC patients who have presented to urologists or gynecologists have been published. The data indicate that approximately 80% of individuals with IC have a positive PST; healthy controls are negative [3,10,26,28–35]. False positive PSTs are rare [10,26,28,29,36–39]. These studies also suggest that a small part of this patient population has no detectable epithelial leak (by current technologies) and may represent some other problem, such as neurological inflammation. A negative PST confirms nothing, however, so it is not currently possible to estimate the actual percentage of "non-leakers".

Role of Urinary Potassium in the Pathogenesis and Diagnosis of IC

One of the most important pieces of the interstitial cystitis puzzle is the identity of the toxic substance in urine that leaks across the epithelium and provokes the symptoms of IC. It has been proposed by Parsons et al. [28] that the principal toxic substance in urine is potassium. In essence, it is rather an obvious toxin in that the urine levels range between 40 and 150 mEq/l with an average of about 90 mEq/l, a concentration that has long been known to be toxic to all mammalian cells. In addition, it has

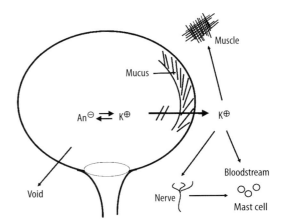

Figure 18.2 The role of the transitional epithelium in regulating potassium metabolism.

been known for many years that potassium at a level of 12–15 mEq/l will depolarize sensory nerves and muscle. Because the kidneys are the main route of excretion of the dietary potassium, the bladder had to develop a method to handle these very toxic levels of potassium. It may well be that the most important role of the relatively impermeable bladder epithelium is to prevent potassium from diffusing into the bladder interstitium and destroying the tissue. The role of the transitional epithelium in regulating potassium metabolism is summarized in Figure 18.2.

If urinary potassium should leak excessively into the bladder interstitium, the rich supply of subepithelial lymphatic and blood vessels could resorb this cation and restore the normal equilibrium [40]. The diffusion of potassium at excessive rates could lead to the destruction of these blood and lymphatic vessels, however, resulting in the acceleration and progression of the disease process. The sequence of events could explain both the presence of symptoms and the gradual progression of disease in most patients.

Toxic levels of interstitial potassium could also induce other neurologically active agents, such as substance P, and lead to upregulation of pain fibers which may be an important feature of IC [41–44]. The potassium hypothesis also explains the lack of any significant inflammatory response in most patients with IC, in either the urine or bladder interstitium [45].

Based on these concepts, several important components in the paradigm of IC pathogenesis can be proposed. For reasons unknown, the regulatory role of mucus in reducing permeability is impaired. Once this impairment takes place, the high levels of urinary potassium will result in increased interstitial levels in the bladder that induce sensory nerves

Table 18.1 Instructions for performing the potassium sensitivity test

Potassium test procedure
Solution 1: 40 ml sterile water Solution 2: 40 ml potassium solution (16 mEq KCl)[a] 1. Ask patient to rate baseline pain and urgency using the scales below. 2. Place small catheter in patient's bladder. 3. Slowly, over 1–2 minutes, instill solution 1 into the bladder. 4. Ask patient to rate current pain and urgency after 5 minutes. 5. Remove solution 1 from the bladder 6. Slowly, over 1–2 minutes, instill solution 2 into the bladder. 7. Ask patient to rate current pain and urgency after 5 mnutes. 8. Remove solution 2 from the bladder and wash once with 40 ml water. 9. Ask patient to compare the solutions using the questionaire below.

Grading scales for symptoms	Questionaire
Pain None Mild Moderate Severe |----------|----------|----------|----------|----------| 0 1 2 3 4 5 **Urgency** None Mild Moderate Severe |----------|----------|----------|----------|----------| 0 1 2 3 4 5	1. Which solution is worse? ____ Solution 1 ____ Solution 2 2. Is the difference between the solutions: ____ None ____ Mild ____ Moderate ____ Severe

[a] For potassium solution, bring 20 mEq KCl ampule up to 50 ml with water.

(and muscle) to depolarize, resulting in pain and urgency, and may destroy tissue, causing progression of the disease. These concepts have also been supported by data from Hohlbrugger [25,46]. Incorporated into the progression may be the upregulation of nerve fibers, mast cells and an ever increasing neurogenic inflammation, which may become an important and perhaps driving force of the disease and one that also has to be dealt with in terms of therapy. In effect, as the disease progresses, patients will become both solute and volume sensitive.

Based on the epithelial permeability model of IC pathogenesis, Parsons developed a test in which the bladder is challenged with separate intravesical instillations of water and potassium [26,28,29] (Table 18.1). In response to the potassium, an individual with an effective urothelial permeability barrier suffers no urinary symptoms of urgency and/or pain. An individual with an abnormally permeable epithelium, however, does experience urgency and/or pain in response to the potassium instillation, as potassium passes through the urothelium and penetrates the bladder muscle, where it can depolarize sensory nerves and cause urgency or pain.

As we have said, published reports indicate that approximately 80% of over 1300 individuals with IC have a positive PST. The PST is helpful in diagnosis, especially in patients with mild IC and when one is unsure of the diagnosis. It is important to recognize that a patient with IC may test PST negative on any given day because of the intermittent nature of IC's symptoms. Therapy should not be withheld from a patient in whom IC is suspected even if the PST is negative.

Neural Upregulation

Pain becomes a prominent factor as IC progresses. This fact suggests the presence of significant upregulation (activation) of sensory nerves in the bladder, a hypothesis that is supported by the results of a number of studies [47,48]. Upregulation of pain fibers can lead to a more substantial and persistent form of interstitial cystitis [41–44]. This aspect of the pathogenesis of IC may be the most difficult part of the disease to treat, as it can persist even if any defect in the epithelium is corrected. As the disease progresses, the increased peripheral and central neuronal activity probably has components of both volume sensitivity and solute (potassium) sensitivity. The volume sensitivity could readily persist even if solute reactivity is controlled.

Mast Cells

The role of mast cells in IC is not fully understood. Mast cells have been reported by a number of investigators to be present in IC bladders while other data suggest that they are also present in non-IC bladders [18,20,49–53]. The central point of confusion is whether or not mast cells play a causative or secondary role. As causative factors, they may be degranulating and producing the symptoms. On the other hand, they may represent a response to whatever is causing IC (e.g. an epithelial leak), and thus may be a type of defense mechanism that may ultimately become part of the problem by degranulating and causing a "leak".

Regardless of how one views the data, most clinical IC researchers believe mast cells play an important role in IC. Clinical impressions are supported by research data in animal models. Saban and coworkers have shown quite well that mast cell activation in guinea pig bladders results in an increase in epithelial permeability [54]. Active allergies will significantly flare IC, as we and others have observed. In light of these observations, the mast cell takes on added significance, especially when one embarks on therapy.

Mast cells also interact with sensory nerves and release transmitters that activate pain, and Sant and others have obtained data to show upregulation of nerves and neurotransmitters [41–44,51,53,55–59]. This is to be remembered when therapy is reviewed because suppression of mast cells appears to be important in successful management of IC.

Diagnosis

For the physician, perhaps one of the greatest challenges associated with IC is recognizing the presence of the disease. Until recently, IC has been diagnosed only in those patients who have the severe symptom complex of urinary urgency, frequency, and pelvic pain. The traditional view of IC recognizes only those patients with advanced-phase disease, however, and probably identifies no more than 5% of the individuals who are afflicted. As such, this view of IC is of little value to the clinician.

In the early phases of IC, patients' complaints are usually intermittent. Until the symptoms become more continuous, it is likely that the disease will be confused with other urologic or gynecologic disorders. In women who consult urologists for their symptoms, IC is often mistaken for recurrent bladder infections or urethral syndrome (which is IC). Women who experience pelvic or perineal pain

as the primary symptom of their IC often present to the gynecologist, who may attribute their pain to endometriosis or various types of vaginitis or vulvodynia. In men, the disease is often confused with prostatitis or with problems associated with bladder outlet obstruction due to prostate enlargement. Recent studies indicate there may be unsuspected numbers of IC patients among women who consult gynecologists for pelvic pain [11] and among men with lower urinary tract symptoms who are being evaluated for possible bladder outlet obstruction [12].

Signs and Symptoms

The principal symptoms of IC are the presence of abnormal sensory urgency and/or pain. From sensory urgency derives urinary frequency. Many patients may experience urgency and frequency with no pain problems, but most will have some combination of urinary frequency and pelvic pain. In addition, there are some patients who have pain and no urgency [10]. One study of over 200 patients [60] showed that approximately 15% of patients presenting with IC have little or no bladder pain, while 85% of patients present with significant pain. The classic description of IC pain increasing with holding of urine and relieved by voiding is in fact a rarity. Bladder pain can increase with holding or voiding, or refer to any location in the pelvis, suprapubically, in the perineum, vulva, scrotum, vaginally or in the low back or even medial in the thighs [10,14]. One-third of patients experience dysuria. Men may experience pain in the scrotum or testes.

Nocturia is variable. Most patients will complain of voiding at least 1–2 times per night, but many patients have no nocturia [60]. As nocturia increases with the severity and duration of the disease, little or no nocturia will be present in the early phases. The average patient with clinically significant and active IC voids approximately 14–15 times a day. A minimum for diagnostic purposes is considered to be 8 voids per day [1]. The average voided volume is 70–90 ml. Between 85% and 90% of individuals with IC are female. Of those who are sexually active (males and females), the majority (71%) will complain of exacerbation of the symptom complex associated with sexual intercourse (during or after) [60]. The increase in symptoms may be felt during sexual activity, immediately after, or within 24 hours. In addition, most women who are still menstruating will complain of a flare of symptoms several days to a week before the onset of the menstrual cycle [60,61].

The median age of diagnosis of IC is quite variable owing to the constantly changing awareness of IC, and is best expressed as a range of 36 to 46 years. At the time of presentation to the urologist, the average patient has had symptoms for 3–4 years, again reflecting the delay in diagnosis [14,60].

Evaluation

The physician has struggled to establish a diagnosis of IC, primarily because no objective "blood test" exists. The evaluation of large numbers of patients with the urgency-frequency syndrome reveals historical and clinical findings that help establish the diagnosis.

The NIH criteria for IC [1], described earlier, defined only those patients with advanced IC. At present, it is generally believed that an individual who voids more than 8 times in 24 hours and/or has associated pain in the bladder, pelvis, or urethra may have IC. The clinician must bear in mind that many, perhaps most, patients with IC do not meet the NIH criteria but do have the disease and will benefit from therapy. The key for diagnosis is that no matter what the frequency is the abnormal urgency and/or pain from which the patient suffers are enough to drive the patient to seek medical care.

Voiding Log

The more accurate assessment of number of daily voidings and average volume can be obtained from a 2-day voiding log in which the patient measures and records each void at home. From voiding log data, it was found that the average patient voids 16 times per day with a capacity of 73 ml. In 97% of patients, voided volume averaged less than 100 ml [1]. The voiding profile is helpful in establishing the diagnosis of IC, and may be used subsequently to create a therapeutic plan and to determine progress in therapy. The clinician should obtain one voiding log initially and one at each subsequent visit. As might be anticipated, patients with a longer disease history have a smaller functional bladder capacity.

The clinician may be quite surprised that many patients have abnormal voiding logs but minimal complaints of frequency. This is because the increase in urgency may be so gradual that patients accept it as normal for them; it is the pain and pain flare cycles that they complain of most.

Physical Examination

There is one important part of the examination that helps confirm the diagnosis of IC. On physical examination, over 95% of patients will complain of a tender bladder base during the pelvic examination. This discomfort is easily demonstrated by palpation of the anterior vaginal wall.

Urine analysis (and certainly cultures) on voided specimens is not useful in these patients because their low voided volumes make midstream collection impossible. One sees only vaginal secretions unless a catheterized specimen is obtained. A catheterized specimen examined under the microscope should show no bacteria, and most will show no red or white blood cells. Urine should be sent for cytological evaluation to rule out the possibility of carcinoma but in actuality, there has never been a positive cytology at our center, but perhaps this is because the patients are usually seen first by other urologists. Patients presenting with hematuria are less common, and when present require a full genitourinary work-up to exclude malignancy. All men and women over 40 probably deserve at least an initial screening to rule out malignancy. This screening should be a cytology and office cystoscopy.

Urodynamics

The cystometrogram (CMG) is a valuable study to perform in patients with this syndrome since a normal study usually excludes the diagnosis of IC. Recently published data by the NIH ICDB Study Group demonstrated that the urodynamics could be substituted for cystoscopy in diagnosis [62]. This study helps substantially to both include and exclude patients in diagnosing IC. Together with the voiding log, the potassium test is quite helpful in diagnosing IC. Since most patients have some degree of urinary urgency, this can usually be documented with cystometry. If gas is employed, they will have a sensation of significant urgency at less than 125 cc and with water <150 ml. If this portion of the CMG is normal, they may not have IC or only a mild form. In 75 patients with cystometrograms reported by Parsons [60], the average bladder capacity was 220 cc, with over 90% of patients having a functional volume of less than 350 cc. In general, patients should have the bladder discomfort they experience provoked by the CMG. But, as noted previously, some patients' bladder pain is not provoked by volume. However, there is an important caveat relative to maximum bladder capacity. A small group of patients with significant IC will develop detrusor myopathy (about 5%) [60,63]. Individuals with this complication will have large atonic bladders with little muscle present. They have moderate to severe sensory urgency, large bladder capacities (>1000 cc), and usually carry residual urines

(>100 cc). Detrusor function is poor or absent. In fact, many patients with IC have poor muscle function as the disease gradually destroys their bladder and hence, empty their bladders only with difficulty. Since most of the patients are women, they are able to void but primarily with a Valsalva maneuver. The myopathy subgroup represents approximately 5% of patients with IC, but the general muscle dysfunction is seen in most patients with advanced disease [60].

Males with advanced IC may require a program of intermittent catheterization (ICP) as part of their treatment. In fact, owing to the generalized atrophy of bladder muscle with this disease, males with low voiding pressure may require ICP. Urodynamics may help differentiate men with IC from those with symptoms secondary to bladder outlet obstruction. If the patient has increased sensory urgency, low volume bladder with low flow and low pressure and positive PST, think IC and not benign prostatic hyperplasia (BPH).

Cystoscopic Evaluation

Cystoscopic evaluation of the bladder under anesthesia is primarily important as a therapeutic maneuver. It is not necessary for diagnosis [62] unless cancer is suspected (in an older male with hematuria, for example). Examination under local anesthesia for the purpose of diagnosing IC is to be discouraged, because it offers little help in diagnosis and causes the patient severe discomfort. To rule out carcinoma in high-risk individuals (those over 40 and those with hematuria), however, cystoscopy under local anesthesia is warranted. When a cystoscopy is performed for therapy, it should be done under anesthesia. Not all patients need cystoscopy. In fact, most patients do not need this unless severe symptoms are present. It is best to omit cystoscopy in milder patients and proceed with other therapies listed below.

The cystoscopy under anesthesia is performed in a manner to both diagnose and treat. The diagnosis depends on discovering one of two findings, a Hunner's ulcer or the presence of glomerulations or petechial hemorrhages. However, at least 40% of patients do not show these changes, so their absence does not exclude the diagnosis.

Pathology

One should keep in mind the concept that IC is a disease in a continuum. The 19-year-old with early disease has significant sensory nerve activation, but no real damage to the bladder. As the disease progresses over 10–20 years, however, the patient may have some significant secondary changes to her bladder at age 40; for example, altered epithelium, adhesion molecules, basement membrane changes, muscle loss, and/or nerve upregulation, but no traditional clinical pathology changes. Consequently, routine pathologic processing of tissue yields neither helpful nor pathognomonic changes in IC; hence biopsy is worthless.

There is no way to rule in or out this disorder by pathological examination of bladder tissue. While it is rare that these patients are confused with those having carcinoma in situ of the bladder, the biopsy may be necessary to rule out cancer (reviewed by Burford and Burford [64]). A combination of cytological evaluation of the urine and bladder washings and biopsy is necessary to exclude malignancy in high-risk patients, that is, men over 40, women over 45, and anyone with hematuria.

Potassium Sensitivity Test

The potassium sensitivity test, discussed above, is a simple method for detecting the abnormal epithelial permeability that is present in most individuals with IC. The PST procedure is presented in Table 18.1.

A positive PST can be regarded as a definitive sign of the presence of IC; false positives are extremely rare [10,26,28,29,36–39]. An individual with IC may test PST negative on any given day, however, owing to the intermittent nature of the symptoms of IC. For this reason, a negative PST does not rule out the presence of IC. Treatment should not be withheld from a patient who has symptoms of IC but is PST negative.

Therapy

As a result of dramatic changes in the therapy of IC in recent years, good disease control can now be achieved in up to 85–90% of patients with this disease. The key principle in the treatment of IC is to use multi-modality therapy to control the various aspects of the disease that are active at causing symptoms. Patients with mild IC may not need much therapy; those with severe disease may require multiple modes of therapy to control their complex of symptoms. A good rule of thumb is that the more active the disease, the more treatment the patient will need.

The range of therapies available for IC has been limited by the fact that many of the compounds that are active in the disease are generic. These generic compounds have not been, and probably never will be, studied in a controlled fashion. Perhaps the only medication that has been studied rigorously in multiple double-blind trials is pentosanpolysulfate (Elmiron), discussed in detail below.

Patients with IC receive the greatest benefit from a treatment program based on three principles:

1. Control the dysfunctional epithelium with heparinoid compounds.
2. Suppress the neural activation with amitriptyline, imipramine, or a selective serotonin reuptake inhibitor (SSRI).
3. Manage allergies.

Recommendations for therapy are discussed in detail below.

Cystoscopy for Therapy

The report by Bumpus in 1930 of bladder hydrodistension improving the symptoms of IC has resulted in this procedure being a mainstay of therapy [65]. Few would question the activity of hydrodistension in ameliorating the symptoms in 60% of IC patients. The procedure must be performed under anesthesia since it is not possible to dilate a painful bladder without it.

Control of Epithelial Dysfunction

Most people who have IC have a bladder epithelial dysfunction, which is reflected in a positive potassium sensitivity test. The cornerstone of treatment for patients with a dysfunctional epithelium is the category of heparin-like drugs, or heparinoids. Heparinoids have revolutionized the treatment of IC because they correct the problem of epithelial dysfunction, which occurs in the majority of patients with the disease. Two such medications are clinically available: heparin and pentosanpolysulfate (Elmiron) (Table 18.2).

Heparin

Although heparin is given intravesically and has the drawback of requiring daily self-administration by

the patient, it can be effective in up to 80–85% of patients [66]. Currently, we use heparin in patients who are potassium sensitive and have failed oral therapy with pentosanpolysulfate, or patients who have very severe disease, and in these individuals we use a combination of oral and intravesical heparinoid therapy.

The patient self-administering heparin at home should utilize a dose of 40 000 units heparin in 20 cc, introducing the solution into the bladder and holding it only for as long as is comfortable. If the patient starts to experience pain, the bladder should be emptied immediately as it is important not to activate the pain cycle. Although the patient may be able to hold the solution in the bladder for only 20 minutes at first, this is a good starting point. Gradually, the patient will be able to hold the heparin solution in the bladder for longer periods of time, with the eventual goal of holding it comfortably for an hour.

On heparin therapy, reasonable improvement of symptoms can be expected between 6 months and 2 years after initiation of therapy. As potassium-sensitive individuals are the patients who are the most likely to respond to heparin, we recommend that they remain on heparin therapy for at least 3–4 years.

Pentosanpolysulfate

Pentosanpolysulfate (Elmiron) is the only IC medication that has been studied rigorously in double-blind trials. Similar results have been obtained in four double-blind trials of pentosanpolysulfate; that is, that IC patients' response to the drug is twice the response to placebo, particularly with regard to pain [36–38,49]. In a longitudinal study that was published in 1997 [67], it was reported that up to 75% of patients will respond to pentosanpolysulfate therapy when the drug is used for 6 months to 3 years. In this particular study, it was also determined that the patients remain better on the medication once improvement has been obtained. Because it basically corrects the major pathology associated with the disease, heparinoid therapy is the only mode of treatment on which the patients improve and stay improved. It has also been reported that if the patients are potassium sensitive, up to 82% will respond. When they are not, only 30% respond [31]. The limitations of the early pentosanpolysulfate trials were that they were done for only 12 weeks on end-stage patients in low dose. Many studies of pentosanpolysulfate are in progress, and new and better dosing regimens will be emerging shortly.

Although the recommended dose of pentosanpolysulfate (100 mg three times a day) is effective,

Table 18.2 Guide to heparinoid therapy for IC

Drug	Dose	Route
Heparin	20 000–40 000 units daily	Intravesical and self-administered
Elmiron (pento-sanpolysulfate)	100–200 mg three times a day	Oral

ongoing trials show that higher doses such as 200 mg or even 300 mg three times a day are more effective. We usually employ, in females, 200 mg twice a day because it works well at this dose and is easier for patients to remember. It is our general recommendation that men be started on a dose of at least 200 mg three times a day. As reported in the double-blind studies mentioned above, the average patient begins to show reasonable improvement in 3–6 months, with good responses seen at 6–12 months. The more active and severe the IC and the longer the disease has been present, the longer it will take for pentosanpolysulfate to work. It is important for the clinician to bear in mind that while pentosanpolysulfate probably corrects the epithelial dysfunction at the bladder surface in a relatively short time, a basic improvement in symptoms will not be seen until neural deactivation takes place, which can be over months or years.

In our experience, approximately 75% of patients who were continuously symptomatic for more than 6–9 months before treatment will relapse with symptoms after 3–4 months if they stop the medication once their symptoms improve. Once our patients have been symptom free for 6–12 months, we give them the choice of continuing or discontinuing the medication. The majority of our patients, at least 80%, elect to stay on therapy. Those who wish may be tapered off of medication and restart should they flare.

Pentosanpolysulfate is safe and non-toxic. The principal side effect appears to be gastrointestinal distress, occurring in about 3–4% of patients. As this side effect may be related to the capsule rather than to the drug itself, we routinely ask patients experiencing gastrointestinal side effects to take the medication with a small snack, or take it out of the capsule and put it into one ounce of water and drink the solution. Another pentosanpolysulfate side effect deserving mention is a rare form of alopecia known as alopecia reata, a patchy baldness. It is important to emphasize to the patient that the alopecia that can be associated with pentosanpolysulfate therapy will not cause complete baldness as in chemotherapy patients; rather, it is a completely reversible process. In those patients who do experience diffuse hair loss with pentosanpolysulfate, I advise continuing the medication because the alopecia tends to resolve. This is probably because the alopecia in many cases is associated with perimenopause rather than with the pentosanpolysulfate.

It has been reported that pentosanpolysulfate affects liver enzymes. This is certainly an unusual event and may be an idiosyncratic reaction. Pentosanpolysulfate does not appear to cause hepatotoxicity and is not metabolized by the liver. We measure liver enzymes once in our patients, at about 6 months after initiation of treatment. In hundreds of patients we have treated with pentosanpolysulfate, we have detected a liver enzyme aberration in only one individual. We stopped the medication for one week and then restarted it; the aberration did not recur.

Neurological Deactivation

Another basic treatment principle in IC concerns a factor that urologists have been addressing for many years in sensory disorders of the bladder; that is, to inhibit the neurological activation that occurs and induces symptoms of urgency, frequency and pain. In a sense, this aspect of therapy treats the symptoms rather than the disease, but it is important to attempt to inhibit the neurological activation while the patient is undergoing heparinoid therapy to repair the epithelium and effect the natural regression of neural upregulation. This neurological aspect is the rate-limiting factor in a patient's response to treatment. It is not that heparinoid agents do not repair the bladder surface relatively quickly, but rather that these patients still have significant bladder volume sensitivity from the neurological activation. Such activation takes months or years to regress, and in some cases the regression never occurs. At the start of treatment, we place all of our patients on heparinoid therapy to address the epithelial dysfunction, plus an antidepressant to address the neural upregulation in perhaps 30–50% of them.

The drugs we have found to be most active in controlling the neural upregulation of IC are amitriptyline [68] and imipramine. The initial dose of either medication is 25 mg at bedtime. After the patient has been on this medication for 1–2 months, the dose can be increased to 50 mg. There is even a 10 mg pill for patients to take until they adjust to the very sedating effects associated with the medication. In an uncontrolled trial, Hanno et al. reported that about 50% of patients will respond to this therapy [68]. In our experience, it is very useful in severely symptomatic IC patients, as it does help alleviate their discomfort.

If the patients are unable to tolerate amitriptyline or imipramine because of the sedative side effects and the appetite stimulation, we recommend using the selective serotonin reuptake inhibitors (SSRIs). We routinely use fluoxetine (Prozac) at doses of 10 or 20 mg per day. Rarely is it necessary to increase the dose. Sertraline (Zoloft) can also be used at doses of 50 mg per day, increasing to 100 mg per day if necessary.

Management of Allergies

Allergies and mast cells play a substantial role in provoking the symptoms of IC. Mast cell activity is present in perhaps up to 70% of the patients with the IC syndrome. If mast cells are not regulated well, they will constantly muddy the waters, stirring up the symptom complex during allergy season or even whenever the patient is exposed to a problematic food allergen. Although a patient's epithelial dysfunction may be under good control (see above), his or her symptoms can activate completely back to the baseline during an allergy attack. Thus, when patients who are successfully managed on heparinoid therapy complain of symptom flares during the allergy season, the heparinoid therapy should not be discontinued, as it is essential to the long-term management of the patient. Instead, the symptom flares should be addressed with additional therapy; that is, antihistamines.

It may be several allergy seasons before this pattern is even recognized so that effective therapies can be undertaken. Nonetheless, this is an important issue to address in the successful long-term management of IC. In our practice, if we had only two medications to treat IC, we would select pentosanpolysulfate (Elmiron) and hydroxyzine (Atarax, Vistaril). With these two medications, we can control the symptoms in up to 85% of our patients quite successfully over the long term.

Up to 70% of IC patients will need antihistamines in addition to heparinoid therapy to regulate the disease. The mast cells have been known to be active in this disease and antihistamines have been used for a number of years to help control symptoms [52, 69–71]. As with other drugs or generics, the antihistamines have never been tried for treatment of IC in a controlled trial, and probably will not be.

The best medication to use to treat mast cell degranulation chronically is a tricyclic compound, the drug hydroxyzine (Atarax, Vistaril) at the same dosing of imipramine and amitriptyline. A dose of 25 mg is more than sufficient to use chronically to inhibit mast cell degranulation. If the sedating effects of the 25 mg dose bother the patient when the medication is started, 10 mg doses are available. After 2–3 months of chronic therapy with this medication, the sedating effects disappear and the most powerful therapeutic effect of this particular antihistamine, the inhibition of mast cell degranulation, starts to become active. Hydroxyzine is the only antihistamine that works in this fashion and we have found it to be the best drug to use [72]. During allergy season, the dose of hydroxyzine can be readily bumped to 50–100 mg per day with minimal sedating effects if the patient is accustomed to the medication. Alternatively, one can use any nonsedating antihistamine to help control the patient's allergy.

Dimethylsulfoxide

Dimethylsulfoxide (DMSO) was approved for use in IC in 1977 based on uncontrolled trials [73]. DMSO appears to induce remission in 34–40% of the patients. The difficulty with DMSO is that it may induce an excellent remission in the first one to three cycles of therapy, but as an individual relapses and requires subsequent treatment, progressive resistance to its beneficial effects is seen in almost all patients for reasons unknown.

For treatment, instill 50 cc of 50% DMSO into the bladder for 5–10 minutes. Longer periods are unnecessary since DMSO rapidly absorbs into the bloodstream. Instillations are performed on an outpatient basis or patients can be taught to perform it themselves. The author recommends that patients receive weekly treatments for a period of 6–8 weeks to determine whether a therapeutic response is achieved. It usually requires 2–3 months to obtain a good clinical response. If the patient has moderate or worse symptoms, continue the therapy for an additional 4–6 months once every other week. It should be remembered that once DMSO is stopped, the patient is likely to become resistant to its use. Some patients will experience a flare of symptoms when DMSO is placed into the bladder. This phenomenon most likely is due to a detergent-like activity with DMSO destroying the superficial bladder umbrella cells and causing a significant increase in the epithelial leak. Nonetheless, DMSO may be very effective at treating these patients. Should the patient experience pain with DMSO, it is recommended that he or she receive intravesically 10 ml of 2% viscous xylocaine jelly 15 minutes before placing DMSO. If this is not successful, then use an injectable narcotic or Toradol 60 mg or meperidine intramuscularly before the intravesical instillation. The flare of symptoms associated with DMSO usually disappears over 24 hours. As these patients receive subsequent treatments, the pain tends to diminish.

Patients may also receive indefinite therapy using DMSO. As originally reported by Stewart et al. [73], patients have used DMSO weekly for several years without problems. DMSO has been reported to be associated with cataracts in animals. However, this complication has not been reported in humans. It seems reasonable, if the patient is on chronic therapy, that he or she has a slit lamp evaluation at 6–12-month intervals, but in fact, we have not found this to be necessary and rarely do it.

Urinary Alkalinizers

Polycitra is a dilation agent that not only alkalinizes the urine, but also binds potassium. Both effects may be beneficial in IC and it is recommended that patients receive a trial of therapy for 3–6 months. Employing two doses of medication a day appears to be sufficient. In general, this drug should be combined with other treatments such as heparin, Elmiron or Elavil to obtain the best effect. The best tolerated salt of Polycitra is potassium, but one does not need to worry about this small amount of potassium. When Polycitra is absorbed and excreted in the urine, it will help chelate urinary potassium so the original salt is not a problem for the bladder.

Surgery

Approximately 2% of patients presenting with IC to the University of California, San Diego Medical Center have ultimately undergone surgery for disease that is severe and refractory to all treatment. The question is the type of surgery to be performed.

Bladder Augmentation

A concept exists that these patients have small bladders and thus, void frequently. Actually the reverse is true. They have sensory urgency, void frequently and subsequently develop a small bladder. Hence, attempts to augment the bladder with a patch of bowel are likely to fail. Patients will then have a capacity that is perhaps large, have more difficulty emptying (usually requiring intermittent catheterization), but still retain all their sensory urgency and pain [74].

Cystectomy and Diversion

The mainstay of therapy for patients with "end-stage bladder" is cystectomy and diversion. It is successful, especially in today's environment of performing continent lower urinary tract diversions. Pelvic pain will present after the procedure in 5% of patients. In general, if the patients have classic bladder pain associated with filling and relieved or partially relieved by emptying and have urinary frequency and urgency and the usual stigmata of IC under anesthesia, they are likely to have relief of their symptoms by cystectomy. Those individuals with severe pelvic pain, not associated with classic parameters of IC and particularly *not* exacerbated by bladder filling, will be less likely to have their pain alleviated.

When continent diversion is performed 40–50% of patients will develop pouch pain 6–36 months after surgery. This can be managed successfully by having the patient instill 10 000 units of heparin in 10 ml water into the pouch after each catheterization. We now routinely place all patients on 300 mg of Elmiron orally and daily heparin to prevent development of pouch pain.

Summary

When IC is recognized as a continuum that may extend over decades of a patient's life, clinicians may detect the disease earlier in its development, and offer effective treatment to the majority of patients before their IC can progress to end-stage disease. A new intravesical test, the potassium sensitivity test, holds promise as a simple diagnostic tool that will be useful in identifying IC patients both in urologic patient populations and in other populations in whom IC rarely has been considered, such as gynecologic pelvic pain patients and men with lower urinary tract symptoms. In most cases, IC responds well to current therapies.

References

1. Gillenwater JY, Wein AJ. Summary of the National Institute of Arthritis, Diabetes, Digestive and Kidney Diseases Workshop on Interstitial Cystitis, National Institutes of Health, Bethesda, Maryland, August 28–29, 1987. J Urol 1988;140(1):203–6.
2. Hanno PM, Landis JR, Matthews-Cook Y et al. The diagnosis of interstitial cystitis revisited: Lessons learned from the National Institutes of Health Interstitial Cystitis Database Study. J Urol 1999;161:553–7.
3. Chambers GK, Fenster HN, Cripps S, Jens M, Taylor D. An assessment of the use of intravesical potassium in the diagnosis of interstitial cystitis. J Urol 1999;162:699–701.
4. Nitze M. Lerbuch der Kystoscopie: Ihre Technik und Klinische Bedeuting. Berlin: JE Bergman, 1907; 410.
5. Oravisto KJ. Epidemiology of interstitial cystitis 1. In: Hanno PM, Staskin DR, Krane RJ et al. Interstitial Cystitis. London: Springer-Verlag, 1990; 25–8.
6. Held PJ, Hanno PM, Pauly MV et al. Epidemiology of interstitial cystitis: 2. In: Hanno PM, Staskin DR, Krane RJ et al. Interstitial Cystitis. London: Springer-Verlag, 1990; 29–48.
7. American Foundation for Urologic Diseases. Research progress and promises. Baltimore: American Foundation for Urologic Diseases, 1980.
8. Jones CA, Nyberg L. Epidemiology of interstitial cystitis. Urology 1997;49(Suppl 5A):2–9.
9. Hamilton-Miller JMT. The urethral syndrome and its management. J Antimicrob Chemother 1994;33(Suppl A):63–73.
10. Parsons CL, Zupkas P, Parsons JK. Intravesical potassium sensitivity in patients with interstitial cystitis and urethral syndrome. Urology 2001;57:428–33.
11. Parsons CL, Bullen M, Kahn BS, Stanford EJ, Willems JJ. Gynecologic presentation of interstitial cystitis as detected by intravesical potassium sensitivity. Obstet Gynecol 2001;98:127–32.

12. Bernie JE, Hagey S, Albo ME, Parsons CL. The intravesical potassium sensitivity test and urodynamics – Implications in a large cohort of patients with lower urinary tract symptoms. J Urol 2001;166:158–61.

13. Oravisto KJ, Alfthan OS, Jokinen EJ. Interstitial cystitis. Clinical and immunological findings. Scand J Urol Nephrol 1970;4:37–42.

14. Hand JR. Interstitial cystitis, a report of 223 cases. J Urol 1949;61:291.

15. Hanash KA, Pool TL. Interstitial and hemorrhagic cystitis: viral, bacterial and fungal studies. J Urol 1970;104:705–6.

16. Oravisto KJ, Alfthan OS. Treatment of interstitial cystitis with immunosuppression and chloroquine derivatives. Eur Urol 1976;2:82–4.

17. Silk MR. Bladder antibodies in interstitial cystitis. J Urol 1970;103:307–9.

18. Holm-Bentzen M, Lose G. Pathology and pathogenesis of interstitial cystitis. Urology 1987;29(4 Suppl):8–13.

19. Oravisto KJ. Interstitial cystitis as an autoimmune disease. A review. Eur Urol 1980;6:10–13.

20. Weaver RG, Dougherty TF, Natoli C. Recent concepts of interstitial cystitis. J Urol 1963;89:377.

21. Eldrup J, Thorup J, Nielsen SL, Hald T, Hainau B. Permeability and ultrastructure of human bladder epithelium. Br J Urol 1983;55:488–92.

22. Parsons CL, Lilly JD, Stein P. Epithelial dysfunction in non-bacterial cystitis (interstitial cystitis). J Urol 1991;145:732–5.

23. Lilly JD, Parsons CL. Bladder surface glycosaminoglycans as a human epithelial permeability barrier. Surg Gynecol Obstet 1990;171:493–6.

24. Parsons CL, Boychuk D, Jones S, Hurst R, Callahan H. Bladder surface glycosaminoglycans: An epithelial permeability barrier. J Urol 1990;143:139–42.

25. Hohlbrugger G, Lentsch P. Intravesical ions, osmolality and pH influence the volume pressure response in the normal rat bladder, and this is more pronounced after DMSO exposure. Eur Urol 1985;11:127–30 .

26. Parsons CL, Stein PC, Bidair M, Lebow D. Abnormal sensitivity to intravesical potassium in interstitial cystitis and radiation cystitis. Neurourol Urodyn 1994;13:515–20.

27. Galloway N, Gabale D, Irwin P. Interstitial cystitis or reflex sympathetic dystrophy of the bladder? Semin Urol 1991;9:148.

28. Parsons CL, Greenberger M, Gabal L, Bidair M, Barme G. The role of urinary potassium in the pathogenesis and diagnosis of interstitial cystitis. J Urol 1998;159:1862–7.

29. Parsons CL. Potassium sensitivity test (1996) Tech Urol 2:171–3.

30. Teichman JMH, Nielsen-Omeis BJ, McIver BD. Modified urodynamics for interstitial cystitis. Tech Urol 1996;3:65–8.

31. Teichman JM, Nielsen-Omeis BJ. Potassium leak test predicts outcome in interstitial cystitis. J Urol 1999;161:1791–6.

32. Payne CK, Browning S. Graded potassium chloride testing in interstitial cystitis. J Urol 1996;155:438A.

33. Chen TY-H, Begin LR, Corcos J. Assessment of potassium chloride test in comparison with symptomatology, cystoscopic findings and bladder biopsy in the diagnosis of interstitial cystitis. J Urol 2001;165(5 Suppl):67–68.

34. Daha L, Riedl CR, Knoll M, Pflüger H, Hohlbrugger G. Comparative (saline vs. 0.2M potassium chloride) assessment of maximum bladder capacity: A well-tolerated alternative to the 0.4M potassium sensitivity test (PST). J Urol 2001;165(5 Suppl):68.

35. Kuo HC. Urodynamic results of intravesical heparin therapy for women with frequency urgency syndrome and interstitial cystitis. J Formos Med Assoc 2001;100:309–14.

36. Parsons CL, Mulholland S. Successful therapy of interstitial cystitis with pentosanpolysulfate. J Urol 1987;138:513–16.

37. Parsons CL, Benson G, Childs SJ et al. A quantitatively controlled method to prospectively study interstitial cystitis and which demonstrates the efficacy of pentosanpolysulfate. J Urol 1993;150:845–8.

38. Mulholland SG, Hanno P, Parsons CL, Sant GR, Staskin DR. Pentosan polysulfate sodium for therapy of interstitial cystitis: A double-blind placebo-controlled clinical study. Urology 1990;35(6):552–8.

39. Parsons CL. Sodium pentosanpolysulfate treatment of interstitial cystitis: An update. Urology 1987;29:14–16.

40. Hohlbrugger G. The vesical blood-urine barrier: a relevant and dynamic interface between renal function and nervous bladder control. J Urol 1995;154:6–14.

41. Spanos C, Pang X, Ligris K, Letourneau R, Alferes L, Alexacos N, Sant GR, Theoharides TC. Stress-induced bladder mast cell activation: Implications for interstitial cystitis. J Urol 1997;157:669–72.

42. Pang X, Boucher W, Triadafilopoulos G, Sant GR, Theoharides TC. Mast cell and substance P-positive nerve involvement in a patient with both irritable bowel syndrome and interstitial cystitis. Urology 1996;47:436–8.

43. Letourneau R, Pang X, Sant GR, Theoharides TC. Intragranular activation of bladder mast cells and their association with nerve processes in interstitial cystitis. Br J Urol 1996;77:41–54.

44. Spanos C, El-Mansoury M, Letourneau R, Minogiannis P, Greenwood J, Siri P, Sant GR, Theoharides TC. Carbachol-induced bladder mast cell activation: Augmentation by estradiol and implications for interstitial cystitis. Urology 1996;48:809–16.

45. Holm-Bentzen J, Sondergaard I, Hald T. Urinary excretion of a metabolite of histamine (1,4-methyl-imidazole-acetic-acid) in painful bladder disease. Br J Urol 1987;59:230–3.

46. Hohlbrugger G, Lentsch P, Pfaller K, Madersbacher H. Permeability characteristics of the rat urinary bladder in experimental cystitis and after over distension. Urologia Internationalis 1985;40:211–16.

47. Sant GR. Interstitial cystitis: Pathophysiology, clinical evaluation and treatment. Ann Urol 1989;3:172–9.

48. Sant GR, Kalaru P, Ucci AA Jr. Mucosal mast cell (MMC) contribution to bladder mastocytosis in interstitial cystitis. J Urol 1988;139:276A.

49. Holm-Bentzen M, Jacobsen F, Nerstrom B et al. Painful bladder disease: Clinical and pathoanatomical differences in 115 patients. J Urol 1987;138:500–2.

50. Hanno P, Levin RM, Monson FC et al. Diagnosis of interstitial cystitis. J Urol 1990;143:278–81.

51. Thoharides TC, Sant GR. Bladder mast cell activation in interstitial cystitis. Semin Urol 1991;9:74–87.

52. Larsen S, Thompson SA, Hald T et al. Mast cells in interstitial cystitis. Br J Urol 1982;54:283.

53. Hofmeister MA, He F, Ratliff TL et al. Mast cells and nerve fibers in interstitial cystitis (IC): An algorithm for histologic diagnosis via quantitative image analysis and morphometry (QIAM). Urology 1997;49(Suppl 5A):41–7.

54. Bjorling DE, Saban MR, Zine MJ, Haak-Frendscho M, Graziano FM, Saban R. In vitro passive sensitization of guinea pig, rhesus monkey and human bladders as a model of noninfectious cystitis. J Urol 1994;152:1603–8.

55. Koziol JA. Epidemiology of interstitial cystitis. Urol Clin North Am 1994;21:7–20.

56. Koziol JA, Clark DC, Gittes RF, Tan EM. The natural history of interstitial cystitis: a survey of 374 patients. J Urol 1993;149:465–9.

57. Hofmeister MA, He F, Ratliff TL, Becich MJ. Analysis of histochemical stains in interstitial cystitis (IC): detrusor to mucosa mast cell ratio is predictive of IC. Lab Invest 1994;70:60A.

58. Christmas TJ, Rode J, Chapple CR, Milroy EJ, Turner-Warwick RT. Nerve fibre proliferation in interstitial cystitis. Virchows Arch A Pathol Anat Histopathol 1990;416:447–51.

59. Lundeberg T, Liedberg H, Nordling L, Theodorsson E, Owzarski A, Ekman R. Interstitial cystitis: correlation with nerve fibers, mast cells and histamine. Br J Urol 1993;71:427–9.

60. Parsons CL. Interstitial cystitis: clinical manifestations and diagnostic criteria in over 200 cases. Neurourol Urodyn 1990;9(3):241–50.

61. Bekturov EA, Bakauova KH, editors. Synthetic Water-Soluble Polymers in Solution. Basel, New York: Hüthig & Wepf, Verlag, 1986; 38–54.

62. Nigro DA, Wein AJ, Foy M et al. Associations among cystoscopic and urodynamic findings for women enrolled in the Interstitial Cystitis Data Base Study. Urology 1997;49(Suppl 5A): 86–92.

63. Holm-Bentzen M, Larsen S, Hainau B, Hald T. Non-obstructive detrusor myopathy in a group of patients with chronic bacterial cystitis. Scand J Urol Nephrol 1985;19(1):21.

64. Burford HE, Burford CE. Hunner ulcer of the bladder: A report of 187 cases. J Urol 1958;79: 952–5.

65. Bumpus HC. Interstitial cystitis. Med Clin North Am 1930;13:1495.

66. Parsons CL, Housley T, Schmidt JD, Lebow D. Treatment of interstitial cystitis with intravesical heparin. Br J Urol 1994;73:504–7.

67. Hanno PM. Analysis of long-term Elmiron therapy for interstitial cystitis. Urology 1997;49 (Suppl 5A):93–9.

68. Hanno PM, Buehler J, Wein AJ. Use of amitriptyline in the treatment of interstitial cystitis. J Urol 1989;141:846–8.

69. Smith BH, Dehner LP. Chronic ulcerating interstitial cystitis (Hunner's ulcer). Arch Pathol 1972;93:76–81.

70. Bohne AW, Hodson JM, Rebuck JW, Reinhard RE. An abnormal leukocyte response in interstitial cystitis. J Urol 1962;88:387.

71. Simmons JL. Interstitial cystitis: an explanation for the beneficial effect of an antihistamine. J Urol 1961;85:149.

72. Theoharides T. Hydroxyzine in the treatment of interstitial cystitis. Urol Clin North Am 1994;21:113–19.

73. Stewart BH, Persky L, Kiser WS. The use of dimethylsulfoxide (DMSO) in the treatment of interstitial cystitis. J Urol 1967;98:671.

74. Nielsen KK, Kromann-Andersen B, Steven K, Hald T. Failure of combined supratrigonal cystectomy and Mainz ileocecocystoplasty in intractable interstitial cystitis: is histology and mast cell count a reliable predictor for the outcome of surgery? J Urol 1990;144 (2 Pt 1):255–8.

19 Vulvodynia and Vestibulitis

Alan H. Gerulath

Introduction

Chronic vulvar pain was first described in the late 1800s as hyperesthesia by Skene [1] with further reports by Thomas and Munde [2] and Kelly in the 1920s [3]. In the 1970s, the terms burning vulvar syndrome, psychosomatic vulvovaginitis and vestibular adenitis became popular.

In 1984 the International Society for the Study of Vulvar Disease (ISSVD) published a standard definition for vulvodynia as a chronic vulvar discomfort characterized by the patient's complaints of burning, stinging, irritation or rawness due to multiple causes [4]. Psychological distress as well as sexual dysfunction could accompany vulvodynia.

Friedrich [5] defined a subset, vestibulitis, as: (1) severe pain on vestibular touch, (2) introital (entry) dyspareunia, and (3) vestibular erythema of various degrees. Woodruff and Parmley [6] were the first to describe a surgical treatment, perineoplasty, for vestibulitis.

McKay [7] coined the term essential or dysesthetic vulvodynia for those patients with non-localizing burning discomfort and normal appearing skin.

Although there is general agreement on the definition of vulvodynia, controversy exists relating to the subsets. Dysesthetic vulvodynia and vestibulitis have gained acceptance; disagreement remains over other subsets. Table 19.1 illustrates the terminology adopted for this chapter.

Data on prevalence and incidence of vulvodynia is sparse. The disease occurs predominantly in Caucasian females. A survey of 150 new consecutive female patients attending a walk-in genitourinary clinic reported twenty patients (13.3%) with vulvar pain, of whom two (1.3%) had vestibulitis [8]. In another general gynecologic practice, vulvar vestibulitis was diagnosed in 15% of patients [9].

Table 19.1 Subsets of vulvodynia

Vulvodynia:
- Generalized vulvar dysesthesia
- Secondary vulvodynia
- Vestibulitis

Pathophysiology

The pathophysiology of vulvodynia has not been well defined. It is generally accepted that multiple factors may play a role. Etiologic hypotheses described in the older literature include allergic responses, contact dermatitis, hormonal dysfunction, early contraceptive use, psychologic disorders, *Candida* antigens, oxalate and responses to infectious agents such as the human papilloma virus (HPV) [10–12]. Current studies have failed to demonstrate a significant association of HPV with vestibulitis [13,14].

Recent progress in neurophysiologic research has improved our understanding of the mechanisms of pain in vulvodynia.

Gracely et al. [15,16] postulate that vulvodynia can be characterized as peripherally-initiated central pain (PICP), in contrast to centrally-initiated central pain (CIPC), which results from a central lesion caused by such conditions as hemorrhage, tumor or mechanical injury. PICP is caused by a peripheral lesion which can produce persistent nociceptive stimuli transmitted to the central nervous system.

Patients with PICP may have both spontaneous and evoked pain abnormalities. They present with allodynia defined as "pain due to a stimulus which does not normally provoke pain", and also suffer from secondary hyperalgesia defined as "an increased response to a stimulus which is normally painful". Altered central processing is present in PICP and maintained by peripheral input.

Neuropathic PICP pain in the vulvar vestibule can vary in extent and spread to the labia majora and minora as well as in the thigh and perineal area. Painful regions are often found in Skene's ducts, the minor vestibular glands and Bartholin's glands. Lidocaine injected at the ducts of Skene's and Bartholin's glands alleviate the pain in injected as well as adjacent areas [16]. Gracely suggests that vulvodynia, especially a subset pudendal neuralgia, is similar to the complex regional pain syndrome type I (CRPS I) [17], which is refractory to conventional analgesics.

Sensitization of normally silent peripheral afferent nerves can occur under the influence of amines such as histamine and serotonin, cytokines, peptides such as substance P, as well as prostanoids and amino acids [18,19]. Sensitization of afferent nerve fibers leads mainly to hyperalgesia; some nerve fibers may even discharge spontaneously with no input at peripheral sites.

De Groat [20] has described "cross talk" between pelvic viscera and striated muscle. Afferents from viscera, muscles, and skin can influence afferent output back to these structures. Vestibular inflammation could thus trigger pelvic muscle spasm. Reflex loops may develop and amplify the pain. Recognition of these loops can lead to interventions such as biofeedback in vestibulitis.

Neuroendocrine factors may play a role in the perception of pain. The main constituents of the stress system are the corticotropin-releasing hormones (CRH) and locus ceruleus norepinephrine (LC/NE) autonomic systems and their peripheral effectors, the pituitary adrenal axis and the autonomic system. Hypo- or hyperactivity of the stress system can occur in pathologic states [21]. Stress generally inhibits the immune response with a decrease in cellular immune response and an increase in humoral response. CRH can be released locally at nerve endings and thus may play a role in regional inflammation [22].

Genetic differences in perception of pain among individual subjects as well as between sexes have recently been demonstrated in studies of mice [23]. Genetic reasons for differences in response to pain are probably multiple rather than being due to involvement of a single gene.

Psychologic factors play a role in perception of pain. Several studies have demonstrated that vulvodynia patients have significant psychological distress, interpersonal disorders and sexual dysfunction [24,25]. Pain consists of both sensory and emotional components, which are further modified by coping mechanisms as well as the depression that can accompany chronic pain syndromes [26]. Depression leads to maladaptive coping mechanisms, which in turn are associated with more disability and decreasing physical activity, sleep disturbances and diminished concentration. In most cases depression is secondary to chronic pain.

Generalized Vulvar Dysesthesia

Signs and Symptoms

Dysesthetic vulvodynia is a symptom with multiple causes of uncertain etiology [27]. Patients present with chronic vulvar pain. It may be constant or intermittent and is primarily described as a burning or occasionally a rawness or irritation of the vulva rather than pruritus, which is more indicative of an inflammatory condition or a vulvar dermatosis.

Patients usually are unable to pinpoint the cause or the onset of pain, although on occasion this may be associated with monilial vaginitis, antibiotic therapy or vulvar surgical procedures. Physical examination in most cases reveals a normal vulva in the absence of recognizable physical signs.

Investigation

An accurate history is the first step in investigation. A concise description of the vulvar pain, namely the location and duration, is obtained. Results of previous investigations and medications given to the patient must be documented. The patient's sexual history, contraceptive practices and hygienic patterns are elicited.

Special attention is paid to medical conditions such as diabetes or inflammatory bowel disease. The history of past health includes neurologic, psychiatric, allergic or dermatologic disease as well as surgical procedures.

It is important to determine if the pain is related to menses or the luteal phase and whether dyspareunia is present on entry or with deep penetration. Pain associated with menses may be due to cyclic vulvovaginitis whereas introital dyspareunia is a symptom of vestibulitis.

On physical examination the vulva is carefully assessed under magnification, ideally with a colposcope or a magnifying lens. Vulvar intraepithelial neoplasia, genital condyloma and vulvar dermatoses are identified. Suspicious areas are biopsied but not tissue showing erythema only.

Vaginal infections must be ruled out by means of a microscopic examination of wet preparations with normal saline or potassium hydroxide as well as appropriate cultures.

Treatment

In the majority of patients with vulvodynia, the investigation will fail to identify the cause. No single therapeutic approach is necessarily valid and different treatment possibilities have to be explored.

Medical Management
The categorization of vulvodynia as neuropathic pain led to the use of drugs that modify nerve impulses. Tricyclic antidepressants are norepinephrine reuptake inhibitors. These drugs, which are effective in the treatment of post-herpetic neuralgia [28] and other cutaneous dysesthesias, were empirically prescribed for patients with vulvodynia at doses insufficient for treatment of depression but effective for pain control [29]. The most widely used agents are amitryptiline and desipramine. Amitryptiline is prescribed at the lowest effective dose, usually 10 mg, which is gradually increased from 20 mg to 100 mg daily. Desipramine is administered at dosages of 50 mg to 200 mg daily, with most responses occurring between 125 mg and 200 mg.

Side effects common with tricyclic antidepressants, drowsiness, dry mouth, or weight gain, may limit the dose required for pain control. Patients unable to tolerate these drugs occasionally respond to newer antidepressants such as trazodone, fluoxetine sertraline or gabapentin.

There are no randomized controlled studies to evaluate drug therapy in this group of patients. McKay [29] published a retrospective analysis of twenty patients with vulvodynia, who were successfully treated with low-dose amitryptiline. The diagnostic profile and symptom pattern were described. Patients most likely to respond had an average age of 66 with vulvodynia present for 3 years.

Supportive Measures
Measures that decrease contact with allergens or irritants to the vulva are recommended. Patients are advised to wear loose-fitting clothing, white cotton underwear, and to eliminate feminine health products or soaps which may be allergenic. Cold compresses may provide pain relief. Coating the labia with a protective layer of vegetable shortening or petrolatum is helpful.

Pain Management Therapy
Recent studies suggest that electromyographic biofeedback of pelvic floor musculature is helpful in some patients with vulvodynia and vestibulitis [30]. Behavior modification, acupuncture and transepidermal nerve stimulation (TNS) as well as physical therapy involving pelvic floor muscle strengthening and relaxation therapy have produced conflicting results [31].

Dietary Therapy
A low oxalate/calcium citrate regimen has shown variable effectiveness in patients with vestibulitis. The original case report [32] of one patient sparked widespread use of this regimen in vulvodynia. Solomons et al. [32] recommend a low oxalate diet combined with oral calcium citrate (200 mg calcium and 950 mg citrate – two tablets 3 to 4 times a day). This regimen was thought to inhibit the formation of calcium oxalate crystals, which may act as an irritant. Baggish et al. [33] were unable to detect a difference in oxalate excretion in vulvodynia patients or controls. He concluded that urinary oxalates may be nonspecific irritants that aggravate vulvodynia; their role as etiologic agents is doubtful.

Psychologic Support
Significant psychologic problems have been reported in vulvodynia. Schover et al. [24] published a study of 45 women with vestibulitis of whom 54% had severe marital conflict, 42% a somatization disorder and 36% depressive symptoms.

The indicators for psychological treatment and the efficacy of psychologic intervention in vulvodynia is unknown. Psychologic counseling and emotional support is often necessary. Patients may benefit from patient support networks.

Pudendal Neuralgia

Pudendal neuralgia is characterized by a stabbing or burning pain extending usually unilaterally over the distribution of the pudendal nerve; the pain can extend from the mons pubis to the upper inner thighs and posteriorly to the ischial tuberosities. Nerve injury, entrapment or compression may follow obstetric trauma, episiotomy, accidents or vaginal surgery [34,35]. Similarly ilio-inguinal and genitofemoral nerve injury has been reported following surgery for urinary stress incontinence and herniorrhaphies [36].

Pain may be relieved by a local nerve block. Therapy consists of tricyclic antidepressants such as amitryptiline, desipramine or alternate drugs such as clonazepam [37].

Surgical procedures for some of the above nerve injuries include removal of sutures around the nerve, decompression procedures and rarely excision of the nerve.

If recurrent herpes zoster is suspected, a course of oral acyclovir is indicated. Other drugs such as phenytoin and carbamazepine may be effective [37].

Related Syndromes

Vulvodynia may be associated with a variety of other regional pain syndromes such as the female urethral syndrome, interstitial cystitis, chronic fatigue syndrome, irritable bowel syndrome and fibromyalgia. Around 10–40% of women with the regional pelvic pain syndrome experience widespread pain such as fibromyalgia and as many as 30–50% of patients with fibromyalgia experience regional genitourinary syndromes [38].

Foster et al. [39] described an increase in urethral pressure variability in patients with vestibulitis compared to asymptomatic controls. Similarly, Drutz et al. [40] showed very high urethral closure pressures in women with the urethral syndrome.

The etiology and pathogenesis of these symptoms is poorly understood. Clauw [41] hypothesizes that these syndromes have aberrant neural processing of pain in common as well as regional or widespread autonomic nervous dysfunction. A genetic predisposition appears to be common.

Secondary Vulvodynia

Vulvar burning and irritation is found in some patients with conditions such as candidiasis or dermatoses. These symptoms can become chronic after the acute onset of vulvar pruritus.

Cyclic Vulvovaginitis

The most common cause of vulvovaginal infections is *Candida*. Symptoms of vulvar burning, pain or irritation are similar to vulvodynia. *Candida* is most accurately diagnosed by fungal culture and treated with the appropriate antifungal agents.

Patients with cyclic vulvitis present with intermittent vulvar pain, worse during the luteal phase of the menstrual cycle and characterized by erythema and inflammation at the introitus [37]. Post-coital pain, either immediate or delayed, is common. Antifungal therapy gives temporary relief but symptoms recur. *Candida* may be cultured consistently in these patients but not during the symptomatic phase.

Localized hypersensitivity to *Candida* antigen is postulated as the cause [11].

The treatment regimen consists of long-term (4–6-month) therapy with systemic antimycotics such as fluconazole or ketoconazole. Vaginal antimycotic creams used during episodic flares may also be effective.

Dermatoses

Vulvar pain with dermatoses is usually pruritic, but occasionally patients may complain of burning.

Dermatoses show visible changes in the vulvar skin with a distinctive histopathology; lesions may be present elsewhere on the body. The major dermatoses are lichen sclerosus (LS), lichen planus (LP) and lichen simplex chronicus (LSC) or squamous hyperplasia, of which lichen sclerosus is the most prevalent [37].

LS presents as an atrophic white change which encircles the vulva, perineum and anus in a figure-eight configuration. Ecchymosis, fissures, ulcerations, erosions and loss of labial architecture may be present. LSC features a nonspecific asymmetric white thickening of vulvar skin. The mucosal presentation of LP varies from a mild inflammatory erythematous change involving the vestibule and vagina to an erosive disease involving the vestibule, vagina and mouth. A biopsy is helpful for a definitive diagnosis.

Topical corticosteroids are the mainstay of therapy for the dermatoses. Superpotent steroids are employed over a short term for the relief of severe symptoms, followed by a maintenance dose of low potency steroids.

Vestibulitis

Vestibulitis, also known as localized vulvar dysesthesia, is the most clearly defined subset of vulvodynia. Friedrich [5] defined the criteria for diagnosis as erythema of the vulvar vestibule, tenderness to pressure in the vestibule, and pain on touch or with intercourse. The etiology and pathophysiology remain unclear.

Histopathology

Biopsy of the vestibule reveals a nonspecific chronic inflammatory reaction, usually in the superficial dermis, consisting mostly of lymphocytes. The minor vestibular glands also show areas of inflammation; metaplastic squamous epithelium may replace the columnar epithelium of the gland.

The Bartholin's duct is occasionally involved with inflammation around the duct [42,43].

Foster and Hasday [19] studied levels of two inflammatory cytokines, interleukin-1-beta and tumor necrosis factor-alpha, in patients with vestibulitis and found elevations in these women compared with asymptomatic controls; a 50% concordance was found between presence of these cytokines and inflammation. The authors theorize that cytokine elevation may contribute to hyperalgesia in the vestibule.

Treatment

The aim of therapy is restoration of normal coital function and a decrease in vulvar pain.

Standard definitions are important in comparing results from various studies; unfortunately, nomenclature differs among investigators. Along with Friedrich's classic definition of vestibulitis, the following terms are useful: Dyspareunia may be primary occurring from first intercourse, or secondary following previous pain-free intercourse. Grading of the severity of dyspareunia is advocated by some authors. Pure vestibulitis may be present, with pain limited to the touch of the vestibule. A mixed form occurs in which pain is present outside the vestibule, and which is occasionally burning, indicative of dysesthetic vulvodynia. Vaginismus (levator ani spasm) is often present, secondary to vestibulitis.

Surgery has the highest success rate in the treatment of pure vestibulitis. Conservative measures are usually employed before surgical intervention is considered.

Conservative Management

A local anesthetic (lidocaine, 4% aqueous solution), applied 15 minutes prior to intercourse is recommended along with a lubricant to relieve discomfort and allow coitus.

If chronic vulvovaginal candidiasis is present, long-term antifungal treatment is prescribed, usually oral fluconazole. Atrophy in the fourchette, seen in the menopausal patient but occasionally in younger women on low-dose oral contraceptives, responds to local application of an estrogen cream; discontinuation of the oral contraceptive is helpful in the younger group. Topical preparations such as aloe vera cream are useful in providing local relief.

Amitryptiline has been suggested for the treatment of vestibulitis. However, its effectiveness is questionable, with best results occurring in the mixed form.

A low oxalate diet with calcium citrate supplementation has been advocated by some. A recent communication by Melmed et al. [44] described a complete response rate of 50% [10 of 20 women). However, Bornstein [45] reports improvement in only 10-20% of women treated with the same protocol.

Glazer et al. [30] described biofeedback-controlled pelvic floor exercises in order to reduce a presumed hypertonicity of pelvic floor muscles. Twenty-two of 28 women were able to resume intercourse after 16 weeks of therapy; 83% reported a subjective decrease of pain. This study suggests that patients with demonstrable vaginismus should be treated with biofeedback before treatment with surgery is contemplated.

Behavior and sex therapy has been reported as beneficial in the resumption of intercourse in patients with vestibulitis [46].

Interferon was initially advocated in patients with vestibulitis at a time when an association with the human papilloma virus was postulated [47]. Recent studies [13,14] have failed to confirm the initial findings. Nevertheless, interferon is still used by some on the basis of immunomodulatory and antiproliferative properties. A report [48] of a focal depression of natural killer lymph cell activity in some patients with vestibulitis supports this practice. Interferon, 1.5 million international units (IU) is injected circumferentially at different areas in the vestibule three times a week for a total of 18 million IU given over 6 weeks. Success rates range from 25 to 80% with an average of 50%. Side effects consist primarily of flu-like symptoms and a low-grade fever.

Surgery

Surgery is carried out on patients who have failed conservative therapy. Surgical procedures are most effective in patients with pure vestibulitis, and may fail in patients with the mixed form. Surgery is ineffective in patients with dysesthetic vulvodynia. The aim of surgery is removal of all sensitive vestibular tissue.

Woodruff [6] originally described a partial vestibulectomy which he referred to as a modified perineoplasty. He excised all of the sensitive areas of the vestibule to a depth of 2 mm, as well as the hymen, with mobilization and advancement of the vaginal mucosa to cover the excised area (Figure 19. 1).

Some surgeons [49] advocate vestibuloplasty, which consists of excision of a localized area of pain such as the posterior, lateral or anterior vestibule without advancement of the vagina. The hymen is excised but perineoplasty is not performed (Figure 19.1).

Others [50–54] advocate a total vestibulectomy, which consists of removal of the entire vestibule starting in the periuretheral area down to the

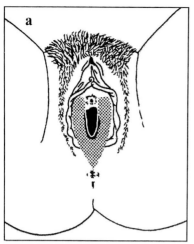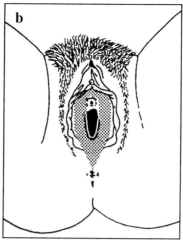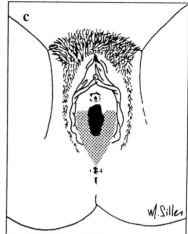

Figure 19.1 Surgical techniques for vestibulitis. Area of excision – shaded. **a** Woodruff's perineoplasty. **b** Total vestibulectomy. **c** Vestibuloplasty.

fourchette, a hymenectomy and perineoplasty with vaginal advancement (Figure 19.1). Some [45,56] advocate removal of Bartholin's glands, which may be involved in vestibulitis; the success rate appears to be increased with the addition of this procedure.

Another technique [24,55] consists of local excision of painful areas which are identified either clinically or colposcopically. The mucosa is excised and margins are undermined sufficiently to allow for primary closure without tension.

Success, as defined in terms of significant improvement, or complete cure, ranges from 50 to 100%; most authors describe pain relief in 80–85% of patients (Table 19.2). Studies are difficult to evaluate and compare because of a variety of methodological flaws, including an absence of control groups, a short follow-up, rudimentary pain measurements and unclear selection criteria [31]. Baggish [10] reports that the initially high success rates with short follow-up decrease by 40–60% with longer observation of one year or more.

Laser therapy for ablation of the vestibule is controversial, with potentially serious side effects [37,57]. Davis [58], utilizing CO_2 laser ablation, reported a 66% success rate; others experienced poor results [37,57]. Reid et al. [56] advocate use of the Flashlamp-Excited Dye laser, which is designed for photocoagulation of small blood vessels within the superficial dermis. The objective of this technique is apparent selective destruction of chroni-

cally inflamed blood vessels adjacent to painful sympathetic nerves. Reid reported a final complete response rate of 62% and a partial response of 30%, usually after re-treatment; these results have not been confirmed.

Summary

Treating patients with vulvar pain is a frustrating and continuing challenge. A systematic approach is necessary, with identification of the subtypes that respond to different therapeutic modalities. Patients with dysesthetic vulvodynia should be treated with medical management utilizing tricyclic antidepressants such as amitryptiline. Vestibulitis responds best to surgical therapy. A multidisciplinary approach involving other health care workers such as nurses, social workers, and psychologists is helpful in the diagnosis and management.

There is a pressing need for epidemiologic studies of vulvodynia. Future directions involve the development of drugs for chronic pain control such as opioids restricted to peripheral action and drugs targeted at spinal cord receptors of neurotransmitters.

Further research is required in the neurophysiology of pain and the neuropathic conditions of the genitourinary system.

Table 19.2 Surgical outcome in vestibulities

Author	Procedure	No.	Successful outcome (%)	Comments	Follow-up (months)
Woodruff and Parmley [6]	Partial vestibulectomy (Woodruff's perineoplastry)	14	100	2/14 – intermittent pain	6–36
Kehoe and Luesley [50]	Woodruff	39	80	31/39 – complete and partial response Some – incision perineal body	3–34 Median: 10
Foster et al. [51]	Woodruff	93	82	47/93 – asymptomatic 29/93 – partial response	48+
Bergeron et al. [52]	Woodruff	38	63	24/38 – positive outcome 14/38 – moderate to no improvement	13–120 Median: 39
Marinoff and Turner [53]	Vestibulectomy	73	82	60/73 – complete relief 11/73 – improvement	Median: 36
Bornstein et al. [54]	Vestibulectomy	11	81	9/11 – complete response 1/11 – partial response	6
Chaim et al. [49]	Vestibulectomy	16	94	15/16 – overall improvement	10–70 Median: 42
Schover et al. [24]	Local excision	32	50	Excision and psychologic counseling 16/32 – much improved 13/32 – somewhat improved	1–24
Goetsch [55]	Local excision	12	83	All – partial hymenectomy 10/12 – complete response 2/12 – improvement	6–72

References

1. Skene AJC. Treatise on the Disease of Women. New York: Appleton, 1889.
2. Thomas TG, Munde PF. A Practical Treatise on the Disease of Women. Philadelphia: Lea Brothers, 1891.
3. Kelly HA. Gynecology. New York: Appleton, 1928.
4. Report of the ISSVD. Burning vulva syndrome. J Reprod Med 1984;29:457.
5. Friedrich EG Jr. Vulvar vestibulitis syndrome. J Reprod Med 1987;32:110–14.
6. Woodruff JD, Parmley TH. Infection of the minor vestibular glands. Obstet Gynecol 1983;62:609–10.
7. McKay M. Vulvodynia: a multifactorial clinical problem. Arch Dermatol 1989;125:256–62.
8. Denbow ML, Byrne MA. Prevalence, causes and outcome of vulvar pain in a genitourinary medicine clinic population. Int J STD AIDS 1998;9(2):88–91.
9. Goetsch MF. Vulvar vestibulitis: Prevalence and historic features in a general gynecologic practice population. Am J Obstet Gynecol 1991;164:1609–16.
10. Baggish SM, Miklos JR. Vulvar pain syndrome: A review. Obstet Gynecol Surv 1995;50:618–27.
11. Ashman RB, Ott AK. Autoimmunity as a factor in recurrent vaginal candidosis and the minor vestibular gland syndrome. J Reprod Med 1989;4:264–6.
12. Turner MLC, Marinoff SC. Association of human papillomavirus with vulvodynia and the vulvar vestibulitis syndrome. J Reprod Med 1988;33:533–7.
13. Wilkinson EJ, Guerrero E, Daniel R, Shah K, Stone IK, Hardt NS, Friedrich EG, Jr. Vulvar vestibulitis is rarely associated with human papillomavirus infection types 6, 11, 16 or 18. Int J Gynecol Pathol 1993;12(4):344–9.
14. Bergeron C, Moyal-Barracco M, Pelisse M, Lewin P. Vulvar vestibulitis. Lack of evidence for a human papillomavirus etiology. J Reprod Med 1994;39(12):936–8.
15. Gracely RH, Lynch SA, Bennett GJ. Painful neuropathy: Altered central processing maintained dynamically by peripheral input. Pain 1992;51:175–94.
16. Turner MLC, Marinoff SC, Gracely RH. Vulvodynia: Altered central processing maintained dynamically by focal peripheral input. American Pain Society Abstracts 1995.
17. Merskey H, Bodduk N, editors. Classification of Chronic Pain, 2nd edn. Seattle: IASP Press, 1994.
18. Gebhart GF. (1997) Pharmacologic agents for chronic pain. In: Vulvodynia Workshop. Bethesda, MD: National Institutes of Health, 68–73.
19. Foster DC, Hasday JD. Elevated tissue levels of interleukin-1 beta and tumor necrosis factor-alpha in vulvar vestibulitis. Obstet Gynecol 1997;89(2):291–6.
20. de Groat WC. Neurophysiology of micturition and its modification in animal models of human disease. In: Maggi CA, editor. The Autonomic Nervous System, Vol. 3, Chapter 8, Nervous Control of the Urogenital System. London: Harwood Publishers, 1993; 227–347.
21. Tsigos C, Chrousos GP. Stress, endocrine manifestations and diseases. In: Cooper CL, editor. Handbook of Stress Medicine. Boca Raton, FL: CRC Press, 1995; 61–5.
22. Chrousos GP. The hypothalamic-pituitary-adrenal axis and immune-mediated inflammation. N Engl J Med 1995;332:1351–62.
23. Mogil JS, Sternberg WF, Marek P, Sadowski B, Belknap JD, Liebeskind JC. The genetics of pain and pain inhibition. Proc Natl Acad Sci USA 1996;93:3048–55.
24. Schover LR, Youngs DD, Cannata R. Psychosexual aspects of the evaluation and management of vulvar vestibulitis. Am J Obstet Gynecol 1992;167:630–6.
25. Stewart DE, Reicher AE, Gerulath AH, Boydell KM. Vulvodynia and psychological distress. Obstet Gynecol 1994;84:587–90.
26. Slocumb JC, Kellner R, Rosenfeld RC, Pathak D. Anxiety and depression in patients with abnormal pelvic pain syndrome. General Hospital Psychiatry 1989;11:48–53.
27. McKay M. Vulvodynia: A multifactorial problem. Arch Dermatol 1989;125:256–62.
28. Watson CP, Evans RJ, Reed K et al. Amitriptyline versus placebo in postherpetic neuralgia. Neurology 1982;32:671.
29. McKay M. Dysesthetic ('essential') vulvodynia. Treatment with amitriptyline. J Reprod Med 1993;38:9–13.
30. Glazer HI, Rodke G, Swencionis C, Hertz R, Young AW. The treatment of vulvar vestibulitis syndrome by electromyographic biofeedback of pelvic floor musculature. J Reprod Med 1995;40:283–90.
31. Bergeron S, Binik YM, Khalife S, Pagidas K. Vulvar vestibulitis syndrome: a critical review. Clin J Pain 1997;13(1):27–42.
32. Solomons CC, Melmed MH, Heitler SM. Calcium citrate for vulvar vestibulitis: a case report. J Reprod Med 1991;36:879–82.
33. Baggish MS, Sze EH, Johnson R. Urinary oxalate excretion and its role in vulvar pain syndrome. Am J Obstet Gynecol 1997;177(3):507–11.
34. Sangwan YP, Coller JA, Barrett RC, Murray JJ, Roberts PJ, Schoetz DJ. Unilateral pudendal neuropathy. Dis Colon Rectum 1996;39:249–51.
35. Alevizon SJ, Finan MA. Sacrospinous colpopexy: management of postoperative pudendal nerve entrapment. Obstet Gynecol 1996;88:713–15.
36. Monga M, Ghoniem G. Ilioinguinal nerve entrapment following needle bladder suspension procedures. Urology 1994;44:447–50.
37. McKay M. Vulvodynia: diagnostic patterns. Dermatol Clin 1992;10:423–33.
38. Clauw DJ. Fibromyalgia: more than just a musculoskeletal disease. Am Fam Phys 1995;52(3):843–51.
39. Foster DC, Robinson JC, Davis KM. Urethral pressure variation in women with vulvar vestibulitis. Am J Obstet Gynecol 1993;169:107–12.
40. Drutz HP, Mainprize TC, Tremblay P. Baker KR. Detrusor sphincter dyssynergia, detrusor instability, and urethral sphincter spasticity as the urodynamic findings in the urethral syndrome: role of treatment with a combined anticholinergic and alpha blocking agent, bladder drill, and antibiotics. Int Urogynecol J 1991;2:10–15.
41. Clauw DJ. The pathogenesis of chronic pain and fatigue syndromes, with special reference to fibromyalgia. Med Hypothesis 1995;44(5):369–78.
42. Pyka RE, Wilkinson EJ, Friedrich EG, Jr, Croker BP. The histopathology of vulvar vestibulitis syndrome. Int J Gynecol Pathol 1988;7(3):249–57.
43. Furlonge CB, Thin RN, Evans BE, McKee PH. Vulvar vestibulitis syndrome: a clinico-pathological study. Br J Obstet Gynaecol 1991;98:703–6.
44. Melmed MH, Solomons CC. (1993) Low oxalate diet and calcium citrate for vulvar vestibulitis. Proceedings of the 12th Congress of the ISSVD. Book of Abstracts: 35.
45. Bornstein J, Goldik Z, Alter Z, Zarfati D, Abramovici H. Persistent vulvar vestibulitis: the continuing challenge. Obstet Gynaecol Surv 1998;53(1):39–44.
46. Weijmar Schultz WC, Gianotten WL, van der Meijden WI et al. Behavioural approach with or without surgical intervention to the vulvar vestibulitis syndrome: a prospective randomized and non-randomized study. J Psychosom Obstet Gynaecol 1996;17(3):143–8.
47. Marinoff SC, Turner ML, Hirsch RP et al. Intralesional alpha interferon: cost-effective therapy for vulvar vestibulitis syndrome. J Reprod Med 1993;38:19.

48. Masterson BJ, Galask RP, Ballas ZK. Natural killer cell function in women with vestibulitis. J Reprod Med 1996;41(8):562–8.

49. Chaim W, Meriwether C, Gonik B, Qureshi F, Sobel JD. Vulvar vestibulitis subjects undergoing surgical intervention: a descriptive analysis and histopathological correlates. Eur J Obstet Gynecol Reprod Biol 1996;68(1–2):165–8.

50. Kehoe S, Luesley D. An evaluation of modified vestibulectomy in the treatment of vulvar vestibulitis: preliminary results. Acta Obstet Gynecol Scand 1996;75(7):676–7.

51. Foster DC, Butts E, Shah KV, Woodruff JD. Long-term outcome of peri-neoplasty for vulvar vestibulitis. J Women's Health 1995;4:669–75.

52. Bergeron S, Bouchard C, Fortier M, Binik YM, Khalife S. The surgical treatment of vulvar vestibulitis syndrome: a follow-up study. J Sex Marital Ther 1997;23(4):317–25.

53. Marinoff SC. Surgical treatment of vulvar vestibulitis. In: Vulvodynia Workshop Bethesda, MD: National Institutes of Health, 1997; 28–32.

54. Bornstein J, Zarfati D, Goldik Z, Abramovici H. Perineoplasty compared with vestibuloplasty for severe vulvar vestibulitis. Br J Obstet Gynaecol 1995;102(8):652–5.

55. Goetsch MF. Simplified surgical revision of the vulvar vestibule for vulvar vestibulitis. Am J Obstet Gynecol 1996;174(6):1701–5.

56. Reid R, Omoto KH, Precop SL et al. Flashlamp-excited dye laser therapy of idiopathic vulvodynia is safe and efficacious. Am J Obstet Gynecol 1995;172:1684–701.

57. Marinoff SC, Turner MLC. Vulvar vestibulitis syndrome. Dermatol Clin 1992;10:435–44.

58. Davis GD. The management of vulvar vestibulitis syndrome with the carbon dioxide laser. J Gynecol Surg 1989;5:87–91.

20 Urogenital Atrophy

Gloria A. Bachmann and Lisa Aptaker-Stirling

Introduction

Because of the rapid increase in the aging population and the plethora of new pharmacologic treatment options, urogenital atrophy disorders have become a more commonly recognized problem in the female population. With the large number of "baby boomers" reaching the menopausal years, by the year 2000 over one-third of the female population in the US were over the age of 50. Up to 43% of this older population will suffer from symptoms of vaginal dryness and 41% will report dyspareunia. However, it is not only gonadal hormonal changes that impact on the anatomic and physiologic alterations that occur in the urogenital tract and characterize urogenital atrophy; many other factors including chronologic aging, parity, genetic and environmental also impact on pelvic health. The fact that disorders related to urogenital atrophy such as cystocele, rectocele and uterine prolapse are frequently a challenge to correct either hormonally or surgically or to ameliorate with estrogen or pessary use suggests that the etiology is often multifactorial. The hormonal changes that occur with the menopause transition have a significant effect on the pelvic vasculature, neurologic and connective tissue, and data clearly indicate that estrogen loss has the greatest impact on the development of pelvic atrophy.

Because vaginal changes associated with urogenital atrophy are so obvious, senile changes in the urogenital area are often discussed from a vaginal point of view with descriptions of vaginal epithelial thinning, loss of vaginal lubrication, decrease vaginal rugation, compromised blood flow and pH elevation to above 7.0. In addition, many of these adverse vaginal changes associated with hypoestrogenism are often exaggerated in intensity because of other chronic conditions. For instance, women with severe arthritic changes and atrophic vaginitis may be unable to maintain perineal hygiene because of their decreased flexibility. However, although vaginal changes are often highlighted when urogenital atrophy is discussed, urinary tract changes are just as important and at times even more troublesome than vaginal changes. Hypoestrogenism in addition to causing anatomic and physiologic vaginal changes also has an adverse impact on collagen, which can contribute to the development of urinary incontinence.

Prior pregnancy and vaginal childbirth also adversely affect the functioning of the urogenital tract and these changes usually are exacerbated with menopause and aging. Poor diet and chronic urogenital infection are other factors that the scant data available suggest may have an adverse effect on urogenital tract function. However, regular exercise and continued sexual activity have been correlated with preservation of urogenital tissue.

Menopausal women present with a spectrum of clinical complaints as the urogenital tract changes with loss of estrogen. In the past, with limited treatment options, these urogenital symptoms were often not addressed because therapies were often not effective and many women were embarrassed to discuss symptoms with their physician. With a greater understanding of the etiology of urogenital changes and the emergence of effective treatments and the increased patient acceptance of open discussion with their clinicians about such issues, including the reporting of malodorous vaginal discharge, urine leakage and coital pain, more older women are being helped. Women are reporting not only urinary and vaginal problems associated with estrogen loss to their clinicians, but rectal symptoms as well.

Common presenting complaints include recurrent urinary tract and vaginal infections, vaginal dryness and pruritus, urinary and rectal incontinence and urinary frequency and urgency. In addition, many patients report sexual problems, such as decreased vaginal lubrication, dyspareunia, vaginal irritation and post-coital bleeding. The most common and efficacious intervention for urogenital atrophy in menopausal women is either systemic or local estrogen replacement therapy. In addition to estrogen replacement being used for the prevention of osteoporosis and menopausal symptoms and for the benefits to cardiovascular and central nervous system (CNS) functions, it is extremely efficacious for both the treatment and prevention of urogenital atrophy. By the reversal of urogenital atrophy with estrogen use, vaginal flora normalizes with an increase in *Lactobacillus*, and vaginal pH decreases to below 5. In addition to physical symptoms improving, emotional and psychological symptoms markedly ameliorate as urogenital problems abate.

Anatomy of the Urogenital Tract and Changes That Occur with Menopause

The proper functioning of the vaginal and urinary tracts depends upon the integrity of the muscular, neurologic and vascular tissue. These tissues are important not only for the maintenance of the urinary tract and vagina, but also for the pelvic floor. For example, in addition to estrogen loss, muscle denervation seen with chronological aging contributes to the development of stress urinary incontinence and genital organ prolapse. Moreover, the common embryologic origin of the female reproductive and urinary tracts also explains the similar tissue atrophy that is seen in these regions with hypoestrogenism. During the fourth week of embryonic growth, the cloaca divides into an anterior and a posterior portion. The anterior portion is the primitive urogenital sinus. The mesonephric ducts, urethra and bladder mucosa are of mesodermal origin but the remaining part of the bladder is derived from the urogenital sinus and is endodermal in origin. With continued embryo growth and differentiation, the mesodermal lining of the trigone of the bladder is replaced by endodermal epithelium and ultimately, the inside of the bladder is completely lined with epithelium of the endodermal origin. It is believed that the upper four-fifths of the vagina is derived from the urogenital canal where the lower one-fifth has its origin in the urogenital

sinus. In the fully developed fetus, the bladder and proximal urethra are endodermal in origin and the vestibule of the vagina and the distal urethra are ectodermal in origin.

Estrogen receptors can be found in the vaginal epithelium, stroma cells and smooth muscle cells and the urethra bladder, trigone and posterior bladder neck. Not all tissues have the same concentration of estrogen receptors. For example, in the urinary tract, receptor concentrations are lower in the trigone and bladder than in the urethra. With loss of estrogenic stimulation to the receptors that occur with menopause, senile changes occur: the vaginal barrel shortens and narrows, blood flow decreases so that the vaginal epithelium becomes pale and dry and loses its rugation, and tissue pliability decreases. The epithelium deposits collagen in the stroma and ultimately the vagina loses its glycogen content. With loss of glycogen, the normal flora made up of different types of *Lactobacillus* is replaced by pathogenic bacteria and vaginal pH increases from 5.5 to over 7.0. With continued estrogen deprivation over time, the vaginal epithelial surface continues to flatten and in some instances superficial keratinization may occur. As a result of these anatomic changes, the urethral orifice comes into closer proximity to the vaginal introitus which further contributes to both vaginal and urethral irritation and inflammation. This is especially detrimental to the female since the urethra is only 3–4 cm in length. Estrogen has a significant impact on the distal third of the urethra as this portion of the urinary tract behaves in the same manner to estrogen deprivation as the vaginal barrel. In addition, atrophy of the pelvic floor tissues also affects urinary tract function since the vesicle neck and proximal urethra are partially supported by these tissues.

Pelvic Floor Changes Related to Atrophy

The levator ani, the pelvic floor ligaments and the fascia make up the muscles of the pelvic floor. The levator ani are composed of a diaphragmatic division made up of the iliococcygeus muscle and the pubovisceral division. The pubovisceral inserts into the vagina and rectum and also forms a "sling" that supports the rectum. Urogenital atrophy leading to denervation of these muscles as a result of estrogen loss, injury and aging plays a role in the development of pelvic floor dysfunction. Not only does muscle degeneration occur with urogenital atrophy but also the integrity and structure of the supporting ligaments and fascia are often weakened by these same processes. With both menopause and aging the connective tissue, made up of collagen and elastin fibers embedded in a ground substance of proteoglycans glycoproteins, is adversely affected. Collagen loses its tensile strength and elastin from estrogen loss. The effects of menopause and aging directly impact on tissue integrity and contribute to the higher percentage of urinary incontinence and pelvic floor prolapse seen in older women. With continued aging, there is progressive tissue trauma, tissue thinning, loss of fat deposition, and decreased smooth muscle tone. In addition, the greater number of cross-linking fibers inhibit collagen tissue remodeling and compromise tissue pliability. Cartilage changes and arthritis in the bony pelvis also add to urogenital symptoms in the geriatric patient. Atrophy-related tissue denervation to pelvic floor muscles has been documented by electromyographic (EMG) studies and has been shown to be an important cause of fecal incontinence. However, it has not been as easy to study the role of muscle denervation as the etiology of stress urinary incontinence and genital organ prolapse. However, data suggest that prior pelvic floor injuries that result in muscle denervation do result in more bladder and genital prolapse problems [1].

Hormonal Influences on Urogenital Function

Estrogen deficiency and its subsequent role in causing adverse urogenital changes is widely recognized as the primary etiology of urogenital atrophy. Decreased estrogen is a universal event in either natural, surgical or medically induced menopause. However, there are other situations in which there may be a temporary lack of estrogen such as during lactation or from pharmacologic interventions, such as gonadotropin-releasing hormone (GnRH) therapy. Symptoms associated with vaginal atrophy are widely recognized and include dryness, dyspareunia, pruritus and discharge with odor. Recurrent urinary tract infections, urinary frequency and urgency as well as urinary incontinence are also associated with estrogen loss. The maturation index of the estrogen-deprived vagina shows no superficial cells and an abundance of basal and parabasal cells. When estrogen is restored, the vaginal epithelial cells mature and superficial cells replace the parabasal cell types. With estrogen loss during menopause vaginal blood flow is also reduced to a level of relative ischemia, which in part contributes to both vaginal dryness and dyspareu-

nia. When estrogen is replaced, blood flow is increased, the vaginal arteries increase in diameter and the number of small blood vessels increases so that vaginal color returns to pink from a pale white [2,3]. This is clinically important since it improves not only vaginal function but urethral function as well and in so doing decreases urinary symptoms. Estrogen replacement therapy eliminates or ameliorates complaints of dyspareunia by increasing vaginal lubrication and improving vaginal elasticity as well as restoring sensitivity of tissue.

Estrogen therapy also has an effect on symptoms related to the urethra and in some instances gives a full or partial response in cases of urinary incontinence [4]. For over 55 years, data have suggested a positive impact of estrogen on urinary tract function. However, not all research data have pointed to estrogen's beneficial effect on urinary incontinence, such as the report by the Hormone and Urogenital Therapy Committee in 1994, which did not show an overwhelming positive effect of estrogen on urinary tract function [5]. In another recent meta-analysis by the above committee published in 1998, there was more overwhelming evidence showing the beneficial effects of estrogen on vaginal health [6]. The 1998 report noted that although the available studies were too variable to make conclusive determinations on urogenital function and estrogen, the data do point to a positive estrogen effect. The authors noted that in many of the studies reviewed, there was no placebo arm and there were no objective outcomes measures for proving the beneficial effects of estrogen. However, the group did conclude that estrogen, both oral and vaginal and in several dosage regimens, was useful for treating vaginal atrophy. The group also concluded that low-dose local estrogen was as effective as systemic estrogen in reversing changes in the urogenital area.

A small percentage of women on systemic estrogen therapy still report symptoms attributable to urogenital atrophy, suggesting that rather than increasing the systemic dose of estrogen, local vaginal estrogen should be used. In addition, because locally applied vaginal estrogen is as effective as systemic estrogen, physicians have another treatment option for women who are unwilling to use systemic estrogenic replacement therapy or cannot take estrogen replacement therapy because of a medical contraindication. It should be emphasized to patients with urogenital atrophy who request local estrogen that this delivery system will not exert the preventive effects systemic estrogen does on coronary artery disease, osteoporosis, menopausal symptoms and cognitive function. As Semmens and Wagner's work showed, reversal of vaginal atrophy in women on estrogen replacement therapy may take up to 6 months before an optimal response is reached [2].

Estrogen's effect on the urinary tract has not been as well studied and it is not clear whether it is a vascular effect or whether estrogen's benefit is increasing production or decreasing degradation of collagen. In a study by Brincat et al., estrogen replacement therapy was shown to have a prophylactic effect in women with high collagen levels at the start of menopause and a therapeutic effect in menopausal women with lower collagen levels [7]. Brincat and colleagues measured the hydroxyproline content in the skin biopsies of a cohort of postmenopausal women who were treated with four different regiments of estrogen replacement therapy. They demonstrated that postmenopausal women treated with estrogen developed higher total collagen levels, which did not appear to be dependent upon the regiment used. Falconer studied related changes in the paraurethral tissues, especially the loss of tissue elasticity with diminishing estrogen levels [8]. In this menopausal cohort he showed that there was a greater degree of cross-linking of collagen fibers. However, when the women were given estrogen replacement therapy, it was demonstrated that these adverse connective tissue changes were reversed.

Effects of Prior Pregnancy and Childbirth on Urogenital Atrophy

With pregnancy, the urethra becomes more hyperemic and congested and under the influence of higher estrogen levels the transitional epithelium of the bladder changes to a squamous type. The urethra in pregnancy has an increased total and functional length and a higher closing pressure. Stress incontinence seen in pregnancy can be attributed to hormonally induced relaxation of the urethrovesical junction and/or to an increase in intra-abdominal pressure. As pregnancy advances, the bladder moves out of the pelvis, becoming an abdominal organ. The detrusor muscle also responds to the high levels of gonadal hormones characteristic of pregnancy, with estrogen causing hypertrophy of the detrusor and progesterone causing hypotonia of the detrusor. These changes contribute to the increased prevalence of lower urinary tract symptoms such as urgency, frequency and nocturia as well as the increased incidence of urinary tract infection in pregnancy. The long-term effects of pregnancy-related changes on urogenital tissue are not clear.

In addition to pregnancy changes to the urogenital tract, the process of vaginal childbirth also may contribute to long-term adverse changes to the urogenital system that become obvious in the menopausal years. Vaginal delivery may cause injury, leading to tissue denervation as the nerve supply from the sacral plexus to the levator ani may be compromised by the perineal stretching that occurs during childbirth. Although this denervation has been confirmed by EMG studies, these changes are usually reversible within approximately 2 months postpartum. Changes may not be totally reversible for multiparous women or women whose deliveries require instrumentation such as forceps or are accompanied by deep perineal lacerations. Therefore, both physiologic and tissue injury changes associated with pregnancy and childbirth may cause irreversible changes in the urogenital that are exacerbated in the menopausal patient when imposed upon aging changes and hormonal loss.

Trauma, Injury, Exercise, Diet and Other Factors Contributing to Urogenital Atrophy

The long-term effects of hysterectomy, radiation therapy and non-childbirth-related trauma to the pelvis have not thoroughly been elucidated. There may be an increased incidence of urinary incontinence in women undergoing hysterectomy or other pelvic surgery in which pelvic support is disrupted. In addition, radiation effects on the pelvic tissue also may compromise pelvic wall support. Therefore, the early use of estrogen replacement therapy should be considered in women in these risk categories.

Although even less studied, dietary deficiency, leading to poor tissue quality, has been proposed as a possible reason for pelvic support defects that are superimposed upon hormonal deprivation seen in the aging population. Poor nutrition has been found to compromise the integrity of collagen by leading to a deficient blood supply, scar tissue degradation and decreased healing.

On the other hand, exercise has been found to make tissue collagen more flexible. Exercise may not only exert this effect by increasing tissue elasticity but it may also change the actual composition of the tissue. Women who exercise may have less cross-linking of tissue collagen and perhaps the elastin itself may be different in exercisers compared to non-exercisers. These positive effects of exercise may continue into the postmenopausal years and advice about exercise should be included in preventive programs.

The same positive results seen with exercise have also been reported in women who continue to be sexually active. In a study by Leiblum et al., it was shown that menopausal women who continue to be sexually active had better scores on their vaginal health index than women who did not continue to be sexually active into their menopausal years [9]. Although sexual activity is often assumed to be coital activity, in this study the researchers found that any type of sexual activity, including self-stimulation, was beneficial for vaginal health. The conclusion of the authors from this cohort of menopausal women was that the "use it or lose it" phenomenon does exist and that sexual activity does improve urogenital health. Therefore, if atrophy is not corrected in the postmenopausal woman and leads to sexual abstinence, the problems of urogenital atrophy will be compounded. These data reconfirm the importance of continued surveillance of urogenital health and intervention at the earliest signs of symptoms so that sexual activity is not compromised.

The link between urogenital atrophy and connective tissue disorders such as Ehlers–Danlos syndrome, Marfan's syndrome, hernias and aneurysms is not well defined. Joint hypermobility, which has been used as a marker for collagen disorders, has been proposed as a possible marker for pelvic floor support defects [10]. Since 10–30% of adult women have been reported to have joint hypermobility, this suggests that prophylaxis should perhaps be started at an earlier point in the menopause transition. However, Ehlers–Danlos syndrome patients have not been shown to have a higher incidence of genital prolapse than the general population, although this may be due to patient under-reporting of symptoms. In addition to abnormal connective tissue, such as tissue that has a higher proportion of weaker collagen types such as collagen type III, there may be conditions characterized by problems with collagen remodeling. Therefore, more than one type of collagen defect may influence tissue integrity and later contribute to urogenital atrophy leading to pelvic floor displacement.

Treatment and Prevention

Although most clinicians link urogenital atrophy symptoms only to quality of life, in actuality urogenital atrophy can span the entire spectrum of severity, from mild to almost no symptoms in some women to marked clinical pathology such as vaginal stenosis and urinary incontinence in others. In addition, urogenital atrophy has psychological significance since it impairs the ability of many older women to feel sexually fulfilled. Because of our broader understanding of the pathophysiology of urogenital aging and the increasing awareness by women and their willingness to discuss this subject openly with their physicians, as well as physicians being able to actively intervene with effective pharmacologic medical and surgical approaches, the topic is an important one to discuss with every patient to ensure delivery of optimal patient care to the aging population. Clinicians can expect that more than 50% of postmenopausal women will experience lack of vaginal lubrication and frequent vaginal infections. In a study done by Rosen and colleagues, looking at the prevalence of sexual dysfunction in women, it was found that as women progress from premenopausal to perimenopausal to postmenopausal the trend is that they report more postcoital bleeding and irritation, lack of lubrication, dyspareunia and difficulty reaching orgasm [11].

At our facility we use a vaginal health index to screen all women beginning in their perimenopausal years to access the degree of atrophy present [12]. The index looks at overall elasticity, fluid type and consistency, pH, epithelial mucosa and moisture. It is felt that this type of index assesses female urogenital health in a clinically objective manner so that not only can physicians follow urogenital health on a longitudinal basis and share the findings with patients, but they can also use objective data in their decision-making regarding pharmacologic intervention and assessment of effectiveness of prescribed treatment. Assessment of aging changes can be put them the context of other conditions that may be occurring simultaneously such as neurologic problems or diabetes. In one recent study there was a 50% increased risk of urge incontinence in diabetic women over the age of 60 [13]. A past history of urinary tract infection is also important as in this same study there was a 50% increased risk of urge incontinence in women who reported two or more urinary tract infections in the prior year. Other predictors for urinary symptoms in postmenopausal women include white race, higher body mass index (BMI), and higher waist-to-hip ratio.

Lastly, obtaining a thorough sexual history is extremely important. Many women become sexually abstinent because of urogenital atrophy, which only exacerbates symptoms of vaginal dryness and urinary urgency and frequency. Since data suggest that any type of sexual activity is beneficial to urogenital health, counseling the patients regarding non-coital sexual activities can be helpful not only for the couple but for the woman who has no partner or a non-sexually functioning partner. In addition, over-the-counter lubricants are very effective in some instances and should be encouraged when a history of vaginal dryness and dyspareunia is elicited. It is also important to assess the ability of the patient to do Kegel exercises (see Figure 24.1) and using the time during the pelvic examination to teach both the quick Kegel and the slow Kegel is an effective use of office time.

The gold standard of care for urogenital atrophy treatment is estrogen replacement therapy. However, the standard dosage of estrogen (conjugated estrogen 0.625 mg or the equivalent) used for the treatment of menopausal symptoms, prevention of bone loss and reduction of cardiovascular disease risk may not be adequate to reverse or ameliorate urogenital symptoms. In these instances, either increasing the dose of systemic estrogen or supplementing the systemic estrogen with a local vaginal estrogen preparation should be considered. Vaginal estrogen for the treatment of urogenital atrophy has been shown to be effective, which is also useful for women who cannot or will not use systemic estrogen replacement therapy. In the US the local vaginal estrogen used is 17β estradiol and is delivered in either a cream or a ring form. There will soon be a 17β estradiol vaginal tablet that will have the same indication as the cream and ring for the treatment of urogenital atrophy. When the 17β estradiol ring is inserted the T_{max} is reached within 40 minutes and the 12-week post-treatment estrogen levels are similar to the pretreatment levels of estradiol.

Summary

Urogenital atrophy is a common problem in the postmenopausal women that has only recently been recognized as having a great impact on women's health and lifestyle. Many factors in addition to estrogen loss contribute to urogenital atrophy, but by far the most significant is hypoestrogenism in the urogenital area that occurs with the menopause. Changes associated with urogenital atrophy, specifically those due to estrogen loss, have been shown to be preventable and responsive to estrogen replacement therapy. It is important to identify women at risk for urogenital atrophy early in their menopause transition so that appropriate interventions can be instituted as soon as an early problem

is identified. Perineal exercises as well as continued sexual activity, both coital and non-coital, have been shown to prevent many of the symptoms resulting from urogenital atrophy. Other contributors to urogenital atrophy such as pregnancy, childbirth, connective tissue disorders, diabetes, previous surgery, radiation therapy and pelvic trauma have not been as well studied and their specific impact on urogenital atrophy is still not clearly defined. However, although there are many unanswered questions regarding the onset and severity of urogenital atrophy, it is clear that physicians can impact positively on women with this condition using the pharmacologic interventions that are currently available.

References

1. Wall, L. The muscles of the pelvic floor. Clin Obstet Gynecol 1993;36(4):910–25.
2. Semmens JP, Wagner G. Estrogen deprivation and vaginal function in postmenopausal women. JAMA 1982;248:445–8.
3. Sarrel PM. Sexuality and menopause. Obstet Gynecol 1990;75:26S–32S.
4. Hilsson K, Heimer G. Low-dose oestradiol in the treatment of urogenital oestrogen deficiency – pharmacokinetic and pharmacodynamic study, Maturitas 1992;15121–7.
5. Fantl JA, Cordoza L, McClish DK. Estrogen therapy in the management of urinary incontinence in post-menopausal women: a meta-analysis. First report of the hormones and urogenital therapy committee. Obstet Gynecol 1994;83:12–18.
6. Cardozo L, Bachmann G, McClish D et al. Meta-analysis of estrogen therapy in the management of urogenital atrophy in postmenopausal women: second report of the Hormones and Urogenital Therapy Committee. Obstet Gynecol 1998;92:722–7.
7. Brincat M, Versi E, Moniz CF et al. Skin collagen changes in postmenopausal women receiving different regimens of estrogen therapy. Obstet Gynecol 1987;70(1):123–37.
8. Falconer C, Ekman Orbeberg G, Ulmsten G et al. Changes in paraurethral connective tissue at menopause are counteracted by estrogen. Maturitas 1996;24:197–204.
9. Leiblum S, Bachmann G, Kemmann E. Colburn D, Swartzman L. Vaginal atrophy in the menopausal woman: The importance of sexual activity and hormones. JAMA 1983;249(16):2194.
10. Norton A. Peggy. Pelvic floor disorders the role of fascia and ligaments. Clin Obstet Gynecol 1993;36(4):926–38.
11. Rosen RC, Taylor JF, Leiblum SR, Bachmann GA. Prevalence of sexual dysfunction in women: Results of a survey of 329 women in an outpatient gynecological clinic. J Sex Marital Ther 1993;19(3):171–88.
12. Bachmann GA. Urogenital aging: an old problem newly recognized. Maturitas 1995;22:S1–S5.
13. Brown J, Grady D, Ouslander JG et al. Prevalence of urinary incontinence and associated risk factors in postmenopausal women. Obstet Gynecol 1999;94:66–70.

21 Common Anal Problems in Women

Marcus J. Burnstein

Anal problems are common in women and often present special therapeutic challenges, especially during pregnancy and following delivery. Thrombosed external hemorrhoids and anal fissure are frequently seen during and after pregnancy. Prolapsed, strangulated internal hemorrhoids, an uncommon problem in the general population, is a well-recognized complication of vaginal delivery. Anal skin tags are common in multiparous women. These problems will be discussed in this chapter.

Thrombosed External Hemorrhoid

Patients with thrombosed external hemorrhoid present with acute continuous anal pain associated with a tender mass. A discrete, subcutaneous, purple-blue lump is seen at the anal verge. The mass does not extend proximally above the dentate line. Thrombosed external hemorrhoid has been described as a perianal hematoma resulting from rupture of an external hemorrhoidal vein. In fact, pathological examination demonstrates thrombosis of the capillaries that have been stretched to over 1 cm in diameter [1]. Straining at stool or other exertion may play an etiologic role, but this is an inconsistent feature. It is a common lesion in young adults and an increased incidence during and after pregnancy seems likely, but is not well documented. The natural history of thrombosed external hemorrhoid is characterized by sudden, severe pain that peaks within 24–48 hours and then slowly resolves over the next 1–3 weeks. The thrombus is either lysed or extruded. A large thrombosed external hemorrhoid leaves behind a skin tag [1,2].

Treatment depends on the severity of the pain and the timing of presentation. The condition is self-limited, and especially during pregnancy and in the postpartum period, it may be best to treat with warm sitz baths, a high fiber diet, a stool softener, and a non-constipating analgesic. A non-medicated ointment may be soothing. Suppositories are not helpful. If pain is severe, excision should be performed. The entire lump should be removed and this can be readily achieved under local anesthesia in the office setting. An anal canal retractor is not needed as the dissection is not extended into the anal canal. The wound is left open, not packed, and the postoperative care is essentially the conservative treatment described above. Excision provides almost immediate pain relief, and the skin tag is avoided [1,2]. Pregnancy is not a contraindication to this approach. In the second and third trimester, the left anterolateral position can be used.

The severe pain of a thrombosed external hemorrhoid often seems disproportionate to the magnitude of the lesion, and it has been suggested that this is explained by "spasm" of the internal anal sphincter [3]. Topical nitroglycerin has been shown to relax the internal anal sphincter, and a role for nitroglycerin ointment has been suggested in the management of thrombosed external hemorrhoid [3,4]. In a small series, pain relief was achieved within minutes in 92% of patients, and each application relieved pain for 4–6 hours [3]. Thrombus resolution or extrusion followed the usual time course. The safety of nitroglycerin during pregnancy has not been established and should only be given if clearly indicated. It is not known whether nitroglycerin appears in breast milk. A role for topical nitroglycerin in the postpartum period exists if the patient is not breastfeeding; otherwise, the conventional treatment options are more prudent until further information is available regarding the safety of topical nitroglycerin during pregnancy and lactation.

There are two potential pitfalls in managing thrombosed external hemorrhoids. Firstly, the skin-covered thrombosed external hemorrhoid at the anal verge must be distinguished from the columnar mucosa-covered thrombosed internal hemorrhoid prolapsing through the anal canal. In general, the prolapsing internal hemorrhoid should not be operatively managed in the office setting. The second potential error is to incise and evacuate the clot rather than to excise the entire lesion. Simple evacuation is much less effective in relieving symptoms than is excision, and evacuation does not prevent the sequela of tag formation.

Anal Fissure

Anal fissure is a tear in the anal canal, extending from just below the dentate line to the anal verge. Fissure occurs equally in men and women, with a peak incidence in the 20–35-year age group. It is a common lesion, so it is not surprising that anal fissure is often seen in association with pregnancy. However, there may be more than a chance association between fissure and pregnancy. In a recent review of anal fissure, symptoms first appeared after delivery in 10% of the female patients [5]. In a study of over 300 primigravid women, postpartum fissure was diagnosed in 9% [6].

The cardinal symptom of anal fissure is pain during and for minutes to hours after defecation. Bright red blood is common. Less common symptoms include itch, swelling, and discharge. It is primarily a posterior midline lesion, but an unexplained gender difference exists with respect to the frequency of anterior fissure. In men, 5–10% of anal fissures are found in the anterior midline; in women, 20–25% are in the anterior midline position, and in a series of postpartum fissures, one-half were in the anterior midline [5–7]. A fissure can generally be visualized on gentle separation of the buttocks. Tenderness usually precludes digital and proctoscopic examination and complete evaluation must await healing of the fissure.

The acute fissure is a mere crack in the anoderm. Fissures which fail to heal acquire features of chronicity, including a distal "sentinel" tag, a proximal hypertrophied anal papilla, fibrotic edges, and exposed internal anal sphincter fibers (Figure 21.1).

Etiology and Pathogenesis

The hypothesis that anal fissure is a traumatic lesion secondary to the passage of a large, hard stool is attractive. Supporting data include a case control

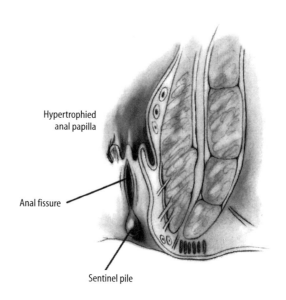

Figure 21.1 Chronic anal fissure. (From Gordon PH, Nivatvongs A. Principles and Practice of Surgery for The colon, Rectum and Anus. Quality Medical Publishing, Inc., St. Louis, Missouri, 1992, with permission.)

study demonstrating risk reduction for anal fissure with increased dietary fruits and vegetables and whole grain bread [8]. Also, a randomized controlled trial of prevention of fissure recurrence demonstrated a decreased recurrence rate with increased dietary fiber [9]. Interestingly, retrospective reviews of bowel habits do not confirm that most fissure patients were constipated when symptoms began [5,7]. On the other hand, in a prospective study of pregnant women, postpartum constipation was significantly more common in those with fissures (62%) than in those without (28%) [6].

Whatever the etiologic mechanism for acute fissure, failure of the acute fissure to heal is the consequence of two interacting factors: resting anal tone and anodermal blood flow. Anal manometry has demonstrated sustained hypertonicity of the internal anal sphincter in patients with chronic anal fissure [10], and laser Doppler flowmetry has revealed an inverse correlation between anodermal blood flow and anal pressure, i.e. the higher the pressure the lower the blood flow [11] (Figure 21.2). Studies of anodermal blood flow indicate lower perfusion of the posterior midline compared to the rest of the anoderm [11–15]. This amounts to strong evidence for the concept that chronic anal fissure is an ischemic ulcer. Whether internal anal sphincter hypertonicity is a cause or effect of anal fissure remains uncertain.

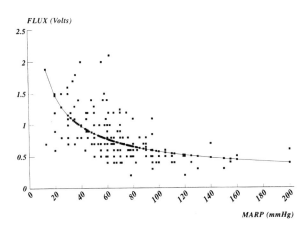

Figure 21.2 Anal pressure and anodermal blood flow in patients with chronic anal fissure (From Schoeten RI, Briel JW, Auwerda JJA. Relationship between anal pressure and anodermal blood flow. Dis Colon Rectum 1994;37:664–669, with permission.)

While it is beyond the scope of this chapter to go into detail, it is important to remember the association between anal fissure and inflammatory bowel disease, especially Crohn's disease. It is also important to remember that not all breaches of the anoderm are typical anal fissures: neoplasms, infections, and AIDS may produce similar lesions. Painless fissures, lateral and multiple fissures, and fissures which cross the dentate line should alert the clinician that further evaluation is indicated.

Treatment

Acute fissure
Warm baths and a diet sufficiently high in fiber to achieve soft, bulky stools allows approximately 80% of acute anal fissures to heal within 3 weeks. Stool softeners and fiber supplements are reasonable additions. Warm baths reduce resting anal pressure by 40%, an effect which persists for approximately 30 minutes [16]. Recurrence is common, but can be reduced by maintaining a high fiber diet [9].

Chronic fissure
Chronic fissures are unlikely to heal with warm baths and a high fiber diet. The key to healing chronic fissures is the reduction of resting anal pressure.

Internal sphincterotomy. Division of the internal anal sphincter is associated with excellent healing rates, but carries a risk of diminished continence. Sphincterotomy in the posterior midline through the base of the fissure has been condemned because of slow wound healing and high rates of soiling,

often associated with a posterior midline gutter or "key hole" deformity [1,2]. Lateral internal sphincterotomy achieves healing in over 95% within several weeks, the key hole deformity is avoided, and the rate and severity of continence problems are reduced, but are not negligible. Continence problems are reported in 0–35% of patients following lateral internal sphincterotomy, and the risk may be highest in women [17,18]. Endoanal ultrasound has revealed that external anal sphincter defects are present in 19% of primiparous and 29% of multiparous women, and has also shown that lateral internal sphincterotomy tends to be more extensive in women than intended, probably related to the shorter female anal canal [19]. Lateral internal sphincterotomy should be applied cautiously in women, and a limited sphincterotomy or a non-sphincterotomy approach should be considered. Traditional practice has been to divide the internal anal sphincter to the level of the dentate line, but excellent healing rates with low rates of incontinence have been achieved with sphincterotomy tailored to the length of the fissure [20].

Where the risk of post-sphincterotomy incontinence is felt to be increased, a V-Y advancement flap can be used with excellent results [21]. This option should be considered in the setting of failed lateral internal sphincterotomy, a history of sphincter trauma, including previous anal operation, and postpartum fissure.

Topical Nitroglycerin. Nitric oxide has been identified as the chemical messenger mediating internal sphincter relaxation. Topical application of nitroglycerin, a nitric oxide donor, causes a transient lowering of resting anal pressure and an increase in anodermal blood flow [11,12]. When used in the treatment of acute fissure, a healing rate of over 90% is expected [22]. Healing of chronic anal fissure was 68% after 8 weeks in a large randomized controlled trial of topical nitroglycerin [23]. There was no incontinence, but half the patients had headache, especially at the start of therapy. The late recurrence rate is not known. The reversible nature of "chemical sphincterotomy" is particularly attractive in patients at increased risk of impaired continence. As mentioned above, the safety of topical nitroglycerin during pregnancy and lactation has not been established.

Internal Hemorrhoids

Internal hemorrhoids are "vascular cushions" in the upper anal canal, above the dentate line, often located in the left lateral, right posterior, and right anterior positions. These are normal structures consisting of venules, arterioles, arteriolar–venular communications, smooth muscle and connective tissue. "Disease" exists when the cushions bleed and/or prolapse. Prolapse may be associated with mucus discharge and local irritation, and if prolapsed tissue becomes incarcerated, edema, thrombosis, and strangulation ensue, a condition characterized by severe pain and tissue necrosis [1,2].

Many factors have been implicated in hemorrhoidal disease, including straining, constipation, vascular engorgement, erect posture, and heredity. Some of the physiologic changes in pregnancy may promote the development of hemorrhoidal symptoms. Constipation, seen in 11–40% of pregnant women, has been attributed to the effects of pregnancy on smooth muscle, to the mechanical effects of the gravid uterus, and to iron supplements [24]. The increase in circulating blood volume and the laxity of connective tissue in pregnancy may also contribute to internal hemorrhoidal disease. Good epidemiologic data on hemorrhoidal disease in pregnancy is lacking, but the incidence of hemorrhoidal symptoms among pregnant women is probably much higher than for age-matched, non-pregnant women. Surveys suggest that about one-third of women report having "hemorrhoids" during pregnancy [24].

Treatment

In the non-pregnant patient, treatment of internal hemorrhoids is determined by the severity of symptoms and the stage of disease (Table 21.1). Most patients with first-degree and some with second-degree internal hemorrhoids can control their symptoms by achieving a daily soft bowel movement through the use of a high fiber diet, a fiber supplement, and increased fluid intake. Stage I and II disease that does not respond to dietary modification and improved bowel habits, and early

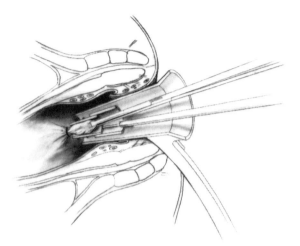

Figure 21.3 Rubber band ligation. (From Gordon PH, Nivatvongs A. Principles and Practice of Surgery for The colon, Rectum and Anus. Quality Medical Publishing, Inc., St. Louis, Missouri, 1992, with permission.)

stage III disease, may be treated in the office with rubber band ligation, infrared photocoagulation, or injection sclerotherapy. These office procedures take advantage of the fact that the internal hemorrhoidal tissue originates above the dentate line and therefore above the zone of sensory innervation. Application of these modalities at the cephalad end of the cushion, 1 cm or more above the dentate line, can be done without the need for local anesthetic and with minimal or no discomfort. The three techniques all work by creating a variable degree of tissue destruction, scarring, and fixation. All three cushions may be treated at a single session, but more commonly one or two hemorrhoids are treated at a time. Long-term efficacy is in the range of 70%. Rubber band ligation is inexpensive and appears to have the best risk: benefit ratio, especially for stage II and early stage III disease [25] (Figure 21.3). Infrared photocoagulation is particularly attractive for small grade I internal hemorrhoids. Injection sclerotherapy is currently less popular. All modalities are extremely safe, although with both injection sclerotherapy and rubber band ligation, infectious complications have been rarely encountered. Late stage III hemorrhoids, stage IV hemorrhoids and "mixed" hemorrhoidal disease (internal hemorrhoids combined with external hemorrhoids and skin tags) may require excisional hemorrhoidectomy [1,2].

Hemorrhoidal symptoms during pregnancy can almost always be managed conservatively. As a result, there is very little data on the use of office procedures during pregnancy [24]. Although the risks associated with injection sclerotherapy and

Table 21.1 Internal hemorrhoids: stage and treatment

	Stage	Treatment
I	Bleeding, no protrusion	Dietary modification Office procedure
II	Protrusion, spontaneous reduction	Dietary modification Office procedure
III	Protrusion, manual reduction	Office procedure Excisional hemorrhoidectomy
IV	Chronic protrusion	Excisional hemorrhoidectomy

rubber band ligation are extremely small, it is most unusual to have to treat uncomplicated early stage hemorrhoidal disease. When this situation does arise, infrared photocoagulation may be best, but there are no data. Injection sclerotherapy has been effectively used during pregnancy, achieving complete symptom control in 86% without complications [26]. Rubber band ligation has also been anecdotally reported to be safe and effective during pregnancy [24].

Acute hemorrhoidal prolapse and strangulation is usually seen postpartum, but may occur during pregnancy. The prolapse cannot be reduced because of massive tissue welling and sphincter spasm. Treatment recommendations for acute hemorrhoidal prolapse include (1) conservative management with Sitz baths, bed rest, stool softeners, and analgesics, (2) field block with a solution of 0.25% bupivacaine with 1:200,000 epinephrine and 150 TRU (1 ml) hyaluronidase to facilitate manual reduction of the prolapse, followed either by conservative management or by rubber band ligation, and (3) immediate hemorrhoidectomy [1,2,27]. Immediate hemorrhoidectomy most efficiently eradicates the disease and restores the patient to good health. In the second and third trimester, hemorrhoidectomy can be done under local anesthesia with the patient in the left anterolateral position. In the postpartum period, the prone jackknife position is preferred. Sedation with intravenous medication is a helpful adjunct to local anesthetic.

The operative principles are the same as for elective hemorrhoidectomy. Excellent lighting is essential. Exposure is achieved with careful attention to avoid a stretch injury of the anal sphincters. The prolapsed mass is reduced and the hemorrhoidal tissue is excised with preservation of anoderm, identification and protection of the underlying internal anal sphincter, extension of the excision above the anal canal, hemostasis, and wound closure. One to three hemorrhoids are excised as indicated.

Saleeby et al. performed closed excisional hemorrhoidectomy under local anesthesia on 25 pregnant women with acute hemorrhoidal disease [28]; 88% of patients were in the third trimester and 80% were multiparous. Symptomatic relief was excellent. Delivery and the foetus were not affected. Six patients required further treatment during follow up. Ruiz-Moreno described 90 patients undergoing emergency hemorrhoidectomy 0–4 days after delivery with excellent symptom relief and no complications. None of the patients who subsequently became pregnant reported anorectal problems [29]. In a report of postpartum hemorrhoidectomy in 98 patients, minor complications occurred in 3 [30].

Only 2 of 21 patients in this series who subsequently became pregnant developed anorectal symptoms, and none of the 98 patients required further operative treatment.

Skin Tags

Skin tags are large folds of skin arising at the anal verge. The exact pathogenesis of tags is not always clear. Tags may be the sequelae of thrombosed external hemorrhoids, may be associated with chronic anal fissure or inflammatory bowel disease, or may have no identifiable cause or association. Skin tags may be seen in association with external hemorrhoids, the dilated vascular plexus below the dentate line [1]. Skin tags are common in multiparous women, and caution must be exercised in ascribing symptoms, especially itch and irritation, to skin tags. Skin tags are more likely to be innocent bystanders [31]. Routine excision is not recommended. Excision may be appropriate when extensive tag formation appears to contribute to poor hygiene or when recurrent edema, thrombosis, and discomfort occur.

References

1. Gordon PH, Nivatvongs A. Principles and Practice of Surgery for the Colon Rectum and Anus. St Louis, MO: Quality Medical Publishing, 1992.
2. Corman ML. Colon and Rectal Surgery, 3rd edn. Philadelphia, PA: JB Lippincott, 1993.
3. Gorfine SR. Treatment of benign anal disease with topical nitroglycerine. Dis Colon Rectum 1995;38:453–7.
4. Schoeten WR, Briel JW, Boerma MO et al. Pathophysiological aspects and clinical outcome of intra-anal application of isosorbide dinitrate in patients with chronic anal fissure. Gut 1996;39:465–9.
5. Hananel N, Gordon PH. Re-examination of clinical manifestations and response to therapy of fissure in ano. Dis Colon Rectum 1997;40:229–33.
6. Corby H, Donnelly VS, O'Herlihy C, O'Connell PR. Anal canal pressures are low in women with postpartum anal fissure. Br J Surg 1997;84:86–8.
7. Lock MR, Thomson JPS. Fissure in ano: the initial management and prognosis. Br J Surg 1977; 64:355–8
8. Jensen SL. Diet and other risk factors for fissure in ano. Prospective case control study. Dis Colon Rectum 1988;31:770–3.
9. Jensen SL. Maintenance therapy with unprocessed bran in the prevention of acute anal fissure recurrence. J R Soc Med 1987;80:296–8.
10. Keck JO, Staninnas RJ, Coller JA et al. Computer generated profiles of the anal canal in patients with anal fissure. Dis Colon Rectum 1995;38:72–9.
11. Schoeten RI, Briel JW, Auwerda JJA, Boerma MO. Anal fissure: new concepts in pathogenesis and treatment. Scand J Gastroenterol 1996;31 Suppl 218:78–81.

12. Lund JN, Scholefield JH. Aetiology and treatment of anal fissure. Br J Surg 1996;83:1335–44.
13. Schoeten WR, Briel JW, Auwerda JJA et al. Ischaemic nature of anal fissure. Br J Surg 1996;83:63–5.
14. Klosterhalfen B, Vogel P, Rixen H et al. Topography of the inferior rectal artery: a possible cause of chronic, primary anal fissure. Dis Colon Rectum 1989;32:43–52.
15. Schoeten WR, Briel JW, Auwerda JJA. Relationship between anal pressure and anodermal blood flow. Dis Colon Rectum 1994;37:664–9.
16. Dodi G, Bogoni F, Infantino A et al. Hot or cold in anal pain? A study of the changes in internal anal sphincter pressure profiles. Dis Colon Rectum 1986;29:248–51.
17. Hananel N, Gordon PH. Lateral internal sphincterotomy for fissure in ano – revisited. Dis Colon Rectum 1997;40:597–602.
18. Garcia-Aguilar J, Belmonte C, Wong WD et al. Open vs closed sphincterotomy for chronic anal fissure. Dis Colon Rectum 1996;39:440–3.
19. Sultan AH, Mann MH, Nicholls, RJ et al. Prospective study of the extent of internal anal sphincterotomy division during lateral sphincterotomy. Dis Colon Rectum 1994;37:1031–3.
20. Littlejohn DRG, Newstead GL. Tailored lateral internal sphincterotomy for anal fissure. Dis Colon Rectum 1997;40:1439–42.
21. Leong AFPK, Seow-Choen F. Lateral sphincterotomy compared to anal advancement flap for chronic anal fissure. Dis Colon Rectum 1995;38:69–71.
22. Bacher H, Mischinger HJ, Werkgartner G et al. Local nitroglycerine for treatment of anal fissures: an alternative to lateral sphincterotomy? Dis Colon Rectum 1997;40:845–9.
23. Lund JN, Scholefield JH. A randomized, prospective, double blind, placebo controlled trial of glyceryl trinitrate ointment in treatment of anal fissure. Lancet 1997;349:11–14.
24. Medich DS, Fazio VW. Haemorrhoids, anal fissure, and carcinoma of the colon, rectum and anus during pregnancy. Surg Clin North Am 1995;75(1):77–88.
25. MacRae, HM, McLeod RS. Comparison of haemorrhoidal treatments: A meta-analysis. Can J Surg 1997;40:14–17.
26. Simmons SC. Anorectal disorders in pregnancy. J Obstet Gynaecol 1964;71:960–2.
27. Salvati EP. Management of acute haemorrhoidal disease. In: Schrock T, editor. Perspectives in Colon and Rectal Surgery. St Louis, MO: Quality Medical Publishing, 1990;(2):309–14.
28. Saleeby RG Jr, Rosen L, Stasik J et al. Hemorrhoidectomy during pregnancy: risk or relief? Dis Colon Rectum 1991;34:260–1.
29. Ruiz-Moreno F. Surgery in the puerperium for painful anorectal disorders. Proc Soc Med 1970;63:102–3.
30. Schottler JL, Balcos EG, Goldberg SM. Postpartum hemorrhoidectomy. Dis Colon Rectum 1973;16:395–6.
31. Berman IR. Mechanisms, diagnosis and management of anal irritation and itching. In: Schrock T, edition: Perspectives in colon and Rectal Surgery. St Louis, MO: Quality Medical Publishing, 1990; 3(1):82–97.

22 Chronic Pelvic Pain

Brenda B. Toner and Taryn N. Tang

Introduction

Chronic pelvic pain (CPP) is defined as a general symptom of persistent pain located in the pelvis of at least 6 months' duration [1]. CPP is considered a confusing entity because the pain is often unrelated to underlying gynecological pathology. Some patients with severe pathology may report little pain while others with mild to moderate tissue deformation may experience severe pain [2,3]. According to several studies of laparoscopy performed for CPP, approximately one-third of patients have endometriosis, one-third have adhesions, and one-third have unclear pathology [4–7]. Moreover, pain experienced by patients can range from the intermittent, such as with dysmenorrhea, to the kind that may be chronic and continuous [8]. Because of the lack of association to organic or physiologic change, CPP is often labeled as a functional somatic syndrome.

Stigma and Myths Associated with Functional Somatic Syndromes

Nearly every medical specialty has identified a functional somatic syndrome. In gynecology, CPP, or a subtype of CPP with "unclear pathology", may be conceptualized as a functional somatic syndrome. These syndromes are usually defined by physical symptoms that are unexplained by organic disease. The term "functional" implies a disturbance of physiological function rather than anatomical structure [9] and is often perceived as psychogenic and less "real" [10]. As a result of the stigma associ-ated with the term "functional" various labels have been used to describe functional somatic syndromes, including somatic disorders, health anxiety, physical syndromes not explained by organic disease, unexplained medical syndromes, and psychophysiological disorders [11].

Western societies in general and Western medicine in particular may attach a moral dimension to functional somatic syndromes. There is metaphysical dualism underlying Western medicine which suggests that either illness is an accident that befalls the patient and can be attributed to impersonal causes, or it has psychological causes that are mediated by and potentially under the person's voluntary control [9]. The morally pejorative connotations associated with functional somatic disorders such as CPP often leave patients believing that their problems are treated as "not real" and due to a psychological and/or moral defect or weakness [9]. Research has found that disorders disproportionately prevalent in women are often trivialized or described as psychological in origin and thus women are especially attentive to the possibility that their symptoms are not being taken seriously [12]. Unfortunately, in our society "psychological" is often equated with "trivialized". Accordingly, it is important to highlight that when people with CPP are referred to health professionals, they may come into the office with the belief that caregivers do not think their symptoms are "real" or serious, but that they are "all in their heads". The therapeutic alliance can be enhanced by validating the reality of the person's symptoms and by challenging the artificial dualism between functional and organic components of illness imposed by our society [13].

As emphasized by Steege and his colleagues [14] in a recent book on CPP, it is important to approach this disorder in an integrated fashion. Such an integrated or biopsychosocial approach avoids the mind/body split by recognizing that the mind and body is one functioning unit rather than separate components of a person. According to Steege [15], this integrated approach has two major goals in the understanding of CPP. The first goal is to determine the subtle interactions among disease states, physical sensations and psychological/emotional processes that currently exist for the patient. The second goal is to assess how the pain problem started and how it gradually reached its present condition in each of these dimensions. The details of this integrated approach are beyond the scope of this chapter and the reader is referred to *Chronic Pelvic Pain: An Integrated Approach*, edited by Steege et al. [14], which details the multitude of factors that contribute to the conceptualization and treatment of CPP.

In addition to the stigma associated with functional somatic syndromes such as CPP, several other myths are unhelpful to both physicians and patients who are experiencing these syndromes. One such myth is that CPP "with unclear pathology" is a psychiatric disorder or that it is masked depression. This myth may persist because several studies have found that a substantial percentage of women in tertiary care settings presenting with CPP also meet criteria for an associated anxiety or depressive disorder. It is unclear why such an association exists but some possible explanations are as follows: (a) Anxiety and depression, like CPP, are common in the general population, and their co-occurrence may simply be due to high frequency. (b) People who also have an associated anxiety/depressive disorder may have more difficulty coping with chronic pain syndromes and may seek specialized help for their pain at higher rates than people with CPP who do not have an associated anxiety or depressive disorder. (c) Depression/anxiety may be a consequence of living with a chronic, debilitating disorder such as CPP [16].

An additional related myth that is an unhelpful formulation for both physicians and patients is that some patients with CPP benefit from the sick role. This myth has pejorative connotations. People with CPP do not want to be ill and do not take any pleasure from this chronic and devastating illness. This myth may have emerged because people with a chronic illness such as CPP often receive more attention than people without an illness, are relieved from some of their usual responsibilities, and may receive social and financial compensation [16]. However, it is important to note that there is no empirical support to validate the notion that patients seek out or wish to benefit from living with a chronic painful syndrome such as CPP. Rather, patients with these disorders are interested in overcoming the disabling consequences of living with a chronic illness that reduces their quality of life.

A final myth is that people with CPP are sometimes difficult patients. Rather than conceptualizing CPP patients as difficult, it is more helpful to conceptualize the disorder as difficult, especially in light of the fact that there is little information and a great deal of stigma associated with these functional somatic disorders [16]. The lack of information coupled with the shame and trivialization associated with having a so-called functional disorder leads to frustration, further distressing patients. Most health care professionals, including physicians, are not adequately trained in the conceptualization and/or treatment of functional somatic syndromes such as CPP. Therefore, treating such patients may elicit uncomfortable feelings that might lead some health care professionals to feel helpless and frustrated in the situation. It is important to recognize that from both the patient and health care provider's perspectives, this is a frustrating disorder with many unanswered questions. A constructive approach would be to engage in an honest and open discussion acknowledging the frustration associated with this chronic and debilitating disorder. It is important for both patient and health care provider to work in a collaborative fashion attempting to understand the most effective strategies in managing the chronic, painful symptoms. As there is no effective medication or cure for CPP at present, the focus needs to be directed at symptom management and coping with this chronic condition. However, improved symptom control requires a shared plan of care between health care professional and patient. Treatment plans tailored to patients' individual needs and concerns will ensure that those with CPP can cope with their condition as comfortably as possible and with minimal disruption to everyday life. This approach has been described in other functional somatic disorders such as irritable bowel syndrome (IBS) [16].

Definition and Subtypes of Chronic Pelvic Pain

Chronic pelvic pain encompasses multiple syndromes [17] and attempts to establish it as a clinical entity are longstanding [18]. Three different operational definitions have been used in the literature: duration, anatomic, and affective-behavioral [19]. Many of the behavioral, emotional and biochemical changes in people with a diagnosis of CPP after 6 months are similar to those in people coping with other types of chronic pain [1].

Many theories have been put forth to attempt to understand the factors associated with CPP, resulting in the description "the disease with 20 different names" [20]. The major reason contributing to this confusion is that the pathophysiology of CPP is poorly understood. Often there is little relationship between the intensity of the pain described and the extent of the observed pathology. Moreover, women with CPP can have normal laparoscopies and women without CPP can have significantly abnormal laparoscopy findings [21]. In a literature review of laparoscopic findings, Gillibrand [22] discovered that in at least two-thirds of women with CPP, there was no obvious identifiable pathology. Another review of the literature, however, stated that the frequency with which perceptible pelvic pathology is diagnosed in women with CPP varies from 8% to 80% [23]. Thus, although the literature is mixed in terms of the percentage of patients with identifiable pathology, the consensus to date is that a sizable core of patients with CPP have "unexplained" pain.

The source and type of chronic pelvic pain can include any of the components of the female reproductive tract as well as those that may involve surrounding viscera, musculoskeletal system and other systems. Moreover, it is not uncommon for more than one type of CPP problem to present in the same person [1]. For example, a woman with vulvar vaginismus may continue to experience pelvic pain even after successful medical or surgical treatment of the original problem. Another such example would be a woman with endometriosis who may later develop IBS or pelvic floor muscle dysfunction.

Prevalence

Although CPP is one of the most common problems seen in gynecological settings, true incidence and prevalence rates are lacking [1]. In a Gallup poll conducted in 1996 involving 5325 women, 16% reported problems with pelvic pain [17]. Of these approximately 850 women who reported pelvic pain, 11% limited home activity, 11.9% limited sexual activity, 15.8% took medication, and 3.9% missed at least one day of work per month. It should also be noted that prevalence rates for CPP reported in the literature often differ depending on the examination setting (i.e., whether it is a tertiary care setting, primary care setting, or community sample). For example, in a study of women attending two non-gynecologic university clinics, 12% of the sample reported current CPP and 33% had experienced it at some point in their lives [24]. By contrast, a survey of 581 women of reproductive age attending primary care private practices found that 39.1% had pelvic pain at least some of the time and 11.7% had pain more than 5 days each month or lasting a full day or more each month [25]. Moreover, when pelvic pain is the primary symptom, gynecologic surgery is frequently performed; this includes 16–40% of laparoscopies [19,26] and 12% of hysterectomies [27,28]. Such procedures are expensive; in the United States alone, CPP accounts for more than US$2 billion annually in direct health care costs.

General Approach to Assessment

In most cases the major contributing factors in CPP can be identified by a history and physical examination. The patient's history should include the description, severity, distribution, and daily chronological pattern of the pain [1]. The pain history should describe the onset of the original pain in addition to the accumulation of components over the course of time. For example, according to Steege [1], women with dysmenorrhea and premenstrual pain attributed to endometriosis may gradually develop problems such as IBS and pelvic floor levator spasms. A detailed and comprehensive pain history chronology will also detect increase in intensity despite stable organic pathology. It is also important to underscore the potential impact of the pain on the patient as an individual, her relationships, and her work experiences. The psychosocial factors associated with CPP may be best measured by a careful clinical history and possibly a psychometric evaluation and consultation with a mental health professional [15].

While the details of a physical examination, which include abdominal and pelvic analysis, are beyond the expertise of the authors, we refer the interested reader to an excellent review by Steege [29] on office assessment of CPP. Rather, this discussion will focus on the approach to the patient, which involves a comprehensive discussion of chronic pain and associated psychosocial factors. Like any medical disorder, it is important to view psychosocial issues as legitimate components of the medical condition. CPP is best conceptualized as a multidimensional condition like other disorders including biological, psychological and social components. Much of this discussion is also appropriate for other functional somatic syndromes including IBS, chronic fatigue syndrome, and fibromyalgia. In particular, there is much ongoing discussion in the IBS literature regarding integrating psychosocial issues into our comprehensive understanding and treatment of chronic pain syndromes [11,13].

Discussion of Chronic Pain

It is important that physicians have a comprehensive understanding of the multifactorial aspects of pain. In this way, both physician and patient can engage in an extensive and meaningful discussion of the psychological, physiological, emotional, cognitive, and behavioral aspects of the pain experience. To begin with, it is important to dispel the common societal myth that if pain is severe, there must be an organic cause. This common myth persists as a function of Western society's false conceptualization of pain (i.e., if the pain is severe, there must be a structural cause) [16]. The experience of pain is a consequence of a complex interaction among physical, cognitive, emotional and behavioral components. We find that the introduction of gate control theory by Melzack [29] provides a good starting point for a discussion of chronic pain [13]. According to Steege [15], the gate control theory of pain remains a useful framework for discussing body/mind synthesis and serves a useful educational function in talking with CPP patients. The gate theory of pain states that pain messages originate at the site of bodily damage, injury, or disease and are then passed through a mechanism that works like a gate to the brain [29]. The brain then interprets the pain message, and it is at this point that pain is experienced. The pain "gate" can be partially or fully opened or closed, determining the amount of pain experienced.

Factors that can open the gate, i.e., make pain more central or more intense, include, for example, thoughts that focus attention on the pain, and boredom because of minimal involvement in life activities. Feelings that can open the gate include depression, anxiety, and anger. Behaviors can also open the gate, such as an inappropriate activity level or lack of pleasant activities [13]. Factors that can close the gate, i.e., make the pain less central or less intense, include coping strategies such as controlling pain thoughts through attention diversion. Examples of attention diversion are distraction, imagery, and relaxation. Gate control theory can be used in cognitive behavioral therapy for patients with CPP. For example, cognitive restructuring strategies, such as altering self-talk to messages such as "I can handle this, I've handled it before" versus "I can't stand another second of this pain" are useful. Pain can also be affected by changing activity patterns [13].

A discussion of the gate control theory as a mechanism to put the mind and body back together is clinically useful. It provides a sound basis for the notion that higher brain centers can modulate spinal cord gating activity. This suggests that information transmitted is bidirectional, and not just in the single direction from damaged tissue up to the brain. This theory also suggests that neurotransmitter states in the brain may have direct chemically mediated effects on the ability of the spinal cord's gating mechanism to block transmission of nociceptive signals [15]. To the degree that this theory is accurate, direct and concrete links are formed between body and mind. Gate control theory allows for the possibility that neurochemical changes associated with pain may alter the client's modulation of pain at a spinal cord level, thus placing an additional burden on the central nervous system in ignoring, blocking, or coping with the pain [15]. It should be noted that although the gate control theory has been debated and discussed in terms of its details, it remains a useful conceptual model for clinicians and clients. The gate control theory of pain also reinforces the notion that the pain cannot simply be assessed based on the amount of tissue damage. As noted by Steege [15], most clinicians, by training, look for some association between pathology and reported pain. With chronic pain patients in general and CPP patients in particular, this association between tissue damage and pain does not exist.

Associated Psychosocial Factors

The role of psychosocial factors within CPP has long been debated in the literature. For two excellent reviews of this literature, the interested reader is referred to an article by Fry et al. [18] entitled "Sociopsychological factors in chronic pelvic pain: A review" and an article entitled "Psychological aspects of chronic pelvic pain" by Savidge and Slade [30]. Taking an overview of this work over the last 50 years, the following relationships between psychosocial factors and CPP have been reported. Studies investigating depression, anxiety, and so-called psychoneurotic profile have shown that depression may be higher in some subgroups of CPP patients [31–34]. Other studies have shown greater degrees of "psychopathology" relative to non-clinical controls [33,35–41]. It has also been proposed that some patients with CPP are more hostile [39] or unable to express hostility [42]. There are some reports suggesting a higher prevalence of family history of depressive spectrum disease [32,41].

Some investigators have found significantly higher levels of childhood sexual abuse or early psychosexual trauma in CPP populations studied [23,41] or subgroups of the CPP populations studied [43]. In contrast, other studies have found no difference in prevalence of childhood sexual abuse in comparison to other chronic pain patients but instead a higher prevalence of childhood physical abuse [44]. Some studies have found that patients may have problems with current sexual relationships [33,34,37,41] and more difficulty with interpersonal relationships [7,23,36].

In terms of specificity, it is noteworthy that other chronic pain syndromes such as IBS have reported similar statistics. For example, approximately 50% of women who have a diagnosis of IBS and who are seen in tertiary care settings also have a history of sexual and physical abuse, a figure which is generally higher than those reported in primary care settings and in the general population. Walker et al. [45] also found that patients who had both IBS and CPP were more likely to have a lifetime history of dysthymic disorder, current and lifetime panic disorder, somatization disorder, and childhood sexual abuse and hysterectomy. Accordingly, the authors concluded that the high rate of psychosocial factors associated with IBS and CPP independently is even higher in women with both syndromes, and suggest that women who present with either chronic pain syndrome should probably be evaluated for these disorders [45]. In fact, Longstreth [46] argues that IBS should be considered in the differential diagnosis of CPP, and collaboration between gynecologists and gastroenterologists is needed in the care of women with CPP and IBS as well as in the conduct of additional research on the relationship between these two disorders.

There are theoretical and methodological problems with studies investigating psychosocial issues in CPP. The main problem is that most of this research has been approached from a traditional biomedical model in which pain has been understood in a dichotomist, organic–psychogenic way and has not been based on reconceptualizations about the role of these factors in the cause of CPP [30]. Within a biopsychosocial framework of illness, however, such dichotomizing in research is unhelpful and unlikely to yield clinically useful results. While issues of psychosocial factors and distress have been reported for women with CPP with and without organic pathology, it is not possible to draw conclusions about the role of these factors in the cause of CPP, particularly given the fact that such findings are common among other chronic pain populations, such as IBS, chronic fatigue syndrome, and fibromyalgia. In addition, most of this research has not considered the possibility that the high levels of psychosocial distress among women with CPP may be a long-term consequence of experiencing chronic pain rather than a specific connection with the disorder itself [30]. More recently, however, research has suggested that the psychosocial characteristics found among women with CPP may be due to the experience of living with chronic pain. As well, although several studies report a relationship between CPP and life events, particularly childhood sexual abuse, it is not clear that such experiences play a straightforward causal role in the development of CPP [30]. Furthermore, studies that have reported a high frequency of sexual and relationship problems in women with CPP have drawn misleading conclusions about the role of sexual anxiety in the development of pain problems rather than as a response to the pain experience. As noted by Savidge and Slade [30], the potential for chronic pain experience to impact on relationships with significant others, especially in terms of sexual difficulties, is hardly surprising given the site of pain.

The relationship between CPP and psychosocial issues is complex and is affected by a multitude of other variables. Researchers looking at psychosocial issues in women with CPP are well advised to take a lead from other areas of chronic pain research by looking at psychosocial issues in a broader based, multidimensional view of pain. Savidge and Slade [30] suggest that a narrow research focus in the area of CPP has left many questions unanswered and it remains a challenge to researchers in this area to begin to understand the psychosocial factors and models involved in CPP.

The multidimensional view of pain in recent years has led to the increasing recognition that chronic pain can affect a person in many ways [30]. A person's beliefs about pain and ways of coping with it have been shown in other pain research to impact upon psychological distress and affect perceptions of what people can do to relieve the pain. For example, research indicates that patients who frequently use comparative self-appraisals to cope with pain tend to be less depressed and more likely to feel in control of their pain [47]. Similarly, beliefs regarding self-efficacy are also important in understanding chronic pain. Nicholas [48] has shown that increased self-efficacy beliefs are associated with improvements in chronic pain, depressed mood, and reduction in medication use.

Overlap Between CPP and IBS

According to Longstreth [46] recent studies indicate that IBS is common in women with CPP and is associated with symptoms normally attributed to disorders of the female organs. In particular, there is considerable overlap of gynecological and gastrointestinal symptoms. One study of CPP patients attending a primary care or obstetrics and gynecology clinic found that 79% of these women also had IBS-type symptoms [24], while another study found that approximately 50% of women having diagnostic laparoscopy for CPP had IBS symptoms [49]. In the latter study, laparoscopic findings did not differ for the women with and without IBS-type symptoms. However, follow-up a year after laparoscopy found patients' overall status and pain improvement ratings to be lower in the group who had IBS-type symptoms. Studies have also found menstruation to be related to bowel symptoms in women without functional bowel disorder and that the association between menstruation and worsening bowel symptoms was more significant among patients with IBS and non-patients with IBS-type symptoms compared to women without IBS-type symptoms [50,51].

Women with IBS undergo hysterectomy more than what would be expected [51] and women with IBS-type symptoms undergo hysterectomy and other surgical abdominal procedures more than women without IBS-type symptoms [52]. In a prospective study of women having elective hysterectomy, Longstreth et al. [49] found increased prevalence of pain and constipation characteristic of IBS relative to a control group. Moreover, chronic or recurrent pelvic pain and abnormal menstrual bleeding were more commonly found among the hysterectomy patients with IBS-type symptoms than those without symptoms. Women who were having hysterectomy for pain were nearly twice as likely to have IBS-type symptoms as the other women. Operative findings did not differ between the two groups with and without IBS-type symptoms, but women with IBS-type symptoms reported lower pain improvement ratings one year after the hysterectomy than women without IBS-type symptoms.

As mentioned earlier, there are overlapping psychosocial issues in the etiology of CPP and IBS. Specifically, research indicates that as with IBS, women with CPP demonstrate a high prevalence of depression, somatization, substance abuse, and childhood sexual and physical abuse [44,53]. Thus, given the multifactorial nature of IBS and CPP, researchers have recommended an integrative approach to both disorders [19,46,54].

Treatment for Chronic Pelvic Pain

Currently, clinicians are confronted with a baffling array of possible treatments for CPP. The majority of these treatments are supported by little data to back up their application, specifically in the area of CPP [1,15]. Treatments for CPP can range from a number of surgical and medical strategies including hysterectomies, operative laparoscopies, oral analgesics, antidepressants (prescribed at lower doses than for major depression), transcutaneous electric nerve stimulation, acupuncture, ovarian cycle suppression, antibiotics, and organ-specific medication such as gastrointestinal agents and medication for bladder irritability, to a full range of psychotherapeutic approaches. As pointed out by Steege [15], many health care providers are not directly involved in mental health fields, and consequently the recommendation of a psychotherapeutic intervention may be discussed as a last resort. However, rather than considering psychotherapeutic interventions as a last resort, it makes sense to include discussion of any psychosocial issues when patients first present with the chronic pain problem. In this way, the multidimensional view of CPP is conveyed early on in the discussion and emotional and psychological concerns are conceptualized as an integral and legitimate part of the formulation of the problem and its effective management. It is desirable to have a psychosocial intervention as one possibility in helping patients cope with the pain rather than as the only decision left after extensive physical work-ups have provided negative results.

As noted by Kames et al. [8], CPP has rarely been discussed in the pain management literature, although it is extremely common in general gynecological practice, and is often refractory to traditional medical and surgical treatments. These investigators demonstrated the effectiveness of an interdisciplinary pain management program for the treatment of CPP relative to a waiting list control group. Kames et al. [8] described their program as one that conceptualized chronic pain as a complicated, multifaceted disorder, requiring both somatic and psychological intervention strategies. This interdisciplinary program included the use of acupuncture and antidepressants, a reduction in narcotic medication, and a broad range of psychological treatments such as stress management, relaxation training, anxiety and depression control, activity management, sex education, and cognitive therapy. Results indicated that there were significant decreases in anxiety and depression as well as a dramatic reduction in recorded levels of pain following treatment. Other benefits included returning to work, improved social activity, and increased sexual activity among people in the pain management program relative to people in the waiting list control group. The outcome suggests that the interdisciplinary pain management approach is an effective treatment for CPP. Moreover, these investigators highlight that their treatment strategy was effective for CPP patients with and without obvious organic pathology.

The effectiveness of multidisciplinary management of CPP was further confirmed by Peters et al. [55] in a randomized clinical trial. The multidisciplinary approach significantly improved pain severity, re-employment, and global somatic symptom scores compared to a traditional medical approach. In a meta-analysis of 65 studies evaluating the efficacy of multidisciplinary pain management, benefits relating to pain severity, mood, increased return to work, and decreased health care use were found to be stable over time [56].

As summarized by Reiter [57], the management of CPP can be greatly facilitated by a multidisciplinary perspective that integrates medical treatment with psychosocial strategies. The majority of the available evidence indicates that multidisciplinary management improves outcomes such as pain severity, general health, functional status, and disability more significantly than traditional, isolated medical or surgical procedures. We need to incorporate such multidisciplinary approaches in both our clinical services and our treatment protocols for women with a diagnosis of CPP.

References

1. Steege JF. Scope of the problem. In: Steege JF, Metzger DA, Levy BS, editors. Chronic Pelvic Pain: An Integrated Approach. Philadelphia: WB Saunders, 1998; 1–4.
2. Guzinski GM. Advances in the diagnosis and treatment of chronic pelvic pain. Adv Psychosom Med 1985;12:124–35.
3. Rapkin AJ. Adhesions and pelvic pain: A retrospective study. Obstet Gynecol 1986;68:13–15.
4. Kresch AJ, Seifer DB, Sachs LB, Barrese I. Laparoscopy in 100 women with chronic pelvic pain. Obstet Gynecol 1984;64:672–4.
5. Lindberg WI, Wall JE, Mathers JE. Laparoscopy in the evaluation of pelvic pain. Obstet Gynecol 1973;42:872–6.
6. Liston WA, Bradford WP, Downie J. Laparoscopy in a general gynecology unit. Am J Obstet Gynecol 1972;113:672–7.
7. Renaer M. Chronic Pelvic Pain in Women. New York: Springer, 1981.
8. Kames LD, Rapkin AJ, Naliboff BD, Afifi A, Ferrer-Brechner T. Effectiveness of an interdisciplinary pain management program for the treatment of chronic pelvic pain. Pain 1990;41:41–6.
9. Kirmayer LJ, Robbins JM. Functional somatic syndromes. In: Kirmayer LJ, Robbins JM, editors, Current Concepts of Somatization. Washington, DC: American Psychiatric Association Press, 1991.
10. Fabrega H Jr. Somatization in cultural and historical perspective. In: Kirmayer L, Robbins JM, editors, Current Concepts of Somatization. Washington, DC: American Psychiatric Association Press, 1991.
11. Toner BB. Cognitive-behavioral treatment of functional somatic syndromes: Integrating gender issues. Cognitive and Behavioral Practice 1994;1:157–78.
12. Lips HM. Sex and Gender: An Introduction. Mountain View, CA: Mayfield, 1997.
13. Toner BB, Segal Z, Emmott S, Myran D. Cognitive-Behavioral Treatment of Irritable Bowel Syndrome: The Brain-Gut Connection. New York: Guilford Publications, 2000.
14. Steege JF, Metzger DA, Levy BS. Chronic Pelvic Pain: An Integrated Approach. Philadelphia: WB Saunders, 1998.
15. Steege JF. Basic philosophy of the integrated approach: Overcoming the mind-body split. In: Steege JF, Metzger DA, Levy BS, editors. Chronic Pelvic Pain: An Integrated Approach. Philadelphia: WB Saunders, 1998; 5–12.
16. Toner BB. Challenging myths associated with IBS. 4 part series published in Participate, newsletter of the International Foundation of Functional Gastrointestinal Disorders, 1998–1999; 7(4); 8(1); 8(2); 8(3).
17. Mathias SD, Kuppermann M, Liberman RF, Lipschutz RC, Steege JF. Chronic pelvic pain: Prevalence, health-related quality of life, and economic correlates. Obstet Gynecol 1996;87:321–7.
18. Fry RPW, Crisp AH, Beard RW. Sociopsychological factors in chronic pelvic pain: A review. J Psychosom Res 1997;42(1):1–15.
19. Steege JF, Stout AL, Somkuti S. Chronic pelvic pain in women: Toward an integrative model. Obstet Gynecol Surv 1993;48:95–110.
20. Renaer M, Vertommen H, Nijs P, Wagemans L, Van Hemelrijck T. Psychological aspects of chronic pelvic pain in women. Am J Obstet Gynecol 1979;134:75–80.
21. Collett BJ, Cordle CJ, Stewart CR, Jagger C. A comparative study of women with chronic pelvic pain, chronic nonpelvic pain and those with no history of pain attending general practitioners. Br J Obstet Gynaecol 1998;105:87–92.
22. Gillibrand PN. The investigation of pelvic pain. In Chronic Pelvic Pain – A Gynaecological Headache. London: RCOG, 1981.
23. Reiter RC, Gambone JC. Demographic and historic variables in women with idiopathic chronic pelvic pain. Obstet Gynecol 1990;75:428–32.
24. Walker EA, Katon WJ, Alfrey H, Bowers M, Stenchever MA. The prevalence of chronic pelvic pain and irritable bowel syndrome in two university clinics. J Psychosom Obstet Gynecol 1991;12:65–75.
25. Jamieson DJ, Steege JF. The association of sexual abuse with pelvic pain complaints in the primary care population. Am J Obstet Gynecol 1997;177(6):1408–12.
26. Hulka JF, Peterson JB, Phillips JM, Surrey MW. Operative laparoscopy: American Association of Gynecologic Laparoscopists 1991 membership survey. J Reprod Med 1993;38:569–71.
27. National Center for Health Statistics, Graves, EJ. National hospital discharge survey: Annual summary, 1990. Vital Health Statistics. Series 13, No. 112. Washington, DC: Government Printing Office, 1992. (DHHS Publication No. (PHS) 92–1773).
28. Steege JF. Office assessment of chronic pelvic pain. Clin Obstet Gynecol 1997;40(3):554–62.
29. Melzack R. Neurophysiologic foundations of pain. In: Sternbach RA, editor. The Psychology of Pain. New York: Raven Press, 1986; 1.
30. Savidge CJ, Slade P. Psychological aspects of chronic pelvic pain. J Psychosom Res 1997;42(5):433–44.
31. Magni C, Andreoli C, de Leo D, Martinotti G, Rossi C. Psychological profile of women with chronic pelvic pain. Arch Gynecol 1986;237:165–8.
32. Magni C, Salmi A, de Leo D, Ceola A. Chronic pelvic pain and depression. Psychopathology 1984;17:132–6.
33. Beard RW, Belsey EM, Lieberman BA, Wilkinson JC. Pelvic pain in women. Am J Obstet Gynecol 1977;128:566–570.

34. Pearce S. A psychological investigation of chronic pelvic pain in women. Unpublished Doctoral Thesis, University of London, 1986.

35. Benson RC, Hanson KH, Matarazzo JD. A typical pelvic pain in women: Gynecologic-psychiatric considerations. Am J Obstet Gynecol 1959;77:806–25.

36. Castelnuovo-Tedesco P, Krout BM. Psychosomatic aspects of chronic pelvic pain. Int J Psychiatry Med 1970;1:109–26.

37. Gidro-Frank L, Gordon T, Taylor HC. Pelvic pain and female identity. Am J Obstet Gynecol 1960;79:1184–202.

38. Grandi S, Fava GA, Trombini G, Orlandi C, Bernardi M, Gubbini G, Michelacci L. Depression and anxiety in patients with pelvic pain. Psychiatr Med 1988;6:1–7.

39. Gross RJ, Doerr H, Caldirola D, Guzinski G, Ripley H. Borderline syndrome and incest in chronic pelvic pain patients. Int J Psychiatry Med 1981;10:79–96.

40. Slocumb JC, Kellner R, Rosenfeld RC, Pathak D. Anxiety and depression in patients with the abdominal pelvic pain syndrome. Gen Hosp Psychiatry, 1989;11:48–53.

41. Walker EA, Katon W, Harrop-Griffiths J, Holm L, Russo J, Hickok L. Chronic pelvic pain: The relationship to psychiatric diagnoses and childhood sexual abuse. Am J Psychiatry, 1988;145:75–80.

42. Duncan CH, Taylor HC. A psychosomatic study of pelvic congestion. Am J Obstet Gynecol 1952;64:1–12.

43. Reiter RC, Shakerin LR, Gambone JC, Milburn AR. Correlation between sexual abuse and somatization in women with somatic and nonsomatic chronic pelvic pain. Am J Obstet Gynecol 1991;165:104–9.

44. Rapkin AJ, Kames LD, Darke LL, Stampler FM, Naliboff BD. History of physical and sexual abuse in women with chronic pelvic pain. Obstet Gynecol 1990;76:92–6.

45. Walker EA, Gelfand AN, Gelfand MD, Green C, Katon WJ. Chronic pelvic pain and gynecological symptoms in women with irritable bowel syndrome. J Psychosom Obstet Gynecol 1996;17:39–46.

46. Longstreth GF. Irritable bowel syndrome and chronic pelvic pain. Obstet Gynecol Surv 1994;49(7):505–7.

47. Jensen MP, Karoly P. Control beliefs, coping efforts and adjustment to chronic pain. J Consult Clin Psychol 1991;59:431–8.

48. Nicholas MK. Self-efficacy and chronic pain. Paper presented at the annual conference of the British Psychological Society, 1989.

49. Longstreth GF, Preskill DB, Youkeles L. Irritable bowel syndrome in women having diagnostic laparoscopy or hysterectomy. Dig Dis Sci 1990;35:1285–90.

50. Heitkemper MM, Jarrett M. Pattern of gastrointestinal and somatic symptoms across the menstrual cycle. Gastroenterology 1992;102:504.

51. Whitehead WE, Cheskin LJ, Heller BR et al. Evidence for exacerbation of irritable bowel syndrome during menses. Gastroenterology 1990;98:1485.

52. Longstreth GF, Wolde-Tsadik G. Irritable bowel-type symptoms in HMO examinees. Dig Dis Sci 1993;38:1581.

53. Harrop-Griffiths J, Katon W, Walker E, Holm L, Russo J, Hickok L. The association between chronic pelvic pain, psychiatric diagnoses, and childhood sexual abuse. Obstet Gynecol 1988;71:589–93.

54. Gambone JC, Reiter RC. Nonsurgical management of chronic pelvic pain. A multidisciplinary approach. Clin Obstet Gynecol 1990;33:205–11.

55. Peters AAW, van Dorst E, Jellis B, van Zuuren E, Hermans J, Trimbos JB. A randomized clinical trial to compare two different approaches in women with chronic pelvic pain. Obstet Gynecol 1991;77:740–4.

56. Flor H, Dydrich T, Turk DC. Efficacy of multidisciplinary pain treatment centers: A meta-analytical flow. Pain 1992;49:221–39.

57. Reiter RC. Evidence-based management of chronic pelvic pain. Clin Obstet Gynecol 1998;41(2):422–35.

5 Conservative Treatment for Pelvic Floor Disorders

23 Pharmacologic Approach to Urinary Incontinence and Voiding Disorders

K.-E. Andersson

Introduction

The main components of the lower urinary tract, i.e. the urinary bladder, urethra, and striated urethral sphincter, constitute a functional unit, which is controlled by a complex interplay between the central and peripheral nervous systems and local regulatory factors [1–3]. Malfunction at various levels may result in bladder control disorders, which roughly can be classified as disturbances of filling/storage or disturbances of emptying [4]. Failure to store urine may lead to various forms of incontinence (mainly urge and stress incontinence), and failure to empty can lead to urinary retention, which may result in overflow incontinence.

Urinary incontinence is as prevalent as or more prevalent than most other chronic diseases, including asthma, coronary artery disease, and peptic ulcer disease, and is associated with considerable direct and indirect costs [5–7]. Appropriate management can significantly reduce both morbidity and costs. Pharmacological treatment has had varying degrees of success, and there is presently no group of drugs which can be used with consistently successful results. Many drugs have been tried, but the results are often disappointing, owing to poor treatment efficacy and/or side effects [8]. There have been many evaluations of the currently used drugs for treating the disorder. The present review is based on the evaluations made by the 2nd International Consultation on Incontinence, held in Paris 2001 [9].

Drugs have been evaluated using different types of evidence (Table 23.1). Pharmacological and/or physiological efficacy evidence means that a drug has been shown to have desired effects in relevant preclinical experiments or in healthy volunteers (or in experimental situations in patients). Clinical drug recommendations are based on evaluations made using a modification of the Oxford system, in which emphasis has been given to the quality of the trials assessed (Table 23.2).

Table 23.1 Types of evidence

Pharmacodynamic
In vitro
In vivo
Pharmacokinetic
Absorption
Distribution
Metabolism
Excretion
Physiological
Animal models
Clinical phase I
Clinical
Oxford guidelines

Table 23.2 ICI assessments: Oxford guidelines (modified)

Levels of evidence
Level 1: Randomized controlled clinical trials
Level 2: Good quality prospective studies
Level 3: Retrospective case-control studies
Level 4: Case series
Level 5: Expert opinion
Grades of recommendation
Grade A: Based on level 1 evidence (highly recommended)
Grade B: Consistent level 2 or 3 evidence (recommended)
Grade C: Level 4 studies or "majority evidence" (recommended with reservation)
Grade D: Evidence inconsistent/inconclusive (not recommended)

Nervous Control of Micturition

The nervous mechanisms for urine storage and bladder emptying involve a complex pattern of efferent and afferent signaling in *parasympathetic*, *sympathetic* and *somatic* nerves (see Figures 23.1 and 23.2). During storage (at low levels of vesical afferent activity) spinal reflexes are active, mediating contraction of urethral sphincter mechanisms through somatic (striated muscle) and sympathetic (smooth muscle) nerves. Sympathetic nerves may also mediate detrusor and ganglionic inhibition. During storage, there is no activity in the sacral parasympathetic outflow. Micturition is initiated by distension of the bladder, activating mechanorecep-

tors in the bladder wall. This triggers a high level of activity in small myelinated afferent nerves (Aδ), which via the dorsal root ganglia reaches the lumbosacral spinal cord. The Aδ afferents connect to a spinobulbospinal reflex consisting of an ascending limb from the lumbosacral spinal cord, integration centers in the rostral brain stem, and a descending limb back to the parasympathetic nucleus in the lumbosacral spinal cord. Afferent information may also be conveyed by small unmyelinated (C-fiber) vesical afferents, which have a high mechanical threshold, but which may be activated by irritation of the bladder mucosa. They may also be active in spinal cord injuries. Efferent micturition reflex pathways reach the bladder through the pelvic nerves.

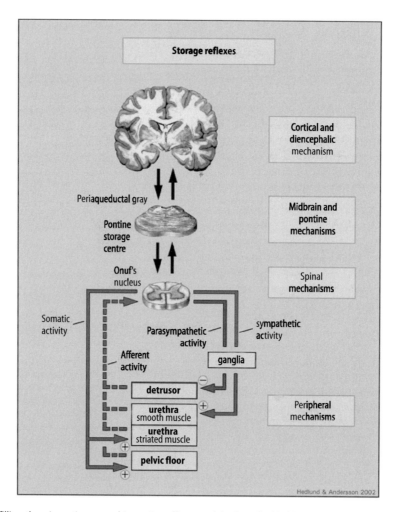

Figure 23.1 During filling, there is continuous and increasing afferent activity from the bladder. There is no spinal parasympathetic outflow that can contract the bladder. The sympathetic outflow to urethral smooth muscle, and the somatic outflow to urethral and pelvic floor striated muscles keep the outflow region closed. Whether or not the sympathetic innervation to the bladder (not indicated) contributes to bladder relaxation during filling in humans has not been established.

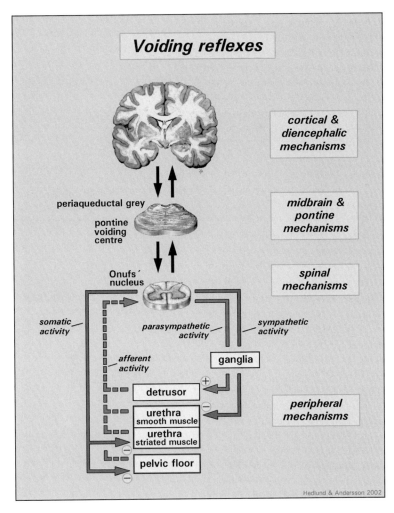

Figure 23.2   Voiding reflexes involve supraspinal pathways, and are under voluntary control. During bladder emptying, the spinal parasympathetic outflow is activated, leading to bladder contraction. Simultaneously, the sympathetic outflow to urethral smooth muscle, and the somatic outflow to urethral and pelvic floor striated muscles are turned off, and the outflow region relaxes.

Bladder Contraction

Normal bladder contraction in humans is mediated mainly through stimulation of muscarinic receptors in the detrusor muscle. Atropine resistance, i.e. contraction of isolated bladder muscle in response to electrical nerve stimulation after pretreatment with atropine, has been demonstrated in most animal species, but seems to be of little importance in normal human bladder muscle [1,10] (Figure 23.3). However, atropine-resistant (non-adrenergic, non-cholinergic: NANC) contractions have been reported in normal human detrusor and may be caused by ATP [1,3]. A significant degree of atropine resistance may exist in morphologically and/or functionally changed bladders (Figure 23.4), and has

been reported to occur in hypertrophic bladders [11,12], interstitial cystitis [13], neurogenic bladders [14], and in the aging bladder [15]. The importance of the NANC component to detrusor contraction in vivo, normally, and in different micturition disorders, remains to be established.

Muscarinic Receptors

Molecular cloning studies have revealed five distinct genes for muscarinic acetylcholine receptors in rats and humans, and it is now generally accepted that five receptor subtypes correspond to these gene products [16,17]. Muscarinic receptors are coupled to G-proteins (Figure 23.5). The signal transduction systems involved varies, but M_1, M_3, and M_5 prefer-

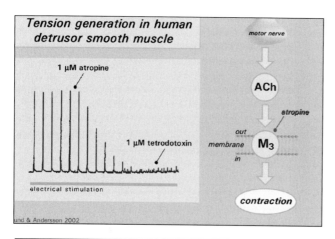

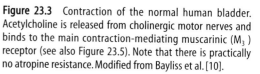

Figure 23.3 Contraction of the normal human bladder. Acetylcholine is released from cholinergic motor nerves and binds to the main contraction-mediating muscarinic (M_3) receptor (see also Figure 23.5). Note that there is practically no atropine resistance. Modified from Bayliss et al. [10].

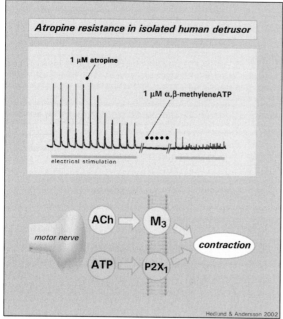

Figure 23.4 Atropine resistance in the human bladder. The contraction remaining after addition of atropine is caused by ATP, and can be abolished by α,β methylene ATP, which causes desensitization of P2X receptors.

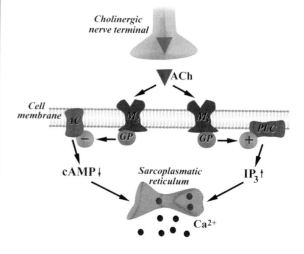

Figure 23.5 Acetylcholine (ACh) is released from cholinergic nerve terminals, and acts on muscarinic receptors (M_2 and M_3) in the detrusor. Both M_2 and M_3 receptors are coupled to G-proteins (GP) and may contribute to bladder contraction, but different signal transduction pathways are involved. M_2 receptors inhibit adenylyl cyclase (AC), which leads to a diminished intracellular level of cyclic AMP (cAMP). cAMP mediates bladder relaxation. Stimulation of M_3 receptors activates phospholipase C (PLC) to generate inositol triphosphate (IP_3). IP_3 can release calcium ions (Ca^{2+}) from the sarcoplasmic reticulum and this Ca^{2+} will activate the contractile machinery within the cell with resulting bladder contraction. The voiding contraction is believed to be mediated mainly through M_3 receptors.

entially couple to phosphoinositide hydrolysis leading to mobilization of intracellular calcium, whereas activation of muscarinic M_2 and M_4 receptors inhibits adenylyl cyclase activity. It has been suggested that muscarinic receptor stimulation may also inhibit K_{ATP} channels in smooth muscle cells from urinary bladder through activation of protein kinase C [18], thereby increasing the open probability of voltage-operated calcium channels and calcium influx.

Bladder Muscarinic Receptors

Detrusor smooth muscle from various species contains muscarinic receptors of the M_2 ($\approx 2/3$) and M_3 ($\approx 1/3$) subtype [19]. The M_3 receptors in the human bladder are believed to cause a direct smooth muscle contraction through phosphoinositide hydrolysis [20], whereas the role for the M_2 receptors has not been clarified. It has been suggested that M_2 receptors may oppose sympathetically (via β-ARs) mediated smooth muscle relaxation, since activation of M_2 receptors (rats) results in an inhibition of adenylyl cyclase [21].

There is general agreement that M_3 receptors are mainly responsible for the normal micturition contraction [19]. On the other hand, in certain disease states, M_2 receptors may contribute to contraction of the bladder [22,23].

Muscarinic receptors may also be located on the presynaptic nerve terminals and participate in the regulation of transmitter release. The inhibitory prejunctional muscarinic receptors have been classified as M_4 in the human [24] urinary bladders. Prejunctional facilitatory muscarinic receptors appear to be of the M_1 subtype and have been detected in human bladders [25].

The muscarinic receptor functions may be changed in different urological disorders, such as outflow obstruction, neurogenic bladders, bladder overactivity without overt neurogenic cause, and diabetes. However, it is not always clear what the changes mean in terms of changes in detrusor function.

Drugs Used for Treatment of Bladder Overactivity

It has been estimated that more than 50 million people in the developed world are affected by urinary incontinence. Even if it affects 30–60% of patients older than 65 years, it is not a disease exclusive to aging. It appears that detrusor overactivity may be the result of several different mechanisms, both myogenic [26] and neurological [27]. Most probably, both factors contribute to the genesis of the disease.

An abundance of drugs has been used for the treatment of the hyperactive detrusor (Table 23.3). However, for many of them, clinical use is based on the results of preliminary, open studies rather than randomized, controlled clinical trials (RCTs).

Antimuscarinic (Anticholinergic) Drugs

Both voluntary and involuntary bladder contractions are mediated mainly by acetylcholine-induced stimulation of muscarinic receptors on bladder smooth muscle. Antimuscarinic drugs will therefore depress both types of contraction, irrespective of how the efferent part of the micturition reflex is activated. In patients with involuntary bladder contractions, the volume to the first contraction is increased, the amplitude of the contraction is decreased, and total bladder capacity is increased [28].

Table 23.3 Drugs used in the treatment of detrusor overactivity. Assessments according to the Oxford system (modified)

	Level of evidence	Grade of recommendation
Antimuscarinic drugs		
Tolterodine	1	A
Trospium	1	A
Propantheline	2	B
Atropine, hyoscyamine	2	D
(Darifenacin, solifenacin)	Under investigation	
Drugs acting on membrane channels		
Calcium antagonists	Under investigation	
Potassium channel openers	Under investigation	
Drugs with mixed actions		
Oxybutynin	1	A
Propiverine	1	A
Dicyclomine	4	C
Flavoxate	4	D
Alpha-adrenoceptor antagonists		
Alfuzosin	4	D
Doxazosin	4	D
Prazosin	4	D
Terazosin	4	D
Tamsulosin	4	D
Beta-adrenoceptor agonists		
Terbutaline	4	D
Clenbuterol	4	D
Salbutamol	4	D
Antidepressants		
Imipramine	2	C[a]
Prostaglandin synthesis inhibitors		
Indomethacin	4	C
Flurbiprofen	4	C
Vasopressin analogues		
Desmopressin	1	A
Other drugs		
Baclofen	2[b]	C[b]
Capsaicin	3	C
Resiniferatoxin	Under investigation	

[a] Should be used with caution.
[b] Intrathecal use.

Atropine and related antimuscarinics are tertiary amines. They are well absorbed from the gastrointestinal tract and pass into the central nervous system (CNS). CNS side effects may therefore limit their use. Quaternary ammonium compounds are not well absorbed, pass into the CNS to a limited extent, and have a lower incidence of CNS side effects [29]. They still produce well-known peripheral antimuscarinic side effects, such as accommodation paralysis, constipation, tachycardia and dryness of mouth. All antimuscarinic drugs are contraindicated in narrow angle glaucoma.

Antimuscarinics are the most widely used treatment for urge and urge incontinence. However, currently used drugs lack selectivity for the bladder [16], and effects on other organ systems may result in side effects which limit their usefulness. One way of avoiding many of the antimuscarinic side effects is to administer the drugs intravesically. However, this is practical only in a limited number of patients.

Several antimuscarinic drugs have been used for treatment of bladder overactivity. For many of them, documentation of effects is not based on RCTs satisfying currently required criteria, and some drugs can be considered as obsolete (e.g. emepronium). Information on these drugs has not been included, but can be found elsewhere [30,31].

Atropine and Scopolamine

Atropine (dl-hyoscyamine) is rarely used for treatment of detrusor overactivity because of its systemic side effects, which preclude its use. However, in patients with detrusor hyperreflexia, intravesical atropine may be effective for increasing bladder capacity without causing any systemic adverse effects, as shown in open pilot trials [32–35]. The pharmacologically active antimuscarinic half of atropine is l-hyoscyamine. Although still used, few clinical studies are available to evaluate the antimuscarinic activity of l-hyoscyamine sulfate.

Scopolamine (l-hyoscine) has been administered transdermally in a randomized, placebo-controlled clinical trial in 20 female patients with detrusor instability [36]. Although the authors concluded that transdermal scopolamine was effective and safe as a treatment of detrusor instability, further investigations are needed to assess its therapeutic value.

Propantheline

Propantheline bromide is a quaternary ammonium compound, non-selective for muscarinic receptor subtypes, which has a low (5–10%) and individually varying biological availability [37]. It is usually given in a dose of 15–30 mg four times daily, but to obtain an optimal effect, individual titration of the dose is necessary, and often higher dosages.

The AHCPR (Agency of Health Care Policy and Research) Clinical Practice Guidelines (Urinary Incontinence Guideline Panel) lists five randomized controlled trials reviewed for propantheline, showing a reduction of urge (percent drug effect minus percent effect on placebo) between 0 and 53%. Controlled randomized trials (n = 6) were also reviewed by Thüroff et al. [38], who confirmed a positive, but varying response.

Although the effect of propantheline on detrusor overactivity has not been well documented in controlled trials satisfying standards of today, it can be considered effective, and may, in individually titrated doses, be clinically useful.

Trospium

Trospium chloride is a quaternary ammonium compound with antimuscarinic actions on detrusor smooth muscle. It has no selectivity for muscarinic receptor subtypes. Its biological availability is low, approximately 5% [39,40], and it does not cross the blood–brain barrier. It seems to have no negative cognitive effects [40–42].

In a placebo-controlled, double-blind study on patients with detrusor hyperreflexia [43], the drug was given twice daily in a dose of 20 mg over a 3-week period. It increased maximum cystometric capacity, decreased maximal detrusor pressure and increased compliance in the treatment group, whereas no effects were noted in the placebo group. Side effects were few and comparable in both groups. In a randomized, double-blind multicenter trial in patients with spinal cord injuries and detrusor hyperreflexia, trospium and oxybutynin were equieffective; however, trospium seemed to have fewer side effects [44].

The effect of trospium in urge incontinence has been documented in placebo-controlled, randomized studies. Allousi et al. [45] compared the effects of the drug with those of placebo in 309 patients in a urodynamic study of 3 weeks' duration. Trospium 20 mg was given twice daily. Significant increases were noted in volume at first unstable contraction and in maximum bladder capacity. Cardozo et al. [46] investigated 208 patients with bladder instability who were treated with trospium 20 mg twice daily for 2 weeks. Also in this study, significant increases were found in volume at first unstable contraction and in maximum bladder capacity in the trospium treated group. Trospium was well tolerated with similar frequency of adverse effects as in the placebo group. Höfner et al. [47] compared the effects of oxybutynin 5 mg twice daily with those of trospium 20 mg twice daily in a double-blind, randomized study over 12 months in 358 patients with urge symptoms or urge incontinence. The urodynamic improvements after the two drugs were comparable, but oxybutynin produced a significantly higher rate of side effects, and the drop-out rate was higher in the oxybutynin group.

Jünemann et al. [48] compared trospium 20 mg twice daily with tolterodine 2 mg twice daily in a placebo-controlled double-blind study on 232 patients with urodynamically proven bladder overactivity, sensory urge incontinence or mixed incontinence. Trospium reduced the frequency of micturition, which was the primary endpoint, more than tolterodine and placebo, and also reduced the number of incontinence episodes more than the comparators. Dry mouth was comparable in the trospium and tolterodine groups (7 and 9%, respectively).

Trospium chloride has a documented effect in detrusor overactivity, and seems to be well tolerated.

Tolterodine

Tolterodine is a new potent and competitive antagonist at muscarinic receptors, developed for treatment of urinary urgency and urge incontinence [49–52]. The drug has no selectivity for muscarinic receptor subtypes, but still shows some selectivity for the bladder over the salivary glands in an animal model [49], and possibly in humans [54]. Tolterodine has a major active metabolite with a similar pharmacological profile as the mother compound [53]. This metabolite contributes significantly to the therapeutic effect of tolterodine [55,56]. Tolterodine is rapidly absorbed and has a half-life of 2–3 h, but the effects on the bladder seem to be more long-lasting than could be expected from the pharmacokinetic data. The main metabolite also has a half-life of 2–3 h [56].

The relatively low lipophilicity of tolterodine implies limited propensity to penetrate into the CNS, which may explain a low incidence of cognitive side effects [52,57].

Several randomized, double-blind, placebo-controlled studies, both on patients with idiopathic detrusor instability and on those with detrusor hyperreflexia, have documented a significant reduction in micturition frequency and number of incontinence episodes [51,52]. Tolterodine immediate release seems to be well tolerated when used in the dose range 1–4 mg a day.

A once daily formulation of tolterodine has been developed, and a large-scale (1529 patients) clinical trial compared the effects of this agent to placebo and the twice daily formulation [58]. Tolterodine extended release (ER) 4 mg once daily and tolterodine immediate release (IR) 2 mg twice daily both significantly reduced the mean number of urge incontinence episodes per week compared with placebo. The median reduction in these episodes as a percentage of the baseline values was 71% for tolterodine ER, 60% for tolterodine IR, and 33% for placebo. Treatment with both formulations of tolterodine was also associated with statistically significant improvements in all other micturition diary variables compared with placebo. The rate of dry mouth (of any severity) was 23% for tolterodine ER, 30% for tolterodine IR, and 8% for placebo. The rates of withdrawal were comparable for the two active groups and the placebo group. No safety concerns were noted.

In a placebo-controlled study, comparing tolterodine 2 mg twice daily and oxybutynin 5 mg three times daily in 293 patients with detrusor instability, both drugs were found to be equally effective in reducing frequency of micturition and number of incontinence episodes. However, tolterodine appeared to have a better efficacy/tolerability profile [59]. These findings were largely confirmed by other investigators [60,61]. These data contrast with those of Appell et al. [62] comparing extended release oxybutynin chloride and immediate release tolterodine in a 12-week randomized, double-blind, parallel-group study in 378 patients with overactive bladder. Participants who had between 7 and 50 episodes of urge incontinence per week and 10 or more voids in 24 hours received extended release oxybutynin, 10 mg once daily, or tolterodine, 2 mg twice daily. The outcome measures were the number of episodes of urge incontinence, total incontinence, and micturition frequency at 12 weeks adjusted for baseline. At the end of the study, extended release oxybutynin was found to be significantly more effective than tolterodine in each of the main outcome measures adjusted for baseline. Dry mouth, the most common adverse event, was reported by 28.1% and 33.2% of participants taking extended release oxybutynin and tolterodine, respectively. Rates of central nervous system and other adverse events were low and similar in both groups. The authors concluded that extended release oxybutynin was more effective than tolterodine and that rates of dry mouth and other adverse events were similar in both treatment groups.

No comparative trials between extended release tolterodine and the extended release form of oxybutynin have been so far been reported. However, comparison of the immediate release forms would seem to indicate that efficacy is no different, whereas the side effect profile of tolterodine is favorable [57,63]. Head to head comparisons between the two extended release preparations are required to adequately compare efficacy and tolerability between the two agents.

Tolterodine, in both the immediate and extended release forms, has a well-documented effect on detrusor overactivity, and the side effect profile seems acceptable.

Drugs in development

Darifenacin. Darifenacin is a selective muscarinic M3 receptor antagonist developed for treatment of bladder overactivity [64]. Published clinical information on its clinical effects is scarce. In a pilot study on patients with detrusor instability, the drug was found to reduce the total number, maximum amplitude, and duration of unstable bladder contractions [65]. A randomized, double-blind trial of 25 patients with detrusor instability compared the effects of darifenacin 15 mg and 30 mg once a day and oxybutynin 5 mg three times daily on ambulatory urodynamic monitoring and salivary flow [66]. Both drugs had similar urodynamic efficacy, but oxybutynin reduced salivary flow significantly more than darifenacin. In another controlled study, on 27 healthy male subjects, the effects of darifenacin 7.5 and 15 mg once a day, dicyclomine 20 mg four times a day, and placebo on cognitive and cardiac functions were investigated [67]. Unlike dicyclomine, darifenacin had no detectable effects on cognitive or cardiovascular function.

Darifenacin is currently being evaluated in a phase III clinical studies.

Solifenacin (YM-905). Solifenacin (YM905) is a long-acting muscarinic receptor antagonist in development for the treatment of overactive bladder. It has some selectivity for M_3 receptors, and it is currently being investigated in phase III clinical studies.

Drugs acting on membrane channels

Calcium antagonists
Activation of detrusor muscle, through both muscarinic receptor and NANC pathways, seems to require influx of extracellular Ca^{2+} through Ca^{2+} channels, as well as via mobilization of intracellular Ca^{2+} [1]. The influx of extracellular calcium can be blocked by calcium antagonists, blocking L-type Ca^{2+} channels, and theoretically, this would be an attractive way of inhibiting detrusor overactivity. However, there have been few clinical studies of the effects of calcium antagonists in patients with detrusor overactivity (see Andersson et al. [31]).

Available information does not suggest that systemic therapy with calcium antagonists is an effective way to treat detrusor overactivity, but controlled clinical trials are lacking. However, the possibility that intravesical therapy with these drugs could be useful should not be ignored, nor the fact that calcium antagonists may enhance the effects of antimuscarinic agents [1].

Potassium Channel Openers
Opening of K^+ channels and subsequent efflux of K^+ will produce hyperpolarization of various smooth muscles, including the detrusor. This leads to a decrease in Ca^{2+} influx by reducing the probability of Ca^{2+} channels opening with subsequent relaxation or inhibition of contraction. Theoretically, such drugs may be active during the filling phase of the bladder, abolishing bladder overactivity with no effect on normal bladder contraction. K^+ channel openers, such as pinacidil and cromakalim, have been effective in animal models [68], but clinically, the effects have not been encouraging.

The first generation of openers of ATP-sensitive K^+ channels, such as cromakalim and pinacidil, were found to be more potent as inhibitors of vascular than of detrusor smooth muscle, and in clinical trials performed with these drugs, no bladder effects have been found at doses already lowering blood pressure. However, new K_{ATP} channel openers have been described, which may be useful for the treatment of bladder overactivity [9].

K^+ channel opening is an attractive way of treating bladder overactivity, since it would make it possible to eliminate undesired bladder contractions without affecting normal micturition. However, at present there is no evidence from controlled clinical trials to suggest that K^+ channel openers represent a treatment alternative.

Drugs with "Mixed" Actions

Some drugs used to block bladder overactivity have been shown to have more than one mechanism of action. They all have a more or less pronounced antimuscarinic effect and, in addition, an often poorly defined "direct" action on bladder muscle. For several of these drugs, the antimuscarinic effects can be demonstrated at much lower drug concentrations than the direct action, which may involve blockade of voltage operated Ca^{2+} channels. Most probably, the clinical effects of these drugs can be explained mainly by an antimuscarinic action.

Oxybutynin
Oxybutynin has several pharmacological effects, some of which seem difficult to relate to its effectiveness in the treatment of detrusor overactivity. It has both an antimuscarinic and a direct muscle relaxant effect, and, in addition, local anesthetic actions. The latter effect may be of importance when the drug is administered intravesically, but probably plays no role when it is given orally. In vitro, oxybutynin was 500 times weaker as a smooth muscle relaxant than as an antimuscarinic agent [69]. Most probably, when given systemically, oxybutynin acts mainly as an antimuscarinic drug.

Oxybutynin has a high affinity for muscarinic receptors in human bladder tissue It was shown to have higher affinity for muscarinic M_1 and M_3 receptors than for M_2 receptors [70], but the clinical significance of this is unclear.

Oxybutynin is a tertiary amine that is well absorbed, but undergoes an extensive first-pass metabolism (biological availability 6% in healthy volunteers). The plasma half-life of the drug is approximately 2 hours, but with wide inter-individual variation [71,72]. Oxybutynin has an active metabolite, N-desethyl oxybutynin, which has pharmacological properties similar to those of the parent compound [73], but which occurs in much higher concentrations [72]. Therefore, it seems reasonable to assume that the effect of oral oxybutynin is exerted to a large extent by the metabolite.

Many controlled studies have shown that oxybutynin is effective in controlling detrusor overactivity, including hyperreflexia (see reviews by Yarker et al. [74], Thüroff et al. [38], Wein [63]). The recommended oral dose of the immediate release form is 5 mg twice daily or four times daily, though lower doses have been used. Thüroff et al. [38] summarized 15 randomized controlled studies on a total of 476 patients treated with oxybutynin. The mean decrease in incontinence was recorded as 52% and the mean reduction in frequency for 24 h was 33%. The overall "subjective improvement" rate was reported as 74% (range 61–100%). The mean percentage of patients reporting side effects was 70 (range 17–93%). Oxybutynin 7.5 to 15 mg/day significantly improved quality of life for patients with overactive bladder in a large open multicenter trial. In this study, patient compliance was 97% and side effects – mainly dry mouth – were reported by only 8% of patients [75].

In nursing home residents (n = 75), oxybutynin did not add to the clinical effectiveness of prompted voiding in a placebo-controlled, double-blind, cross-over trial. On the other hand, in another controlled trial in elderly subjects, oxybutynin with bladder training was found to be superior to bladder training alone. Several open studies in patients with spinal cord injuries have suggested that oxybutynin, given orally or intravesically, can be of therapeutic benefit [9].

The therapeutic effect of immediate release oxybutynin on detrusor overactivity is associated with a high incidence of side effects (up to 80% with oral administration). These are typically antimuscarinic in nature (dry mouth, constipation, drowsiness, blurred vision) and are often dose-limiting [76,77]. Oxybutynin passes the blood–brain barrier and may have effects on the central nervous system [29,41]. The drug can cause cognitive impairment [78,79], and this side effect may be particularly troublesome in the geriatric population [80]. The effects on the electrocardiogram of oxybutynin were studied in elderly patients with urinary incontinence [82]; no changes were found. It

cannot be excluded that the commonly recommended dose 5 mg × 3 is unnecessarily high in some patients, and that a starting dose of 2.5 mg × 2 with following dose-titration would reduce the number of adverse effects [75,81].

Once daily formulations of oxybutynin have been developed. The oxybutynin ER (Ditropan XL) uses an osmotic drug delivery system to release the drug at a controlled rate over 24 h. This formulation overcomes the marked peak to trough fluctuations in plasma levels of both drug and the major metabolite that occur with immediate release oxybutynin [83]. A trend towards a lower incidence of dry mouth with oxybutynin ER was attributed to reduced first-pass metabolism and to the maintenance of lower and less fluctuating plasma levels of drugs. Clinical trials on oxybutynin ER have concentrated primarily on comparing this drug with immediate release oxybutynin [84,85]. Anderson et al. [84] reported on a multicenter, randomized, double-blind study on 105 patients with urge incontinence, or mixed incontinence with a clinically significant urge component. Urge urinary incontinence episodes were the primary efficacy parameter. The number of weekly urge incontinence episodes decreased from 27.4 to 4.8 after controlled release and from 23.4 to 3.1 after immediate release oxybutynin, and total incontinence episodes decreased from 29.3 to 6 and from 26.3 to 3.8, respectively. Weekly urge incontinence episodes from baseline to end of study also decreased to 84% after controlled and 88% after immediate release oxybutynin. Since only patients who had previously responded to treatment with oxybutynin were selected for treatment, these figures do not represent what can be considered normal in clinical practice. Dry mouth of any severity was reported by 68% and 87% of the controlled and immediate release groups, respectively, and moderate or severe dry mouth occurred in 25% and 46%, respectively.

Appell et al. [62] compared extended release oxybutynin chloride 10 mg/day and tolterodine 2 mg twice daily in a 12-week randomized, double-blind, parallel-group study in 378 patients with overactive bladder. Extended release oxybutynin was found to be significantly more effective than tolterodine in each of the main outcome measures (number of episodes of urge incontinence, total incontinence, and micturition frequency at 12 weeks) adjusted for baseline, and the rates of dry mouth and other adverse events were similar in both treatment groups.

Administered intravesically, oxybutynin has in several studies been demonstrated to increase bladder capacity and produce clinical improvement with few side effects, both in hyperreflexia and in other types of bladder overactivity, and in both children and adults [86]. Cognitive impairment can also occur in children treated with intravesical oxybutynin. Since it was reported that these effects may differ from those with oral administration [79], these patients should be closely monitored.

Oxybutynin has a well-documented efficacy in the treatment of detrusor overactivity, and is, together with tolterodine, the drug of first choice in patients with this disorder.

Dicyclomine

Dicyclomine has attributed to it both a direct relaxant effect on smooth muscle and an antimuscarinic action. Favorable results in detrusor overactivity have been demonstrated in several studies, performed more than a decade ago, and which do not satisfy current criteria of good quality RTCs [9].

Even though published experiences of the effect of dicyclomine on detrusor overactivity are favorable, the drug is not widely used, and RTCs documenting its efficacy and side effects are scarce.

Propiverine

Propiverine has been shown to have combined anticholinergic and calcium antagonistic actions [87,88]. The drug is rapidly absorbed, but has a high first-pass metabolism. Several active metabolites are formed, whose pharmacological characteristics remain to be established. It seems most probable that these metabolites contribute to the clinical effects of the drug [89].

Propiverine has been shown in several investigations to have beneficial effects in patients with detrusor overactivity [89]. Thüroff et al. [38] collected 9 randomized studies on a total of 230 patients, and found reductions in frequency (30%) and micturitions per 24 h (17%), a 64 ml increase in bladder capacity, and a 77% (range 33–80%) subjective improvement. Side effects were found in 14% (range 8–42%).

In patients with hyperreflexia, controlled clinical trials have demonstrated propiverine's superiority over placebo [89]. Controlled trials comparing propiverine, flavoxate and placebo [90], and propiverine, oxybutynin and placebo [91,93], have confirmed the efficacy of propiverine, and suggested that the drug may have equal efficacy and fewer side effects than oxybutynin.

Stöhrer et al. [92] reported a double-blind, randomized, prospective, multicenter trial comparing propiverine 15 mg three times a day to placebo in 113 spinal cord injury patients with detrusor hyperreflexia. Maximal cystometric capacity increased significantly in the propiverine group, by an average of 104 ml. Changes in bladder capacity at first contraction and in maximum bladder contraction were likewise statistically significant. Bladder compliance showed a more pronounced increase under propiverine in comparison to placebo. Sixty-three percent of patients experienced subjective improvement with propiverine in comparison with 23% of the placebo group. Dryness of the mouth (37% in the propiverine and 8% in the placebo group), and accommodation disorders (28% and 2% respectively) were reported side effects.

Madersbacher et al. [93] compared the tolerability and efficacy of propiverine (15 mg three times a day) oxybutynin (5 mg twice daily) and placebo in 366 patients with urgency and urge incontinence in a randomized, double-blind placebo-controlled clinical trial. Urodynamic efficacy of propiverine was judged similar to that of oxybutynin, but the incidence and the severity of dry mouth were judged to be less with propiverine than with oxybutynin.

Dorschner et al. [94] investigated, in a double-blind, multicenter, placebo-controlled, randomized study, the efficacy and cardiac safety of propiverine in 98 elderly patients (mean age 68 years), suffering from urgency, urge incontinence or mixed urge–stress incontinence. After a 2-week placebo run-in period, the patients received propiverine (15 mg three times a day) or placebo (twice daily) for 4 weeks. Propiverine caused a significant reduction in micturition frequency (from 8.7 to 6.5) and a significant decrease in episodes of incontinence (from 0.9 to 0.3 per day). Resting and ambulatory electrocardiograms indicated no significant changes. The incidence of adverse events was very low (2% dryness of the mouth with propiverine – 2 out of 49 patients).

Propiverine has a documented beneficial effect in the treatment of detrusor overactivity, and seems to have an acceptable side effect profile. Its complex pharmacokinetics with several active, not very well-characterized metabolites, needs more attention.

Flavoxate

The main mechanism of flavoxate's effect on smooth muscle has not been established. The drug has been found to possess a moderate calcium antagonistic activity, to have the ability to inhibit phosphodiesterase, and to have local anesthetic properties; no anticholinergic effect has been found [95]. It has been suggested that pertussis toxin-sensitive G-proteins in the brain are involved in the flavoxate-induced suppression of the micturition reflex in rats [96]. Its main metabolite (3-methylflavone-8-

carboxylic acid, MFCA) has been shown to have low pharmacological activity [95].

The clinical effects of flavoxate in patients with detrusor instability and frequency, urge and incontinence have been studied in both open and controlled investigations, but with varying rates of success [97]. Stanton [98] compared emepronium bromide and flavoxate in a double-blind, cross-over study of patients with detrusor instability and reported improvement rates of 83% and 66% after flavoxate or emepronium bromide, respectively, both administered as 200 mg three times daily. In another double-blind, cross-over study comparing flavoxate 1200 mg/day with that of oxybutynin 15 mg daily in 41 women with idiopathic motor or sensory urgency, and utilizing both clinical and urodynamic criteria, Milani et al. [99] found both drugs effective. No difference in efficacy was found between them, but flavoxate had fewer and milder side effects. The lack of placebo arm in these studies reduces the value of the efficacy conclusions.

Other investigators comparing the effects of flavoxate with those of placebo, have not been able to show any beneficial effect of flavoxate at dosages up to 400 mg three times daily [100–102].

In general, few side effects have been reported during treatment with flavoxate. On the other hand its efficacy, compared with other therapeutic alternatives, is not well documented.

α-Adrenoceptor antagonists

The normal human detrusor responds to norepinephrine (noradrenaline) by relaxing, probably because of the effect on both α- and β-adrenoceptors (ARs). Stimulation of α_2-ARs on cholinergic neurons may lead to a decreased release of acetylcholine, and stimulation of postjunctional β-ARs to direct relaxation of the detrusor muscle [1].

Drugs stimulating α-ARs have hardly any contractile effects in isolated, normal human detrusor muscle. However, there is evidence that this may change in bladder overactivity associated with, for example, hypertrophic bladder and outflow obstruction and neurogenic bladders [1]. A significant subtype selective α_{1D}-AR mRNA upregulation was found in rats with outflow obstruction [103], but functional correlates were not reported. It cannot be excluded that factors such as the degree and duration of obstruction have an important influence on the α-ARs in the detrusor, but the functional consequences have not been established.

α-AR antagonists have been used to treat patients with neurogenic bladders and bladder overactivity [104–107]; however, the success has been moderate. Abrams [107] reported results from a placebo-controlled study (4 weeks' duration) on the effects of tamsulosin in 263 patients with supra-sacral spinal cord lesions and neurogenic lower urinary tract dysfunction. There was a trend, but no statistically significant reduction of maximum urethral pressure with tamsulosin after 4 weeks. In 134 patients who completed a 1-year open-label treatment, significant positive effects, urodynamic as well as symptomatic, were found. At present no definitive conclusions can be drawn on the efficacy of α_1-AR antagonists in the treatment of neurogenic bladders until further information is available.

Lower urinary tract symptoms in women have been reported to respond favorably to treatment with α-AR antagonists [108,109]. In a prospective open study of 34 women with urgency and frequency, evaluated by an expanded AUA (American Urological Association) symptom score, a combination of doxazosin and hyoscyamine was found to be more effective than either drug given alone [110]. The value of such a combination should be evaluated in a controlled clinical trial.

Although α-AR antagonists may be effective in selected cases of bladder overactivity, convincing effects documented in RCTs are lacking. In women, these drugs may produce stress incontinence [111,112].

β-Adrenoceptor Agonists

In isolated human bladder, non-subtype selective β-AR agonists such as isoprenaline have a pronounced inhibitory effect, and administration of such drugs can increase bladder capacity in humans. However, the β-ARs of the human bladder were shown to have functional characteristics typical of neither β_1-, nor β_2-ARs [1]. On the other hand, receptor binding studies using subtype selective ligands suggested that the β-ARs of the human detrusor are primarily of $\beta_?$ subtype [113]. In a double-blind investigation clenbuterol 0.01 mg three times daily was shown to have a good therapeutic effect in 15 of 20 women with motor urge incontinence [114]. Other investigators, however, have not been able to show that β-ARs agonists represent an effective therapeutic principle in elderly patients with unstable bladder [115], or in young patients with myelodysplasia and detrusor overactivity [116].

Atypical β-AR-mediated responses have been shown to be mediated by a β_3-AR, which has been cloned, sequenced, expressed in model systems, and extensively characterized functionally [117]. Both normal and neurogenic human detrusors were shown to express β_1-, β_2-, and β_3-AR mRNAs, and selective β_3-AR agonists effectively relaxed both types of detrusor muscle [118–120]. Thus, it seems that the atypical β-AR of the human bladder may be the $β_3$-AR. Whether or not this is of importance in humans, and whether $β_3$-AR stimulation will be an effective way of treating the overactive bladder, has yet to be shown in controlled clinical trials.

Antidepressants

Several antidepressants have been reported to have beneficial effects in patients with detrusor overactivity [121,122]. However, imipramine is the only drug that has been widely used clinically to treat this disorder.

Imipramine has complex pharmacological effects, including marked systemic anticholinergic actions [123] and blockade of the reuptake of serotonin and norepinephrine [124], but its mode of action in detrusor overactivity has not been established [125]. Even if it is generally considered that imipramine is a useful drug in the treatment of detrusor overactivity, no good quality RCTs that can document this have been retrieved.

It has been known for a long time that imipramine can have favorable effects in the treatment of nocturnal enuresis in children, with a success rate of 10–70% in controlled trials [125,126].

It is well established that therapeutic doses of tricyclic antidepressants, including imipramine, may cause serious toxic effects on the cardiovascular system (orthostatic hypotension, ventricular arrhythmias). Imipramine prolongs QTc intervals and has an antiarrhythmic (and proarrhythmic) effect similar to that of quinidine [127,128]. Children seem particularly sensitive to the cardiotoxic action of tricyclic antidepressants [123].

The risks and benefits of imipramine in the treatment of voiding disorders do not seem to have been assessed. Very few studies have been performed during the last decade [125], and no good quality RCTs have documented that the drug is effective in the treatment of detrusor overactivity. However, a beneficial effect has been documented in the treatment of nocturnal enuresis.

Prostaglandin synthesis inhibitors

Human bladder mucosa has the ability to synthesize eicosanoids, and these agents can be liberated from bladder muscle and mucosa in response to different types of trauma [129]. Even if prostaglandins cause contraction of human bladder muscle [1], it is still unclear whether prostaglandins contribute to the pathogenesis of unstable detrusor contractions. More important than direct effects on the bladder muscle may be sensitization of sensory afferent nerves, increasing the afferent input produced by a given degree of bladder filling. Involuntary bladder contractions can then be triggered at a small bladder volume. If this is an important mechanism, treatment with prostaglandin synthesis inhibitors could be expected to be effective. However, clinical evidence for this is scarce.

Cardozo et al. [130] performed a double-blind controlled study of 30 women with detrusor instability using the prostaglandin synthesis inhibitor flurbiprofen at a dosage of 50 mg three times daily. The drug was shown to have favorable effects, although it did not completely abolish detrusor overactivity. There was a high incidence of side effects (43%) including nausea, vomiting, headache and gastrointestinal symptoms. Palmer [131] studied the effects of flurbiprofen 50 mg × 4 versus placebo in a double-blind, cross-over trial in 37 patients with idiopathic detrusor instability (27% of the patients did not complete the trial). Active treatment significantly increased maximum contractile pressure, decreased the number of voids and decreased the number of urgent voids compared to baseline. Indomethacin 50–100 mg daily was reported to give symptomatic relief in patients with detrusor instability, compared with bromocriptine in a randomized, single-blind, cross-over study [132]. The incidence of side effects was high, occurring in 19 of 32 patients. However, no patient had to stop treatment because of side effects.

The paucity of controlled clinical trials on the effects of prostaglandin synthesis inhibitors in the treatment of detrusor overactivity, and the limited number of drugs tested, makes it difficult to evaluate their therapeutic value. No new information has been published during the last decade.

Vasopressin Analogues

Desmopressin
Desmopressin (1-desamino-8-D-arginine vasopressin; DDAVP) is a synthetic vasopressin analogue with a pronounced antidiuretic effect, but practically lacking vasopressor actions. It is now widely used as a treatment for primary nocturnal enuresis [133]. Studies have shown that one of the factors that can contribute to nocturnal enuresis in children, and probably in adults, is lack of a normal nocturnal increase in plasma vasopressin, which results in high nocturnal urine production [134–137]. By decreasing the nocturnal production of urine, beneficial effects may be obtained in enuresis and nocturnal polyuria.

Several, controlled, double-blind investigations have shown intranasal administration of desmopressin to be effective in the treatment of nocturnal enuresis in children [126,138,139]. The dose used in most studies has been 20 µg intranasally at bedtime. However, the drug is orally active, even if the bioavailability is low (less than 1% compared to 2–10% after intranasal administration), and its oral efficacy in primary nocturnal enuresis in children and adolescents has been documented in randomized, double-blind, placebo-controlled studies [140,141].

Positive effects of desmopressin on nocturia in adults have been documented. Nocturnal frequency and enuresis due to bladder instability responded favorably to intranasal desmopressin therapy even when previous treatment with "antispasmodics" had been unsuccessful [142]. In patients with multiple sclerosis, desmopressin was shown in controlled studies to reduce nocturia, and micturition frequency [143–146]. Furthermore, desmopressin was shown to be successful in treating nocturnal enuresis in spina bifida patients with diurnal incontinence [147]. Oral desmopressin has proved to be effective in the treatment of nocturia with polyuric origin. In addition to prolonging sleep duration to first void, desmopressin reduced the number and frequency of nocturnal voids and nocturnal urine volume in both men and women [148,149].

Desmopressin is a well-documented therapeutic alternative in pediatric nocturnal enuresis, and seems to be effective also in adults with nocturia with polyuric origin. Even if side effects are uncommon, there is a risk of water retention and hyponatremia during desmopressin treatment [150,151], and due consideration should be given to this potential side effect, particularly in elderly patients.

Other Drugs

Baclofen

Baclofen is considered to depress monosynaptic and polysynaptic motor neurons and interneurons in the spinal cord by acting as a GABA receptor agonist, and has been used in voiding disorders, including detrusor hyperreflexia secondary to lesions of the spinal cord [37]. The drug may also be an alternative in the treatment of idiopathic detrusor overactivity [152]. However, published experience with the drug is limited.

Intrathecal baclofen may be useful in patients with spasticity and bladder dysfunction [153].

Capsaicin and Resiniferatoxin

Capsaicin, the pungent ingredient of red peppers, has identified a pharmacological classification of subpopulations of primary afferent neurons innervating the bladder and urethra, the "capsaicin-sensitive nerves". Capsaicin exerts a biphasic effect on sensory nerves: initial excitation is followed by a long-lasting blockade which renders sensitive primary afferents (C-fibers) resistant to activation by natural stimuli [154]. It is believed that capsaicin exerts these effects by acting on specific receptors, "vanilloid" receptors [155]. It is possible that capsaicin at high concentrations (mM) has additional, nonspecific effects [156].

Intravesical capsaicin has been used with success in bladder overactivity caused by neurological disorders such as multiple sclerosis, or traumatic chronic spinal lesions. The effect of treatment may last for 2 to 7 months [157–159]. However, negative results have also been reported [160].

Side effects of intravesical capsaicin include discomfort and a burning sensation at the pubic/urethral level during instillation, an effect that can be overcome by prior instillation of lidocaine, which does not interfere with the beneficial effects of capsaicin [161]). No premalignant or malignant changes in the bladder have been found in biopsies of patients who had repeated capsaicin instillations for up to 5 years [159].

Resiniferatoxin is a phorbol related diterpene, isolated from some species of *Euphorbia*, a cactus-like plant. It has effects similar to those of capsaicin. Given intravesically, resiniferatoxin has been shown to be approximately 1000 times more potent than capsaicin in stimulating bladder activity [162].

Lazzeri et al. [163] instilled resiniferatoxin intravesically in 15 subjects, including 8 normal subjects and 7 with bladder over activity (6 with hyperreflexia). Resiniferatoxin (10 nM concentration) did not produce any warm or burning sensation suprapubically. In the patients with bladder overactivity, but not in the normal subjects, the mean bladder capacity increased significantly immediately after resiniferatoxin treatment. However, this effect remained in only 2 out of the 7 patients 4 weeks after the instillation. Higher doses (50 and 100 nM) were used by Cruz et al. [164], who treated 7 patients with hyperreflexia with intravesical resiniferatoxin. They found no temporary deterioration of urinary symptoms, as seen with capsaicin, and found improvement in urinary frequency in 5 of the patients that lasted up to 3 months. The beneficial effect of resiniferatoxin has been confirmed in other studies [165,166]. These observations make resiniferatoxin an interesting alternative to capsaicin, but further investigations are needed to explore its clinical potential. Currently it is not in clinical development owing to formulation problems.

Table 23.4 Drugs used in the treatment of stress incontinence. Assessments according to the Oxford system (modified)

	Level of evidence	Grade of recommendation
Alpha-adrenoceptor agonists		
Ephedrine	3	C
Norephedrine (phenylpropanolamine, PPA)	2	NR
Other drugs		
Imipramine	4	C[a]
Clenbuterol	4	C
(Duloxetine)	Under investigation	
Hormones		
Estrogens	2	D

NR, not recommended.
[a] Should be used with caution.

Drugs Used for Treatment of Stress Incontinence

Factors which may contribute to urethral closure include urethral smooth muscle tone and the passive properties of the urethral lamina propria, in particular the vascular submucosal layer. The relative contribution to intraurethral pressure of these factors is still subject to debate. However, there is ample pharmacological evidence that a substantial part of urethral tone is mediated through stimulation of α-ARs in the urethral smooth muscle by released norepinephrine [1]. A contributing factor to stress incontinence, mainly in elderly women with lack of estrogen, may be lack of mucosal function. The role of striated urethral and pelvic floor muscles has not yet been established.

The pharmacological treatment of stress incontinence (Table 23.4) aims at increasing intraurethral pressure by increasing tone in the urethral smooth muscle, or by affecting tone of the striated muscles in the urethra and pelvic floor (see below). Although several drugs may contribute to such an increase in intraurethral pressure, including β-AR antagonists and imipramine, only α-AR agonists and estrogens (see below), alone or together, have been more widely used.

α-Adrenoceptor Agonists

Although several drugs with agonistic effects on α-ARs have been used in the treatment of stress incontinence, for example midodrine [167,168] and norfenefrine [169], ephedrine and norephedrine seem to be the most widely used drugs. Ephedrine,

pseudoephedrine (a stereoisomer of ephedrine), and norephedrine (phenylpropanolamine, PPA) directly stimulate α- as well as β-ARs, but can also release norepinephrine from adrenergic nerve terminals. They have all been reported to be effective in stress incontinence, as found in open and controlled clinical trials, ephedrine at a dose of 25 to 50 mg 3–4 times daily, and PPA at a dose of 50 to 100 mg 2–3 times daily. These drugs lack selectivity for urethral α-ARs, and may increase blood pressure. They also can cause sleep disturbances, headache, tremor and palpitations. Long-term experience with the drugs is lacking. It has been pointed out that individuals taking PPA might have an initial increase in blood pressure that can be dangerous, and it should be noted that the FDA has asked manufacturers to voluntarily stop selling PPA-containing drugs and replace the ingredients with a safer alternative. Judging from the clinical benefit documented with PPA and the possible risks, this drug (and probably drugs with similar action) should not be used [9].

Radley et al. [170] evaluated the effect of the selective α_1-AR agonist, methoxamine, in a randomized, double-blind, placebo-controlled, cross-over study on a group of women with genuine stress incontinence while measuring maximum urethral pressure (MUP), blood pressure, heart rate, and symptomatic side effects. Methoxamine evoked nonsignificant increases in MUP and diastolic blood pressure, but caused a significant rise in systolic blood pressure and significant fall in heart rate at maximum dosage. Systemic side effects including piloerection, headache, and cold extremities were experienced in all subjects. The authors suggested that the clinical usefulness of direct, peripherally acting subtype-selective α_1-AR agonists in the medical treatment of stress incontinence may be limited by side effects.

α-AR agonists has been used in combination with estrogens, and with other nonsurgical treatments of stress incontinence, such as pelvic floor exercises and electrical stimulation. Even if this type of treatment can be effective in women with mild stress incontinence or in those not suitable for surgery, the risks with PPA and related compounds (see above) do not seem to warrant their use as single drug therapy or in combination with estrogen. In carefully selected patients, selective α_1-AR agonists may be used on an "on demand" basis in certain situations known to provoke leakage.

β-Adrenoceptor Antagonists

The theoretical basis for the use of β-AR antagonists in the treatment of stress incontinence is that blockade of urethral β-ARs may enhance the effects of norepinephrine on urethral α-ARs. Even though propranolol has been reported to have beneficial effects in the treatment of stress incontinence [171,172], there are no RCTs supporting such an action.

Imipramine

Imipramine, among several other pharmacological effects, inhibits the reuptake of norepinephrine and serotonin in adrenergic nerve ending. In the urethra, this can be expected to enhance the contractile effects of norepinephrine on urethral smooth muscle. Theoretically, such an action may also influence the striated muscles in the urethra and pelvic floor by effects at the spinal cord level (Onuf's nucleus).

Gilja et al. [173] reported in an open study on 30 women with stress incontinence that imipramine, 75 mg daily, produced subjective continence in 21 patients and increased mean maximal urethral closure pressure (MUCP) from 34 to 48 mmHg. Lin et al. [174] assessed the efficacy of imipramine (25 mg imipramine three times a day for 3 months) as a treatment for genuine stress incontinence in 40 women with genuine stress incontinence. A 20-minute pad test, uroflowmetry, filling and voiding cystometry, and stress urethral pressure profile were performed before and after treatment. The efficacy of successful treatment was 60% (95% CI 44.8–75.2). No RCTs on the effects of imipramine seem to be available.

Clenbuterol

Since β-AR antagonists have been used as a treatment for stress incontinence, it seems paradoxical that the selective β$_2$-AR agonist, clenbuterol, was found to cause significant clinical improvement and increase in MUCP in 165 women with stress incontinence [175]. The study was double-blind and placebo-controlled. The number of patients reporting any degree of improvement was 56 (out of 77) in the clenbuterol group and 48 (out of 88) in the placebo group, and the changes in MUCP was 3.3 cmH$_2$O in the clenbuterol and –1.5 cmH$_2$O in the placebo group. The positive effects were suggested to be the result of an action on urethral striated muscle and/or the pelvic floor muscles.

Ishiko et al. [176] investigated the effects of clenbuterol on 61 female patients with stress incontinence in a 12-week randomized study, comparing drug therapy to pelvic floor exercises and a combination of drug therapy and pelvic floor exercises. The frequency and volume of stress incontinence and the patient's own impression were used as the basis for the assessment of efficacy. The improvement of incontinence was 76.9%, 52.6%, and 89.5% in the respective groups. Further well-designed RTCs documenting the effects of clenbuterol are needed to adequately assess its potential as a treatment for stress incontinence as it is possible that this agent may have a novel, as yet undefined mechanism of action.

Duloxetine

Duloxetine, a combined norepinephrine and 5-HT reuptake inhibitor, has been shown, in animal experiments, to increase the neural activity to the external urethral sphincter, and increase bladder capacity through effects on the central nervous system [177]. In a double-blind, placebo-controlled study in women with stress (n = 140) or mixed (n = 146) incontinence, duloxetine (20–40 mg four times a day) was shown to cause significant improvements in several efficacy measures (ICS 1 h stress pad test, 24 h pad weight, number of incontinence episodes, quality of life assessment [178]). The drug was well tolerated and there were few discontinuations due to side effects (8% for duloxetine, 3% for placebo).

The drug is still undergoing clinical trials.

Drugs Used for Treatment of Overflow Incontinence

According to the definition of the ICS (1997), overflow incontinence is "leakage of urine at greater than normal bladder capacity. It is associated with incomplete bladder emptying due to either impaired detrusor contractility or bladder outlet obstruction". Two types of overflow incontinence are recognized, one as a result of mechanical obstruction, and the other secondary to functional disorders. Occasionally both types can coexist.

The clinical presentation of overflow incontinence may vary depending on the age of the patient and the cause of the incontinence. In children, overflow incontinence can be secondary to congenital obstructive disorders (e.g. urethral valves) or to neurogenic vesical dysfunction (myelomeningocele, Hinman syndrome). In adults, overflow incontinence may be associated with outflow obstruction secondary to benign prostatic hyperplasia (BPH) or can be a consequence of diabetes mellitus. Mixed

Table 23.5 Drugs used in the treatment of overflow incontinence. Assessments according to the Oxford system (modified)

	Level of evidence	Grade of recommendation
Alpha-adrenoceptor antagonists		
Alfuzosin	4	C
Doxazosin	4	C
Prazosin	4	C
Terazosin	4	C
Tamsulosin	4	C
[a](Phenoxybenzamine)	4	NR
Muscarinic receptor agonists		
Bethanechol	4	D
Carbachol	4	D
Anticholinesterase inhibitors		
Distigmine	4	D
Other drugs		
Baclofen	4	C
Benzodiazepines	4	C
Dantrolene	4	C

NR, not recommended.
[a] Should be used with caution.

forms may be seen in disorders associated with motor spasticity (e.g. Parkinson's disease).

Pharmacologic treatment (Table 23.5) should be based on previous urodynamic evaluation. The aim of treatment is to prevent damage to the upper urinary tract by normalizing voiding and urethral pressures. Drugs used for increasing intravesical pressure, i.e. "parasympathomimetics" (acetylcholine analogues such as bethanechol, or acetylcholine esterase inhibitors), or β-AR antagonists, have not been documented to have beneficial effects (see Finkbeiner [179], Wein [4]). Stimulation of detrusor activity by intravesical instillation of prostaglandins has been reported to be successful; however, the effect is controversial and no RCTs are available [4].

The "autonomous" contractions in patients with parasympathetic decentralization are probably mediated by α-AR mediated bladder activity, since they can be inhibited by α-AR antagonists [180]. The α-AR antagonist that has been most widely used is probably phenoxybenzamine [181–183]. However, uncertainties about the carcinogenic effects of this drug, and its side effects, have focused interest on selective α_1-AR antagonists such as prazosin [184].

Other means of decreasing outflow resistance in these patients, particularly if associated with spasticity, are baclofen, benzodiazepines (e.g. diazepam) and dantrolene sodium (see Wein [4]).

Hormonal Treatment of Urinary Incontinence

Estrogens and the Continence Mechanism
The estrogen-sensitive tissues of the bladder, urethra and pelvic floor all play an important role in the continence mechanism. For a woman to remain continent the urethral pressure must exceed the intravesical pressure at all times except during micturition. The urethra has four estrogen-sensitive functional layers which all play a part in the maintenance of a positive urethral pressure: (1) epithelium, (2) vasculature, (3) connective tissue, (4) muscle.

Estrogens in the Treatment of Urinary Incontinence
There are a number of reasons why estrogens may be useful in the treatment of women with urinary incontinence. As well as improving the "maturation index" of urethral squamous epithelium [185], estrogens increase urethral closure pressure and improve abdominal pressure transmission to the proximal urethra [186–188]. The sensory threshold of the bladder may also be raised [189].

Lose and Englev [190] evaluated the effect of estrogens in 251 postmenopausal women, with a mean age of 66 years, reporting at least one bothersome lower urinary tract symptom in an open, randomized, parallel group, controlled trial. One hundred and thirty-four women were treated with the estradiol-releasing ring for 24 weeks; 117 women were treated with estriol pessaries 0.5 mg every second day for 24 weeks. Subjective scores of urgency, frequency, nocturia, dysuria, stress incontinence and urge incontinence were evaluated. The two treatments were equally efficacious in alleviating urinary urgency (51% versus 56%), urge incontinence (58% versus 58%), stress incontinence (53% versus 59%) and nocturia (51% versus 54%). The authors concluded that low dose vaginally administered estradiol and estriol are equally efficacious in alleviating lower urinary tract symptoms which appear after the menopause. The lack of a placebo group makes the improvement rates difficult to evaluate.

Estrogens for Stress Incontinence
The role of estrogen in the treatment of stress incontinence has been controversial, even though there are a number of reported studies (see Hextall [191]). Some have given promising results but this may be because they were observational, not randomized, blinded or controlled. The situation is

further complicated by the fact that a number of different types of estrogen have been used with varying doses, routes of administration and durations of treatment. Fantl et al. [192] treated 83 hypoestrogenic women with urodynamic evidence of genuine stress incontinence and/or detrusor instability with conjugated equine estrogens 0.625 mg and medroxyprogesterone 10 mg cyclically for 3 months. Controls received placebo tablets. At the end of the study period the clinical and quality if life variables had not changed significantly in either group. Jackson et al. [193] treated 57 postmenopausal women with genuine stress incontinence or mixed incontinence with estradiol valerate 2 mg or placebo daily for 6 months. There was no significant change in objective outcome measures although both the active and placebo group reported subjective benefit.

There have been two meta-analyses performed which have helped to clarify the situation further. In the first, a report by the Hormones and Urogenital Therapy (HUT) committee, the use of estrogens to treat all causes of incontinence in postmenopausal women was examined [194]. Of 166 articles identified which were published in English between 1969 and 1992, only 6 were controlled trials and 17 uncontrolled series. The results showed that there was a significant subjective improvement for all patients and those with genuine stress incontinence. However, assessment of the objective parameters revealed that there was no change in the volume of urine lost. Maximum urethral closure pressure did increase significantly, but this result was influenced by only one study showing a large effect. In the second meta-analysis, Sultana and Walters [195] reviewed 8 controlled and 14 uncontrolled prospective trials and included all types of estrogen treatment. They also found that estrogen therapy was not an efficacious treatment of stress incontinence, but may be useful for the often associated symptoms of urgency and frequency.

Estrogen when given alone, therefore, does not appear to be an effective treatment for stress incontinence. However, several studies have shown that it may have a role in *combination* with other therapies (for combination with a-AR agonists, see above). In a randomized trial, Ishiko et al. [196] compared the effects of the combination of pelvic floor exercise and estriol (1 mg/day) in 66 patients with postmenopausal stress incontinence. Efficacy was evaluated every 3 months based on stress scores obtained from a questionnaire. They found a significant decrease in stress score in mild and moderate stress incontinence patients in both groups 3 months after the start of therapy and concluded that combination therapy with estriol plus pelvic floor exercise was

effective and capable of serving as first-line treatment for mild stress incontinence.

Estrogens for Urge Incontinence

Estrogen has been used to treat postmenopausal urgency and urge incontinence for many years, but there are few controlled trials confirming that it is of benefit [191].

A double-blind multicenter study of 64 postmenopausal women with the "urge syndrome" has failed to confirm its efficacy [197]. All women underwent pre-treatment urodynamic investigation to establish that they had either sensory urgency or detrusor instability. They were then randomized to treatment with oral estriol 3 mg daily or placebo for 3 months. Compliance was confirmed by a significant improvement in the maturation index of vaginal epithelial cells in the active but not the placebo group. Estriol produced subjective and objective improvements in urinary symptoms, but it was not significantly better than placebo. Grady et al. [198] determined whether postmenopausal hormone therapy improves the severity of urinary incontinence. in a randomized, blinded trial among 2763 postmenopausal women younger than 80 years with coronary disease and intact uteri. The report included 1525 participants who reported at least one episode of incontinence per week at baseline. Participants were randomly assigned to 0.625 mg of conjugated estrogens plus 2.5 mg of medroxyprogesterone acetate in one tablet daily (n = 768) or placebo (n = 757) and were followed for a mean of 4.1 years. Severity of incontinence was classified as improved (decrease of at least two episodes per week), unchanged (change of at most one episode per week), or worsened (increase of at least two episodes per week). The results showed that incontinence improved in 26% of the women assigned to placebo compared with 21% assigned to hormones, while 27% of the placebo group worsened compared with 39% of the hormone group (p = 0.001). This difference was evident by 4 months of treatment and was observed for both urge and stress incontinence. The number of incontinent episodes per week increased an average of 0.7 in the hormone group and decreased by 0.1 in the placebo group (p < 0.001). The authors concluded that daily oral estrogen plus progestin therapy was associated with worsening urinary incontinence in older postmenopausal women with weekly incontinence, and did not recommend this therapy for the treatment of incontinence. It cannot be excluded that the progestagen component had a negative influence on the outcome of this study.

Estrogen has an important physiological effect on the female lower urinary tract and its deficiency is an etiological factor in the pathogenesis of a number of conditions. However, the use of estrogens alone to treat urinary incontinence has given disappointing results.

References

1. Andersson K-E. The pharmacology of lower urinary tract smooth muscles and penile erectile tissues. Pharmacol Rev 1993;45:253–308.
2. de Groat WC, Downie JW, Levin RM, Long Lin AT, Morrison JFB, Nishizawa O, Steers WD, Thor KB. Basic Neurophysiology and Neuropharmacology. In: Abrams P, Khoury S, Wein A, editors. Incontinence, 1st International Consultation on Incontinence, Plymouth, UK: Plymbridge Distributors, 1999; 105–54.
3. de Groat WC, Yoshimura N. Pharmacology of the lower urinary tract. Annu Rev Pharmacol Toxicol 2001;41:691–721.
4. Wein AJ. Neuromuscular dysfunction of the lower urinary tract and its treatment. In: Campbell's Urology, 8th edn. Philadelphia: WB Saunders, 2001.
5. Hampel C, Wienhold D, Benken N, Eggersmann C, Thüroff JW. Definition of overactive bladder and epidemiology of urinary incontinence. Urology 1996;50 (Supplement 6A):4–14.
6. HuT, Wagner TH. Economic considerations in overactive bladder. Am J Manag Care 2000;6:S591–8.
7. Milsom I, Abrams P, Cardozo L, Roberts RG, Thuroff J, Wein AJ. How widespread are the symptoms of an overactive bladder and how are they managed? A population-based prevalence study. BJU Int 2001;87:760–6.
8. Kelleher CJ, Cardozo LD, Khullar V, Salvatore S. A medium-term analysis of the subjective efficacy of treatment for women with detrusor instability and low bladder compliance. Br J Obstet Gynaecol 1997;104:988–93.
9. Andersson K-E, Appell R, Awad S, Chapple C, Drutz H, Fourcroy J, Finkbeiner A, Haab F, Wein A. Pharmacological treatment of urinary incontinence. In: Abrams P, Khoury S, Wein A, editors. Incontinence, 2nd International Consultation on Incontinence. Plymouth, UK: Plymbridge Distributors, 2002; 481–511.
10. Bayliss M, Wu C, Newgreen D, Mundy AR, Fry CH. A quantitative study of atropine-resistant contractile responses in human detrusor smooth muscle, from stable, unstable and obstructed bladders. J Urol 1999;162:1833–9.
11. Sjögren C, Andersson K-E, Husted S, Mattiasson A, Møller-Madsen, B. Atropine resistance of the transmurally stimulated isolated human bladder. J Urol 1982;128:1368–71.
12. Smith DJ, Chapple CR. In vitro response of human bladder smooth muscle in unstable obstructed male bladders: a study of pathophysiological causes? Neurourol Urodyn 1994;134:14–15.
13. Palea S, Artibani W, Ostardo E, Trist DG, Pietra C. Evidence for purinergic neurotransmission in human urinary bladder affected by interstitial cystitis. J Urol 1993;150:2007–12.
14. Wammack R, Weihe E, Dienes H-P, Hohenfellner R. Die Neurogene Blase in vitro. Akt Urol 1995;26:16–18.
15. Yoshida M, Homma Y, Inadome A, Yono M, Seshita H, Miyamoto Y, Murakami S, Kawabe K, Ueda S. Age-related changes in cholinergic and purinergic neurotransmission in human isolated bladder smooth muscles. Exp Gerontol 2001;36:99–109.
16. Eglen RM, Hegde SS, Watson N. Muscarinic receptor subtypes and smooth muscle function. Pharmacol Rev 1996;48:531–65.
17. Caulfield MP, Birdsall NJM. International Union of Pharmacology: XVII. Classification of muscarinic acetylcholine receptors. Pharmacol Rev 1998;50:279–90.
18. Bonev AD, Nelson MT. Muscarinic inhibition of ATP-sensitive K^+ channels by protein kinase C in urinary bladder smooth muscle. Am J Physiol 1993;265:C1723–8.
19. Hegde SS, Eglen RM. Muscarinic receptor subtypes modulating smooth muscle contractility in the urinary bladder. Life Sci 1999;64:419–28.
20. Harriss DR, Marsh KA, Birmingham AT, Hill SJ. Expression of muscarinic M3-receptors coupled to inositol phospholipid hydrolysis in human detrusor cultured smooth muscle cells. J Urol 1995;154:1241–5.
21. Hegde SS, Choppin A, Bonhaus D, Briaud S, Loeb M, Moy TM, Loury D, Eglen RM. Functional role of M_2 and M_3 muscarinic receptors in the urinary bladder of rats in vitro and in vivo. Br J Pharmacol 1997;120:1409–18.
22. Braverman A, Legos J, Young W, Luthin G, Ruggieri M. M2 receptors in genito-urinary smooth muscle pathology. Life Sci 1999;64:429–36.
23. Braverman, AS, Ruggieri MR, Pontari MA. The M2 muscarinic receptor subtype mediates cholinergic bladder contractions in patients with neurogenic bladder dysfunction. J Urol 2001;165 Suppl:36 (abstract 147).
24. D'Agostino G, Bolognesi ML, Lucchelli A, Vicini D, Balestra B, Spelta V, Melchiorre C, Tonini M. Prejunctional muscarinic inhibitory control of acetylcholine release in the human isolated detrusor: involvement of the M4 receptor subtype. Br J Pharmacol 2000;129:493–500.
25. Somogyi GT, de Groat WC. Function, signal transduction mechanisms and plasticity of presynaptic muscarinic receptors in the urinary bladder. Life Sci 1999;64:411–18.
26. Brading AF. A myogenic basis for the overactive bladder. Urology 1997;50(Suppl 6A):57–67.
27. de Groat WC. A neurological basis for the overactive bladder. Urology 1997;50(Suppl 6A):36–52.
28. Jensen D Jr. Pharmacological studies of the uninhibited neurogenic bladder. II. The influence of cholinergic excitatory and inhibitory drugs on the cystometrogram of neurological patients with normal and uninhibited neurogenic bladder. Acta Neurol Scand 1981;64:175–95.
29. Pietzko A, Dimpfel W, Schwantes U, Topfmeier P. Influence of trospium chloride and oxybutynin on quantitative EEG in healthy volunteers. Eur J Clin Pharmacol 1994;47:337–43.
30. Andersson K-E, Appell R, Cardozo L, Chapple C, Drutz H, Finkbeiner A, Haab F, Vela Navarrete R. Pharmacological treatment of urinary incontinence. In: Abrams P, Khoury S, Wein A, editors. Incontinence, 1st International Consultation on Incontinence. Plymouth, UK: Plymbridge Distributors, 1999; 447–86.
31. Andersson KE, Appell R, Cardozo LD, Chapple C, Drutz HP, Finkbeiner AE, Haab F, Vela Navarrete R. The pharmacological treatment of urinary incontinence. BJU Int 1999;84:923–47.
32. Ekström B, Andersson K-E, Mattiasson A. Urodynamic effects of intravesical instillation of atropine and phentolamine in patients with detrusor hyperactivity. J Urol 1992;149:155–8.
33. Glickman S, Tsokkos N, Shah PJ. Intravesical atropine and suppression of detrusor hypercontractility in the neuropathic bladder. A preliminary study. Paraplegia 1995;33:36–9.
34. Deaney C, Glickman S, Gluck T, Malone-Lee JG. Intravesical atropine suppression of detrusor hyperreflexia in multiple sclerosis. J Neurol Neurosurg Psychiatry 1998;65:957–8.

35. Enskat R, Deaney CN, Glickman S. Systemic effects of intravesical atropine sulphate. BJU Int 2001;87:613–16.

36. Muskat Y, Bukovsky I, Schneider D, Langer R. The use of scopolamine in the treatment of detrusor instability. J Urol 1996;156:1989–90.

37. Andersson K-E. Current concepts in the treatment of disorders of micturition. Drugs 1988;35:477–94.

38. Thuroff JW, Chartier-Kastler E, Corcus J, Humke J, Jonas U, Palmtag H, Tanagho EA. Medical treatment and medical side effects in urinary incontinence in the elderly. World J Urol 1998;16(Suppl 1):S48–61.

39. Schladitz-Keil G, Spahn H, Mutschler E. Determination of bioavailability of the quaternary ammonium compound trospium chloride in man from urinary excretion data. Arzneimittel Forsch/Drug Res 1986;36:984–7.

40. Fusgen I, Hauri D. Trospium chloride: an effective option for medical treatment of bladder overactivity. Int J Clin Pharmacol Ther 2000;38:223–34.

41. Todorova A, Vonderheid-Guth B, Dimpfel W. Effects of tolterodine, trospium chloride, and oxybutynin on the central nervous system. J Clin Pharmacol 2001;41:636–44.

42. Wiedemann A, Füsgen I, Hauri D. New aspects of therapy with trospium chloride for urge incontinence. Eur J Geriatr 2001;3:41–5.

43. Stöhrer M, Bauer P, Giannetti BM, Richter R, Burgdorfer H, Murtz G. Effect of trospium chloride on urodynamic parameters in patients with detrusor hyperreflexia due to spinal cord injuries: a multicentre placebo controlled double-blind trial. Urol Int 1991;47:138–43.

44. Madersbacher H, Stöhrer M, Richter R, Burgdorfer H, Hachen HJ, Murtz G. Trospium chloride versus oxybutynin: a randomized, double-blind, multicentre trial in the treatment of detrusor hyper-reflexia. Br J Urol 1995;75:452–6.

45. Allousi S, Laval K-U, Eckert R. Trospium chloride (Spasmolyt) in patients with motor urge syndrome (detrusor instability): a double-blind, randomised, nulticentre, placebo-controlled study. J Clin Res 1998;1:439–51.

46. Cardozo L, Chapple CR, Toozs-Hobson P, Grosse-Freese M, Bulitta M, Lehmacher W, Strosser W, Ballering-Bruhl B, Schafer M. Efficacy of trospium chloride in patients with detrusor instability: a placebo-controlled, randomized, double-blind, multicentre clinical trial. BJU Int 2000;85:659–664.

47. Höfner K, Halaska M, Primus G, Al Shukri S, Jonas U. Tolerability and efficacy of Trospium chloride in a long-term treatment (52 weeks) in patients with urge-syndrome: a double-blind, controlled, multicentre clinical trial. Neurourol Urodyn 2000;19:487–8.

48. Jünemann KP, Al-Shukri S. Efficacy and tolerability of trospium chloride and tolterodine in 234 patients with urge-syndrome: a double-blind, placebo-controlled multicentre clinical trial. Neurourol Urodyn 2000;19:488–9.

49. Nilvebrant L, Andersson K-E, Gillberg P-G, Stahl M, Sparf B. Tolterodine – a new bladder selective antimuscarinic agent. Eur J Pharmacol 1997;327:195–207.

50. Nilvebrant L, Hallén B, Larsson G. Tolterodine – A new bladder selective muscarinic receptor antagonist: preclinical pharmacological and clinical data. Life Sci 1997;60:1129–36.

51. Hills CJ, Winter SA, Balfour JA. Tolterodine. Drugs 1998;55:813–20.

52. Clemett D, Jarvis B. Tolterodine a review of its use in the treatment of overactive bladder. Drugs Aging 2001;18:277–304.

53. Nilvebrant L, Gillberg PG, Sparf B. Antimuscarinic potency and bladder selectivity of PNU-200577, a major metabolite of tolterodine. Pharmacol Toxicol 1997;81:169–72.

54. Stahl MMS, Ekström B, Sparf B, Mattiasson A, Andersson K-E. Urodynamic and other effects of tolterodine: a novel antimuscarinic drug for the treatment of detrusor overactivity. Neurourol Urodyn 1995;14:647–55.

55. Brynne N, Stahl MMS, Hallén B, Edlund PO, Palmér L, Höglund P, Gabrielsson J. Pharmacokinetics and pharmacodynamics of tolterodine in man: a new drug for the treatment of urinary bladder overactivity. Int J Clin Pharmacol Ther 1997;35:287–95.

56. Brynne N, Dalen P, Alvan G, Bertilsson L, Gabrielsson J. Influence of CYP2D6 polymorphism on the pharmacokinetics and pharmacodynamics of tolterodine. Clin Pharmacol Ther 1998;63:529–39.

57. Chapple CR. Muscarinic receptor antagonists in the treatment of overactive bladder. Urology 2000;(Suppl 5A):33–46.

58. Van Kerrebroeck P, Kreder K, Jonas U, Zinner N, Wein A. Tolterodine once-daily: superior efficacy and tolerability in the treatment of the overactive bladder. Urology 2001;57:414–21.

59. Abrams P, Freeman RN, Anderström C, Mattiasson A. Tolterodine, a new antimuscarinic agent: as effective but better tolerated than oxybutynin in patients with overactive bladder. Br J Urol 1998;81:801–10.

60. Drutz HP, Appell RA, Gleason D, Klimberg I, Radomski S. Clinical efficacy and safety of tolterodine compared to oxybutynin and placebo in patients with overactive bladder. Int Urogynecol J Pelvic Floor Dysfunct 1999;10:283–9.

61. Malone-Lee J, Shaffu B, Anand C, Powell C. Tolterodine: superior tolerability than and comparable efficacy to oxybutynin in individuals 50 years old or older with overactive bladder: a randomized controlled trial. J Urol 2001;165:1452–6.

62. Appell RA, Sand P, Dmochowski R, Anderson R, Zinner N, Lama D, Roach M, Miklos J, Saltzstein D, Boone T, Staskin DR, Albrecht D. Prospective randomized controlled trial of extended-release oxybutynin chloride and tolterodine tartrate in the treatment of overactive bladder: results of the OBJECT Study. Mayo Clin Proc 2001;76:358–63.

63. Wein AJ. Pharmacological agents for the treatment of urinary incontinence due to overactive bladder. Exp Opin Invest Drugs 2001;10:65–83.

64. Alabaster VA. Discovery and development of selective M_3 antagonists for clinical use. Life Sci 1997;60:1053–60.

65. Rosario DJ, Leaker BR, Smith DJ, Chapple CR. A pilot study of the effects of multiple doses of the M3 muscarinic receptor antagonist darifenacin on ambulatory parameters of detrusor activity in patients with detrusor instability. Neurourol Urodyn 1995;14:464–5.

66. Mundy AR, Abrams P, Chapple CR, Neal DE. Darifenacin, the first selective M_3 antagonist for overactive bladder: comparison with oxybutynin on ambulatory urodynamic monitoring and salivary flow. Proceedings of the International Continence Society, Seoul, Korea abstract 221, 2001.

67. Nichols D, Colli E, Goka J, Wesnes K. Darifenacin demonstrates no effect on cognitive and cardiac function: results from a double-blind, randomised, placebo controlled study. Proceedings of the International Continence Society, Seoul, Korea, abstract 354, 2001.

68. Andersson K-E. Clinical pharmacology of potassium channel openers. Pharmacol Toxicol 1992;70:244–54.

69. Kachur JF, Peterson JS, Carter JP, Rzeszotarski WJ, Hanson RC, Noronha-Blob L. R and S enantiomers of oxybutynin: pharmacological effects in guinea pig bladder and intestine. J Pharmacol Exp Ther 1988;247:867–72.

70. Norhona-Blob L, Kachur JF. Enantiomers of oxybutynin: in vitro pharmacological characterization at M1, M2 and M3 muscarinic receptors and in vivo effects on urinary bladder

contraction, mydriasis and salivary secretion in guinea pigs. J Pharmacol Exp Ther 1991;256:562–7.

71. Douchamps J, Derenne F, Stockis A, Gangji D, Juvent M, Herchuelz A. The pharmacokinetics of oxybutynin in man. Eur J Clin Pharmacol 1988;35:515–20.

72. Hughes KM, Lang JCT, Lazare R, Gordon D, Stanton SL, Malone-Lee J, Geraint M. Measurement of oxybutynin and its N-desethyl metabolite in plasma, and its application to pharmacokinetic studies in young, elderly and frail elderly volunteers. Xenobiotica 1992;22:859–69.

73. Waldeck K, Larsson B, Andersson K-E. Comparison of oxybutynin and its active metabolite, N-desethyl-oxybutynin, in the human detrusor and parotid gland. J Urol 1997;157:1093–7.

74. Yarker YE, Goa KL, Fitton A. Oxybutynin. A review of its pharmacodynamic and pharmacokinetic properties, and its therapeutic use in detrusor instability. Drugs Aging 1995;6:243–62.

75. Amarenco G, Marquis P, McCarthy C, Richard F. Qualité de vie des femmes souffrant d'impériosité mictionelle avec ou sans fuites: étude prospective après traitement par oxybutinine (1701 cas). Presse Med 1998;27:5–10.

76. Baigrie RJ, Kelleher JP, Fawcett DP, Pengelly AW. Oxybutynin: is it safe? Br J Urol 1988;62:319–22.

77. Jonville AP, Dutertre JP, Autret E, Barbellion M. Effets indésirables du chlorure d'oxybutynine (Ditropan®). Therapie 1992;47:389–92.

78. Katz IR, Sands LP, Bilker W, DiFilippo S, Boyce A, D'Angelo K. Identification of medications that cause cognitive impairment in older people: the case of oxybutynin chloride. J Am Geriatr Soc 1998;46:8–13.

79. Ferrara P, D'Aleo CM, Tarquini E, Salvatore S, Salvaggio E. Side-effects of oral or intravesical oxybutynin chloride in children with spina bifida. BJU Int 2001;87:674–8.

80. Ouslander JG, Shih YT, Malone-Lee J, Luber K. Overactive bladder: special considerations in the geriatric population. Am J Manag Care 2000;6(11 Suppl):S599–606.

81. Malone-Lee J, Lubel D, Szonyi G. Low dose oxybutynin for the unstable bladder. Br Med J 1992;304:1053.

82. Hussain RM, Hartigan-Go K, Thomas SHL, Ford GA. Effect of oxybutynin on the QTc interval in elderly patients with urinary incontinence. Br J Clin Pharmacol 1994;37:485P–6P.

83. Gupta SK, Sathyan G. Pharmacokinetics of an oral once-a-day controlled-release oxybutynin formulation compared with immediate-release oxybutynin. J Clin Pharmacol 1999;39:289–96.

84. Anderson RU, Mobley D, Blank B, Saltzstein D, Susset J, Brown JS. Once daily controlled versus immediate release oxybutynin chloride for urge urinary incontinence. OROS Oxybutynin Study Group. J Urol 1999;161:1809–12.

85. Versi E, Appell R, Mobley D, Patton W, Saltzstein D. Dry mouth with conventional and controlled-release oxybutynin in urinary incontinence. The Ditropan XL Study Group. Obstet Gynecol 2000;95:718–21.

86. Lose G, Norgaard JP. Intravesical oxybutynin for treating incontinence resulting from an overactive detrusor. BJU Int 2001;87:767–73.

87. Haruno A. Inhibitory effects of propiverine hydrochloride on the agonist-induced or spontaneous contractions of various isolated muscle preparations. Arzneim-Forsch /Drug Res 1992;42:815–17.

88. Tokuno H, Chowdhury JU, Tomita T. Inhibitory effects of propiverine on rat and guinea-pig urinary bladder muscle. Naunyn-Schmiedeberg's Arch Pharmacol 1993;348:659–662.

89. Madersbacher H, Mürz G. Efficacy, tolerability and safety profile of propiverine in the treatment of the overactive

bladder (non-neurogenic and neurogenic). World J Urol 2001;19:324–35.

90. Wehnert J, Sage S. Comparative investigations to the action of Mictonorm (propiverin hydrochloride) and Spasuret (flavoxat hydrochloride) on detrusor vesicae. Z Urol Nephrol 1989;82:259–63.

91. Wehnert J, Sage S. Therapie der Blaseninstabilität und Urge-Inkontinenz mit Propiverin hydrochlorid (Mictonorm®) und Oxybutynin chlorid (Dridase®) – eine randomisierte Cross-over-Vergleichsstudie. Akt Urol 1992;23:7–11.

92. Stohrer M, Madersbacher H, Richter R, Wehnert J, Dreikorn K. Efficacy and safety of propiverine in SCI-patients suffering from detrusor hyperreflexia – a double-blind, placebo-controlled clinical trial. Spinal Cord 1999;37:196–200.

93. Madersbacher H, Halaska M, Voigt R, Alloussi S, Hofner K. A placebo-controlled, multicentre study comparing the tolerability and efficacy of propiverine and oxybutynin in patients with urgency and urge incontinence. BJU Int 1999;84:646–51.

94. Dorschner W, Stolzenburg JU, Griebenow R, Halaska M, Schubert G, Murtz G, Frank M, Wieners F. Efficacy and cardiac safety of propiverine in elderly patients – a double-blind, placebo-controlled clinical study. Eur Urol 2000;37:702–8.

95. Guarneri L, Robinson E, Testa R. A review of flavoxate: pharmacology and mechanism of action. Drugs Today 1994;30:91–8.

96. Oka M, Kimura Y, Itoh Y, Sasaki Y, Taniguchi N, Ukai Y, Yoshikuni Y, Kimura K. Brain pertussis toxin-sensitive G proteins are involved in the flavoxate hydrochloride-induced suppression of the micturition reflex in rats. Brain Res 1996;727:91–8.

97. Ruffmann R. A review of flavoxate hydrochloride in the treatment of urge incontinence. J Int Med Res 1988;16:317–30.

98. Stanton SL. A comparison of emepronium bromide and flavoxate hydrochloride in the treatment of urinary incontinence. J Urol 1973;110:529–32.

99. Milani R, Scalambrino S, Milia R, Sambruni I, Riva D, Pulici D, Avaldi F, Vigano R. Double-blind crossover comparison of flavoxate and oxybutynin in women affected by urinary urge syndrome. Int Urogynecol J 1993;4:3–8.

100. Briggs KS, Castleden CM, Asher MJ. The effect of flavoxate on uninhibited detrusor contractions and urinary incontinence in the elderly. J Urol 1980;123:665–6.

101. Chapple CR, Parkhouse H, Gardener C, Milroy EJG. Double-blind, placebo-controlled, cross-over study of flavoxate in the treatment of idiopathic detrusor instability. Br J Urol 1990;66:491–4.

102. Dahm TL, Ostri P, Kristensen JK, Walter S, Frimodt-Møller C, Rasmussen RB, Nohr M, Alexander N. Flavoxate treatment of micturition disorders accompanying benign prostatic hypertrophy: a double-blind placebo-controlled multicenter investigation. Urol Int 1995;55:205–8.

103. Schwinn DA, Michelotti GA. Alpha1-adrenergic receptors in the lower urinary tract and vascular bed: potential role for the alpha1d subtype in filling symptoms and effects of ageing on vascular expression. BJU Int 2000;85(Suppl 2):6–11.

104. Jensen D. Uninhibited neurogenic bladder treated with prazosin. Scand J Urol Nephrol 1981;15:229–33.

105. Petersen T, Husted S, Sidenius P. Prazosin treatment of neurological patients with detrusor hyperreflexia and bladder emptying disability. Scand J Urol Nephrol 1989;23:189–94.

106. A[o]mark P, Nerga[o]rdh A. Influence of adrenergic agonists and antagonists on urethral pressure, bladder pres-

sure and detrusor hyperactivity in children with myelodysplasia. Acta Paediatr Scand 1991;80:824–32.

107. Abrams P and The European Tamsulosin NLUTD Study Group. Tamsulosin efficacy and safety in neurogenic lower urinary tract dysfunction (NLUTD). J Urol 2001;165 Suppl:276 (abstract 1137).

108. Jollys JV, Jollys JC, Wilson J, Donovan J, Nanchamel K, Abrams P. Does sexual equality extend to urinary symptoms? Neurourol Urodyn 1993;12:391–2.

109. Lepor H, Machi G. Comparison of the AUA symptom index in unselected males and females between 55 and 79 years of age. Urology 1993;42:36–40.

110. Serels S, Stein M. Prospective study comparing hyoscyamine, doxazosin, and combination therapy for the treatment of urgency and frequency in women. Neurourol Urodyn 1998;17:31–6.

111. Dwyer PL, Teele JS. Prazosin: a neglected cause of genuine stress incontinence. Obstet Gynecol 1992;79:117–21.

112. Marshall HJ, Beevers DG. Alpha-adrenoceptor blocking drugs and female urinary incontinence: prevalence and reversibility. Br J Clin Pharmacol 1996;42:507–9.

113. Levin RM, Ruggieri MR, Wein AJ. Identification of receptor subtypes in the rabbit and human urinary bladder by selective radio-ligand binding. J Urol 1988;139:844.

114. Grüneberger A. Treatment of motor urge incontinence with clenbuterol and flavoxate hydrochloride. Br J Obstet Gynaecol 1984;91:275–8.

115. Castleden CM, Morgan B. The effect of ß-adrenoceptor agonists on urinary incontinence in the elderly. Br J Clin Pharmacol 1980;10:619–20.

116. Naglo AS, Nerga[o]rdh A, Boréus LO. Influence of atropine and isoprenaline on detrusor hyperactivity in children with neurogenic bladder. Scand J Urol Nephrol 1981;15:97-102

117. Lipworth BJ. Clinical pharmacology of ß$_3$-adrenoceptors. Br J Clin Pharmacol 1996;43:291–300.

118. Igawa Y, Yamazaki Y, Takeda H, Hayakawa K, Akahane M, Ajisawa Y, Yoneyama T, Nishizawa O, Andersson KE. Functional and molecular biological evidence for a possible beta3-adrenoceptor in the human detrusor muscle. Br J Pharmacol 1999;126:819–25.

119. Igawa Y, Yamazaki Y, Takeda H, Kaidoh K, Akahane M, Ajisawa Y, Yoneyama T, Nishizawa O, Andersson KE. Relaxant effects of isoproterenol and selective beta3-adrenoceptor agonists on normal, low compliant and hyperreflexic human bladders. J Urol 2001;165:240–4.

120. Takeda M, Obara K, Mizusawa T, Tomita Y, Arai K, Tsutsui T, Hatano A, Takahashi K, Nomura S. Evidence for beta3-adrenoceptor subtypes in relaxation of the human urinary bladder detrusor: analysis by molecular biological and pharmacological methods. J Pharmacol Exp Ther 1999;288:1367–73.

121. Martin MR, Schiff AA. Fluphenazine/nortriptyline in the irritative bladder syndrome: a double-blind placebo-controlled study. Br J Urol 1984;56:178–9.

122. Lose G, Jorgensen L, Thunedborg P. Doxepin in the treatment of female detrusor overactivity: A randomized double-blind crossover study. J Urol 1989;142:1024–6.

123. Baldessarini KJ. Drugs in the treatment of psychiatric disorders. In: Gilman AF, Goodman LS, Rall TW, Murad F, editors. The Pharmacological Basis of Therapeutics, 7th edn. McMillan Publishing, 1985; 387–445.

124. Maggi CA, Borsini F, Lecci A, Giuliani S, Meli P, Gragnani L, Meli A. The effect of acute and chronic administration of imipramine on spinal and supraspinal micturition reflexes in rats. J Pharmacol Exp Ther 1989;248:278–85.

125. Hunsballe JM, Djurhuus JC. Clinical options for imipramine in the management of urinary incontinence. Urol Res 2001;29:118–25.

126. Miller K, Atkin B, Moody ML. Drug therapy for nocturnal enuresis. Drugs 1992;44:47–56.

127. Bigger JT, Giardina EG, Perel JM, Kantor SJ, Glassman AH. Cardiac antiarrhythmic effect of imipramine hydrochloride. N Engl J Med 1977;296:206–8.

128. Giardina EG, Bigger JT Jr, Glassman AH, Perel JM, Kantor SJ. The electrocardiographic and antiarrhythmic effects of imipramine hydrochloride at therapeutic plasma concentrations. Circulation 1979;60:1045–52.

129. Jeremy JY, Tsang V, Mikhailidis DP et al. Eicosanoid synthesis by human urinary bladder mucosa: pathological implications. Br J Urol 1987;59:36.

130. Cardozo LD, Stanton SL, Robinson H, Hole D. Evaluation on flurbiprofen in detrusor instability. Br Med J 1980;280:281–2.

131. Palmer J. Report of a double-blind crossover study of flurbiprofen and placebo in detrusor instability. J Int Med Res 11 Supplement 2:11-17

132. Cardozo LD, Stanton SL (1980) A comparison between bromocriptine and indomethacin in the treatment of detrusor instability. J Urol 1983;123:399–401.

133. Neveus T, Lackgren G, Tuvemo T, Hetta J, Hjalmas K, Stenberg A. Enuresis – background and treatment. Scand J Urol Nephrol Suppl 2000;206:1–44.

134. Rittig S, Knudsen UB, Norgaard JP, Pedersen EB, Djurhuus JC. Abnormal diurnal rhythm of plasma vasopressin and urinary output in patients with enuresis. Am J Physiol 1989;256:F664–71.

135. Matthiesen TB, Rittig S, Norgaard JP, Pedersen EB, Djurhuus JC. Nocturnal polyuria and natriuresis in male patients with nocturia and lower urinary tract symptoms. J Urol 1996;156:1292–9.

136. Norgaard JP, Djurhuus JC, Watanabe H, Stenberg A, Lettgen B. Experience and current status of research into the pathophysiology of nocturnal enuresis. Br J Urol 1997;79:825–35.

137. Hjalmas K. Desmopressin treatment: current status. Scand J Urol Nephrol Suppl 1999;202:70–2.

138. Moffat ME, Harlos S, Kirshen AJ, Burd L. Desmopressin acetate and nocturnal enuresis: how much do we know? Pediatrics 1993;92:420–5.

139. Neveus T, Lackgren G, Tuvemo T, Olsson U, Stenberg A. Desmopressin resistant enuresis: pathogenetic and therapeutic considerations. J Urol 1999;162:2136–40.

140. Janknegt RA, Zweers HMM, Delaere KPJ, Kloet AG, Khoe SGS, Arendsen HJ. Oral desmopressin as a new treatment modality for primary nocturnal enuresis in adolescents and adults: a double-blind, randomized, multicenter study. J Urol 1997;157:513–17.

141. Skoog SJ, Stokes A, Turner KL. Oral desmopressin: a randomized double-blind placebo controlled study of effectiveness in children with primary nocturnal enuresis. J Urol 1997;158:1035–40.

142. Hilton P, Stanton SL. The use of desmopressin (DDAVP) in nocturnal frequency in the female. Br J Urol 1982;54:252–5.

143. Hilton P, Hertogs K, Stanton SL. The use of desmopressin (DDAVP) for nocturia in women with multiple sclerosis. J Neurol Neurosurg Psychiatry 1983;46:854–5.

144. Kinn A-C, Larsson PO. Desmopressin: a new principle for symptomatic treatment of urgency and incontinence in patients with multiple sclerosis. Scand J Urol Nephrol 1990;24:109–12.

145. Eckford SD, Swami KS, Jackson SR, Abrams PH. Desmopressin in the treatment of nocturia and enuresis in patients with multiple sclerosis. Br J Urol 1994;74:733–5.

146. Fredrikson S. Nasal spray desmopressin treatment of bladder dysfunction in patients with multiple sclerosis. Acta Neurol Scand 1996;94:31–4.

147. Horowitz M, Combs AJ, Gerdes D. Desmopressin for nocturnal incontinence in the spina bifida population. J Urol 1997;158:2267–8.

148. Weiss J, Blaivas JG, Abrams P, Mattiasson A, Robertson G, van Kerrebroeck P, Walter S. Oral desmopressin (Miririn, DDAVP) in the treatment of nocturia in men. J Urol 2001;165 Suppl:250 (abstract 1030).

149. Van Kerrebroeck P, Bäckström T, Blaivas JG, Freeman R, Lose G, Robertson G. Oral desmopressin (Miririn, DDAVP) in the treatment of nocturia in women. J Urol 2001;165 Suppl:250 (abstract 1031).

150. Robson WL, Nørgaard JP, Leung AK. Hyponatremia in patients with nocturnal enuresis treated with DDAVP. Eur J Pediatr 1996;155:959–62.

151. Schwab M, Ruder H. Hyponatraemia and cerebral convulsion due to DDAVP administration in patients with enuresis nocturna or urine concentration testing. Eur J Pediatr 1997;156:668.

152. Taylor MC, Bates CP. A double-blind crossover trial of baclofen – a new treatment for the unstable bladder syndrome. Br J Urol 1979;51:504–5.

153. Bushman W, Steers WD, Meythaler JM. Voiding dysfunction in patients with spastic paraplegia: urodynamic evaluation and response to continuous intrathecal baclofen. Neurourol Urodyn 1993;12:163–70.

154. Maggi CA. The dual, sensory and "efferent" function of the capsaicin-sensitive primary sensory neurons in the urinary bladder and urethra. In: Maggi CA, editor, The Autonomic Nervous System, vol. 3, Nervous Control of the Urogenital System, Chapter 11. Harwood Academic Publishers, Chur, Switzerland, 1993; 383–422.

155. Szallasi A. The vanilloid (capsaicin) receptor: receptor types and species differences. Gen Pharmacol 1994;25:223–43.

156. Kuo H-Cm. Inhibitory effect of capsaicin on detrusor contractility: Further study in the presence of ganglionic blocker and neurokinin receptor antagonist in the rat urinary bladder. Urol Int 1997;59:95–101.

157. Fowler CJ, Jewkes D, McDonald WI, Lynn B, de Groat WC (1992) Intravesical capsaicin for neurogenic bladder dysfunction. Lancet 339:1239.

158. De Ridder D, Baert L. Vanilloids and the overactive bladder. BJU Int 2000;86:172–8.

159. Fowler CJ. Intravesical treatment of overactive bladder. Urology 2000;55(Suppl 5A):60–4.

160. Petersen T, Nielsen JB, Schroder HD. Intravesical capsaicin in patients with detrusor hyper-reflexia – a placebo-controlled cross-over study. Scand J Urol Nephrol 1999;33:104–10.

161. Chandiramani VA, Peterson T, Duthie GS, Fowler CJ. Urodynamic changes during therapeutic intravesical instillations of capsaicin. Br J Urol 1996;77:792–7.

162. Ishizuka O, Mattiasson A, Andersson K-E. Urodynamic effects of intravesical resiniferatoxin and capsaicin in conscious rats with and without outflow obstruction. J Urol 1995;154:611–16.

163. Lazzeri M, Beneforti P, Turini D. Urodynamic effects of intravesical resiniferatoxin in humans: preliminary results in stable and unstable detrusor. J Urol 1997;158:2093–6.

164. Cruz F, Guimaraes M, Silva C, Reis M. Suppression of bladder hyperreflexia by intravesical resiniferatoxin. Lancet 1997;350:640–1.

165. Lazzeri M, Beneforti P, Spinelli M, Zanollo A, Barbagli G, Turini D. Intravesical resiniferatoxin for the treatment of hypersensitive disorder: a randomized placebo controlled study. J Urol 2000;164:676–9.

166. Silva C, Rio ME, Cruz F. Desensitization of bladder sensory fibers by intravesical resiniferatoxin, a capsaicin analog: long-term results for the treatment of detrusor hyperreflexia. Eur Urol 2000;38:444–52.

167. Jonas D. Treatment of female stress incontinence with midodrine: preliminary report. J Urol 1982;118:980–2.

168. Gnad H, Burmucic R, Petritsch P, Steindorfer P. Conservative therapy of female stress incontinence. Double-blind study with the alpha-sympathomimetic midodrin. Fortschr Med 1984;102:578–80 (in German).

169. Lose G, Lindholm D. Clinical and urodynamic effects of norfenefrine in women with stress incontinence. Urol Int 1984;39:298–302.

170. Radley SC, Chapple CR, Bryan NP, Clarke DE, Craig DA. Effect of methoxamine on maximum urethral pressure in women with genuine stress incontinence: a placebo-controlled, double-blind crossover study. Neurourol Urodyn 2001;20:43–52.

171. Gleason DM, Reilly SA, Bottacini MR, Pierce MJ. The urethral continence zone and its relation to stress incontinence. J Urol 1974;112:81–8.

172. Kaisary AV. Beta-adrenoceptor blockade in the treatment of female stress urinary incontinence. J d'Urol (Paris) 1984;90:351–3.

173. Gilja I, Radej M, Kovacic M, Parazajdes J. Conservative treatment of female stress incontinence with imipramine. J Urol 1984;132:909–11.

174. Lin HH, Sheu BC, Lo MC, Huang SC. Comparison of treatment outcomes for imipramine for female genuine stress incontinence. Br J Obstet Gynaecol 1999;106:1089–92.

175. Yasuda K, Kawabe K, Takimoto Y, Kondo A, Takaki R, Imabayashi K, Toyoshima A, Sato A, Shimazaki J, and the Clenbuterol Clinical Research Group. A double-blind clinical trial of a b₂-adrenergic agonist in stress incontinence. Int Urogynecol J 1993;4:146–51.

176. Ishiko O, Ushiroyama T, Saji F, Mitsuhashi Y, Tamura T, Yamamoto K, Kawamura Y, Ogita S. beta(2)-Adrenergic agonists and pelvic floor exercises for female stress incontinence. Int J Gynaecol Obstet 2000;71:39–44.

177. Thor KB, Katofiasc MA. Effects of duloxetine, a combined serotonin and norepinephrine reuptake inhibitor, on central neural control of lower urinary tract function in the chloralose-anesthetized female cat. J Pharmacol Exp Ther 1995;274:1014–24.

178. Zinner N, Sarshik S, Yalcin I, Faries D, DeBrota D, Riedl P, Thor KB. Efficacy and safety of duloxetine in stress urinary incontinent patients: double-blind, placebo-controlled multiple dose study. ICS 28th Annual Meeting, Jerusalem, Israel, September 14–17, 1998.

179. Finkbeiner AE. Is bethanechol chloride clinically effective in promoting bladder emptying: a literature review. J Urol 1985;134:443–9.

180. Sundin T, Dahlström A, Norlén L, Svedmyr N. The sympathetic innervation and adrenoreceptor function of the human lower urinary tract in the normal state and after parasympathetic denervation. Invest Urol 1977;14:322–8.

181. Hachen HJ. Clinical and urodynamic assessment of alpha adrenolytic therapy in patients with neurogenic bladder function. Paraplegia 1980;18:229–38.

182. Krane RJ, Olsson CA. Phenoxybenzamine in neurogenic bladder dysfunction, part II: clinical considerations. J Urol 1973;104:612–15.

183. McGuire EJ, Wagner FM, Weiss RM. Treatment of autonomic dysreflexia with phenoxybenzamine. J Urol 1976;115:53–5.

184. Andersson K-E, Ek A, Hedlund H, Mattiasson A. Effects of prazosin on isolated human urethra and in patients with lower motor neuron lesions. Invest Urol 1981;19:39–42.
185. Bergman A, Karram MM, Bhatia NN. Changes in urethral cytology following estrogen administration. Gynecol Obstet Invest 1990;29:211.
186. Hilton P, Stanton SL. The use of intravaginal oestrogen cream in genuine stress incontinence. Br J Obstet Gynaecol 1983;90:940–4.
187. Bhatia NN, Bergman A, Karram MM. Effects of estrogen on urethral function in women with urinary incontinence. Am J Obstet Gynecol 1989;160:176–81.
188. Karram MM, Yeko TR, Sauer MV, Bhatia NN. Urodynamic changes following hormone replacement therapy in women with premature ovarian failure. Obstet Gynecol 1989;74:208–11.
189. Fantl JA, Wyman JF, Anderson RL, Matt DW, Bump RC. Postmenopausal urinary incontinence: comparison between non-estrogen and estrogen supplemented women. Obstet Gynecol 1988;71:823–8.
190. Lose G, Englev E. Oestradiol-releasing vaginal ring versus oestriol vaginal pessaries in the treatment of bothersome lower urinary tract symptoms. Br J Obstet Gynaecol 2000;107:1029–34.
191. Hextall A. Oestrogens and lower urinary tract function. Maturitas 2000;36:83–92.
192. Fantl JA, Bump RC, Robinson D, McClish DK, Wyman JF. Efficacy of estrogen supplementation in the treatment of urinary incontinence. Obstet Gynecol 1996;88:745–9.
193. Jackson S, Shepherd A, Abrams P. The effect of oestradiol on objective urinary leakage in postmenopausal stress incontinence; a double blind placebo controlled trial. Neurourol Urodyn 1996;15:322–3.
194. Fantl JA, Cardozo L, McClish DK. Estrogen therapy in the management of urinary incontinence in postmenopausal women: a meta-analysis. First report of the Hormones and Urogenital Therapy Committee. Obstet Gynecol 1994;83:12–18.
195. Sultana CJ, Walters MD. Estrogen and urinary incontinence in women. Maturitas 1990;20:129–38.
196. Ishiko O, Hirai K, Sumi T, Tatsuta I, Ogita S. Hormone replacement therapy plus pelvic floor muscle exercise for postmenopausal stress incontinence. A randomized, controlled trial. J Reprod Med 2001;46:213–20.
197. Cardozo L, Rekers H, Tapp A, Barnick C, Shepherd A, Schussler B, Kerr-Wilson R, van Geelan J, Barlebo H, Walter S. Oestriol in the treatment of postmenopausal urgency: a multicentre study. Maturitas 1993;18:47–53.
198. Grady D, Brown JS, Vittinghoff E, Applegate W, Varner E, Snyder T. Postmenopausal hormones and incontinence: the Heart and Estrogen/Progestin Replacement Study. Obstet Gynecol 2001;97:116–20.

24 Behavioral Strategies for the Treatment of Urinary Incontinence in Women

K.N. Moore and A. Saltmarche

Introduction

Urinary incontinence is estimated to affect nearly 40% of older women. While it is widely accepted that the prevalence of urinary incontinence is high in older women [1], the few longitudinal studies that included younger women have shown a surprising prevalence in younger age groups, with only minimal increases in prevalence as age increases (peaking in the fifth decade) [2–5]. Further, in studies comparing gender differences, women older than 60–65 years have urinary incontinence prevalence rates 1.5 to 2 times that of same aged men [6,7]; the gender difference is even greater (3 to 7 times) in younger women, 25 to 64 years old [4]. The earlier age of onset magnifies the potential impact that urinary incontinence has on years of healthy life in women compared to men. Women are not only much more likely to become incontinent than men, but will also live a much larger portion of their life with urinary incontinence than will men.

Psychological Impact of Urinary Incontinence

Incontinence may impact on both men and women to varying degrees, ranging from a minor nuisance to a severe limitation. Restrictions in physical activity [8,9], stress, frustration, thoughts of suicide [10], confusion, depression, anger, decreased well-being [11], low self-esteem, social isolation, and impaired sleep [12,13] have all been reported by incontinent individuals. Despite health care professionals' awareness of the negative impact of incontinence on quality of life, treatment of the problem may be less than optimum, partly due to misunderstandings about the significant effect that simple behavioral interventions may have. In many cases, non invasive conservative treatment initiated by family physicians, specialist nurses or physiotherapists is highly effective and long-lasting [14–16].

Current Status of Behavioral Research and Urinary Incontinence

Behavioral strategies include a variety of approaches intended to change continence status and require a degree of willingness on the part of the woman to incorporate lifestyle adjustments into her daily routine. The most frequently recommended strategies include fluid adjustment, caffeine elimination, bowel management, pelvic floor muscle exercises (PFME), and bladder training. The research to date addressing behavioral strategies (also called conservative strategies or lifestyle adjustments) is limited by several design issues, including subjective outcome measures, no standardized protocols, lack of control groups, and small heterogeneous samples. Thus, it is difficult to state unequivocally that behavioral strategies for urinary incontinence are highly effective. Nevertheless, continence experts across disciplines agree that, in nearly all cases, conservative treatment provides some benefit and should be the first-line approach to urinary incontinence treatment in all women, except those with severe prolapse [17–20].

Assessment at the Primary Care Level

History

Women who overcome the embarrassment and shame associated with urinary incontinence will usually approach their family physician as a first step in treatment. There is good evidence that initial assessment and conservative intervention by the family physician is very effective, long-lasting, and significantly reduces the psychosocial impact of incontinence [14,16,21,22]. All programs of behavioral intervention begin with a detailed history about all medical or associated conditions. Sensitive questioning about symptoms, a detailed history, and a focused physical examination including a pelvic assessment, rectal examination, and brief neurological examination are required to make an initial diagnosis.

The most useful classification of incontinence for initial management is symptom-based: overactive bladder (urge incontinence), stress urinary incontinence, or overflow incontinence. Note that a definitive diagnosis requires a detailed, expert assessment, including urodynamics, and is described in detail in other chapters of this book.

Overactive Bladder

Typically, women with overactive bladder describe nocturia more than twice a night, as well as urgency and an inability to delay the urge more than just a few minutes. Such symptoms, however, should not be confused with urinary tract infection; urethritis; atropic vaginitis; or stress, mixed, or overflow incontinence. Behavioral strategies combined with anticholinergic/antimuscarinic drug therapy can be highly effective in the treatment of overactive bladder.

Stress Urinary Incontinence

Women suffering from pure stress incontinence usually describe incontinence with increased abdominal pressure but no leakage at night and no nocturia. A 24-hour bladder diary is an effective tool for discriminating between stress and urge incontinence in women with incontinence. The number of night-time voids is the best factor in separating the two groups [23]. Strategies to increase the ability of the pelvic floor muscles to withstand increases in abdominal pressure, possibly combined with alpha agonists, are the choice of management of stress urinary incontinence.

Overflow Incontinence

Overflow incontinence or incomplete emptying may also present with mixed symptoms of urgency, a feeling that the bladder is never empty, and/or leakage with increased abdominal pressure. The most effective treatment for overflow incontinence is clean intermittent self-catheterization. Pharmacologic therapy with cholinergic stimulators is rarely effective.

Table 24.1 outlines the symptom presentation, presumed etiology, and usual treatment strategies at the primary care level. Note that more than one type of incontinence may be present (for example, mixed urge and stress urinary incontinence). As the bladder can be an "unreliable witness" [24,25], if the initial strategies discussed in this chapter are not effective, referral to a specialist and urodynamic testing are warranted.

Assessment

As well as a physical examination to assess pelvic muscle tone, sensation, and contractile ability, the initial incontinence assessment should include urinalysis and post-void residual. A clinical rating scale for pelvic floor muscle strength such as that shown in Table 24.2 can help in the initial and follow-up documentation of progress [26]. In addition, a fluid volume chart (also called a frequency volume chart, voiding diary, bladder diary, bladder record) is part of the initial continence assessment (Table 24.3). The fluid volume chart is a reliable tool for assessing voiding patterns and fluid intake over 24 hours to 7 days (average 48 hours), even without detailed instruction from the health care provider [27,28]. Over a set period, the subject records the amount of fluid consumed (in ml), the amount of each void (in ml), and the situations in which leakage occurred. A 7-day dietary and stool record will be helpful if constipation is identified as a problem.

For a cognitively able and motivated person, the frequency/volume chart poses little problem. For people with cognitive limitations, obtaining a true estimate of the frequency and volume of micturitions may be a challenge. Another limitation is that individuals may put down what they "think" the practitioner wants to know, rather than what the real situation is, or they may guess at the amounts rather than measuring them. Finally, the chart is limited by the activities in which the individual engages, such as sitting in an armchair or digging in the garden. Such limitations can be minimized by fully explaining the purpose of the chart, providing the person with an easy-to-read measuring receptacle, and keeping the record for more than one day to capture

Table 24.1 Symptom presentation and usual treatment strategies at the primary care level

Presumed etiology	Description	Treatment options at the primary care level
Overactive bladder (urge incontinence)	Loss of urine associated with a strong desire to void; may be accompanied by frequency and nocturia; nocturia is typically described by women with overactive bladder but not by those with stress urinary incontinence	medication review Bladder training, timed toileting, fluid management, Constipation management. Pelvic muscle exercises (PFME) PFME + biofeedback Electrical stimulation (10–20 Hz) Estrogen therapy Anticholinergic/antimuscarinic medications Incontinence pads Environmental modifications such as bedside commodes, night lights and clearly marked toilets
Stress	Loss of urine on physical exertion or increases in abdominal pressure due to laughing, coughing, sneezing, etc., due to sphincter deficiency; women with stress incontinence are usually dry at night and do not complain of nocturia.	Weight loss, fluid increase/decrease, smoking cessation Constipation management PFME PFME + biofeedback Electrical stimulation (>30 Hz) Pessary (occasionally) Alpha agonists
Mixed	Loss of urine with urge and also with increases in abdominal stress; symptoms are mixed with urgency, frequency, nocturia, leaking with increased abdominal pressures	Combination of above conservative measures, with an initial focus on the dominant symptom
Overflow	Leakage associated with bladder distension; leak with increased abdominal pressure; may be confused with stress incontinence; due to acontractile or poorly contractile detrusor or outlet obstruction; chronic retention is usually painless	Refer Intermittent catheterization Relief of obstruction Medication review Alpha adrenergic antagonists Last resort: indwelling catheter

the individual's typical urine flow, leakage patterns, and activities that provoke leakage.

Finally, assessment should include some determination of cognitive ability, ability to adhere to a behavioral regimen, and the impact of urinary incontinence on the woman's quality of life.

Behavioral Strategies

Frequently recommended conservative or behavioral strategies include: fluid adjustment, caffeine reduction, smoking cessation, weight reduction,

Table 24.2 Clinical rating scale for pelvic floor muscle strength

0	No palpable muscle contraction
1	Flicker (barely able to detect)
2	Weak but clearly perceived
3	Moderate
4	Good
5	Strong

regular moderate physical exercise, bowel management, bladder training, and pelvic floor muscle exercises [20,29].

Fluid Adjustment

Frequency and incontinence may not be related to fluid intake, although fluid intake is related to voided volume [30,31]. A relationship between evening fluid intake and night-time incontinence or voiding in elderly people with urge incontinence suggests that evening fluid restriction and night-time toileting may help [30]. In a study to evaluate the effects of fluid intake on urine loss, Dowd and colleagues [32] randomized women to one of three groups – increase fluid by 500 ml, reduce fluid by 300 ml, or remain the same. Small sample size (n = 32) and poor adherence to the fluid volume record resulted in non-significant results. Subjectively, however, the authors reported that women who increased their fluid intake reported fewer incidents of leakage.

Table 24.3   Fluid volume chart

Date:_____Name:_____

Time	Amount urinated	Leakage? (Yes or No)	Liquid intake	Comments
6–8 a.m.				
8–10 a.m.				
10–12 a.m.				
12–2 p.m.				
2–4 p.m.				
4–6 p.m.				
6–8 p.m.				
8–10 p.m.				
10–12 p.m.				
Overnight (Just make a check mark for night-time voids – no need to measure)				
Total in 24 hours	*Voids*	*Wet pads*	*Fluid intake*	

Caffeine Reduction

There are drugs such as caffeine that can directly affect the partially decompensated lower urinary tract and precipitate urgency or incontinence. The relationship between caffeine intake and incontinence remains unclear. While some have identified caffeine as a factor in daytime urinary incontinence [31], others have been unable to identify a clear association between caffeine and urinary incontinence in community-dwelling women [33] or the disabled [34]. Creighton and Stanton [35] demonstrated that 200 mg of caffeine exacerbated unstable contractions in those individuals with an unstable bladder, but made no difference in subjects whose bladders were stable. This oft cited study on the effect of caffeine on individuals with an unstable bladder has not been replicated.

Reduction or Cessation of Cigarette Smoking

The relationship between cigarette smoking and chronic respiratory problems is irrefutable. Two large epidemiological studies have demonstrated a significant risk of incontinence in women over 60 years of age with chronic obstructive pulmonary disease and chronic respiratory symptoms (coughing and sneezing) [36,37]. Although epidemiological studies have not confirmed a significant association between smoking and urinary incontinence in younger women [33], men aged 50 to 70 who were smokers and former smokers had a significantly increased risk of lower urinary tract symptoms (odds ratio 1.47 and 1.38 respectively) when compared to those who had never smoked [38].

Moreover, two case-control studies have demonstrated a relationship between cigarette smoking and both stress and urge incontinence [39]. In another case-control study comparing 71 smokers and 118 non-smokers (all with pure stress incontinence), smokers had stronger urethral sphincters, a lower risk profile (younger and less often hypoestrogenic), and significantly stronger coughs than non-smokers [40]. It was concluded that more violent coughing by smokers promoted the earlier development of the anatomic and pressure transmission defects that contribute to stress urinary incontinence and overcame any protective advantage of a stronger urethral sphincter.

Weight Reduction

Obesity is a commonly cited risk factor in the development and recurrence of urinary incontinence in women and is independent of obstetric history, surgery, smoking, and family history [41]. Defined as greater than 120% of the average weight for height and age, obesity is significantly more prevalent both in women with genuine stress incontinence and in those with detrusor instability than in the normal population [42]. Women with a positive stress test on urodynamics may have a significantly higher body mass index (BMI) than subjects with a negative stress test [43]. However, the relationship between weight loss and improvement in symptoms is unclear. Although women with profound weight loss after bypass surgery reported a significant improvement in incontinence [44], more modest weight loss programs have not led to notable improvement [20].

Encouraging women to maintain or attain their ideal weight or to stop smoking are credible health maintenance goals that might also prevent urinary incontinence. Women should be made aware of this potential health benefit. A weight loss or smoking cessation strategy combined with other behavioral strategies should be incorporated when reasonable into a comprehensive treatment plan.

Physical Activity/Regular Exercise

An area that has attracted little research related to etiology of urinary incontinence is physical activity associated with repeated or excessive increases in abdominal pressure. Amongst nulliparous or elite athletes, incontinence occurs in as many as 33% [45,46]. What is unclear from the limited literature is whether exercise or activities exceed the physiological threshold of the lower urinary tract, or whether vigorous exercise represents the insult that causes

those thresholds to degenerate and decompensate. In terms of prevention of incontinence, there are no studies of women assessing the impact of regular (not high impact) exercise. Men aged 40 to 75 who undertake moderate exercise (walk 2 to 3 hours a week) have a 25% lower risk of total benign prostatic hyperplasia [47], but whether lower urinary tract symptoms in women are delayed by exercise is unknown. Many women limit their activities or stop exercising because of incontinence, thereby increasing the risk of other weight-related problems. As exercise has significant health benefits, it should be encouraged as part of every woman's healthy routine.

Bowel Management

Data linking constipation and urinary incontinence in women relate to the growing body of evidence linking urinary incontinence, fecal incontinence, and pelvic organ prolapse to each other and each of these conditions, in turn, to pelvic floor denervation and pudendal neuropathy [48–50]. Stretching of the pudendal nerve is felt to be a major cause of nerve damage; excessive straining in conjunction with perineal descent is felt to be the major cause of nerve stretch. While vaginal childbirth has been implicated as a major contributing event for urinary incontinence and pelvic neuropathy [50,51], chronic constipation with repeated prolonged straining related to defecation may also contribute to progressive neuropathy and dysfunction [52].

Questioning the woman about bowel and flatus incontinence, information which people do not willingly volunteer unless directly asked, gives a general idea of the ability to control the pelvic floor muscles. In one study, 24% of women had urinary incontinence plus fecal incontinence. The majority stated that stool leakage, although less frequent, was significantly more devastating than the urinary incontinence [53]. Discussing fecal incontinence provides an opportunity to discuss an embarrassing issue with even more stigma than urinary incontinence, and the information obtained provides the practitioner and woman with a discussion point on which to base collaborative goals and expectations for conservative treatment.

Older women with urinary incontinence have been shown to be significantly more likely to have both constipation and fecal incontinence than women without urinary incontinence, lending further evidence to the association [36], and constipation is one of several associated risk factors for incontinence along with obesity, gynecologic surgery, and parity [54]. Chronic constipation has a known effect on the bladder outlet causing obstruction-like symptoms of reduced urinary flow rate, increased voiding time, and increased bladder capacity [55]. The evidence identifying chronic constipation as a risk factor for urinary incontinence may be sufficient to warrant efforts to identify young continent women with severe constipation. As with urinary incontinence, a specialist referral is required if initial dietary and non-stimulant bowel preparations are not effective.

Bladder Training

The purpose of bladder training (also called bladder retraining urge suppression or scheduled voiding) is to increase the length of time between voiding by adherence to a particular schedule (usually based on an individual fluid volume chart). Ultimately continence and an interval of 3 to 4 hours between voids should be achieved. The treatment is recommended for individuals with urgency and urge incontinence. Bladder training generally comprises three components: patient education, scheduled voiding, and positive reinforcement [17]. Bladder training may be more effective if combined with other behavioral methods and anticholinergic or antimuscarinic medications [56].

Despite having received the most research attention of all the behavioral strategies, the evidence to strongly support bladder training as an effective protocol is moderate at best. Currently, seven randomized controlled trials that included a total of 259 participants have been published [57]. The studies were of moderate quality and lacked details concerning teaching methods, patient education materials, fluid intake, and concomitant medications. The trials did not address the importance of ongoing follow-up, nor were subjects followed on a long-term basis. Despite the shortcomings of the studies, the authors (Roe, Williams and Palmer) conclude that bladder retraining is a useful management strategy for urge incontinence. Key to success are good sensation of bladder fullness, adequate pelvic muscle tone (assessed by a pelvic examination), and motivation.

Bladder training is effective in many women, but 3 or more months of commitment may be required before the desired voiding goal is achieved. During that time, women require ongoing support and encouragement from the health care professional. Table 24.4 outlines a protocol for assisting a woman with a bladder training protocol [58].

Pelvic Floor Muscle Exercises (PFME)

Pelvic floor muscle exercises remain the mainstay of therapy, especially for stress urinary incontinence. The purpose of pelvic floor muscle exercises is to increase the woman's awareness of pelvic muscle function and to strengthen the voluntary muscles to withstand increases in abdominal pressure. Women without prolapse who follow an intensive exercise regimen led by a physiotherapist or nurse report

Table 24.4 Scheduled (timed) voiding for bladder training

1. *Establish a voiding pattern* by using a "bladder diary" (frequency/volume chart) to record volume of voids, incontinence episodes, and fluid intake.

2. *Determine a voiding interval* based on the voiding pattern of the individual. If frequency is more than every 60 minutes, have the person void every 60 minutes; if less than 60 minutes, start with a 30-minute interval.

3. *Teach urge suppression.* Pelvic muscle exercises and distraction techniques may help dissipate the urge to void when it is felt.

To control the urge, take a deep breath and relax. Stand still or sit down. Contract your pelvic floor muscles 5 or 6 times. Count backwards from 100. Wait until the urge passes and then resume your activities. If it is longer than 2 hours since you last used the toilet, proceed slowly to the toilet to empty your bladder. Rushing to the toilet will make the symptoms of urgency much worse.

Practice pelvic floor muscle exercises. Pelvic muscles form a muscle support system for your bladder and urethra. A physiotherapist or nurse specializing in continence care can show you the correct method for doing pelvic muscle exercises.

4. *Gradually increase the length of time* between voids as continence is achieved.

5. *Record progress by bladder diary.* A daily or weekly bladder diary helps to track progress.

6. *Follow up regularly.* Bladder retraining requires a lot of work and commitment on the part of the person. Encouragement is important for success.

Scheduled voiding is successful in many cases. It requires a very motivated, cognitively able individual and a committed nurse. The goal is to reach normal voiding patterns by increasing bladder capacity. Scheduled voiding should be combined with an adequate intake of non-caffeinated fluids (approximately 2 liters per day).

significant benefit from pelvic floor muscle exercises [59–61].

Moreover, at least 70% of women who have an initial successful outcome from PFME will report a durable benefit 4 or more years after cessation of formal exercise training [62,63]. Primiparas randomized to pelvic floor muscle exercises or routine care had significantly fewer incontinence episodes during pregnancy and postpartum than the control group [26]. Pelvic floor muscle exercises have been compared to vaginal cones, electrical stimulation [59] and bladder training [61]. In both studies women who practiced exercises did as well or better than those following other treatment protocols. Critical to success of pelvic floor muscle exercises is teaching, support, and ongoing follow-up by an experienced health care professional, usually a physiotherapist or nurse. Without adequate instruction, there is good evidence that between 30 and 70% of women will be unable to perform an adequate pelvic muscle contraction [64].

Teaching pelvic floor muscle exercises involves a pelvic examination with instruction on identifying the correct muscles and timing of the contractions. It also involves teaching the woman how to do a self-vaginal examination so that she may assess her progress. Experts have also begun to systematically teach women to contract their pelvic floor muscles before the leak-provoking event. Older women with mild to moderate stress incontinence, randomized to pre-event contractions (also called the "Knack") reported significantly reduced urine loss from a medium and deep cough compared to the control group [65]. Variation is found between practitioners about the frequency, type, and duration of each exercise session with ranges between 45 and 400 times per day [29]. The Canadian Continence Foundation recommends 3 sets of exercises per day, totaling no more than 50 contractions per day, based on the work of Bø, Kvarstein, Hagan and Larsen [66]. Figure 24.1 shows the basic pelvic floor muscle instruction sheet that the Canadian Continence Foundation provides. This basic information is best combined with physiotherapy or nursing expertise.

Adjuncts to Pelvic Floor Muscle Exercises

There is also modest evidence from case series or non-controlled studies that continence is regained more rapidly when PFME are augmented with electrical stimulation, biofeedback, or transcutaneous electrical nerve stimulation (TENS). Vaginal cones are also promoted as an adjunct to enhance the performance of pelvic muscle contractions. However, recent reviews have questioned the use of cones as a treatment modality, finding that pelvic floor muscle exercises were equally effective [67–69]. In practice, the foreign feel of the cone in the vagina may be useful for certain women who have difficulty isolating the pelvic floor muscles (a Foley catheter with a balloon inflated 20 to 30 ml may also serve the purpose). Other studies considering adjunct therapies such as biofeedback and electrical stimulation are described in detail in Chapter 25.

Intermittent Catheterization

Traditional behavioral strategies for women with overflow incontinence or incomplete emptying include double voiding, voiding on a regular basis, Valsalva maneuver, external compression, trigger points, and sitting in or having warm water poured over the perineum. None of these methods have been systematically tested for their effectiveness for incomplete emptying. There is good evidence that bladder health and complete emptying can be achieved with intermittent catheterization. In the community, the procedure is clean, with catheters being reused after washing with soap and water [17]. It is currently recommended that sterile single use catheters be used by immunocompromised patients, pregnant women, diabetics, or any individuals at high risk of systemic infection [70].

Conclusion

Urinary incontinence is a common health problem among women. Behavioral interventions are safe, effective, and can be actively implemented at the primary care level by the family physician, nurse or physiotherapist. Structured interventions with support, individualized care, and regular follow-up will go far to enhance treatment success. The strategies suggested in this chapter may not be applicable to all women and specialist referral may be required. Even complex cases requiring referral to a specialist can still afford an opportunity for teaching the woman good bladder habits (Table 24.5) [19]. Initial assessments such as urinalysis, post-void residual, and fluid volume chart are important at both primary and specialist level of care and the family physician is pivotal in ensuring continuity of care.

The Canadian continence foundation

Continence facts • **Kegel exercises** •

Pelvic Muscle exercises • for urinary incontinence

Introduction

Pelvic muscle exercises are a therapy used for treating incontinence in both women and men of all ages. They do not involve surgery or medication, and pose little risk for side effects. Similar to any other exercises, they are a series of repeated contractions of one set of muscles - the pelvic muscles. The exercises are commonly called Kegal exercises, named after Dr. Kegal, who developed them over 40 years ago. Your healthcare professional may have recommended Kegal exercises for you. The following information may be helpful as you begin to do the exercises.

How Pelvic Muscle Exercises may Help

The pelvic muscles support the bladder like a hammock. We can tighten, and relax these muscles. When tightened or contracted, the urethra, the tube which passes urine from the bladder to outside the body is squeezed so that urine is held in. If the muscles are strong, urine will not leak. But if the muscles are weak, they cannot close off the urethra, and urine may leak. Pelvic muscle exercises help to strengthen the "hammock" so that the urethra can be kept closed, to keep urine in.

Consult a Healthcare Professional

Incontinence can almost always be cured, treated or managed successfully. Pelvic muscle exercises are only one method for retraining the muscles. Consult a healthcare professional who is interested and experienced in the area of incontinence. If you have any questions or concerns about these exercises ask your healthcare professional for help.

The Canadian continence foundation

How to do Pelvic Muscle Exercises

Teach yourself to relax and focus on the pelvic muscle exercises. This will become easier with practise.

1. Stand sit or lie down with your knees slightly apart (about 25 cm or 10 in apart). **Relax.**

2. Find your pelvis muscles. Imagine that you are trying to hold back urine, or a bowel movement. Squeeze the muscles you would use to do that.

• Women

To check that you are tightening the correct muscles, you can insert your finger into the vagina and tighten the muscle. You should feel a tightening around the finger.

• Men

To check that you are tightening the correct muscles, when you tighten, you should see your penis twitch and contract in. In both cases, you should feel the rectal muscle (the one you use to hold back bowel movements and passing gas) tighten. You can check this by touching the opening at the rectum as you are tightening the muscle - you should feel the opening contract at the same time.

3. Tighten the muscles for 5 to 10 seconds. Do not hold your breath - breathe normally. Do not tighten your stomach or buttocks - keep them relaxed.
4. Now relax the muscle for about 10 seconds.
5. Repeat.

Your Schedule

• Repeat the contractions 12 to 20 times.
• Do the set of 12 to 20 contractions and relaxations three times per day.
• Schedule the times you exercise with activities that you do every day, so that you remember to do them consistently.

Tips

• Do them properly - check often to be sure that you are using the correct muscles.
• Do them regularly - at least three times per day.
• Do them when you need them most - learn to do them just before sneezing, coughing, or straining.
• Keep on doing them - Do not become discouraged. You should start to see results after a few weeks. However, like any muscle of the body, the pelvic muscles will only stay strong as long as you exercise them. Once you have reached your goal, continue your exercises at least every other day.

Some Other Techniques which may be presented to you

If you find it difficult to identify the correct muscles to exercise, your healthcare professional can help. Your healthcare professional may recommend the use of biofeedback equipment to help you identify and exercise your pelvic muscles. Biofeedback allows you to see the effects of your muscle contractions on a monitor, so that you can more easily know if you are contracting the right muscles.

For women there are devices called vaginal cones, which can be inserted into the vagina, again to help identify and strengthen the pelvic muscles. Once a cone is inserted, you would try to hold it in, by contracting the pelvic muscle for a short period of time, before removing the cone.

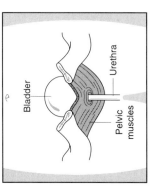

Before

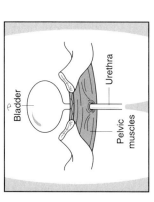

After

Figure 24.1 Kegel exercises for urinary incontinence. (Reproduced by permission of The Canadian Continence Foundation.)

Table 24.5 Healthy bladder habits

Drink adequately:
- 6–8 cups of fluids per day, more when it is hot or when exercising.

Drink enough fluids to keep your urine a very pale yellow color. In general 6 to 8 glasses of fluids a day is recommended, especially water. To calculate the approximate number of ounces of fluid you require a day divide your weight in pounds by 2. Avoid caffeine, which is found in tea, coffee, colas, and chocolate. Some people find that their bladder symptoms improve by reducing or eliminating caffeine.

Recognize that:
- most people empty their bladder about every 3–4 hours during the day (4–8 times in 24 hours)
- getting up in the night to empty the bladder is not abnormal
- being awakened more than twice is abnormal

Relax:
- don't strain to empty the bladder or bowels
- practice pelvic floor muscle exercises

Practice urge suppression if the urge to empty your bladder is happening more than every 2 hours. *To control the urge, take a deep breath and relax. Stand still or sit down. Contract your pelvic floor muscles 5 or 6 times. Count backwards from 100. Wait until the urge passes and then resume your activities. If it is longer than 2 hours since you last used the toilet, proceed slowly to the toilet to empty your bladder.* Rushing to the toilet will make the symptoms of urgency much worse.

Practice pelvic floor muscle exercises. Pelvic muscles form a muscle support system for your bladder and urethra. A physiotherapist or nurse specializing in continence care can show you the correct method for doing pelvic muscle exercises.

Try to keep bowel movements regular:
- don't ignore feelings that the bowels need emptying

Keep the bowels regular for overall health and well-being. For some people, bladder symptoms are more severe if they are constipated.

Seek professional help when:
- any leakage of urine from the bladder occurs (incontinence)
- pain is experienced when passing urine
- any blood is seen in urine

The Future

Research opportunities abound in the area of behavioral strategies and the treatment of urinary incontinence in women [20]. This review provides a strong basis for further randomized controlled trials: current evidence and recommendations for research for most behavioral strategies are equivocal. Research is required to explore the effect of lifestyle interventions, the impact of weight loss and bowel management, the effect of pelvic floor muscle exercises, and the effect of bladder training. Detailed descriptions of subjects who succeeded with treatment and those who did not, and the number and duration of pelvic floor muscle exercises, will go far to assist in the initial management of urinary incontinence. Expert opinion obtained at consensus meetings strongly endorses behavioral management as the first-line approach to urinary incontinence. Health care professionals have a responsibility to encourage further randomized controlled trials for a ubiquitous health problem and improved practice based on the best evidence.

References

1. Bø K, Stien R, Kulseng-Hanssen S, Kristofferson M. NIH Consensus Development Panel: urinary incontinence in adults. JAMA 1989;261:2685–90.
2. Jolleys JV. Reported prevalence of urinary incontinence in women in a general practice. BMJ 1988;296:1300–2.
3. Rekers H, Drogendijk AC, Valkenburg H, Riphagen F. Urinary incontinence in women from 35 to 79 years of age: prevalence and consequences. Eur J Obstet Gynecol Reprod Biol 1992;43:229–34.
4. Thomas TM, Plymat KR, Blannin J, Meade TW. Prevalence of urinary incontinence. BMJ 1980;281:1243–5.
5. Yarnell JWG, Voyle GJ, Richards CJ, Stephenson TP. The prevalence and severity of urinary incontinence in women. J Epidemiol Community Health 1981;35:71–4.
6. Diokno AC, Brock BM, Brown MB, Herzog RA. Prevalence of urinary incontinence and other urological symptoms in the noninstitutionalized elderly. J Urol 1986;136:1022–5.
7. Herzog AR, Diokno AC, Brown MB, Normolle DP, Brock BM. Two-year incidence, remission and change patterns of urinary incontinence in noninstitutionalised older adults. J Gerontol 1990;45:M67–M74.
8. Herr H. Quality of life in incontinent men after radical prostatectomy. J Urol 1994;151:652–4.
9. Jønler M, Madsen FA, Rhodes PR, Sall M, Messing EM, Bruskewitz RC. A prospective study of quantification of urinary incontinence and quality of life in patients undergoing radical retropubic prostatectomy. Urology 1996;48:433–40.

10. Moore KN, Estey A. The early post-operative concerns of men after radical prostatectomy. J Adv Nurs 1999;29:1121–9.

11. Braslis KG, Santa-Cruz C, Brickman AL, Soloway MS. Quality of life 12 months after radical prostatectomy. Br J Urol 1995;75:48–53.

12. Grimby A, Milsom I, Molander U, Wiklund I, Ekelund P. The influence of urinary incontinence on the quality of life of elderly women. Age Ageing 1993;22:82–9.

13. Hunskaar S, Visnes A. The quality of life in women with urinary incontinence as measured by the Sickness Impact Profile. J Am Geriatr Soc 1991;39:378–82.

14. Lagro-Janssen AL, Debruyne FM, Smits AJ, van Weel C. The effects of treatment of urinary incontinence in general practice. Fam Pract 1992;9:284–9.

15. Lightner DJ, Itano NM. Treatment option for women with stress urinary incontinence. Mayo Clin Proc 1999;74:1149–56.

16. Seim A, Hermstad R, Hunskaar S. Management in general practice significantly reduced psychosocial consequences of female urinary incontinence. Qual Life Res 1997;6:257–64.

17. Agency for Health Care Policy and Research. Urinary incontinence in adults: acute and chronic management. A clinical practice guideline. Update. Rockville, MD: US Department of Health and Human Services, 1996, Publication 96–0862 (http://text.nlm.nih.gov/ftrs/tocview).

18. Canadian Continence Foundation. Canadian Continence Foundation consensus conference on clinical practice guidelines and models for delivery of continence care in Canada. Sponsored by Canadian Continence Foundation, Montreal, Quebec, Canada, May 2000.

19. Consensus Statement: 1st International Conference for the Prevention of Incontinence. Co-sponsored by Simon Foundation for Continence, USA, Continence Foundation, UK, in association with the International Continence Society, Continence Promotion Committee, Danesfield House, UK, June 1997.

20. Wilson PD, Bø K, Bourcier A, Hay-Smith J, Staskin D, Nygaard I, Wyman J, Shepherd A. Conservative management in women. In: Abrams P, Khoury S, Wein A, editors. Incontinence: 1st International Consultation on Incontinence, Monaco, 1998. Plymouth, UK: Plymbridge Distributors, 1999; 581–636.

21. Holtedahl K, Verelst M, Schiefloe A. A population based, randomised, controlled trial of conservative treatment for urinary stress incontinence in women. Acta Obstet Gynecol Scand 1998;77:671–7.

22. Lagro-Janssen AL, van Weel C. Long-term effect of treatment of female incontinence in general practice. Br J Gen Pract 1998;48:1735–8.

23. Fink D, Perucchini D, Schaer GN, Haller U. The role of the frequency-volume chart in the differential diagnostic of female urinary incontinence. Acta Obstet Gynecol Scand 1999;78:254–7.

24. Blaivas JG. The bladder is an unreliable witness. Neurourol Urodyn 1996;15:443–5.

25. Ding YY, Lieu PK, Choo PW. Is the bladder "an unreliable witness" in elderly males with persistent lower urinary tract symptoms? Ger Nephrol Urol 1997;7:17–21.

26. Laycock, J. Clinical evaluation of the pelvic floor. In: Schüssler B, Laycock J, Norton P, Stanton S, editor. Pelvic Floor Re-education: Principles and Practice. London: Springer-Verlag, 1994; 42–8.

27. Nordling J, Abrams P, Ameda K, Andersen JT, Donovan J, Griffiths D, et al. Outcome measures for research in treatment of adult males with symptoms of lower urinary tract dysfunction. Neurourol Urodyn 1998;17:263–71.

28. Robinson D, McClish DK, Wyman JF, Bump RC, Fantl JA. Comparison between urinary diaries completed with and without intensive patient instructions. Neurourol Urodyn 1996;17:143–8.

29. Wilson D, Herbison P. Conservative management of incontinence. Curr Opin Obstet Gynecol 1995;7:386–92.

30. Griffiths DJ, McCracken PN, Harrison GM, Gormley EA. Relationship of fluid intake to voluntary micturition and urinary incontinence in geriatric patients. Neurourol Urodyn 1993;12:1–7.

31. Tomlinson BU, Dougherty MC, Pendergast JF, Boyington AR, Coffman MA, Pickens SM. Dietary caffeine, fluid intake and urinary incontinence in older rural women. Int Urogynecol J Pelvic Floor Dysfunct 1999;10:22–8.

32. Dowd TT, Campbell JM, Jones JA. Fluid intake and urinary incontinence in older community-dwelling women. J Community Health Nurs 1996;13:179–86.

33. Burgio KL, Matthews KA, Engel BT. Prevalence, incidence and correlates of urinary incontinence in healthy, middle-aged women. J Urol 1991;146:1255–9.

34. Fried GW, Goetz G, Potts-Nulty S, Cioschi HM, Staas WE Jr. A behavioral approach to the treatment of urinary incontinence in a disabled population. Arch Phys Med Rehabil 1995;76:1120–4.

35. Creighton SM, Stanton SL. Caffeine: does it affect your bladder? Br J Urol 1990;66:613–14.

36. Diokno AC, Brock BM, Herzog AR, Bromberg J. Medical correlates of urinary incontinence in the elderly. Urology 1990;36:129–38.

37. Brown JS, Seeley DG, Fong J, Black DM, Ensrud KE, Grady D. Urinary incontinence in older women: who is at risk? Obstet Gynecol 1996;87:715–21.

38. Koskimaki J, Hakama M, Huhtala H, Tammela TL. Association of smoking with lower urinary tract symptoms. J Urol 1998;159:1580–2.

39. Bump RC, McClish DK. Cigarette smoking and urinary incontinence in women. Am J Obstet Gynecol 1992;167:1213–18.

40. Bump RC, McClish DK. Cigarette smoking and pure genuine stress incontinence of urine: a comparison of risk factors and determinants between smokers and nonsmokers. Am J Obstet Gynecol 1994;170:579–82.

41. Wingate L, Wingate MB, Hassanein R. The relation between overweight and urinary incontinence in postmenopausal women: a case control study. J North Am Menopause Soc 1994;1:199–203.

42. Dwyer PL, Lee ETC, Hay DM. Obesity and urinary incontinence in women. Br J Obstet Gynaecol 1988;95:91–6.

43. Kolbl H, Riss P. Obesity and stress urinary incontinence: significance of indices of relative weight. Urol Int 1988;43:7–10.

44. Bump RC, Sugerman HJ, Fantl JA, McClish DK. Obesity and lower urinary tract function in women: effect of surgically induced weight loss. Am J Obstet Gynecol 1992;167:392–9.

45. Bø K, Stien R, Kulseng-Hanssen S, Kristofferson M. Clinical and urodynamic assessment of nulliparous young women with and without stress incontinence symptoms: case-control study. Obstet Gynecol 1994;84:1029–32.

46. Nygaard I, Thompson F, Svengalis S, Albright J. Urinary incontinence in elite nulliparous athletes. Obstet Gynecol 1994;84:183–7.

47. Platz EA, Kawachi I, Rimm EB, Colditz GA, Stampfer JF, Willett WC, Giovannucci E. Physical activity and benign prostatic hyperplasia. Arch Intern Med 1998;158:2349–56.

48. Jackson, SL, Weber AM, Hull TL, Mitchinson AR, Walters MD. Faecal incontinence in women with urinary incontinence and pelvic organ prolapse. Obstet Gynecol 1997;89:423–7.

49. Pannek J, Haupt G, Sommerfeld H-J, Schulze H, Senge T. Urodynamic and rectomanometric findings in urinary incontinence. Scand J Urol Nephrol 1996;30:457–60.

50. Smith ARB, Hosker GL, Warrell DW. The role of pudendal nerve damage in the aetiology of genuine stress incontinence in women. Br J Obstet Gynaecol 1989;96:29–32.

51. Snooks SJ, Swash M, Henry MM, Setchel M. Risk factors in childbirth causing damage to the pelvic floor innervation. Int J Colorectal Dis 1986;1:20–4.

52. Lubowski DZ, Swash M, Nichols J, Henry MM. Increase in pudendal nerve terminal motor latency with defecation straining. Br J Surg 1988;75:1095–7.

53. Saltmarche A, Reid DW, Linton L. Rural continence management project. Research report submitted to the Assistive Devices Program, Ontario Ministry of Health, Ottawa, Canada, 1992.

54. Chiarelli P, Brown WJ. Leaking urine in Australian women: prevalence and associated conditions. Women Health 1999;29:1–13.

55. MacDonald A, Shearer M, Paterson PJ, Finlay IG. Relationship between outlet obstruction, constipation and obstructed urinary flow. Br J Surg 1991;78:693–5.

56. Szonyi G, Collas DM, Ding YY, Malone-Lee JG. Oxybutynin with bladder retraining for detrusor instability in elderly people: a randomized controlled trial. Age Ageing 1995;24:287–91.

57. Roe B, Williams K, Palmer M. Bladder training for urinary incontinence in adults (Cochrane Review). In: The Cochrane Library, Issue 4, 1999. Oxford: Update Software.

58. Wyman JF, Fantl JA. Bladder training in ambulatory care management of urinary incontinence. Urol Nurs 1991;11:11–17.

59. Bø K, Talseth T, Holme, I. Single blind randomized controlled trial of pelvic floor exercises, electrical stimulation, vaginal cones or no treatment in management of genuine stress incontinence in women. BMJ 1999;318:487–93.

60. Sampselle C, Wyman J, Thomas K, Newman D, Gray M, Dougherty M, Burns P. Continence for women: evaluation of AWHONN's evidence-based protocol. J Obstet Gynecol Neonatal Nurs 2000;29:18–26.

61. Wyman J, Fantl A, McClish D, Bump R. Comparative efficacy of behavioral interventions in the management of female urinary incontinence. Am J Obstet Gynecol 1998;179:999–1007.

62. Bø K, Talseth T. Long-term effect of pelvic floor muscle exercise 5 years after cessation of organized training. Obstet Gynecol 1996;87:261–5.

63. O'Brien J. Evaluating primary care interventions for incontinence. Nursing Standard 1996;10:40–3.

64. Bø K, Larson S, Oseid S, Kvarstein B, Hagen R, Jørgensen J. Knowledge about and ability to correct pelvic floor muscle exercises in women with urinary stress incontinence. Neurourol Urodyn 1988;7:261–2. (abstract)

65. Miller J, Aston-Miller J, Delancey J. A pelvic muscle precontraction can reduce cough-related urine loss in selected women with mild SUI. J Am Geriatr Soc 1998;46:870–4.

66. Bø K, Kvarstein B, Hagan R, Larsen S. Pelvic floor muscle exercise for the treatment of female stress urinary incontinence: effects of two different degrees of pelvic floor muscle exercises. Neurourol Urodyn 1990;9:489–502.

67. Bø K. Vaginal weight cones. Theoretical framework, effect on pelvic floor muscle strength and female stress urinary incontinence. Acta Obstet Gynecol Scand 1995;74:87–92.

68. Herbison P, Plevnik S, Mantle J. Weighted vaginal cones for urinary incontinence (Cochrane Review). In: The Cochrane Library, Issue 2, 2000. Oxford: Update Software.

69. Pieber D, Zivkovic F, Tamussino K, Ralph G, Lippitt G, Fauland B. Pelvic floor exercises alone or with vaginal cones for the treatment of mild to moderate stress urinary incontinence in premenopausal women. Int Urogynecol J 1995;6:14–17.

70. Wein AJ. Neuromuscular dysfunction of the lower urinary tract. In: Walsh PC, Retik AB, Stoney TA, Vaughn ED Jr, editors. Campbell's Urology, 6th edn. Philadelphia: WB Saunders, 1992; 573–642.

25 Biofeedback and Functional Electrical Stimulation

Magali Robert and Thomas C. Mainprize

Introduction

Despite a high prevalence of urinary incontinence in society, its pathophysiology is not yet fully understood. A complex interaction between the pelvic structures and the nervous system is required to maintain continence. By providing support to the abdomino-pelvic viscera, the pelvic floor plays a pivotal role in the continence mechanism. Thus a weak pelvic floor may promote urinary stress and/or urge incontinence. This chapter will address the role of the pelvic floor and the therapies developed to improve its function.

The pelvic floor is composed of connective tissue, the levator ani muscles and the perineal membrane. The levator ani muscles are further subdivided into the coccygeus, iliococcygeus and pubococcygeus (puborectal, pubovaginal) muscles. The urethra, vagina and rectum traverse it through the urogenital hiatus. The innervation of the levator ani is via the pudendal nerve. The muscle is normally under continual tonic contraction but modulated by voluntary contraction and relaxation. Pelvic floor pathology can impair normal function by diminishing the resting tone and/or impairing contractility.

As the pelvic floor muscles are connected to the immobile pelvis, contraction and relaxation move the urethra and bladder neck. With normal pelvic floor relaxation, the urethra and bladder neck descend caudally and posteriorly [1]. This facilitates urethral opening and allows normal voiding. With pelvic floor contraction the urethra is elongated and brought anteriorly and cephalad against the precervical arch, thereby increasing urethral closure pressure [1] and maintaining continence (Figure 25.1). Further increase in urethral closure pressure is mediated by a reflex contraction of the periurethral striated muscles [2]. The muscles contract synergis-

tically with the abdominal, gluteal and adductor muscles [3]. The role of these muscles in providing increased pelvic stability is not fully understood. Excitation of the pudendal nerve causes reflex bladder relaxation via two reflex arcs: (1) the pelvic floor efferents (parasympathetic) cause bladder inhibition at high urethral pressures and (2) the hypogastric efferents (sympathetic) cause bladder inhibition at low urethral pressures [4].

For these reasons pelvic floor rehabilitation has been advocated to treat both stress and urge incontinence. Pelvic floor contraction prior to an increase

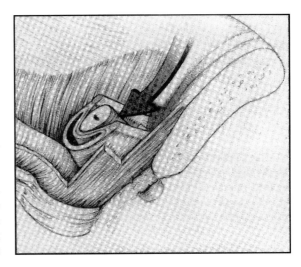

Figure 25.1 The hammock hypothesis: Lateral view of pelvic floor with urethra, vagina and fascial tissues transected at level of vesical neck drawn from three-dimensional reconstruction indicating compression of urethra by downward force (arrow) against supportive tissues indicating influence of abdominal pressure on urethra (arrow). (From DeLancey J (1994) Structural support of the urethra as it relates to stress urinary incontinence: The hammock hypothesis. Am J Obstet Gynecol 170:1713–23.)

in abdominal pressure will increase urethral closure pressure and thereby maintain continence at times of stress. Pelvic floor contraction will reinforce bladder inhibitory reflexes causing bladder relaxation, thereby decreasing urge incontinence. If the bladder still contracts, leaking may be further minimized by working against a higher pressure urethra.

Different regimens of pelvic floor exercises have been developed. As the levator ani is a striated muscle, composed of a combination of slow twitch (type I) and fast twitch (type II) fibers, it follows the same training principles as any striated muscle. Depending on the intensity, frequency and load of exercise, the pelvic floor will respond with muscle fiber hypertrophy and increased fiber recruitment. Most of the improvement will be seen in the early treatment phase and depend on baseline muscle strength and endurance. This early improvement is due to more effective recruitment of motor units [5] brought about by increased awareness. Further increase in strength is seen by muscle hypertrophy and requires a longer period of exercise. For these reasons, exercise should be maintained for 15 to 20 weeks to provide adequate evaluation [6].

Since Kegel first described the importance of exercising the pelvic floor through biofeedback [7] other methods have been advocated; ranging from simple verbal and written instructions, to physiotherapy, vaginal cones and functional electrical stimulation. These methods are all aimed at strengthening the pelvic floor. The merits and successes of these therapies will be further discussed.

Simple Instruction

Simple verbal and written instructions for exercising the pelvic floor are often given as the sole conservative treatment for GSI (genuine stress incontinence). Unfortunately Bo et al. [8] showed that 31.7% of women could not contract the levator ani muscle after simple verbal instruction. Bump et al. [9] showed that 25% of women actually promoted incontinence with their efforts. Since awareness of the pelvic floor is not taught with simple instruction, this group of women cannot be expected to exercise successfully.

After 3 months, 6% (3–13%) of women reported being completely dry and 31% (18–54%) were significantly improved with simple instructions (Table 25.1). This low success rate has led women to seek other treatment modalities.

Physiotherapy and Biofeedback

Exercising the pelvic floor under supervision of a physiotherapist allows a woman to gain awareness of the pelvic floor and improve her ability to contract it. A successful program will follow muscle training physiology. A minimum of 8–10 exercises, sustained for 6–8 seconds, with 8–12 repetitions to fatigue, two times a week is recommended [6]. The motivation of the woman and the enthusiasm of the physiotherapist are the key to any successful program [10]. Adherence to the exercise regime will provide optimal results. Unfortunately, over time compliance decreases. Hahn et al. [11] showed that after 2 years, 15% of women continued to follow the exercise program prescribed initially, while 6% did not exercise at all. Glavind et al. [12] reported 50% of women were still "exercising regularly" after 2 years following a physiotherapy program.

Studies have only addressed the role of physiotherapy to correct GSI. After 3 months of training the average subjective cure rate is 21% (9–36%) while the significant improvement rate is 69% (55–85%) (Table 25.1) Only two studies [11,12] have assessed women beyond 2 years, with a combined cure rate of 8% (0–9%) and significant improvement rate of 40% (20–42%).

To improve the success rate, biofeedback has been advocated. Auditory or visual representation of pelvic floor recruitment allows increased awareness and facilitates learning (Figure 25.2). This is accomplished by placing a probe in the vagina or rectum. During exercise, the probe is squeezed and this increased pressure is translated into a graphic cue. Learning and motivation is improved by providing direct, immediate feedback on the effort. The overall 3-month success rate is 29% (15–55%) and improvement rate 78% (68–95%) (Table 25.1). After 2 years the success rate remains high at 26% with a 42% improvement rate [12]. This difference in success compared to physiotherapy may result from the fact that only 50% of women with physiotherapy alone were still exercising the pelvic floor after 2 years compared with 89% of women who initially had biofeedback [12]. Randomized trials comparing biofeedback and physiotherapy show that biofeedback is superior: success rate 22% (16/73) versus 15% (11/74) and significant improvement rate 79% (58/73) versus 66% (49/74) at 3 months [13–15]. Biofeedback shows increased promise especially in the early treatment period [15]. This allows increased awareness of the pelvic floor and therefore improved muscle recruitment.

Heterogeneity amongst the different studies has not allowed a standardized approach to be devel-

Table 25.1 Subjective results following 3 months of treatment for genuine stress incontinence

Author	Simple instruction		Physiotherapy		Biofeedback		Vaginal cones		FES[a]	
	Cure	Improv[b]	Cure	Improv	Cure	Improv	Cure	Improv	Cure	Improv
Kujansu [20]	3/24	13/24								
Burgio [13]			1/11	6/11	2/13	12/13				
Plevnik [31]									25/80	38/80
Klarskov [45]			3/24	17/24						
Wilson [46]	–	4/15			–	11/15				
Henalla [47]			–	39/58						
Olah [25]							4/24	19/24		
Bent (4)									1/14	10/14
Tapp [52]			4/21	13/21						
Moore [29]							6/10	7/10		
Don Wilson [50]							–	16/34		
Castleden [48]					–	14/19				
Peattie [24]							–	21/29		
Lagro-Janssen [19]			7/33	28/33						
Cammu [49]			12/52	38/52						
Kato [28]							–	21/30		
Elia [16]			13/36	20/36						
Hahn [11]			39/170	120/170						
Burns [14]	1/39	7/39	7/43	26/43	9/40	27/40				
Wrigley [26]							4/14	8/14		
Sand [36]									0/35	13/35
Glavind [12]	3/20	–	11/20	–						
Luber [32]									2/20	5/20
Wilson [51]									–	11/30
Yamanishi [37]									8/25	19/25
Berghmans [15]			3/20	17/20	5/20	19/20				
Total	4/63	24/78	92/430	324/468	27/93	83/107	14/48	92/151	36/174	96/204
Percentage	6%	31%	21%	69%	29%	78%	29%	61%	21%	47%
Range (%)	(3–13)	(18–54)	(9–36)	(55–85)	(15–55)	(68–95)	(17–60)	(47–79)	(6–17)	(18–29)

[a] Functional electrical stimulation.
[b] >50% improvement in leaking or not requiring further treatment (includes cure).

oped. For example; physiotherapy has been prescribed for three 30-minute sessions a week for 4 weeks in one study [15] compared to one 1.5 hour session every 2 weeks for 6 weeks in another [16]. Continued pelvic floor contractions range from 8 to 12 daily contractions [17] to ten contractions every hour [18]. Lagro-Janssen [19] found a direct correlation between decreased incontinent episodes and women who performed more than 50 contractions a day. Therefore the most important factor for successful treatment is the motivation of the woman and her continued participation in the exercise program [11].

Although therapy may be successful, the urodynamic changes before and after treatment have been conflicting. Increases in maximal urethral closure pressure have been reported [16,18], while others have failed to demonstrate this [14,20]. Functional

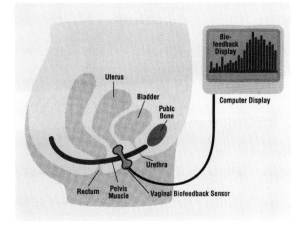

Figure 25.2 Biofeedback: Visual representation of pelvic floor recruitment. (Courtesy of Medtronic of Canada, Mississauga, Ontario, Canada.)

urethral length also shows inconsistent change [14,16,20].

There are no factors that can predict who will respond to pelvic floor exercises [19–21]. Age, parity, degree or duration of incontinence, prolapse and psychological features are not predictive [21]. Elia and Bergman [16] showed that a pressure transmission ratio of greater than 80% had a 90% positive predictive value for success. No other urodynamic parameters have been predictive.

Despite differences in therapy prescription it is reasonable to accept that both physiotherapy and biofeedback provide a low-risk alternative for the treatment of GSI. By increasing pelvic floor awareness and/or motivation, biofeedback appears to be somewhat superior to physiotherapy alone in increasing success in the short and long term.

Vaginal Cones

The ancient Chinese used "stone eggs" to strengthen the pelvic floor and improve sexual satisfaction [22]. Plevnik in 1985 [23] introduced vaginal cones to strengthen the pelvic floor and treat GSI. The cones are similarly shaped but have varying weights (Figure 25.3). The cones are placed in the vagina above the levator plate. Theoretically, the pelvic floor contracts to prevent the cones from slipping out. This immediate sensory biofeedback improves both awareness and strength of the pelvic floor. The program begins with the maximum passive weight, i.e.: the heaviest weight that can be held for one minute without pelvic floor contraction. The most commonly prescribed regimen consists of 15-minute sessions, twice a day [24–26]. Once a weight can be held on two separate occasions then the woman progresses to a heavier weight [24–26]. The weights vary from 20 g to 100 g.

After a 3-month session the average cure rate is 29% (17–60%) and the significant improvement rate is 61% (47–79%) (Table 25.1). Olah et al. [25] found that the cure rate from 3 to 6 months increased from 17% (4/24) to 42% (10/24) while the improvement rate remained unchanged at 79% (19/24) versus 71% (17/24). No long-term results have been published.

Vaginal cones have been criticized for not following basic muscle training philosophies [27]. It is felt that prolonged isometric exercises can cause muscle ischemia and therefore muscle damage [27]. Depending on the vaginal shape and degree of prolapse, the cones may not be held appropriately [25]. The cones cannot be used by 13% (9/69) of women because of discomfort or a narrow vagina [25]. The drop-out rate due to discomfort and irritation ranges from 10% [28] to 27% [25]. Despite these criticisms the short-term results compare favorably with the other treatment modalities (Table 25.1). In addition, cone therapy is easily taught and can be practiced in privacy without the need of a physiotherapist. As with other pelvic floor training modalities, motivation is critical to insure ongoing success [29].

Functional Electrical Stimulation

Stimulation of the pudendal nerve by electrical impulses causes contraction of the levator ani and activation of the inhibitory bladder reflex. Activation of the sacral autonomic reflex (S2–S4) causes bladder relaxation. This has been exploited to treat urge incontinence. Activation of the somatic part of the pudendal nerve causes somatic muscle contraction (external urethral sphincter and levator ani) and can be used to treat GSI. Functional electrical stimulation is accomplished through interferential therapy or faradism (direct nerve stimulation). Interferential therapy works by placing two electrodes on the abdomen and two on the inner thighs. Alternating currents interact to produce a low-frequency current at the point where they meet [25]. This method bypasses skin resistance. Owing to the cumbersome nature of the application, this method is not used as often as faradism. Electrical stimulation to the pudendal nerve is best obtained when the electrodes are placed in close proximity to the nerve trunk. As the nerve courses around the ischial spine it is easily accessible by vaginal or anal probe

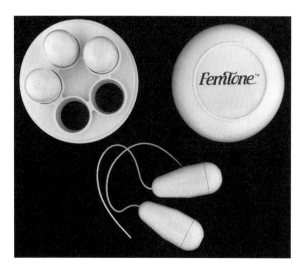

Figure 25.3 Example of a set of vaginal cones. (Courtesy of Femtone, ConvaTec North Pacific, a Bristol-Myers-Squibb Company, Princeton, NJ.)

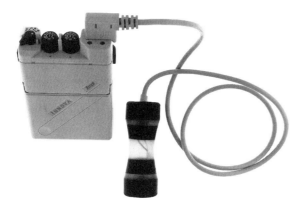

Figure 25.4 Example of a portable functional electrical stimulation device. (Courtesy of Innovative Outcome Solutions, Laguna Hills, CA.)

(Figure 25.4). The placement of the probe is essential in providing optimal stimulation: the closer to the nerve trunk the more specific the action. A partially innervated pelvic floor is required but the central nervous system does not need to be intact. Therefore functional electrical stimulation provides a passive muscle contraction not requiring active conscious control.

The optimal parameters for stimulation have not yet been clearly defined. Frequencies of 50–100 Hz are required to achieve maximal urethral closure by contracting the external sphincter and the levators [30]. Meanwhile, frequencies of 5–10 Hz have provided reflex bladder inhibition [30]. Functional electrical stimulation can thus be used to treat GSI (high frequencies, high amperage) and urge incontinence (low frequencies, moderate amperage) depending on the parameters used. With mixed symptoms two strategies have been employed: (1) a compromised frequency of 20 Hz or (2) alternating low and high frequencies [30]. Both intermittent and continual stimulation have been advocated. With intermittent stimulation the probes are used for 15–20 minutes once or twice a day [30–32]. A carry-over effect allows for less therapy time. Seigel et al. [33] were unable to show a difference between daily and every-other-day treatment for urge and mixed incontinence. Continual stimulation requires the probes to be held for as long as possible (6–8 hours a day) [34]. This stimulation occurs below sensory threshold. Short-term electrical stimulation is more popular and increases compliance [35].

When used for less than 3 months for the treatment of GSI the overall cure rate is 21% (0–32%) and the significant improvement rate is 47% (25–76%) (Table 25.1). This compares to an 11% (6/54) cure rate and 24% (13/54) improvement rate with a sham device [32,36,37]. The sham device may improve incontinence by working as a "vaginal cone" [32]. Two studies have followed patients up to one year with a cure rate of 11% and improvement rate of 68% [38,39]. Eriksen and Eik-Nes [34] reported a 36% cure rate and 56% improvement rate after more than 2 years of treatment.

When combined with physiotherapy, the 3-month cure rate is 6% (1/18) and the improvement rate is 89% (16/18) [40]. Although the study had few patients, this treatment regime may be superior to functional electrical stimulation alone. The belief is that the pelvic floor muscles are "jump started" in women unable to perform the exercises [32]. Since voluntary pelvic floor muscle contraction increases urethral closure pressure by approximately 10 cmH$_2$O more than by vaginal electrical stimulation only [41], additional benefit should be seen with active pelvic floor exercises.

Functional electrical stimulation is the only pelvic floor treatment modality which has been evaluated for the treatment of urge incontinence. The 3-month cure rate is 27% (10–30%) and the improvement rate is 57% (49–70%) [4,31,33,42]. The success remains high at 30% (22–33%) and the improvement is 73% (72–73%) up to one year after initiation of treatment. When Smith [39] compared functional electrical stimulation to propantheline bromide, it was found to be superior, with a cure rate of 22% (4/18) versus 15% (3/20) and improvement rate of 72% (13/18) versus 50% (10/20).

The results for women with mixed incontinence are very similar: success 23% (0–28%) and improvement 49% (47–64%) [4,31,33]. Sand [43] studied a cohort of women with mixed incontinence and a low pressure urethra. In this difficult-to-treat group of women, the cure rate was 8% (2/26) and improvement rate was 27% (7/26).

Functional electrical stimulation is a passive treatment and therefore does not require the same motivation as physiotherapy or biofeedback. The treatments can be unsupervised and done in private once instructions are given and understood. The initial drop-out rate is approximately 20% [32,38]. Home devices have been marketed to make this treatment modality widely accessible. Despite different treatment protocols, functional electrical stimulation has been successfully used to treat GSI urge incontinence and mixed incontinence. For the treatment of GSI, the results are more conflicting with wider variations amongst the studies than with other treatment modalities (Table 25.1). When combined with active muscle contraction the improvement is increased. This results from passive contractions being less powerful then active contractions. The reflex sacral arc is stimulated at lower frequency and does not require somatic muscle contraction. For urge incontinence the success is similar or superior to behavioral and medical therapy with the advantage of having minimal to no side effects. This has made functional electrical stimulation very attractive for the treatment of urge incontinence.

Conclusion

Pelvic floor rehabilitation is important in managing genuine stress incontinence. In the short term, no therapy appears to be greatly superior to the others (Table 25.1). This is seen despite the heterogeneity amongst the different studies. Long-term studies are few but provide encouraging results. "Demand for use is the most important factor in restoring functional capacity of any skeletal muscle."[7]. Therefore any successful rehabilitation program requires ongoing participation. The motivation of the woman is the most important factor to ensure success [11,12,29]. This is partially dependent on the physiotherapist or caregiver involved in her care. Continued exercise is crucial for success: the specific therapy prescribed is important in maximizing the pelvic floor performance, but will only work if the program is followed. A decrease in motivation to exercise the pelvic floor may explain why different exercise modalities have similar outcomes.

A successful program will result in a woman regaining autonomy of her pelvic floor [44]. This requires (1) evaluation and assessment of the pelvic floor, (2) training awareness of the pelvic floor so that it can be under voluntary control, (3) improving strength and endurance of the pelvic floor muscles and (4) teaching muscle recruitment at times of need (stress and urge) [44]. For these reasons simple verbal or written information is insufficient. If a woman is able to contract her pelvic floor, she may benefit from physiotherapy alone. However, if she is unable to isolate the pelvic floor muscles, awareness can be achieved through the use of biofeedback, vaginal cones or functional electrical stimulation. If the muscles are very weak then functional electrical stimulation may help initiate recruitment and "jump start" the muscles [32]. Any program should therefore provide supervised pelvic floor exercises and have the ability to individualize the program to suit the needs of a woman.

Functional electrical stimulation has proved to be superior to propantheline bromide in treating urge incontinence [39]. It appears similar or superior to medical and behavioral therapy. There are minimal side effects and it is acceptable to most patients [38]. Because of the "carry-over effect" stimulation may not be required as often as previously prescribed

[33]. This would provide increased compliance and ongoing participation. Other pelvic floor rehabilitation programs have not been evaluated although Moore and Metcalf [29] showed two of four patients cured with the use of vaginal cones.

Although exercising the pelvic floor has been advocated since Kegel first described it in 1948 [7], it has not yet been critically evaluated. Long-term, randomized trials are required to further evaluate and optimize the role of different pelvic floor rehabilitation programs in the treatment of GSI and urge incontinence. However, the success of this low risk, non-invasive conservative approach cannot be overlooked. Despite a lower success rate than surgery for GSI, 2 years after a physiotherapy program 42% of women had declined surgical intervention [45]. The success cannot be predicted by age, parity, severity or duration of incontinence [19–21]. Therefore pelvic floor exercises should be prescribed for every woman presenting with stress and/or urge incontinence.

References

1. DeLancey J. Structural support of the urethra as it relates to stress urinary incontinence: The hammock hypothesis. Am J Obstet Gynecol 1994;170:1713–23.
2. Trontelj JV, Janko M, Godec C et al. Electrical stimulation for urinary incontinence: A neurophysiologic study. Urol Int 1974;29:213–20.
3. Bo K. Pelvic floor muscle exercise for the treatment of stress urinary incontinence: An exercise physiology perspective. Int Urogynecol J 1995;6:282–91.
4. Bent AE, Sand PK, Ostergard DR, Brubaker LT. Transvaginal electrical stimulation in the treatment of genuine stress incontinence and detrusor instability. Int Urogynecol J 1993;4:9–13.
5. Norton P. Treatment of stress urinary incontinence. In: Schussler B, Laycock J, Norton P, Stanton S, editors. Pelvic Floor Re-Education. London: Springer-Verlag, 1994.
6. American College of Sports Medicine. The recommended quantity and quality of exercise for developing and maintaining cardiorespiratory and muscular fitness in healthy adults. Med Sci Sports Exerc 1990;22:265–74.
7. Kegel AH. Progressive resistance exercise in the functional restoration of the perineal muscles. Am J Obstet Gynecol 1948;56(2):238–48.
8. Bo K, Larsen S, Oseid S, Kvarstein B, Hagen R, Jorgensen J. Knowledge about and ability to correct pelvic floor muscle exercises in women with urinary stress incontinence. Neurourol Urodyn 1988;7(3):261–2.
9. Bump RC, Hurt WG, Fantl JA, Wyman JF. Assessment of Kegel pelvic muscle exercise performance after brief verbal instruction. Am J Obstet Gynecol 1991;165:322–9.
10. Brown C. Pelvic floor rehabilitation: Conservative treatment for incontinence. Ostomy/Wound Manage 1998;44(6):72–6.
11. Hahn I, Milsom I, Fall M, Ekelund P. Long-term results of pelvic floor training in female stress urinary incontinence. Br J Urol 1993;72:421–7.
12. Glavind K, Nohr SB, Walter S. Biofeedback and physiotherapy versus physiotherapy alone in the treatment of genuine stress urinary incontinence. Int Urogynecol J 1996;7:339–43.

13. Burgio K, Robinson JC, Engel BT. The role of biofeedback in Kegel exercise training for stress urinary incontinence. Am J Obstet Gynecol 1986;154:58–64.

14. Burns PA, Pranikoff K, Nochajski TH, Hadley EC, Levy KJ, Ory MG. A comparison of effectiveness of biofeedback and pelvic muscle exercise treatment of stress incontinence in older community-dwelling women. J Gerontol 1993;48:167–74.

15. Berghmans LCM, Frederiks CMA, de Bie RA et al. Efficacy of biofeedback, when included with pelvic floor muscle exercise treatment, for genuine stress incontinence. Neurourol Urodyn 1996;15:37–52.

16. Elia G, Bergman A. Pelvic muscle exercises: When do they work? Obstet Gynecol 1993;81:283–6.

17. Bo K. Physical activity, fitness and bladder control. In: Bouchard C, Shephard RJ, Stephens T, editors. Physical Activity, Fitness and Health. Champaign, IL: Human Kinetics Publishers, 1994; 774–95.

18. Benvenuti F, Caputo GM, Bandinelli S, Mayer F, Biagini C, Sommavilla A. Reeducative treatment of female genuine stress incontinence. Am J Phys Med 1987;66(4):155–68.

19. Lagro-Janssen T, Debruyne F, Smits A, Van Weel C. Controlled trial of pelvic floor exercises in the treatment of urinary stress incontinence in general practice. Br J Gen Pract 1991;41:445–9.

20. Kujansuu E. The effect of pelvic floor exercises on urethral function in female stress urinary incontinence and urodynamic study. Ann Chirurg Gynaecol 1983;72:28–32.

21. Theofrastous JP, Wyman JF, Bump RC et al. Relationship between urethral and vaginal pressures during pelvic muscle contraction. Neurourol Urodyn 1997;16:553–8.

22. Chia M, Chia M. Cultivating Female Sexual Energy, vol. 9. New York: Healing Tao Books, 1987; 180–204.

23. Plevnik S. New method for testing and strengthening of pelvic floor muscles. Proceedings of the 15th Annual General Meeting, International Continence Society, 1985; 267–8.

24. Peattie AB, Plevnik S, Stanton SL. Vaginal cones: A conservative method of treating genuine stress incontinence. Br J Obstet Gynaecol 1988;95:1049–53.

25. Olah KS, Bridges N, Denning J, Farrar DJ. The conservative management of patients with symptoms of stress incontinence: A randomized, prospective study comparing weighted vaginal cones and interferential therapy. Am J Obstet Gynecol 1990;162:87–92.

26. Wrigley T. The effect of training with vaginal weighted cones and pelvic floor exercises on the strength of the pelvic floor muscles: A pilot study. Int Urogynecol J 1995;6:4–9.

27. Bo K. Vaginal weight cones. Theoretical framework, effect on pelvic floor muscle strength and female stress urinary incontinence. Acta Obstet Gynecol Scand 1995;74:87–92.

28. Kato K, Kondo A, Hasegawa S et al. Pelvic floor muscle training as treatment of stress incontinence. The effectiveness of vaginal cones. Jpn J Urol 1992;83:498–504.

29. Moore K, Metcalfe JB. Effectiveness of vaginal cones in treatment of urinary incontinence. Urol Nurse 1992;12(2):69–72.

30. Appell RA. Electrical stimulation for the treatment of urinary incontinence. Urology 1998;51 (s 2A):24–6.

31. Plevnik S, Janez J, Vrtacnik P, Trsinar B, Vodusek DB. Short-term electrical stimulation: Home treatment for urinary incontinence. World J Urol 1986;4:24–6.

32. Luber KM, Wolde-Tsadik G. Efficacy of functional electrical stimulation in treating genuine stress incontinence: A randomized clinical trial. Neurourol Urodyn 1997;16:543–51.

33. Siegel SW, Richardson DA, Miller KL et al. Pelvic floor electrical stimulation for the treatment of urge and mixed urinary incontinence in women. Urology 1997;50:934–40.

34. Eriksen BC, Eik-Nes SH. Long-term electrostimulation of the pelvic floor: Primary therapy in female stress incontinence? Urol Int 1989;44:90–5.

35. Bourcier AP, Juras JC. Nonsurgical therapy for stress incontinence. Urol Clin North Am 1995;22:613–27.

36. Sand PK, Richardson DA., Staskin DR et al. Pelvic floor electrical stimulation in the treatment of genuine stress incontinence: A multicenter, placebo-controlled trial. Am J Obstet Gynecol 1995;173:72–9.

37. Yamanishi T, Yasuda K, Sakakibara R, Hattori T, Ito H, Murakami S. Pelvic Floor Electrical Stimulation in the treatment of stress incontinence: An investigational study and a placebo controlled double-blind trial. J Urol 1997;158:2127–31.

38. Fall M, Ahlstrom K, Carlsson C et al. Pelvic floor stimulation for female stress-urge incontinence. Urology 1986;27(3):282–7.

39. Smith JJ. Intravaginal stimulation randomized trial. J Urol 1996;155:127–30.

40. Meyer S, Dhenin T, Schmidt N, De Grandi P. Subjective and objective effects of intravaginal electrical myostimulation and biofeedback in patients with genuine stress urinary incontinence. Br J Urol 1992;69:584–8.

41. Bo K, Talseth T. Change in urethral pressure during voluntary pelvic floor muscle contraction and vaginal electrical stimulation. Int Urogynecol J 1997;8:3–7.

42. Brubaker L, Benson JT, Bent A, Clark A., Shott S. Transvaginal electrical stimulation for female urinary incontinence. Am J Obstet Gynecol 1997;177:536–40.

43. Sand P. Pelvic floor stimulation in the treatment of mixed incontinence complicated by a low-pressure urethra. Obstet Gynecol 1996;88:757–60.

44. Schussler B, Prince S. Concept of an individualised combined pelvic floor re-education programme. In: Schussler B, Laycock J, Norton P, Stanton S, editors. Pelvic Floor Re-education. London: Springer-Verlag, 1994; 169–75.

45. Klarskov P, Belvind D, Bischoff N et al. Pelvic floor exercise versus surgery for female urinary stress incontinence. Urology 1986;42:129–32.

46. Wilson PD, Al Samarrai T, Deakin M, Kolbe E, Brown ADG. An objective assessment of physiotherapy for female genuine stress incontinence. Br J Obstet Gynaecol 1987;94:575–82.

47. Henalla SM, Kirwan P, Castleden CM, Hutchins CJ, Breeson AJ. The effect of pelvic floor exercises in the treatment of genuine urinary stress incontinence in women at two hospital. Br J Obstet Gynaecol 1988;95:602–6.

48. Castleden CM, Duffin HM, Mitchell EP. The effect of physiotherapy on stress incontinence. Age Ageing 1984;13:235–7.

49. Cammu H, Van Nylen M, Derde M, DeBruyne R, Amy J. Pelvic physiotherapy in genuine stress incontinence. Urology 1991;38(4):332–7.

50. Don Wilson P, Borland M. Vaginal cones for the treatment of genuine stress incontinence. Aust NZ J Obstet Gynaecol 1990;30:157–60.

51. Wilson PD, George M, Imrie JJ. Vaginal electrostimulation for the treatment of genuine stress incontinence. Aust NZ J Obstet Gynaecol 1997;37:446–9.

52. Tapp AJS, Hills B, Cardozo LD. Randomised study comparing pelvic floor physiotherapy with the Burch colposuspension. Neurourol Urodyn 1989;8:356–7.

26 Supportive Devices

Cathy Flood and Lesley-Ann Hanson

Pessaries

Pessaries were developed many centuries ago to manage troublesome genital prolapse in an era when surgical management was not an option. In 1867, according to the American Medical Association, there were 123 types of pessaries available [1]. During the last century, the improved safety of surgical intervention for the treatment of prolapse resulted in the decline of pessary use. Pessaries were even viewed as dangerous as they were known to cause the occasional fistula when left unattended. Pessaries are currently experiencing a rebirth in both design and in indications for use. Pessaries and related supportive devices are now viewed as an excellent conservative management alternative for the treatment of urinary incontinence and pelvic floor prolapse, as well as a useful diagnostic tool to determine the appropriate surgical procedure for pelvic floor reconstruction.

Historical Perspective

Pessaries are some of the oldest known medical devices. Conservative means previously used to correct uterine prolapse included repositioning, douches, salves and concoctions, herbal therapy, leeching, sitz baths, abdominal supports with or without vaginal attachments, and pessaries of multiple shapes and materials. The first mention in literature of the oval and ring pessaries was in the late sixteenth century. Pessaries fashioned from wood, leather, glass, ivory, sea sponges, fabric, whalebone, metal, rubber, plastics, and purified dried latex (from trees) have been discovered [2]. A cone-shaped bronze vaginal pessary was found among the ruins of Pompeii. Brass, gold and silver inventions were held in place by a waist belt [3]. Pessaries achieved a peak of popularity in the 1800s when uterine retroversion was believed to be the cause of multiple gynecological "evils" including menorrhagia and infertility. The ring, Smith, and Hodge pessaries were developed to correct this condition [4,5].

Most pessaries currently available are of medical grade silicone construction. The advantages of silicone include a long shelf life, the lack of odor absorption, the ability to be autoclaved or boiled, and the non-allergic nature. A wide range of sizes and shapes are available (Figure 26.1).

Indications for Pessary Use

Genital Prolapse

All types and stages of genital prolapse can potentially be managed with pessaries. There is a prevailing myth that pessaries are not useful if the prolapse is large, or if the uterus is absent [6]. In reality, vaginal vault prolapse can be very successfully managed with a pessary, and degree of prolapse is irrelevant. In these patients a Gellhorn or Shaatz pessary may be more successful than a ring. Pessaries are the only treatment options for the patient who desires a non-surgical option for prolapse. They are an alternative for the patient who is a high surgical risk, desires more children, has to put off surgery for personal reasons or is on a waiting list for surgery.

Urinary Incontinence

Pessaries are a relatively new conservative option for the treatment of urinary incontinence [7]. There are several pessary styles available specifically designed for this purpose (Figure 26.2). These are useful not only for the woman with a presenting complaint of incontinence, but also for the woman

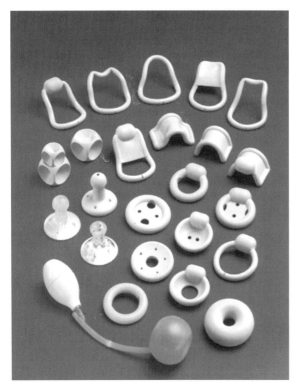

Figure 26.1 Pessary devices available from Milex Products Inc. (Courtesy of Milex Products Inc., Chicago, Illinois.)

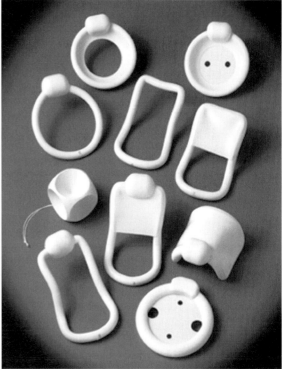

Figure 26.2 Incontinence devices available from Milex Products Inc. (Courtesy of Milex Products Inc., Chicago, Illinois.)

who develops stress incontinence once her prolapse is reduced by more traditional pessaries. The incontinence dish and the incontinence ring are useful devices for these purposes. One of the more recent and surprising discoveries is that urgency incontinence can often be successfully managed with a pessary. In a review of patients who experienced both incontinence and prolapse 12 out of the 18 (67%) experiencing urgency incontinence had successful relief with a pessary. Pessaries corrected 17 of 28 (61.5%) with stress incontinence. This was prior to the introduction of the devices specifically designed for incontinence [6]. The addition of these designs to a pessary armamentarium will likely improve these statistics. Pessaries may alleviate stress and urge incontinence by elevating the bladder neck. A urodynamic evaluation of women with stress incontinence relieved after placement of a pessary resulted in an increase in urethral closure pressure and functional urethral length, and diminished the mobility of the urethra and urethrovesical junction without causing obstruction [8].

Preoperative Diagnosis

A number of researchers have proposed the use of the pessary as a preoperative assessment tool. Stress incontinence develops in up to 22% of patients after vaginal surgery for genital prolapse [9,10]. Pessaries are useful in reduction of prolapse to assess for the development of underlying stress incontinence, undetected prior to reduction by the obstructive effect of the prolapse. In a group of 70 continent women with prolapse, 27% developed stress incontinence after insertion of a pessary. The detection of "latent incontinence" often changes the surgical procedure offered with the addition of an anti-incontinence operation to the procedure of choice for prolapse management [11].

Pessaries can help predict whether urgency incontinence will be relieved after surgery. In the woman with mixed stress incontinence, the relief of overactive bladder symptoms with pessary support may indicate that bladder neck stability with surgery may give a positive result. Pessaries are also useful in predicting whether surgery will correct problems such as pelvic and back pain, which may be due to prolapse. Urodynamic evaluation done with and without a pessary in place can also help to determine which surgical approach is optimal. However, patients must be counseled that surgery may not achieve the same effect as the pessary.

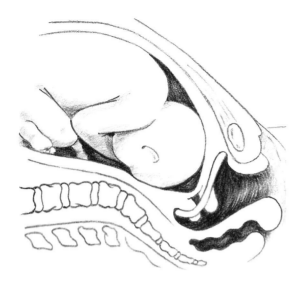

Figure 26.3 Lever pessary in place during pregnancy to direct the cervix posteriorly as in a normal pregnancy. (Courtesy of Milex Products Inc., Chicago, Illinois.)

Pregnancy

The woman who develops prolapse or disabling incontinence during pregnancy can safely wear a pessary for symptom control. Uterine prolapse in pregnancy can be associated with the complications of cervical ulceration, infection, and uterine rupture [3]. It is essential to check the post-void residual after the fitting of a pregnant woman. The patient may require several different sizes as her pregnancy progresses.

Uterine incarceration is a rare complication in pregnancy. The retroverted uterus becomes trapped in the sacral hollow as the uterus enlarges. Insertion of the Hodge pessary prior to 15 weeks may prevent a recurrence in subsequent pregnancies [12]. The prevention of habitual abortion due to the incompetent cervix is another potential use for the pessary. Insertion is at 14 weeks with removal at 38 weeks. Pessaries have not been compared to cervical cerclage in a clinical trial, but may be an alternative for the patient who cannot be treated with cerclage [5]. Reported success rates for both the Hodge and Smith pessaries in the alleviation of cervical incompetence range up to 86%. These lever pessaries direct the cervix posterior and reduce pressure on the cervix [3] (Figure 26.3).

Other Uses

Uterine retroversion was one of the most popular indications for pessary use in the 1950s. It was felt that 50% of women with retroversion had symptoms due to this condition. A pessary to correct retroversion relieved abdominal and back pain in 75%, dys-

menorrhea in 60%, menstrual disorders, abortion and infertility in 10%, and endometriosis in 75% [13]. The modern use of the pessary for these conditions has not been explored, as retroversion is not currently recognized as a condition requiring treatment.

Pessary Fitting

One of the reasons physicians avoid the pessary is a lack of familiarity with their fitting and management. From a survey done in 1993, only half of the senior residents in Obstetrics and Gynecology programs across Canada had ever seen or fitted a pessary [14]. The manufacturers' guidelines for pessary fitting, care and follow-up are quite time-consuming and, if followed to the letter, costly to the health care system. In clinical practice, practitioners use more relaxed guidelines, which have been evaluated and published [15]. Limiting factors are time and cost. Most private practitioners cannot afford the time it takes to fit and evaluate properly nor afford to have an unlimited number of pessaries in their office for a patient to try before purchasing. Most provinces do not currently have a separate fee for pessary fitting.

To size a pessary properly, the index and middle fingers are inserted into the vagina. The fingers are spread into the fornices and the diameter and depth estimated. The covered ring pessary with corresponding diameter is a good initial choice for prolapse. It is successful in correcting most types of prolapse and is simple for the patient and caregiver to remove and insert. If the rings are unsuccessful for prolapse then the Shaatz or Gellhorn pessaries can be tried. These pessaries are particularly helpful in the patient presenting with post-hysterectomy vault prolapse. With the Gellhorn, removal usually needs to be done by a caregiver or health care professional. If there is stress or urge incontinence associated with the prolapse, or if the pessary is being used primarily for urinary incontinence, an incontinence ring or dish is the pessary of choice.

The following is an explanation of the fitting of the covered ring (this can be modified slightly to fit most other types of pessaries). With the patient supine, in lithotomy position, the examiner's non-dominant hand separates the labia. Lubricant is placed at the insertion point of the pessary. The pessary is inserted folded, and kept folded, until the pessary is well into the vagina. It is then tilted so that the anterior portion is behind the symphysis pubis (Figures 26.4 and 26.5). If the patient has a uterus, the ring should be below the cervix in the posterior fornix. A quarter turn once the pessary is in place helps to prevent the pessary from dislodg-

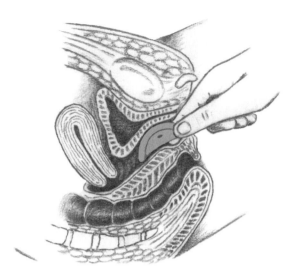

Figure 26.4   Insertion of the Ring with Support pessary. (Courtesy of Milex Products Inc., Chicago, Illinois.)

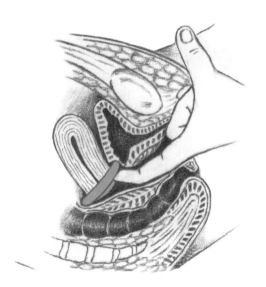

Figure 26.5   Ring with Support pessary in place. (Courtesy of Milex Products Inc., Chicago, Illinois.)

ing. For the appropriate fit, there should be approximately a finger's-breadth of room between the vaginal walls and the device. The patient is then asked to perform a Valsalva maneuver. If the pessary stays in place, the patient is asked to walk around to determine comfort. Assessing the correct size is fairly simple: if the pessary hurts or is noticeable by the patient, it is the wrong shape or too big; if it falls

out, it is the wrong shape or too small. The patient should then void and have a post-void residual checked to ensure that this is less than 100 cc or one-third of voided volume. The patient is reassessed within a short time. There are no ideal guidelines for reassessment, but between 24 hours and 2 weeks is reasonable. This allows the patient to try out the pessary with her usual activity pattern to see if it is comfortable and corrects the problem. Sometimes several reassessments and fittings are necessary until the ideal device is found. Once the patient is fitted with the appropriate device, she can often be taught to insert and remove it.

Pessary Clinics

One of the difficulties with offering the pessary as a treatment option is having the availability of an appropriate range of pessary sizes and shapes to accommodate a wide range of pelvic shapes and associated pelvic dysfunction. A centralized, nurse-run clinic is an ideal solution. In Edmonton, we currently have such a system in operation. Gynecologists and family doctors screen the patients for suitability for pessary use and then refer the patient on to the clinic. The nurse assesses the patient and may recommend to the referring physician that local estrogen support (or alternative lubrication) be initiated prior to fitting. The nurse takes a focused history and examines the patient for sizing. Various pessaries are fitted until the pessary stays in place without discomfort. After voiding and having her post-void residual checked, the patient is sent home with instructions to phone if problems such as pain, bleeding, or difficulty voiding are encountered. The patient is re-examined within a week or two. If the pessary is effective, comfortable and no erosions are seen, the patient is instructed on removal, insertion, and care for the pessary or alternative arrangements are made for a caregiver to do it. For difficult cases, the on-site urogynecologist can review the patient for additional suggestions. When the patient is satisfied with the pessary for both comfort and treatment of the presenting complaint she purchases the pessary. Pessaries that are tried and found to be unsuitable are sterilized and used again.

A review was conducted of 1216 patients referred to the nurse-run pessary clinic at the Royal Alexandra Hospital in Edmonton, Alberta. The median age of the patients was 63 years (range 22–95). Gynecologists referred 41%, urogynecologists 35%, family physicians 21%, and nurse continence advisors 3%. The presenting diagnoses were 54% with prolapse, 30% with stress incontinence,

9% with mixed incontinence, and 6% with urgency incontinence. A median number of two pessary-fitting sessions were required (range 1–7). Successful pessary fitting was accomplished in 75% of patients with prolapse, 67% of patients with mixed incontinence, 64% of patients with stress incontinence and 58% of patients with urge incontinence. Of a subgroup of patients on both systemic and local hormone replacement therapies, 78% were successfully fitted. Also the addition of local estrogen appeared to be important to successful fitting, independent of the use of systemic estrogen. The incontinence dish, Shaatz and ring with support were the most frequently used pessaries found comfortable by the patients (L. Hanson, C. Flood, J. Schulz and B. Cooley, unpublished work).

Pessary Care and Follow-up

Prior to leaving the office, it is important to ensure the patient can properly empty her bladder. By history, she should not have to strain excessively to void. Objectively, she should have a low post-void residual, determined either by bladder scanner or in and out catheterization. Pessaries can lead to urinary retention and subsequent recurrent urinary tract infections. This has not been found to be a problem as long as the post-void residual is less than 100 cc. A patient may develop urinary retention after she leaves the office as the pessary may shift position during activity. The patient is informed prior to leaving the office of the possibility of this happening, with the subsequent need for urgent removal. Two important messages to emphasize to patients once successfully fitted are (1) the importance of regular removal and cleaning of the pessary with soap and water and (2) the necessity for regularly scheduled visits to the health care professional for vaginal examination. The frequency of pessary removal and cleaning varies depending on the patient's views on personal hygiene, the amount of vaginal discharge the patient experiences, the age of the patient, the need for removal for sexual intercourse, and the ease of removal. Some younger patients choose to remove the pessary nightly to allow the vagina to "rest". In this situation, once the patient is fitted properly and comfortable with the device, it is reasonable to have a visual inspection of the vagina annually during pelvic examination. The time frame between the removal and cleaning of a pessary in someone who cannot remove their own pessary is no more than 3 months. Women who develop erosions from the pessary require more frequent follow-up.

In an ideal situation, the patients, once successfully fitted, can be returned to their family physician with appropriate follow-up instructions. An excellent published regime recommends the following: initial follow-up in 2 weeks, subsequent follow-up after successful fitting every 3 months for the first year, and subsequent follow-up visits after the first year of successful visits, yearly [6]. At each visit the pessary is removed, washed with soap and water, and the vagina inspected for erosions. The patient is examined for proper fit as pessary shape and size requirements may change over time. Sterilization is not necessary if the pessary is being returned to the same patient. The pessary is then reinserted. Annual Pap smears should be done.

The perimenopausal and postmenopausal woman should be on some form of estrogen replacement if they are to wear a pessary. The added vaginal lubrication eases fitting and removal of the device. Estrogen also thickens the vaginal wall, increases elasticity and prevents erosions. Pessaries left in without estrogen support of the vagina can become embedded, making removal difficult if not impossible. In the patient who is reluctant to begin systemic hormone replacement, vaginal estrogen alone works well. Vaginal estrogen cream, 0.5–1 g into the vagina three times per week, is often enough to prevent erosions. In the woman who still has her uterus, higher doses of estrogen cream will likely require the addition of systemic progesterone every few months. The patient should be instructed to observe and report any vaginal bleeding, and the usual vaginal bleeding work-up initiated.

The estrogen ring, "Estring" (Pharmacia & Upjohn), which has minimal systemic absorption, is an alternative for the patient in whom systemic estrogen therapy is contraindicated. The estrogen ring is inserted first, with the pessary beneath it. The estrogen ring is changed every 3 months. In most patients, the Estring does not interfere with the fitting of the pessary. Currently, there is only one size available, which somewhat limits their use. Long-lasting lubricants such as Replens (Roberts Pharmaceutical), Gyne-Moistrin (Schering-Plough) or K-Y Long Lasting (Johnson & Johnson) can be substituted for local estrogen support if necessary.

Silicone pessaries can last for years before needing replacement. Discoloration is not an indication for replacement. As long as the device continues to provide symptomatic relief, it need not be exchanged. Patients have used the same device for 10 years or more. The postmenopausal woman, despite the use of estrogen, may experience vaginal and pelvic structure shrinkage and require a smaller size over time.

Basic Pessary Shapes

Ring Pessaries

Ring pessaries are available in open and covered forms. The covered forms have perforations for drainage. Rings work by replacing the pelvic diaphragm. A spring mechanism elevates the vagina above the pelvic outlet. The covered model helps protect against prolapse through the center of the ring. The Shaatz pessary is stiffer, adding more support, and a good alternative to try if the ring models fall out. The incontinence dish and incontinence ring pessaries have an elevated knob to support the bladder neck. They fit in a similar manner to the ring with the bladder neck support anterior in the midline. The incontinence ring is more flexible and easier to remove than the dish. The dish provides better overall support because of its shape and stiffness. Both pessaries work well for stress incontinence with or without intrinsic sphincter deficiency. If a patient develops stress incontinence after the insertion of a pessary that does not have bladder neck support, a switch to one of the incontinence pessaries may solve the problem.

Doughnut Pessaries

The silicone doughnut pessary works by taking up slack in the vagina and supporting the cervix. The design is meant for advanced uterine prolapse with accompanying cystocele and rectocele. It is inserted edgewise and then turned perpendicularly to the axis of the vagina. A variation on the doughnut is the Inflatoball pessary, suitable for a capacious vagina with a narrower pelvic outlet. The patient must deflate it daily for removal, which limits its practical use.

Stem Pessaries

The Gellhorn, or stem, pessary is often successful in correcting severe prolapse, particularly vaginal vault prolapse. This pessary cannot be used in the sexually active patient. The Gellhorn pessary works like the rings, but also creates suction between the pessary and the vaginal walls. The stem helps to keep the pessary from shifting position. To insert, the base is inserted parallel to the introitus, then rotated over the perineal body. To remove these pessaries, the suction must be released by inserting a finger between the base and the vaginal wall. Occasionally, a Kelly forceps is required to grasp the stem in order to assist removal. These pessaries can be difficult to remove and are often the "last resort". It is usually impossible for patients to remove these by themselves. The flexible silicone models have less chance of becoming impacted than the stiff lucite version.

Cube Pessaries

The cube pessary also works by suction. Each of the six sides is concave and functions as a suction cup on the vaginal wall. It is effective when other pessaries have failed because of inadequate pelvic tone. Original models that do not have drainage holes require daily removal for cleaning. A newer version has holes, which may decrease the suction ability but eliminates the need for daily removal. Removal requires breaking the suction by inserting a finger between the cube and the vaginal wall. There is a string attached to the cube to aid in removal. However, pulling on the string only increases the suction. If left in place too long, the odor can be foul. These pessaries may also work well for vault prolapse.

Lever Pessaries

The lever pessaries – Smith–Hodge, Hodge, Risser, and Gehrung – are all variations of Hodge's design from the 1860s [3]. The broad anterior part of the Hodge prevents urethral compression and pessary turning. The Smith has a narrower anterior end for the patient with a narrow suprapubic angle. The Risser is designed for a flatter pubic arch. To insert, the retroverted uterus is elevated and the pessary inserted folded until the posterior bar rests behind the cervix and the anterior bar behind the pubic arch. The anterior portion rests below the urethrovesical junction. Versions of the lever pessaries are now available to treat stress incontinence. An elevated bar or knob on the anterior part is designed for support of the bladder neck.

The Gerhung pessary is rarely used. Although also a lever pessary, it is designed for a cystocele and rectocele. It is inserted on its side and then rotated so the curved bar follows the vaginal curve. It resembles a covered bridge, and rests in the vagina with the cervix supported between two curved arches. When properly inserted, the back arch is in the anterior fornix and the front arches behind the symphysis, creating a "bladder bridge". It may be difficult to keep this pessary in position.

Pessary Trouble-shooting

Erosions

Erosions of the vaginal wall are a common problem. Erosions usually start as redness where the pessary is resting. If left untreated they may progress to actual ulceration. Diligent observation for erosions with early intervention is vital to pessary care. To prevent erosions, it is best if perimenopausal and menopausal women are offered local estrogen therapy, even if on systemic estrogen. This is particularly important if there is evidence of estrogen deficiency on vaginal examination or if the patient complains of vaginal dryness with intercourse. Ideally local estrogen therapy should be started several weeks before fitting, as this will prevent tearing and discomfort with multiple insertions and removals. A fit that is too big may also contribute to erosion development. The patient who develops erosions and/or vaginal bleeding from pessary use should be given a reprieve from pessary use for several weeks and then re-examined. An increase in vaginal estrogen cream as well as the addition of clindamycin or metronidazole cream during this period can be helpful to   ed up the healing. The addition of Trimo-San (Milex Products Inc., Chicago, Illinois) lubricating gel inserted alternately from the local hormone cream at bedtime may also speed up healing and when used long term may decrease the likelihood of developing further erosions. The erosions should be healed prior to reinsertion of the pessary. Alternative sources of vaginal bleeding, such as endometrial cancer or cervical pathology, should be ruled out. A pessary that is too large and has caused an erosion needs to be downsized. If possible, a switch to the nightly removal and cleaning of the pessary can allow the vagina to "rest" and prevent the recurrence of erosions.

Patients who do develop erosions require more vigilant follow-up with regular vaginal inspection to observe for further development of erosions. In rare instances, the erosions recur no matter what is attempted and pessary use must be abandoned. Of the patients seen in our pessary clinic in a 6-month period 6% developed erosions (Figure 26.6).

Difficulty with Fit

The ability to successfully fit a pessary decreases if there has been previous pelvic surgery – from 79% to 67% [6]. A woman who has had previous vaginal surgery or who has had pelvic radiation may have a vaginal vault that is too narrow and shortened to even attempt a pessary. On examination, the examiner's index and middle fingers cannot be spread wider than the introitus. The vagina's shape is a narrow tube instead of a cone. To keep a pessary in position, the examiner's fingers should be able to spread to a wider diameter in the upper vagina than the widest diameter of the introitus.

The other patient who can be difficult to fit is the patient with the wide pubic arch in conjunction with prolapse beyond the hymenal ring. Several attempts will likely reveal that a pessary will not stay in. The patient with a wide pelvis but a narrow

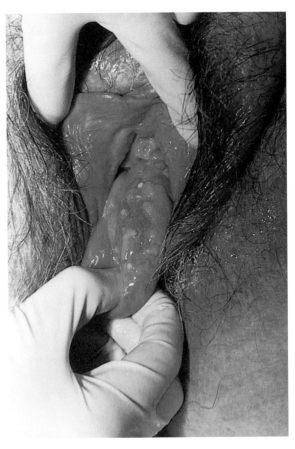

Figure 26.6 Vaginal vault erosion from short-term pessary use without local estrogen support.

vaginal opening and the patient with previous vaginal surgery may benefit from several months of local estrogen therapy prior to attempting a fit.

Device Irritation

When a patient experiences irritation from a pessary, it is often the accompanying local estrogen preparation or lubricant that is the culprit. A switch in estrogen preparation or lubricant can correct the problem. Patients have been known to develop a contact dermatitis from pessaries.

Interference with Bowel and Bladder Function

At follow-up visits, the patient should be questioned about change in bowel or bladder function. An improvement in function is usually the rule. If this is not the case, the health care professional should make an effort to ensure the device is not causing the problem. In the patient who develops difficulty evacuating her bowels, a rectal examination should be done. If the pessary is found to be obstructing the rectum, the pessary will have to be removed and either re-fitted or discontinued. Despite an often-voiced concern about pessary use resulting in bladder infections, this has not been reported as a reason to discontinue pessary use [6].

The Sexually Active Woman
Sexually active women can leave the pessary in place during intercourse if it does not bother either partner. Alternative forms of treatment should be considered in the woman who would like to have vaginal intercourse, with which the device interferes or is contraindicated (Gellhorn pessary).

Vaginal Discharge
An increase in vaginal discharge is to be expected with the insertion of a foreign body into the vagina, especially if estrogen replacement is initiated. The patient should be counseled to expect this. If accompanied by pruritus or an odor, cultures should be taken and antibiotic/antifungal treatment initiated if appropriate. A common concern of patients and their physicians prior to beginning pessary use is the worry of recurrent vaginal infections. The need to discontinue pessary use for this reason is unusual. If the pessary is difficult for the patient to remove and the patient has had a hysterectomy, the patient may douche with warm water between visits. Trimo-San gel (Milex Products Inc., Chicago, Illinois) inserted twice weekly into the vagina at night can help to keep odor to a minimum. Urinary tract infections are an unusual complication of pessaries. In the patient with a cystocele contributing to high post-void residuals and subsequent urinary tract infections, pessaries can actually cure the problem by repositioning the bladder and allowing the bladder to empty.

The Impacted Pessary
Occasionally, a pessary is placed into a woman and forgotten, only to be discovered impacted years later. This usually happens in the patient who develops dementia, or other medical problems that result in an inability to do self-care. Impacted pessaries may lead to severe infections including cellulitis, peritonitis, or the formation of a fistula or sinus tract. The worst complications reported are urethral erosion, or the formation of a vesicovaginal or rectovaginal fistula [16]. Although previously thought to be a problem primarily with rigid pessaries, a vesicovaginal fistula has also been reported with a silicone Gellhorn pessary in a 98-year-old woman who was not taking estrogen and had neglected the pessary for several years [17]. The discovery of a forgotten pessary usually occurs when nursing home personnel, health care workers, or family members notice a foul vaginal discharge, with or without

bleeding. Pelvic examination will reveal the device lodged in the vagina. The physician should use great caution in removing the device in the office. Extreme pelvic discomfort and occasional brisk vaginal bleeding can accompany an attempt at office removal. This bleeding can require surgical control. If the device is difficult to remove, starting the patient on a nightly dose of 1 g of vaginal estrogen cream for a month may facilitate removal. If this does not ease removal, then removal in an operating room with general anesthetic or intravenous sedation is the next step, allowing for repair of any vaginal lacerations. In the woman who is not a good surgical candidate the device may be left alone, especially if the patient is not expected to live long. Discharge and odor in this situation may be managed with daily estrogen cream application and weekly Betadine douches.

An impacted Gellhorn can be removed with the assistance of an endometrial biopsy cannula attached to a syringe filled with saline. The Gellhorn stem is grasped with a ring forceps and a cannula inserted into the stem and irrigated until the saline breaks the vacuum. The Gellhorn is then removed by grasping the stem using a ring forceps or single tooth tenaculum.

Pessaries are not for everyone. Life-table analysis reveals that the highest rate of pessary discontinuation occurs in the first 12 months [6]. The most common reasons for discontinuation of pessary use were failure to successfully support the prolapse, urinary incontinence, vaginal discharge, pelvic pain, and vaginal erosions [6]. Reviews of patients wearing pessaries have not reported major complications [6,18].

New Horizons for Supportive Devices

Research is in its infancy regarding new frontiers of pessary use. A number of physicians have independently observed that after a few years of pessary use, prolapse may resolve and a pessary is no longer required. There are intriguing questions to be answered. Is the pessary holding the vagina and uterus in place, thereby decreasing the stretching and allowing connective tissue remolding to occur? If so, then can pessaries be used as an attempt at cure, rather than as a temporizing situation? Should we encourage the younger woman with prolapse, especially the women who desire more children, to wear the pessary as a prophylactic measure even if her symptoms are not troublesome? Future research may address this issue.

The pessary is a safe and effective method of correcting genital prolapse, and managing stress, mixed, and urge incontinence. Contraindications to the modern pessary are rare. Ideally a postmenopausal woman should have local estrogen support added to help prevent vaginal erosions. Difficulty with fitting a pessary can preclude their use.

Alternate Devices

Numerous devices are being developed for the treatment of incontinence and prolapse. Because of the female anatomy collective devices are not easily fitted. However, a short urethra and a vagina allowing a place for exertion of pressure on the bladder neck is an advantage over the male for the treatment of urinary incontinence. Some devices already available for other uses are also employed to treat incontinence. The contraceptive diaphragm has been used to treat incontinence. It appears to work by causing mild urethral obstruction in that the urethral pressure doubles, and the flow rate decreases with the device in place [19]. Most models lack the support that the pessaries have. A tampon can be inserted for short periods of time during exercise. In women with mild forms of incontinence, this is sometimes useful. It cannot be left in place for an extended period of time because of odor and the risk of toxic shock syndrome. Tampons may be difficult to retain with an associated cystocele. They can also be irritating and dry, causing discomfort with insertion and removal in the non-menstruating woman. Moistening the tip of the tampon with water or lubricant prior to insertion may facilitate insertion and removal [20].

The urethral plug is another device (not currently available in Canada). This disposable device inserts into the urethra and is removed for voiding. It comes in five sizes from 3 to 5 cm in length and is sized to fit the patient. An inflated balloon anchors the device. A small string permits deflation of the balloon for removal. The Reliance Urinary control Insert (Uromed Inc., Needham MC) was tested over a 4-month period. Of the 215 women entered into the study, only 63% completed the study. Eighty-nine percent were subjectively dry or improved. Twenty percent developed urinary tract infections and 21% had gross hematuria. In 5 women the device migrated into the bladder [21]. A similar device is FemSoft (Rochester Medical Corp., Stewartville, MN), a soft jelly-like insert.

Another device available through a toll-free number in Canada is the Fem-Assist (Insight Medical, Boulton, Covington, GA). This device is an external seal device that fits over the urethral meatus between the labia. A small amount of suction secures it in place with a paste to provide a watertight seal. It has not yet gained mass popularity. The device is reused for a week and does not require sterilization. Three sizes are available. Fourteen women were assessed using this device. The device decreased pad weights by 47%. There was subjective and objective improvement [22].

The Continence Guard is a polyurethane foam product with American FDA approval for use. It comes in three sizes and is placed in the vagina by means of an applicator. It can be worn all day, or for lesser periods of time, depending on patient need. In a study of 22 women employing the device for a one-year period, 68% were subjectively dry, and 26% improved. There were no signs of vaginal irritation, and minimal subjective complaints [23,24]. Objective improvement in women with detrusor instability was 56.7%. The theory supplied is that the device may prevent the entrance of urine into the urethra; which might be the triggering factor of uninhibited contractions and urgency incontinence [25].

The Conti-Ring is a soft doughnut-shaped hollow polyurethane ring with protrusions that lie on either side of the urethra and support the urethra similar to a bladder suspension. Air can be added or removed to help with fitting. Various sizes are available (Calmia Medical Inc., Toronto).

There is currently a great deal of interest in devices and further designs are likely to be seen in great numbers in the future.

Conclusion

Vaginal pessaries are an important device to be familiar with when caring for the patient with pelvic floor dysfunction. They have been available longer than any other treatment for prolapse and still have an important role to play. They are useful in short- and long-term treatment of genital prolapse and incontinence, and have a role to play in deciding surgical approach to repair. They are easy to become familiar with, and should be an essential part of a gynecologist's armamentarium.

References

1. Zeitlin MP, Lebherz TB. Pessaries in the geriatric patient. J Am Geriatr Soc 1992;40:635–9.
2. Wood NJ. The use of vaginal pessaries for uterine prolapse. Nurse Pract 1992;17(7):31–8.

3. Miller DS. Contemporary use of the pessary. In: Sciarra JJ, editor. Gynecology and Obstetrics: Clinical Gynecology, Vol. 1, Rev edn. Philadelphia: Lippincott, 1999; 1–13.

4. Speert H. A pictorial history of gynecology and obstetrics. Iconographia Gyniatrica. Philadelphia: Davis, 1973; 463–9.

5. Deger RB, Menzin AW, Mikuta JJ. The vaginal pessary: past and present. Postgrad Obstet Gynecol 1993;13(18):1–8.

6. Wu V, Farrell SA, Baskett TF, Flowerdew G. A simplified protocol for pessary management. Obstet Gynecol 1997;90(6):990–4.

7. Moore KN, Flood CG, Griffiths DJ. Pessary use for stress urinary incontinence. J Soc Obstet Gynaecol Can 1994;16:2231–7.

8. Bhatia NN, Bergman A, Gunning JE. Urodynamic effects of a vaginal pessary in women with stress urinary incontinence. Am J Obstet Gynecol 1983;147:876–84.

9. Bergman A, Koonings PP, Ballard CA. Predicting post operative urinary incontinence development in women undergoing operation for genitourinary prolapse. Am J Obstet Gynecol 1988;158:1171–5.

10. Fianu S. Preoperative screening for latent stress incontinence in women with cystocele. Neurourol Urodyn 1985;4:3–7.

11. Hextall A, Boos K, Cardoza L, Tooz-Hobson P, Anders K, Khullar V. Videocystourethrography with a ring pessary in situ. A clinically useful pre-operative investigation for continent women with urogenital prolapse? Int Urogynecol J 1998;9:205–9.

12. Gibbons JM, Paley WB. The incarcerated pessary. Obstet Gynecol 1969;33:842.

13. Colmer WM, Hattiesburg MD. Use of the pessary. Am J Obstet Gynecol 1953;65(1):170–4.

14. Flood CG, Drutz HP, DelaCruz A, Brown D. Urogynecology training in obstetrics and gynaecology programs across Canada. J Soc Obstet Gynaecol Can 1997;19:51–7.

15. Farrell S. Practical advice for ring pessary fitting and management. J Soc Obstet Gynaecol Can 1997;19:625–32.

16. Buckley P, McInerey PD, Stephenson TP. Actinomycotic vesicuterine fistula from a wishbone pessary contraceptive device. Br J Urol 1991;68:206–7.

17. Grody MH, Nyirjesy P, Chatwani A. Intravesical foreign body and vesicovaginal fistula: A rare complication of a neglected pessary. Int Urogynecol J 1999;10:407–8.

18. Sulek P, Kuehl T, Shull B. Vaginal pessaries and their use in pelvic relaxation. J Reprod Med 1993;38(12):919–23.

19. Suarez G, Baum NH, Jacobs J. Use of the standard contraceptive diaphragm in management of stress incontinence. Urology 1991;37:119–22.

20. Nygaard I. Prevention of exercise incontinence with mechanical devices. J Reprod Med 1995;40(2):89–94.

21. Staskin D, Bavendam T, Miller J, Davila G, Diokno A, Knapp P, Rappaport S, Sand P, Sant G, Tutrone R. Effectiveness of a urinary control insert in the management of stress urinary incontinence: Early results of a multi-center study. Urology 1996:47:629–36.

22. Versi E, Harvey MA. Efficacy of an external urethral device in women with genuine stress urinary incontinence. Int Urogynecol J 1998;9:271–4.

23. Thyssen HH, Lose G. Long-term efficacy and safety of a disposable vaginal device (Continence Guard) in the treatment of female stress incontinence. Int Urogynecol J 1997;8:130–3.

24. Sander P, Thyssen H, Lose G, Andersen JT. Effect of a vaginal device on quality of life with urinary stress incontinence. Obstet Gynecol 1999;93(3):407–11.

25. Thyssen H, Sanders P, Lose G. A vaginal device (Continence Guard) in the management of urge incontinence in women. Int Urogynecol J 1999;10:219–22.

27 Sacral Nerves Neurostimulation

Magdy M. Hassouna

Outline of the Chapter

This chapter discusses the concept of neurostimulation of the sacral nerve roots in treating voiding dysfunction. Voiding dysfunction could be divided into two categories according to the underlying cause:

1. Neurogenic voiding dysfunction usually occurs following damage to the central or peripheral innervation of the bladder. A typical example of neurogenic bladder occurs following a suprasacral spinal cord injury. The primary function of the sacral stimulation is to enhance bladder evacuation.

2. Non-neurogenic voiding dysfunction affects a larger group of patients who have no apparent lesion in bladder innervation. These patients present with voiding dysfunction very similar to those with neurological lesions. A typical example of non-neurogenic voiding dysfunction is encountered in urge-frequency syndromes, chronic unobstructed urinary retention and patients with refractory urge incontinence. These patients respond to sacral "neuromodulation" of the pelvic floor musculature.

The chapter will describe the two modalities of sacral neurostimulation for different causes of voiding dysfunction.

Sacral Root Neurostimulation for Voiding in Patients with Spinal Cord Injury

Historical Background

The interest in electric stimulation as a means of controlling bladder function dates back to the 1950s. The first attempt to develop an electrical stimulator to treat the paralyzed human bladder was made in 1960 [1]. Since then several reports have been published which describe different systems of neurostimulation to induce voiding.

Direct detrusor stimulation received an initial interest, which faded with time. The advantage of this technique was the simplicity of the procedure of electrode placement. The electrodes were implanted directly on the bladder wall. Nevertheless, the effect was not durable owing to electrode displacement, production of fibrosis or even electrode erosion through the bladder. The need for current densities above the physiological levels was another major drawback [2].

Direct sacral cord stimulation was another possibility that was extensively addressed in the literature during the 1970s. Jonas and co-workers tried to stimulate the spinal cord at the level of the spinal micturition center by surface electrodes. These early trials proved to be a failure because of the proximity of both the micturition and the pudendal nuclei making it practically impossible to stimulate the parasympathetic nucleus without stimulating the pudendal nucleus. Nevertheless, these experiments conceived the concept of post-stimulus voiding which was later used in sacral root electrostimulation (see below) [3,4].

Pelvic nerve stimulation was then tried, but likewise proved to be a failure. Many factors were involved since the pelvic nerves were shown not to tolerate the stimulation for long periods of time. Vesico-sphincteric dyssynergia was a problem because of the simultaneous activation of the external urinary sphincter resulting in an increase in the outflow resistance. In humans, the early division of the pelvic nerve to form a broad pelvic plexus made it practically unsuitable for electrode placement [2].

The use of sacral roots electrical stimulation to induce voiding attracted attention in the 1960s. Habib reported his experience with sacral root electrical stimulation in 1967 [5]. Since then several reports has been published on this subject.

Sacral Root Electrical Stimulation

Since the early reports of the use of sacral root electrical stimulation, it was apparent that although this technique is by far superior to the other techniques such as direct bladder and spinal cord stimulation, it was still associated with potential drawbacks. The major drawback was the dyssynergic voiding due to simultaneous contraction of the sphincter during bladder evacuation. Nevertheless, the sacral nerve roots were found to be suitable for implanting with cuff electrodes around the nerve roots. Other practical solutions for handling the dyssynergic pattern of voiding made this sacral root electrical stimulation the procedure of choice to induce voiding in paraplegic subjects [2]. Researches on experimental animals conducted in the universities of California and McGill and Toronto Research Laboratories shed light on almost all the practical aspects of sacral root electrical stimulation.

Dyssynergia Induced by Sacral Root Stimulation

The S2 root was shown to be the major root supplying the urinary bladder while S1 is the one supplying the external sphincter in canine models. Unfortunately, the S2 root does not contain autonomic bladder supply exclusively. Stimulation of the S2 root will result in simultaneous contraction of the bladder and sphincter leading to dyssynergic voiding [6]. Two major contributing factors were shown to induce dyssynergic voiding with sacral

root electrical stimulation: reflex and direct recruitment of the external urethral sphincter musculature. Stimulation of the dorsal root of the S2 sacral nerve, which contains primarily afferent fibers from the pelvic organs, induced a similar response to stimulation of the whole S2 nerve. This response was only eliminated by dorsal rhizotomies proximal to the stimulation electrode, indicating that the mechanism here is through reflex recruitment of the bladder and the external sphincter. On the other hand, stimulation of the ventral root of the S2 nerve induced bladder and sphincteric contraction even after cutting the root proximally, indicating that the mechanism here is through direct recruitment. Cutting the pudendal nerve peripherally while stimulating the ventral root produced bladder contraction without dyssynergic sphincteric contraction. Stimulation of the ventral root proximal cut end did not induce any response [7].

Several studies have been conducted to address the detrusor sphincter dyssynergia induced by sacral root electrical stimulation. Post-stimulus voiding [8], dorsal rhizotomy [9], selective stimulation of the sacral rootlets [10], selective sectioning of the pudendal branches of the S2 root [11], pudendal neurotomy and sphincterotomy [9] were proposed over the years with variable success, morbidity and disadvantages. High frequency stimulation of the pudendal nerve to induce fatigue of the external sphincter prior to the stimulation of the sacral root with low frequency current was tested in our institute with good results. The experimental animals were able to void with a minimal post-void residual of urine [12]. Anodal blockade to the somatic contribution in the sacral root with a simultaneous application of a stimulating current allowed selective stimulation of the autonomic efferent branches supplying the detrusor [13].

In a limited clinical trial, Tanagho and co-workers implanted five patients with sacral root pulse generator. They used different combinations of electrode placement. In none of these cases was voiding possible using sacral root electrical stimulation owing to the severe dyssynergia. In another group of seven patients limited dorsal rhizotomy was performed to one or two roots. Only two patients were able to void effectively with the stimulation, one of them after bilateral pudendal neurotomy and levatorotomy. When dorsal rhizotomy was done extensively and combined with pudendal neurotomy all patients were able to void (5/5) compared to 4 patients who underwent extensive rhizotomies without pudendal neurotomies and were not able to void with stimulation [9]. From this study it became clear that it is practically impossible to induce voiding by sacral root electrical stimulation without dorsal rhizotomies and pudendal neurotomy with or without levatorotomy.

Extensive dorsal rhizotomy is an essential part of the procedure for patients implanted with a Fintech–Brindley stimulator. This was not sufficient alone to induce voiding since it has to be combined with a specific stimulation protocol to induce a post-stimulus voiding [8,14].

Post-stimulus voiding is possible by applying the principle that the striated muscles of the sphincter relax more rapidly than the detrusor after turning off the stimulation current. Hence, intermittent bursts of stimulation can be timed to produce more or less stable intravesical pressure with intermittent sphincteric relaxation leading to voiding in the form of bursts of interrupted urinary flow [8].

In a recent study, 47 patients underwent extensive dorsal rhizotomy (S2–S4/5). Forty-two of them were evacuating the bladder effectively using the stimulator without considerable residual urine. This occurred with minimal residual urine and with no effect on the upper tract. Posterior rhizotomies resulted in increased bladder capacity, stabilization of the renal function and resolution of the vesicoureteral reflux in two cases. On the other hand, complications included nerve damage in two patients, one of whom recovered after 6 months while the other did not, implant infection in one case, and clear CSF leakage which was treated conservatively. The authors did not discuss the effect of the rhizotomies on erectile function in patients who otherwise were potent [14].

Although the previous study was very successful, some authors contest the results of dorsal rhizotomies and the post-stimulus voiding. Many reports demonstrated the recurrence of the bladder spasticity and hyperreflexia after dorsal rhizotomies, making this extremely risky and invasive procedure of limited value [15]. Creasey has also pointed out some drawbacks to sacral rhizotomy: the loss of reflexogenic potency, reflex micturition and bladder neck function with increased possibility of stress incontinence. Although micturition by stimulation is more effective than that induced reflexly, the loss of reflex micturition after rhizotomy would be a major drawback if the patient is not able to use his stimulator [8]. Furthermore, some authors raised concern about the non-physiological nature of voiding using the post-stimulus voiding. In this type of voiding too an excessively high intravesical pressure is generated that may result in damage to the upper urinary tract.

Hohenfellner and associates have reported their results of selective stimulation of the ventral rootlets supplying the sphincter. By intradural dissection and stimulation of different rootlets composing the S2 nerves in a canine animal model, they were able to identify different components of the S2 root. Selective stimulation of these rootlets resulted in a bladder contraction with relatively less sphincteric activity. The method did not eliminate sphincteric activity totally and was done on an acute basis only [10].

Synchronized electrical stimulation of the sympathetic trunk and S2 root in dogs has been tried. The investigators reported that voiding was possible in 83.3% of stimulations when the sympathetic trunk was stimulated 5–10 seconds prior to the stimulation of the S2 root compared to 7.4% without sympathetic system stimulation [16].

Li and associates applied the principle of sphincteric fatigue during sacral root stimulation in order to decrease the urethral resistance. This was accomplished by stimulating the pudendal nerve with high frequency current ranging from 100 to 300 Hz for 20 seconds prior to stimulation of the S2 nerve. Using this stimulation protocol, bladder evacuation was possible in 5–7 cycles with each cycle inducing voiding of 40–100 ml urine [12]. Long-term studies have shown structural changes in the external sphincter that rendered it more resistant to the fatigue [17].

Haleem and colleagues used a different approach. They selectively sectioned the somatic contribution of the S2 root to the pudendal nerve preserving only the autonomic branches to the detrusor. This was done before stimulation of the main trunk of S2 root. They compared this technique to another group in which they did not section the somatic branches of S2. Their approach resulted in the ability to stimulate the detrusor selectively with no associated sphincteric activity [11].

Selective Sacral Root Stimulation

S2 comprises mixed nerves containing both autonomic fibers supplying the bladder and somatic fibers to the sphincter. Autonomic fibers are the Ad type, thin lightly myelinated fibers. Somatic fibers are the Aa type, thick and heavily myelinated fibers. The difference between these two types of fibers is not limited to the size of the fibers. The difference extends to the conduction velocity and, more importantly, to the current threshold. The stimulation threshold of the somatic fibers is lower than that of autonomic fibers. Stimulation of these fibers with a gradually increasing current intensity leads to activation of the somatic fibers before the autonomic fibers. This phenomenon is termed "reversed recruitment". According to this phenomenon it is practically impossible to stimulate the autonomic fibers without activation of the somatic ones. Barata and colleagues demonstrated that this phenomenon could be reversed by blocking the large diameter fibers, leaving the smaller fibers to be activated with the stimulation current. This phenomenon was termed "orderly recruitment" [18].

The following paragraphs describe two of the methods used for orderly stimulation that have shown potential clinical application.

Selective Sacral Root Stimulation Using Anodal Blockade

The idea was first suggested by Brindley and Craggs [19] for selective sacral root neurostimulation and popularized by Koldewijn and colleagues [20]. The principle of the anodal blockade is that the axon becomes hyperpolarized at the site of the anode. If the hyperpolarization is sufficient, no action potential will pass this point. With the increase of the anodal current, large fibers become blocked first, followed by small diameter fibers, leading to selective blockade of the large diameter fibers. Rijkhoff and co-workers used a tripolar cuff electrode for anodal blockade and were able to deliver both the stimulating and the blocking current through it. The design of the electrode was done so as to have one cathode in the middle and two asymmetrically placed anodes on each side of the cathode. The electrode was controlled by two electric circuits in such a way as to control each anode independently. The theory behind this is to accomplish (1) excitation at the cathode for all fibers, (2) blocking of all fibers at the proximal anode to prevent reflex recruitment and finally (3) blocking of large diameter fibers only distally leaving the small diameter autonomic fibers able to conduct action potential. The authors used a computer modeling technique to optimize the procedure. They concluded from this computer modeling that it is possible to generate unidirectional action potential down the autonomic fibers with simultaneous blocking of the somatic fibers [13]. During the application of this principle on an acute animal model the authors were able to block the sphincteric activity totally but unfortunately no bladder activity was recorded. They explained this by the effect of the anesthesia. Another major point of concern is the very large pulse width ranging between 600 and 800 ms that they used to block the sphincteric activity, generating very high charge injection rates. Whether this is applicable in a chronic animal model is not known and the long term effect on nerve integrity is yet to be determined.

Selective Neurostimulation Using High Frequency Blockade

This was first described by Wedensky in the nineteenth century. He used a 20 kHz current to block skeletal muscle contraction. Tanner demonstrated that this high frequency current if increased gradually could block first the conduction in large diameter fibers followed by a block of small diameter fibers if the current is further increased [21]. Solomonow showed that the most efficient blocking frequency is 600 Hz. He used 100 ms rectangular pulses rather than sinusoidal ones. In this work, he was able to show that the use of this high frequency current for up to 9 hours did not alter the muscle properties. He theorized with reasonable proof that the mechanism of action of blockade is putting the motor neurons and the endplates in a temporary refractory period, thus preventing the muscle from contracting [22]. Barata and colleagues used a tripolar cuff electrode to stimulate the skeletal muscles motor unit through stimulation of the sciatic nerve. They used two anodes symmetrically placed around a centrally placed cathode. They again used two independent circuits but for a different reason than anodal blockade. One circuit was used to deliver the low frequency current while the other circuit was used to deliver the high frequency current. Using this technique they were able to specifically stimulate small diameter fibers without the recruitment of the large diameter fiber [18].

Clinical Results of Sacral Root Stimulation for Voiding in Paraplegic Patients

Surgical Procedure

Two different techniques were developed for sacral root electrical stimulation for the purpose of bladder evacuation in paraplegic subjects. Brindley used extensive laminectomy from L4 to S2. Posterior sacral rhizotomy was performed intradurally for roots of S2 to S5 followed by intradural electrode placement on the sacral anterior roots supplying the bladder. These roots can be identified by peroperative stimulation and simultaneous recording of intravesical pressure. Electrodes are then brought out from a grommet in the dura, which is then closed. The electrodes are tunneled subcutaneously to be connected to a radio receiver placed subcutaneously on the front of the chest or abdomen [8]. The technique of Tanagho and colleagues uses a slightly different approach. This involves intradural rhizotomy with extradural placement of the electrodes. The rootlets are dissected and separated at the very distal end of the dura [12].

Clinical Results

Out of 184 implanted patients, 85% are using the stimulator alone to evacuate their bladders. The rest are using it in conjunction with intermittent catheterization. Residual urine was less than 60 ml in 95% of patients using it. Urinary tract infection dropped as well [8]. McDonagh and colleagues reported that 13 patients out of 15 became continent after receiving the Brindley stimulator. They emphasized the importance of having a closed bladder neck preoperatively [23].

Urodynamically, there has been a tremendous increase in the cystometric capacity of the bladder of these patients. It has been shown to be the result of the dorsal rhizotomy. MacDonagh and colleagues reported the disappearance of the hyperreflexia in 14 of 15 undergoing dorsal rhizotomy. Voiding pressure was extremely high, reaching up to 125 cmH2O with a mean voiding pressure of 89 cmH2O. Surprisingly, this did not affect the upper tract.

Neurapraxia or axonotmesis was the commonest complication in this group of patients, but recovery occurred in less than a month. Other reported complications included pain, CSF leakage, implant infection, cable failure, loss of reflexogenic erection and loss of reflex voiding [8].

Sacral Root Neuromodulation

Sacral root neuromodulation is on of the relatively recent concepts for treatment of various voiding and storage dysfunctions in patients with intact spinal cord. The modality is gaining wide acceptance among the urology community. Tanagho and Schmidt laid the principles of this modality early in 1988 [2,24]. Since then hundreds of patients have been implanted with neuroprostheses for treatment of various dysfunctions. Several reports have been published addressing different aspects. Indications have expanded to included urge incontinence and sensory urgency [25,26], idiopathic chronic urinary retention [27,28], pelvic pain [25,28] and interstitial cystitis [29].

Procedure

Patients in any of the previously mentioned categories have to go through a screening test called "Percutaneous nerve evaluation (PNE)". In this test a temporary wire electrode is put in the S3 foramen. The patient is sent home with a mobile pulse gener-

ator for the next few days. Responders are then implanted with a permanent sacral foramen implant and an implantable pulse generator (IPG).

Percutaneous Nerve Evaluation

This test was first described as a clinical test to evaluate detrusor innervation [30]. The technique that was used was quite different in the early publications. The procedure was performed under spinal anesthesia and the patient was positioned laterally. The aim was to test the response of the urinary bladder, manifested in pressure changes, to S3 electrical stimulation in patients who might be candidates for implantation of a neuroprosthesis for bladder evacuation. The procedure that is currently used for PNE is described by Thon and colleagues [28]. The patient is positioned prone with slight flexion of the hips. Bolsters under the chest and abdomen are used to maintain this position. After preparing the skin in a sterile fashion, the patient is draped in a way allowing access to the sacrum, perineum and feet. The S3 foramen is located one finger breadth off the midline at the level of the greater sciatic notch (Figure 27.1). Local anesthetic is used to infiltrate all planes down to the sacral bone. In their description, Thon et al. used an angiocatheter with a finder needle to probe the foramen. Currently this has been replaced with a relatively atraumatic needle supplied with the PNE kit from Medtronic® (Minneapolis MN). The angle recommended by the

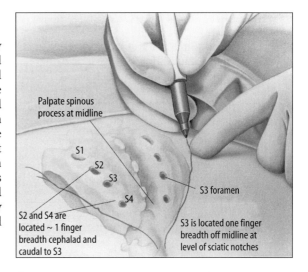

Figure 27.1 Determining the sacral landmarks. Palpate the bony topography or use fluoroscopy to find and identify the sacral landmarks with a sterile marker. One finger width on each side of the midline level with the sciatic notches marks the approximate sites of the S3 foramina. One finger width cephalad of these S3 marks approximately locates the S2 foramina. One finger width caudal to S3 approximates the S4 foramina.

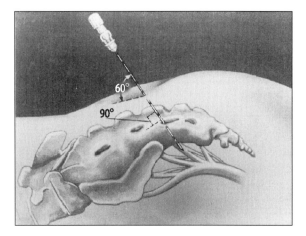

Figure 27.2 Test stimulation procedure. Insert the insulated foramen needle at an angle perpendicular to the bony surface (approximately 60° angle relative to the skin for the S3 site) using the needle tip to palpate the rime of the foramen and identify superior/inferior and medial/lateral margins.

authors was 60∞ to the skin (Figure 27.2). The more tangential the angle is the narrower the contact with the nerve. Stimulation of the nerve was done with an insulated spinal needle. Current used was 3–5 mA, 15 Hz and 200 ms pulse duration. Each foramen is separated with one finger within the vertical plane from adjacent foramina. Once the desirable somatic response is found, a 3-0 electrode wire supplied in the kit (Medtronic") is passed through the insulated needle and secured in place on the skin by means of adhesive tapes.

Hassouna and Elhilali reported a slightly different technique. The main difference was in the angle of the probing needle. They used a 30–40∞ angle to the skin [31].

Somatic Responses to Sacral Roots Neurostimulation

Sacral roots S2–4 are responsible for nervous supply of most of the pelvic organs. They give rise to both the pelvic nerve and pudendal nerve. The pelvic nerve is the one carrying the autonomic innervation while the pudendal nerve carries the somatic innervation. In addition, a few somatic fibers arise from the S2 and S3 and run in close proximity to the pelvic nerve to supply the levator muscle and the striated rhabdosphincter around the membranous urethra [2].

The sacral root of interest is the S3 root. The typical response of stimulating this nerve is seen in the perineum and the foot. Electrical stimulation of this root will result in contraction of the detrusor, levator ani and to a lesser extent the urethral sphinc-

ter in addition to the big toe muscles. During percutaneous nerve evaluation this response is visualized as a bellow movement of the perineum, that is, inwards movement of the anus and deepening of the gluteal cleft. Subjectively the patient feels a pulling sensation in the rectum with variable sensation in the scrotum and tip of the penis in men and labia and vagina in females. Stimulation of S2 produces contraction of more superficial perineal muscles causing a clamping-like effect. It may cause some sphincteric contraction but no detrusor response. Furthermore, it causes planter flexion of the foot and lateral rotation of the leg. Stimulation of S4 causes below-like action without any foot movement. Occasionally there is an overlap between these dermatomes [28,31].

Complications of PNE

Very minor complications have been reported in the large experience at the North American and European centers of more than 2000 cases who underwent PNE. These complications included some local discomfort and skin irritation at the puncture site during the trial period and wire displacement. There were no reports of infection or nerve damage in any cases following PNE [28,31].

Subchronic PNE Test

After obtaining the desired response and securing the wire in place the patient is sent home with the wire coupled to a portable pulse generator (Medtronic Screener") for a 5–7-day period of outpatient stimulation. Responders are those patients that show considerable improvement of their symptoms during the subchronic testing period. The choice of implant side depends on which side that gave the best response [28,31].

Results of the PNE

Out of fifty patients tested by PNE for various voiding and storage problems, Elabbady et al. reported a satisfactory response to the subchronic testing in 17 patients. It has to be mentioned that the response criteria in this study were rather strict as only patients who showed more than 70% improvement in their main baseline symptoms were considered to be qualifiers. The rest of the patients either did not show any response or the response was suboptimal [25]. Siegel has reported a 51% response rate in 49 patients who underwent PNE. In his series, four patients had a sustained improvement of their baseline symptomatology long after the PNE [32]. When 50% improvement was used as a cutoff value in patients undergoing PNE results improved to 61% [26].

Hasan and colleagues compared the results of transcutaneous electrical stimulation (TENS) of the sacral roots and PNE of S3 roots in patients with idiopathic detrusor instability. They reported that the symptomatic relief of patients undergoing PNE was more pronounced than that of patients having TENS. Both tests showed favorable responses on the ambulatory urodynamics. It has to be mentioned that the duration of the TENS was 2–4 weeks compared with 4–8 days for PNE, reflecting the superior direct specific stimulation of the S3 root in the PNE [33].

Implantation of the Permanent Neuroprosthesis

Patients who show a satisfactory response to the PNE will receive a permanent implant of the neuroprosthesis. In the prone position, under intubated general anesthesia, an incision is made in the skin over the lower two-thirds of the sacrum and is carried down to the thoracolumbar fascia (Figure 27.3). The fascia is incised and the gluteal and the paraspinous muscles are retracted over the side that demonstrated a satisfactory response during the PNE testing. The foramen is identified and a quadripolar electrode (lead electrode model 3080 Medtronic®) is then inserted in the foramen and

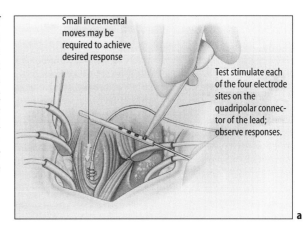

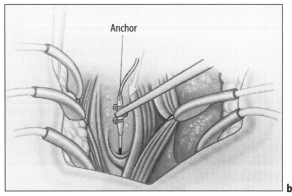

Figure 27.4 Device implantation procedure. **a** Implant lead and test for response. Place foramen needle and apply stimulation. If necessary, turn stimulation off and then reinsert foramen needle and retest until response is confirmed. Remove foramen needle. Gently insert the distal end of the lead into the foramen. Depth is usually 1.0–1.5 inches (2.5–4.0 cm). The lead should maneuver easily until the lead anchor (3080) contacts the periosteum. Test stimulate on various electrodes of the quadripolar connector and reposition as necessary until the desired response is observed. Positive motor responses should be observed at two or more electrodes of the 3886 lead. **b** Anchor lead and partially close the sacral incision site. Anchor the lead in place by suturing to the sacral bone or periosteum, then close the fascia or sacral incision and, if desired, suture a second anchor to tissue using non-absorbable sutures.

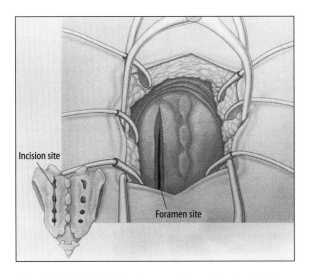

Figure 27.3 Device implantation procedure: performing the dissection. Make a midline incision appropriate to the size of the patient from approximately half a finger width below S4 up to S1; clean off the fascia lateral to the midline and divide in the direction of the incision; split paraspinal muscle fibers sharply and retract; expose the sacral foramen, preserving the periosteum; locate the desired foramen by observing anatomical landmarks and palpating for marble-board-like depression.

secured in place by non-absorbable material sutured to the periosteum (Figure 27.4). The direction of the electrode insertion is inferolaterally towards the greater trochanter to follow the course of the sacral root. The four contact points of the electrode are checked at this point. An ideal response is the one obtained with a current of 0.5–2 mA. Lower current denotes a very close position and higher current indicates that the electrode is too far away. If a less than ideal response is demonstrated, the electrode is removed and then replaced. The lead is then tunneled subcutaneously to be brought out just above the iliac crest, or more recently in the gluteal area.

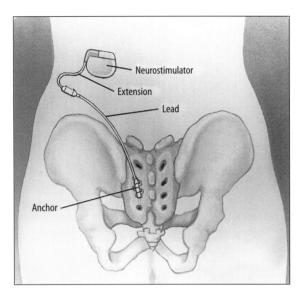

Figure 27.5 The implantable pulse generator (neurostimulator) in place.

The patients are then positioned on their flank. The implantable pulse generator (IPG model 3023 Interstim, Medtronic") is implanted in a pouch fashioned for this purpose medial to and above the anterior-superior iliac spine or in the gluteal region (Figure 27.5). The implantable pulse generator is then connected to the electrode by an extension cable (Model 7495 extension Medtronic") tunneled subcutaneously. Patients are placed under antibiotic coverage. The pulse generator is activated on the second postoperative day and patient discharged on the third postoperative day [31].

Results of Sacral Neuromodulation

Several studies have been conducted on the subject of sacral neuromodulation. The two main indications for sacral root neuromodulation will be discussed separately and other minor indications will be discussed collectively.

Urge Incontinence and Bladder Instability

Urge incontinence and bladder instability are one of the primary indications for this form of therapy. The principle of this indication stems from observation of the possibility of restoring the reservoir function of the bladder in patients with suprasacral spinal cord injury with sacral root neurostimulation [9]. In that study, the primary aim of sacral root stimulation was to induce voiding. It has to be mentioned that most the patients in this study have undergone extensive dorsal rhizotomy, which may be the main reason for restoration of continence in them.

Bosch and Groen reported their results in 18 implanted patients with urge incontinence secondary to detrusor instability. The voiding diaries of these patients showed a highly significant drop in the leakage episodes and frequency with a significant increase in the average voided volume. The number of protective pads/day dropped significantly as well. The effect was durable as 13 patients who have been followed up for more than 2 years maintained their initial improvement. Urodynamically, the bladder instability disappeared in 8 of the 18 patients while the other 10 showed an increased infused volume to first uninhibited contraction and to the maximum uninhibited contraction. This was associated with increased bladder volume at capacity and at first sensation. There was no complete correlation between the urodynamic findings and the patient symptomatology. Three of the nine patients who were completely dry showed persistence of the uninhibited contractions while two of the nine who were not completely dry showed a stable bladder [26].

Thon and colleagues provided similar results. Out of 20 patients with urge urinary incontinence, 17 showed an improvement of more than 50% compared with the baseline, which persisted for more than a year of follow-up [28]. Elabbady and colleagues presented their results in patients with urgency frequency and/or urge incontinence. Frequency improved by 73%, urgency by 42% and incontinence by 50%. Urodynamically, bladder instability disappeared in one patient and bladder volume at first sensation increased by 50% [25]. In a more recent study Shaker and Hassouna showed the long-term efficacy of sacral neuromodulation in 18 patients with urge incontinence. They followed the patients for 4 years. The results were consistent as shown in the significant decrease in the number and degree of urge incontinence with the help of treatment modality [34].

Idiopathic Non-obstructive Chronic Urinary Retention

This is another major indication for sacral root neuromodulation. Very few reports have peen published on this issue. Thon and colleagues reported their results in seven patients within this category. Thirty-three patients with chronic urinary retention were implanted with permanent neuroprosthetic implants. Twenty-three of them showed a long-lasting significant improvement [28]. Vapnek and Schmidt reported their experience in seven patients with chronic retention. Five of the seven patients are voiding normally, one is voiding with hesitancy and straining, and the last was doing well but lost the implant because of infection [27]. Elabbady and colleagues presented their data in eight implanted patients. All patients were able to void postoperatively. Average voided volume improved significantly and was associated with marked reduction in the residual urine. This was associated with significant improvement in the uroflowmetry data [25]. In another more recent study, Shaker and Hassouna presented their results on 20 patients with chronic retention. They showed that all patients were able to void with minimal residual urine with the help of the neurostimulator [35].

Miscellaneous Indications

Pelvic pain or discomfort is a very common symptom associated with other storage or voiding dysfunctions. In many of the publications for sacral root neuromodulation, associated pelvic pain has improved remarkably. This improvement ranged from 85% to 90% when post-implant status was compared with the baseline [26,28].

Tanagho presented his data concerning the use of sacral root neuromodulation in various voiding dysfunctions and storage problems in children. Nineteen patients with meningomyelocele have been tested with PNE. Eleven have shown good response. Seven of them have been implanted. Six of these seven demonstrated a very good response while one failed. Children with voiding dysfunction with no apparent cause all responded to PNE (6/6). And they all showed fair to good response postoperatively. Two patients with neonatal hypoxia have been treated with neuroprosthetic implants. One failed owing to behavioral problems [36].

Complications

Complications in general were minimal and within expectations. These included electrode migration, electrode failure and pain at the IPG site [25,26]. Cessation of the response with time is another problem that some investigators encountered. Thon et al. theorized that this is due to an electrode–nerve interface problem resulting from high charge injection. The reason for this is electrode placement far from the nerve. The close proximity of the electrode to the nerve prevents the use of high current amplitude, thus preventing nerve damage [28]. Pain whether referred or at the IPG site constituted a problem in 8 out of 17 implanted patients. This was dealt with by adjustment of parameters in seven patients. Since the relocation of the IPG in the gluteal area, the incidence of pain has been eliminated. No cases of nerve damage have been reported [25].

Theories of Mechanisms of Action

The mechanism of action of this modality is not well understood. There is not any solid evidence of the mechanism of action and not much basic research has been done to address this issue. The theories explaining the results of the sacral root neuromodulation are all derived from the clinical observations. It has been shown that activation of the afferent input of the S3 root inhibits the spinal micturition reflex. This could explain the suppression of the sense of urgency and urge incontinence [37–39].

An additional observation with sacral neuromodulation is the substantial improvement of the pelvic pain associated with urgency and urge incontinence. This could be explained by the gate theory proposed by Melzack and Wall [40]. According to their theory, pain perceived from visceral origin such as pelvic organs can be blocked by converging impulses arising from a somatic origin such as the S3 nerve root and supplied by the same dermatome (S3). Another finding following sacral neuromodulation was the change in the expression of the *c-fos* protein in the spinal cord. The increase in the *c-fos* protein was found to be very specific in the spinal segment supplied by the pelvic or the pudendal nerves when the latter have been stimulated electrically [41]. This finding proves that neuromodulation of the sacral nerve roots causes physiologic changes in the spinal cord that are responsible for the micturition reflexes.

Summary

The application of sacral nerve root neuromodulation and stimulation has gained wide acceptance as a tool to enhance the control of voiding. The simplicity of the technique has made this therapy appealing for refractory cases of voiding dysfunction. The percutaneous screening test is mandatory for the success of the therapy. Long-term follow-ups have shown its efficacy and safety in patients with voiding dysfunction.

Voiding dysfunction affects more than 20 million Americans. The major problem facing these patients is urinary incontinence. Eighty percent of the incontinent population are female. It is estimated that half of nursing home patients are suffering from urinary incontinence. Bladder dysfunction has significant economic and social impacts, such as the estimated US$1 billion annual turnover in the pad and appliances industry [42], and the social reclusion affecting incontinent patients.

The function of the bladder is twofold: a reservoir to hold urine at low pressure and voiding to evacuate the urine. Disturbances in one or both of these functions will result in urinary voiding dysfunction.

The urinary bladder and outlet are under neural control from the sacral nerves. The latter are under influence from higher centers, particularly the pontine micturition center (PMC). The PMC receives neural input from the frontal lobe cortex, the cerebellum and the basal nuclei, to mention a few. Any neurological disturbances inflicted on one or more of these nerve structures result in voiding dysfunction secondary to neurogenic bladder.

Voiding dysfunction can occur also in the absence of an overt neurologic lesion. It is estimated that urinary incontinence represents 80% of non-neurologic bladder dysfunction. These patients suffer from different forms of incontinence, namely urge in conjunction with stress incontinence. Patients are also known to have pelvic floor dysfunction that results in lower urinary tract malfunction. The association between urinary bladder and the musculature of the pelvic floor has been proven in repeated studies [43,44].

Treatment of patients with conventional pharmacological therapy usually does not achieve satisfactory results. Repeated surgical intervention aimed at denervating or augmenting the bladder is usually insufficient to control urge incontinence. Other techniques used to treat urinary voiding dysfunction that involve the use of stimulation include: pelvic floor stimulation (either with or without biofeedback), sacral root stimulation, direct bladder stimulation, and sacral neuromodulation.

Pelvic Floor Stimulation and Biofeedback

Pelvic floor stimulation with or without biofeedback (BFB) has been used with 20–60% success in treating patients with urinary urgency and frequency. The principle of treatment relies on educating patients to contract the pelvic muscles in order to achieve a better control of bladder contractility. By recruiting the pelvic musculature into contraction, the patient may be able to inhibit unwanted bladder contractions and suppress the sense of urgency and hence the incontinence.

The treatment involves the use of recording probes that are inserted inside the vagina or the anal canal. These probes convert the pelvic floor contractility into signals perceived by the patients either by visual or auditory means. The patient is requested to contract and relax the pelvic muscle according to those signals.

Pelvic floor stimulation either with or without biofeedback involves repeated office visits to train the patients. Once the patient becomes familiar with the devices, he/she is requested to perform those exercises at home repeatedly. The latter involves long-term commitment and dedication on the part of the patient towards the therapy. The results available in the literature vary in the degree of cure from 17 to 60% [45,46].

Disadvantages of pelvic floor stimulation and biofeedback include:

1. An early, good result fades with time.
2. Commitment and motivation of the patient are crucial to the success of the therapy.
3. Patients need continuous reminder of the therapy in order to maintain success.

Sacral Root Stimulation

This modality has been advocated for patients with spinal cord injury in order to drive the bladder to evacuate. The treatment involves exposure of the sacral nerve roots in the sacral neural canal. This involves a laminectomy that extends to the upper two-thirds of the sacrum. The sacral nerve roots are separated into dorsal and ventral. The dorsal roots of the 2nd, 3rd and 4th sacral nerves are cut in order to facilitate the bladder evacuation with the least sphincter contraction during stimulation. Electrodes connected to an implantable receiver device are wrapped around the ventral nerve roots. The latter is activated by radiofrequency signals to stimulate the bladder to evacuate. This treatment is limited to patients with complete suprasacral spinal cord lesions (i.e. paraplegic and quadriplegic). It is not recommended for:

1. Patients with incomplete spinal cord injury, since they show poor tolerance to the stimulation.
2. Male patients who desire to keep their erectile function intact. The dorsal rhizotomy of S2, 3 and 4 risks denervating the penis and hence causes erectile dysfunction.

Direct Bladder Stimulation

Direct stimulation of the bladder or electrical vesical stimulation to facilitate urinary evacuation in patients with lower motor neuron lesions (spinal cord injury) was performed during the 1970s by surgical implantation of electrodes on the detrusor muscle of the bladder. The electrodes were attached to an implanted receiver, and an external stimulating device used radio-frequency signals to transmit electrical signals to the electrodes. Stimulation resulted in contraction of the detrusor muscle with subsequent emptying of the bladder.

Use of bladder stimulation for the treatment of incontinence has not been adopted by the medical community because of the low documented efficacy rate of 20–50%, risk of adverse events including pain and high pressure urine storage, and technical problems with the implanted devices such as lead wire breakage [47–50].

Sacral Nerve Stimulation (Neuromodulation)

Treatments for urge incontinence as described above either act on the bladder directly or act on the neural reflexes that influence detrusor (muscle of the bladder) behavior. Pharmacological treatments for urge incontinence are intended to act directly on the bladder to calm or relax detrusor activity. Treatments that act on the neural reflexes influencing lower urinary tract behavior consist of behavioral techniques, such as bladder training, urge suppression, pelvic muscle exercises, biofeedback, and electrical stimulation (vaginal or anal). These treatments are intended to condition the pelvic floor and to suppress detrusor contraction by modulating neural reflexes that have an inhibitory effect on the bladder. Sacral nerve stimulation also acts on neural reflexes but does so internally at the level of the sacral nerve.

Sacral nerve stimulation therapy consists of electrical stimulation of the sacral nerves via a lead implanted adjacent to a targeted sacral nerve, an implantable pulse generator (IPG) implanted in the lower abdomen, and an extension that connects the lead to the IPG. Electrical pulses from the IPG are transmitted through the extension and lead, and to the targeted sacral nerve via electrodes located at the distal end of the lead. It is thought that sacral nerve stimulation induces reflex-mediated inhibitory effects on the detrusor through either afferent and/or efferent stimulation of the sacral nerves [25,27,28,51–55].

Sacral nerve stimulation therapy is delivered in two stages: test stimulation and surgical implantation. Test stimulation is an office-based procedure that allows the patient to experience the effects of sacral nerve stimulation on voiding behavior over a trial period of several days. Patients who demonstrate improvement during the test stimulation phase may be considered candidates for surgical implantation of the sacral nerve stimulation system (Medtronic, Inc., Minneapolis MN).

In a prospective, randomized trial, urge incontinent patients implanted with the sacral nerve stimulation system significantly reduced incontinent episodes/day, severity of incontinence, and absorbent pads/diapers replaced/day due to incontinence (all p < 0.0001) at 6 months, compared with control group patients who did not receive stimulation therapy. Forty-seven percent (16 of 34) demonstrated a greater than 50% reduction in incontinent episodes at 6 months post-implantation. Sustained clinical benefit was documented through 18 months post-implant.

The most commonly reported adverse events associated with use of the device or therapy included pain at the implantable pulse generator site (15.9% of patients); pain at the implant site (19.1% of patients); and lead migration (7.0% of patients). There were no reports of nerve damage or permanent injury associated with use of the sacral nerve stimulation system [56].

Conclusion

Various stimulation treatments are available for patients suffering from lower urinary tract dysfunction and incontinence. Based upon review of the scientific literature, each stimulation therapy should be viewed as unique in its application, mode of action, and risk/benefit profile (Table 27.1).

In comparing sacral neuromodulation with other treatment modalities, it is imperative to delineate the following:

1. Sacral neural modulation is a less invasive therapy than stimulation of the sacral nerve roots and direct bladder stimulation. It offers treatment to patients who are neurologically intact yet are suffering from refractory urinary voiding dysfunction. The latter are more numerous than patients with spinal cord injury.

2. Sacral neuromodulation offers continuous low-grade stimulation to the sacral nerve which influences voiding function.

3. Patients are not required to continuously wear or interact with intravaginal or anal devices to achieve efficacy in the therapy.

4. Sacral neuromodulation improves significantly (greater than 75% of patients) bladder control in patients with urge incontinence.

Acknowledgment

This work has been supported by a grant from the Paralyzed Veterans of America and Medtronic Inc., MN.

Table 27.1   Comparison of different therapies for bladder dysfunction

	Sacral neuromodulation	Pelvic floor stimulation[a]	Sacral root stimulation	Direct bladder stimulation
Indications	Urge incontinence	Urge and stress incontinence	Neurogenic bladder	Neurogenic bladder
Nerve integrity	Present	Present	Absent	Absent
Localization of stimulation	Precise	Diffuse	Precise	Precise
Efficacy	>75%	17–60%	70%	20–50%
Safety	Safe	Safe	Risk of denervation	Risk of pain, technical problems
Stimulation	Low frequency and amplitude	Low frequency and amplitude	High amplitude	High amplitude

[a] With or without biofeedback.

References

1. Boyce WH, Lathem JE, Hunt LD. Research related to the development of an artificial electrical stimulator for paralyzed human bladder. J Urol 1964;91:41–50.
2. Tanagho EA, Schmidt RA. Electrical stimulation in the management of neurogenic bladder. J Urol 1988;140:1331–3.
3. Jonas U, Tanagho EA. Studies on the feasibility of urinary bladder evacuation by direct spinal cord stimulation. I. Parameters of most effective stimulation. Invest Urol 1975;13:142–5.
4. Jonas U, Tanagho EA. Studies on the feasibility of urinary bladder evacuation by direct spinal cord stimulation. II. Post-stimulus voiding a way to overcome outflow resistance. Invest Urol 1975;13:151–5.
5. Habib HN. Experience and recent contribution in sacral nerve stimulation for voiding in both human and animal. Br J Urol 1967;39:73–5.
6. Schmidt RA, Bruschini H, Tanagho EA. Urinary bladder and sphincter responses to stimulation of dorsal and ventral sacral roots. Invest Urol 1979;16:300–4.
7. Schmidt RA, Bruschini H, Tanagho EA. Sacral root stimulation in controlled micturition : peripheral somatic neurotomy and stimulated voiding. Invest Urol 1979;17:130–5.
8. Creasey GH. Electrical stimulation of sacral roots for micturition after spinal cord injury. [Review] Urol Clin North Am 1993;20(3):505–15.
9. Tanagho EA, Schmidt RA, Orvis BR. Neural stimulation for control of voiding dysfunction: a preliminary report in 22 patients with serious neuropathic voiding disorders. J Urol 1989;142(2 Pt 1):340–5.
10. Hohenfellner M, Paick JS, Trigo-Rocha F, Schmidt RA, Kaula NF, Thuroff JW, Tanagho EA. Site of deafferentation and electrode placement for bladder stimulation: clinical implications. J Urol 1992;147(6):1665–70.
11. Haleem AS, Boehm F, Legatt AD, Kantrowitz A, Stone B, Melman A. Sacral root stimulation for controlled micturition: prevention of detrusor-external sphincter dyssynergia by intraoperative identification and selective section of sacral nerve branches. J Urol 1993;149(6):1607–12.
12. Li JS, Hassouna M, Sawan M, Duval F., Elhilali MM. Electric stimulation induced sphincteric fatigue during voiding. J Urol 1992;148:949–52.
13. Rijkhoff N, Holsheimer J, Koldewijn E, Struijk JJ, van Kerrebroeck PEV, Debruyne FMJ, Wijkstra H. Selective stimulation of sacral nerve for bladder control: a study by computer modeling. IEEE Transactions on Biomedical Engineering 1995;41(5):413–24.
14. Van Kerrebroeck PE, Koldewijn EL, Rosier PF, Wijkstra H, Debruyne FM. Results of the treatment of neurogenic bladder dysfunction in spinal cord injury by sacral posterior root rhizotomy and anterior sacral root stimulation. J Urol 1996;155(4):1378–81.
15. Toczek SK, McCullough DC, Gragour GW, Kachman R, Baker R, Luessenhop AJ. Selective sacral rootlet rhizotomy for hypertonic neurogenic bladder. J Neurosurg 1975;42:567–70.
16. Bosch RJLH, Aboseif SR, Benard F, Stief CG, Schmidt RA, Tanagho EA. Synchronized electrical stimulation of the sympathetic and parasympathetic innervation of the bladder: facilitation of the initiation of micturition in the dog. J Urol 1990;144:1252–5.
17. Juenemann KP, Lue TF, Schmidt RA,, Tanagho EA. Clinical significance of sacral and pudendal nerve anatomy. [Review]. J Urol 1988;139(1):74–80,
18. Barata R, Ichie M, Hwang S, Solomonow M. Orderly stimulation of skeletal muscles motor units with tripolar nerve cuff electrode. IEEE Trans Biomed Eng BME 1989;36:836–40.
19. Brindley GS, Craggs, MD. A technique for anodally blocking large nerve fibers through chronically implanted electrodes. J Neurol Neurosurg Psychiatry 1980;43:1083–5.
20. Koldewijn E, Rijkhoff N, Holsheimer J, van Kerrebroeck PEV, Debruyne FMJ, Wijkstra H. Selective sacral root stimulation for bladder control: Acute experiments in an animal model. J Urol 1994;151:1674–7.
21. Tanner J. Reversible blocking of nerve conduction by alternating current excitement. Nature 1962;195:712–14.
22. Solomonow M. External control of the neuromuscular system. IEEE Transactions Biomed Engineering 1984;317–22.
23. MacDonagh R, Forster DM, Thomas DG. Urinary continence in spinal injury patients with spinal injury patients following complete sacral posterior rhizotomy. Br J Urol 1990;66:618–22.
24. Schmidt RA. Applications of neurostimulation in urology. Neurourol Urodyn 1988;7:585–7.
25. Elabbady AA, Hassouna MM, Elhilali MM. Neural stimulation for chronic voiding dysfunctions. J Urol 1994;152:2076–80.
26. Bosch J, Groen J. Sacral (S3) segmental nerve stimulation as a treatment for urge incontinence in patients with detrusor instability: results of chronic electrical stimulation using an implantable neural prosthesis. J Urol 1995;154:504–9.

27. Vapnek JM, Schmidt RA. Restoration of voiding in chronic urinary retention using neuroprosthesis. World J Urol 1991;9:142–5.

28. Thon WF, Baskin LS, Jonas U, Tanagho EA, Schmidt RA. Neuromodulation of voiding dysfunction and pelvic pain. World J Urol 1991;9:138–40.

29. Fall M. Conservative management of chronic interstitial cystitis: Transcutaneous electrical nerve stimulation and transurethral resection. J Urol 1985;133:774–9.

30. Markland C, Merrill D, Chou S, Bradley W. Sacral nerve root stimulation: A clinical Test of detrusor innervation. Br J Urol 1971;43:453–6.

31. Hassouna, MM, Elhilali MM. Role of the sacral root stimulator in voiding dysfunctions. World J Urol 1991;9:145–8.

32. Siegel S. Management of voiding dysfunction with an implantable neuroprosthesis. In: Novick A, editor. Urol Clin North Am 1992;19:163–6.

33. Hasan ST, Robson WA, Pride AK, Neal DE. Transcutaneous electrical nerve stimulation and temporary S3 neuromodulation in idiopathic detrusor instability. J Urol 1996;155:2005–10.

34. Shaker HS, Hassouna MM. Sacral nerve root neuromodulation: effective treatment for refractory urge incontinence. J Urol 1998;159:1516–19.

35. Shaker HS, Hassouna MM. Sacral root neuromodulation in idiopathic nonobstructive chronic urinary retention. J Urol 1998;159:1476–9.

36. Tanagho EA. Neuromodulation in the management of voiding dysfunction in children. J Urol 1992;148:655–8.

37. Vadusek DB, Light JK, Liddy JM. Detrusor inhibition induced by stimulation of pudendal nerve afferents. Neurourol Urodyn 1986;5:381–4.

38. Ohlson BL, Fall M, Frankeberg-Sommar S. Effects of external and direct pudendal nerve maximal electrical stimulation in the treatment of the uninhibited overactive bladder. Br J Urol 1989;64:374–8.

39. Wheeler JS, Walter JS, Zaszczyrynsji PJ. Bladder inhibition by penile nerve stimulation in spinal cord injury patients. J Urol 1992;147:100–3.

40. Melzack R, Wall PD. Pain mechanisms: a new theory. Science 1965;150:971.

41. Birder LA, de Groat WC. Induction of c-fos gene expression of spinal neurons in the rat by nociceptive and non-nociceptive stimulation of the lower urinary tract. Am J Physiol. 265:326–30.

42. Blaivas JG. A modest proposal for the diagnosis and treatment of urinary incontinence in women. J Urol 1987;138:597–8.

43. Fall M, Erlandson BE, Nilson AE, Sundin T. Long-term intravaginal electric stimulation in urge and stress incontinence. Scand J Urol Nephrol Suppl. 1997;44:55–63.

44. Jonasson A, Larsson B, Pschera H, Nylund L. Short-term maximal electrical stimulation: a conservative treatment of urinary incontinence. Gynecol Obstet Invest 1990;30:120–3.

45. Payne CK, Kunkle JC, Whitmore KE. Combined biofeedback and electrical stimulation for the treatment of female incontinence. J Urol 1991;145:222A:Abstract 40.

46. Hirakawa S, Hassouna M, Deleton R, Elhilali M. The role of combined pelvic floor stimulation and biofeedback in female urinary incontinence. Can J Urol 1994;1:72–7.

47. Halverstadt DB. Electrical stimulation of the human bladder: 3 years later. J Urol 1971;106:673–6.

48. Merrill DC, Conway CJ. Clinical experience with the mentor bladder stimulator. I. Patients with upper motor neuron lesions. J Urol 1974;112:52–4.

49. Merrill DC. Clinical experience with the mentor bladder stimulator. II. Meningomyelocele patients. J Urol 1974;112:823–6.

50. Coffman LM, Finkelstein LH. Twenty-year experience with the Mentor bladder pacemaker. JAOA No. 11, 1995.

51. Dijkema HE, Weil EHJ, Mijs PT, Janknegt RA. Neuromodulation of sacral nerves for incontinence and voiding dysfunctions. Eur Urol 1993;24:72–6.

52. Bosch R, Groen J. Effects of sacral segmental nerve stimulation on urethral resistance and bladder contractility: how does neuromodulation work in urge incontinence patients? Neurourol Urodyn 1995;14:502–4.

53. Koldewijn EL, Fosier PRWM, Meuleman EJS, Koster JHM, Debruyne FMH, Van Kerrebroeck PEVV. Predictors of success with neuromodulation in lower urinary tract dysfunction: results of trial stimulation in 100 patients. J Urol 1994;152:2071–5.

54. Melzack R. Folk medicine and the sensory modulation of pain. In: Wall PD, Melzack R, editors. Textbook of Pain. Edinburgh: Churchill Livingstone, 1994; 1191–208.

55. Collins JJ, Imhoff TT, Grigg P. Noise-enhanced information transmission in rat SA1 cutaneous mechanoreceptors via a periodic stochastic resonance. J Neurophysiol 1996; 76:642–5.

56. Medtronic, Inc. Data on file.

Further Reading

(Recent articles related to sacral neuromodulation)

Benson. Sacral nerve stimulation results may be improved by electrodiagnostic techniques. Int Urogynecol J 2000; 11:352–7.

Bosch J, Groen J. Sacral nerve neuromodulation in the treatment of patients with refractory motor urge incontinence: long-term results of a prospective longitudinal study. J Urol 2000;163:1219–22.

Chai, Zhang, Arren, Keay. Percutaneous sacral third nerve root neurostimulation improves symptoms and normalizes urinary HB-EGF levels and antiproliferative activity in patients with interstitial cystitis. Urology 2000:55:643–6.

Chai, et al. Sacral nerve stimulation in interstitial cystitis patients. Urology 2000;55:643–6.

Chancellor, Chartier-Kastler. Principles of sacral nerve stimulation (SNS) for the treatment of bladder and urethral sphincter dysfunction. Neuromodulation 2000; 3:15–26.

Chartier-Kastler, Bosch J et al. Long-term results of sacral nerve stimulation (S3) for the treatment of neurogenic refractory urge incontinence related to detrusor hyperreflexia. J Urol 2000;164(5).

Costa, Kreder. Spinal cord neuromodulation for voiding dysfunction. Clin Obstet Gynecol 2000;September: 43.

Das, White, Longhurst. Sacral nerve stimulation for the management of voiding dysfunction. Rev Urol 2000;1:43–60.

Edlund, Hellstom, Peeker et al. First Scandinavian experience of electrical stimulation in the treatment of the overactive bladder. Scand J Urol Nephrol 2000; 366–376.

Everaert, Devulder, DeMuynck et al. The pain cycle: implications for the diagnosis and treatment of pelvic pain syndromes. Int Urogynecol J 2001;12:9–14.

Hassouna MM, Siegel S et al. Sacral neuromodulation in the treatment of urgency-frequency symptoms: a multicenter study on efficacy and safety. J Urol 2000;163:1849–54.

Hassouna M. Implantable electrostimulator of sacral root for refractory urinary problems. Mature Medicine Canada 2000:100–104.

Jonas, Fowler, Chancellor, et al. Efficacy of sacral nerve stimulation for urinary retention: Results 18 months after implantation. J Urol 2001:15–19.

Leroi, Michot, et al. Effect of sacral nerve stimulation in patients with fecal and urinary incontinence. Dis Colon Rectum 2001;44(6):779–89.

Maher, Carey, Dwyer et al. Percutaneous sacral nerve root neuro-modulation for intractable interstitial cystitis. J Urol 2001;165:884–6.

Siegel S. Long-term results of a multicenter study on sacral nerve stimulation for treatment of urinary urge incontinence, urgency-frequency and retention. Urology 2000;56:87–91.

Weil et al. Novel test lead designs for SNS: improved passive fixation in an animal model. J Urol 2000;164:551–5.

28 Biofeedback for Anorectal Disorders

Kenneth R. Jones, Steven Heymen and William E. Whitehead

Introduction

Fecal incontinence and constipation are common disorders: Fecal incontinence is reported to occur "often" in 2.2% [1] to 6.9% [2] of adults in the United States, with frequent, large volume fecal incontinence occurring in an estimated 0.7% of the population [2]. Constipation occurs in an estimated 4% of US adults [3], with pelvic floor dyssynergia type constipation making up an estimated 25–50% of this group [4,5]. Neither disorder is life-threatening, although both have an adverse effect on quality of life and are associated with significant morbidity and costs (e.g. cost of care and work absenteeism). Functional rectal pain is reported by an estimated 11.3% of adults, including 7.9% who have proctalgia fugax (fleeting sharp pain) and 6.6% who have levator ani syndrome (chronic or recurring episodes of dull, aching pain) [2].

Biofeedback is frequently employed to treat both chronic fecal incontinence and pelvic floor dyssynergia type constipation when these symptoms do not respond to conservative interventions such as dietary recommendations, bowel scheduling, and medications. Because uncontrolled trials suggest that biofeedback is associated with outcomes as good as medical management or surgery for fecal incontinence and constipation, and because it has a low incidence of adverse effects, biofeedback is often recommended as the first-line treatment for these conditions [6]. Less is known about the effectiveness of biofeedback for the treatment of rectal pain; biofeedback is one of many treatments that have been recommended but there exists no consensus on what is the best treatment for this condition [7].

Although biofeedback is frequently recommended for the treatment of these disorders, several factors have limited the widespread use of biofeedback: (1) There are no adequate controlled trials (comparison to placebo or comparison to standard treatment) to demonstrate biofeedback's effectiveness in any of these disorders. (2) There have been no uniform protocols for conducting biofeedback training; different clinics vary widely in how this training is done. (3) There is no consensus on what criteria should be used to select patients for treatment. For example, should fecally incontinent patients with an anatomical defect be tried on biofeedback or should they be referred to surgery? Are patients with rectal prolapse likely to benefit?

The goals of this chapter are (1) to explain the rationale for biofeedback for fecal incontinence, constipation, and pelvic pain; (2) to describe the treatment protocols used in each of these areas; and (3) to evaluate the effectiveness of treatment based on a systematic review of the literature.

Fecal Incontinence

Epidemiology

Prevalence

Estimates of the prevalence of fecal incontinence range from 2% ([1] to 7% [2]. Severe or large volume fecal incontinence occurs in 0.8% to 1.5% of US adults [1,2]. The incidence is high in children up to about age 9 years [8,9] but then decreases to a low level in adolescents and young to middle-aged adults, and increases again after about age 60, achieving a prevalence of about 7–9.5% in adults over the age of 65 [2,10].

Impact on Quality of Life

Fecal incontinence, in combination with urinary incontinence, is the second most common reason for elderly institutionalization [11]. Fecal incontinence is present in an estimated 47% of nursing homes patients [12] and 56% of psychogeriatric ward patients [13]. Among community-dwelling adults, fecal incontinence has a marked inhibitory effect on sexual behavior and may lead to social isolation as a result of embarrassment [14]. In a random sample of 704 Olmsted County, Minnesota, residents who were 65 years or older, incontinent subjects showed impairment on the role-functioning and current-health subscales of the SF-36 (short-form health survey) even after statistical adjustment for the presence of chronic illness, number of medications taken, and impact on activities [15]. Similarly, incontinent patients seen in an outpatient medical clinic had impairments on the SF-36 scales for Bodily Pain, Role Physical, Mental Health, and Social Functioning [16]. These are generic scales for the assessment of quality of life. A new disease-specific instrument for assessing quality of life in patients with fecal incontinence has recently been described [17].

Morbidity and Economic Burden

There is no increase in mortality specifically attributable to fecal incontinence, but there is a significant morbidity attributable to skin breakdown and urinary tract infections [11]. In addition to the cost of institutionalization, more than US$400 million is spent each year on fecal incontinence appliances in the United States [18].

Pathothysiology

Figure 28.1 shows the anatomy of the pelvic floor and illustrates the physiological mechanisms which are critical to the preservation of continence. The first of these factors is the motility (contractile activity) of the distal colon: Constipation associated with decreased peristaltic motility, and diarrhea associated with patterns of motility that promote the delivery of liquid stool to the rectum, are the most common causes of fecal incontinence. However, these forms of incontinence are rarely treated with biofeedback.

The rectum has two characteristics that are important to continence: compliance and sensation.

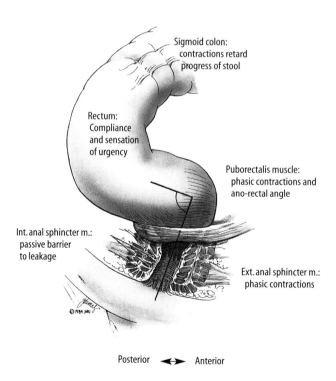

Figure 28.1   Anatomy of the anal canal and rectum showing the physiologic mechanisms important to continence and defecation. See text for details. (Reproduced with permission from Whitehead WE, Schuster MM. Gastrointestinal Disorders: Behavioral and Physiological Basis for Treatment. Orlando, FL: Elsevier Science, 1985.)

The rectum normally relaxes to store stool just prior to defecation, and decreased compliance (seen in inflammation of the rectum or radiation injury) contributes to incontinence by causing rapid transit through the rectum with insufficient time to contract the pelvic floor muscles to avoid incontinence. At the other extreme, an overly compliant rectum may promote the development of a fecal impaction, which decreases perception of rectal filling with new stool, dilates the internal anal sphincter, and allows liquid stool to leak out [19]. Abnormal compliance is not thought to be modifiable with biofeedback training.

The second characteristic of the rectum important to continence is sensation: People are normally able to perceive very small distensions of the rectum, and this is a critical cue to tell them when to contract the pelvic floor muscles to avoid incontinence [20]. Impaired ability to sense rectal distension, which is common in diabetics with peripheral neuropathies [21] as well as in patients with brain and spinal cord injuries [22], may cause patients to fail to contract at appropriate times, resulting in incontinence. Biofeedback training in the form of sensory discrimination training may be useful for this type of incontinence.

The anal canal is surrounded by the striated muscles of the pelvic floor and by the external anal sphincter. The puborectalis is a sling muscle which loops around the posterior aspect of the rectum to form the anorectal angle and anchors anteriorly to the symphysis pubis. The puborectalis muscle normally stays partially contracted and is responsible for maintaining the approximately 90-degree angle between the rectum and the anal canal. It is innervated by the pudendal nerve, originating from the sacral spinal cord. This muscle can be voluntarily contracted further to pinch off the rectum and prevent any loss of solid stool. However, because it is a sling muscle, the puborectalis is less effective for preventing the loss of liquid and gas than it is for solid stool.

The external anal sphincter is a purse-string muscle which surrounds the anal canal (no bony attachments) and which is able to close the anal canal very effectively when it is voluntarily contracted. This striated muscle, like the puborectalis, is innervated by the pudendal nerve and is under voluntary control. Obstetrical tears or other traumas to this muscle [23], or injuries to the pudendal nerve which innervates it, are common causes of fecal incontinence. Weakness of the external anal sphincter due to pudendal nerve injury is thought to be more responsive to biofeedback training than are other types of fecal incontinence [24].

Types of Biofeedback Training

Theory of Biofeedback Learning

The type of learning on which biofeedback training is based is motor skills learning: the patient attempts to perform some action and uses feedback from the success or failure of his/her attempt to learn how to refine their performance [25]. A good example is learning to throw a basketball: the individual throws repeatedly and learns from the successful shots how to throw the ball more accurately. In the case of physiological responses such as sphincter contractions, however, feedback on the success or failure of attempts to control the pelvic floor muscles may be difficult to perceive, especially if the muscle is initially quite weak. Consequently, biofeedback training involves detecting and transforming small changes in the muscle response to visual or auditory signals, which the patient can use to refine his/her motor skills. Biofeedback training sessions are usually supplemented by home practice (Kegel exercises), the purpose of which is to increase muscle strength by increasing the number of muscle fibers innervated by existing nerves. Biofeedback is not thought to repair or generate new neural pathways.

Biofeedback for fecal incontinence was first described more then 25 years ago [26]. The goal of biofeedback is to improve the ability of the patient to voluntarily contract the external anal sphincter in response to rectal filling either by improving the strength of the sphincter or by increasing the patient's ability to perceive weak distensions of the rectum, or by a combination of these two mechanisms. We have systematically reviewed the 36 studies in which biofeedback was used to treat fecal incontinence, limiting our review to those studies in which there were at least five patients treated and in which the technique was described in sufficient detail to confirm that biofeedback was the primary treatment. We found that biofeedback protocols could be divided into three basic types: pressure biofeedback, electromyographic (EMG) biofeedback, and sensory discrimination training (described below).

Pressure Biofeedback

Biofeedback training to improve the strength of the external anal sphincter has most frequently been done by recording anal canal pressures and providing a visual or auditory signal that is proportional to anal canal pressure. The patient is asked to squeeze as if preventing defecation and is given visual feedback and verbal guidance on how to accomplish this. He/she may also be taught to inhibit inappropriate responses such as contraction of the rectus abdominis or gluteal muscles, which may accompany the contraction of the external anal sphincter. In many laboratories, patients have been asked to squeeze in response to distension of the rectum (accomplished by inflating a balloon in the rectum) [27,28], but in other laboratories, the patient is asked to squeeze without rectal distension [29].

EMG Biofeedback

Biofeedback training to strengthen pelvic floor muscles may also be done by showing the patient a recording of the average EMG activity recorded from the striated muscles surrounding the anal canal [29]. In EMG biofeedback training, the patient is usually asked to squeeze and relax repeatedly without the rectum being distended. Information on inappropriate abdominal wall contraction is usually not provided with this type of biofeedback training. Home exercises in which the patient is asked to repeatedly squeeze the pelvic floor muscles (Kegel exercises) to further strengthen these muscles are usually requested whether the biofeedback training employs anal canal pressure or pelvic floor EMG.

Sensory Discrimination Training

Biofeedback training directed at increasing the patient's ability to perceive and respond to rectal distension [21,30] is based on sensory discrimination training. A catheter with a balloon attached to its tip is introduced into the rectum, and the balloon is distended with different volumes of air. The patient may be asked to report when he/she feels the distension, or may be asked to respond to the balloon distension by contracting the pelvic floor muscles. In either case, large distensions which the patient can easily perceive are presented first, and then the volume of rectal distension is gradually reduced until the patient has difficulty detecting when the balloon was distended. By repeatedly distending the balloon slightly above and then slightly below the patient's sensory threshold, and by providing feedback on accuracy of detection, the patient is taught to recognize weaker and weaker distensions. In many laboratories, this type of sensory training is combined with sphincter strengthening training by having the patient always contract in response to rectal distension and encouraging the patient to contract as strongly as possible while providing feedback on the strength of contraction as well as the accuracy of detection [22,30].

Biofeedback Treatment of Fecal Incontinence in Geriatric Patients

In the early 1980s, our laboratory undertook a study of the biofeedback treatment of fecal incontinence in patients over 65 years of age [30]. In this study, we sought to control for the nonspecific effects of behavioral and medical management by providing a behavioral management program in which patients attempted defecation at a routine time every day, for 4 weeks prior to the start of biofeedback. Only patients who continued to be incontinent progressed to biofeedback training. In addition, we sought to show that Kegel exercises, which are usually prescribed in combination with biofeedback training for fecal incontinence, are not sufficient to establish continence without biofeedback (i.e., visual or auditory feedback) training. Half of the patients were randomly selected to perform Kegel exercises during this 4-week run-in period but were not provided with any biofeedback information to help them learn how to perform Kegel exercises appropriately; the other half of patients waited until the end of the 4-week run-in before beginning Kegel exercises, and did these exercises in conjunction with biofeedback training. All patients were tested for voluntary anal canal squeeze pressures at the beginning of the run-in period, at the onset of biofeedback training, and again at the end of biofeedback training.

Principal findings were: (1) Behavioral training, with or without Kegel exercises, was associated with a non-significant trend towards reduced frequency of incontinence, with two patients achieving continence with behavioral training alone. (2) Patients who performed Kegel exercises during the 4-week run-in showed greater increases in sphincter squeeze pressures from before to after the run-in period when compared to the patients who did not perform Kegel exercises. However, the Kegel group did not show significantly greater improvements in bowel control as compared to the patients who did not perform Kegel exercises during the run-in. (3) Biofeedback was associated with a significant increase in the strength of the external anal sphincter squeeze pressure from before to after biofeedback training, and this was associated with a significant improvement in bowel control when compared to the run-in period. Thus, it appeared from this study that biofeedback was superior to Kegel exercises alone, but the experiment did not provide a definitive test of this hypothesis because the sample size was small and because biofeedback plus Kegel exercises was not compared to Kegel exercises alone in a parallel group design.

One of the authors (SH) compared four types of biofeedback training to determine whether one could be shown to be superior to the others [31]. The four training methods were (1) EMG biofeedback training, (2) EMG plus rectal balloon training, (3) EMG biofeedback plus daily use of a home biofeedback trainer, and (4) EMG, balloon training, and use of a home biofeedback trainer. There were 8–10 subjects in each group, and all completed weekly one-hour training sessions in the clinic. All four groups showed significant reductions in the frequency of fecal incontinence, but there were no significant differences between groups.

Literature Review on Outcomes of Biofeedback Training

As previously noted, we have systematically reviewed published studies in which biofeedback was used to treat fecal incontinence. To be included, studies had to meet minimal criteria (i.e., minimum of five patients studied, biofeedback technique described, biofeedback effects not confounded with surgery). The following is a summary of this literature review:

1. The median success rate for the 36 studies we reviewed was 75% of patients who achieved at least a 75% reduction in the frequency of fecal incontinence. However, only approximately 50% of patients achieved complete continence.

2. Only two studies employed prospective, randomized, parallel group experimental designs [22,32]: (a) The study by Whitehead and colleagues [22] compared biofeedback plus behavioral management to behavioral management alone in children with fecal incontinence secondary to myelomeningocele. They found a significant improvement in both groups, suggesting that biofeedback is not superior to behavioral management for most children with myelomeningocele. (b) Miner and colleagues [32] employed a complex crossover design which made interpretation of results difficult. Their 25 adult patients were first randomized to receive either three sessions of sensory discrimination training (feedback on accuracy of perceiving threshold volumes of distension) or a control treatment involving exposure to similar distensions without instructions or feedback on accuracy of perception. The sensory training group showed significant reductions in frequency of incontinence and the control group did not, but between-group differences were not statistically significant due to small samples. Patients in the control group were subsequently provided with sensory training and showed improved continence. Then all 25 patients were randomized again to receive either sphincter strengthening exercises without rectal distensions, or they were taught to squeeze in response to rectal distension with feedback (which the investigators termed coordination training). As a group, patients showed further improvements in continence with this second phase of training, but there were no significant differences between the groups, due perhaps to the confounding from multiple crossovers and small sample sizes. This study suggested that sensory training was important to the elimination of incontinence, but the results were not definitive owing to limited statistical power. (c) A third study [33] employed a parallel group design comparing 16 patients who received pressure biofeedback to 8 patients who received medications, but in a major design flaw, patients were not randomly assigned (they were allowed to select the treatment they preferred). These investigators found significant improvements relative to baseline in the biofeedback group but not in the medication control group. However, between-group comparisons were not reported and are presumed not to have been statistically significant.

3. Most published studies have used recordings of pressure from the anal canal rather than pelvic floor EMG as the basis for biofeedback. In the majority of these studies, patients were taught to squeeze in response to rectal distension with a balloon. However, comparisons between studies do not show any clear superiority for pressure versus EMG feedback.

4. Several studies suggest that sensory discrimination training (i.e., training directed at reducing the threshold for perception of rectal distension) is important to the success of biofeedback training [21,28,32,34,35]. However, sensory training is not essential for a successful outcome, as is shown by the good outcomes in several studies which employed EMG biofeedback and did not include any sensory training.

5. Nonspecific components of treatment including education, attention from health care providers, and sometimes the use of laxatives or anti-diarrheal agents, clearly contribute to the successful outcomes which have been reported [[30–32,34].

Others have reviewed this literature: Enck [36] reviewed 13 biofeedback studies published between 1974 and 1990 and found an overall improvement rate of 80% (range: 50–90% improved). A subsequent review of 14 biofeedback studies done between 1988 and 1997 reported that 40–100% of patients were improved [37]. However, these impressive outcomes should be considered cautiously because: (1) there have been no uniform criteria for defining improvement or assessing outcome; (2) only three of the studies used parallel group designs, and these studies lacked statistical power due to small samples and did not control for placebo effects; (3) inclusion criteria differed; and (4) treatment protocols varied.

Constipation Caused by Pelvic Floor Dyssynergia

Epidemiology

The prevalence of pelvic floor dyssynergia in the population is unknown because the diagnosis requires laboratory testing (anorectal manometry, pelvic floor EMG, and/or radiological studies) [7]. However, the prevalence of the symptoms believed to be associated with pelvic floor dyssynergia has been studied: In a random sample of 10 018 US adults, Stewart and colleagues [38] reported that 12% had difficulty letting go of a stool on at least 25% of bowel movements, 19% experienced a blockage on more than 25% of bowel movements, and 12% reported pressing with fingers on the perineum or in the vagina to facilitate defecation at least 25% of the time. The proportion of patients with chronic constipation who have been referred to an academic medical center has been reported to be as low as 8% [39] and as high as 74% [40], but more typically it is 25–50% [5,41].

Pathophysiology

Normally, during the act of defecation the puborectalis sling muscle and the external anal sphincter (Figure 28.1) relax to permit defecation, as can be demonstrated by recording EMG activity from the pelvic floor muscles or anal canal pressures during defecation (Figure 28.2). However, some chronically constipated patients inappropriately contract [4] or fail to relax the external anal sphincter or puborectalis muscle, or both muscles, which obstructs defecation [42,43] (Figure 28.3). Pelvic floor dyssynergia (also called anismus) is defined by paradoxical contraction or failure to relax the pelvic floor during attempts to defecate.

Preston and Lennard-Jones [4] first described the association of paradoxical contraction of the pelvic floor with constipation, and subsequent investigators confirmed their observation [44]. This abnormality is not attributable to a neurological lesion

since at least two-thirds of patients can learn to relax the external anal sphincter and puborectalis muscles appropriately when provided with biofeedback training [36].

Recent reports suggest that the finding of pelvic floor dyssynergia is variable from one occasion of testing to another [45] and is less likely to be seen when the patient is at home when ambulatory monitors are used to record the response to straining, as compared to laboratory testing. Pelvic floor dyssynergia is also observed in some asymptomatic controls and fecally incontinent patients [46], causing some investigators to question whether this is a distinct abnormality causing constipation [47]. However, most believe that, while current diagnostic criteria may lead to false positive diagnoses, there exists a subgroup of patients whose symptoms of chronic constipation and/or fecal impaction occur as a result of inability to relax the pelvic floor when straining to defecate [7].

Psychological Contributions to Etiology

Anxiety and/or psychological stress may also contribute to the development of pelvic floor dyssynergia by increasing the level of skeletal muscle tension. Heymen and colleagues [48] found clinically significant elevations on the Minnesota Multiphasic Personality Inventory (MMPI) scales for hypochondriasis and depression, and an elevation which was nearly two standard deviations above normal for scale 3 (hysteria) in these patients; and Burnett et al. [16] (1998) reported that they had significantly higher scores on the SCL-90R (symptom checklist 90, revised) scales for anxiety, depression, hostility, interpersonal sensitivity, obsessive compulsive traits, phobic anxiety, and somatization. Similar studies showing elevated levels of psychological distress in patients with symptoms of difficult defecation were reviewed by Whitehead [49]. However, other studies suggest that children with pelvic floor dyssynergia do not have any more behavior problems than children without pelvic floor dyssynergia [50,51].

Inappropriate learning may contribute to the development of pelvic floor dyssynergia in children, as suggested by the fact that the defect may be rapidly reversed with biofeedback training (see below). Some investigators have speculated that the pain associated with attempting to defecate large, hard stools may result in inadvertent learning by children to contract the sphincters in order to avoid or terminate pain during defecation [50,52,53]. This could result in a spiral of harder stools and further fear of defecation.

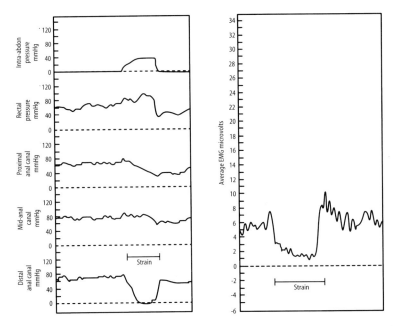

Figure 28.2 The left panel shows normal anal canal pressure in response to straining to defecate in a patient with colonic inertia type constipation. Top channel shows pressure in a 10 ml air-filled rectal balloon used to detect increases in intra-abdominal pressure during straining. The next four channels show pressures in the anal canal. In the most distal channel, which is in the high pressure zone of the anal canal, straining is associated with a decrease in anal canal pressure, which is the normal response. The right panel, taken from the same patient, shows the averaged EMG recorded from a perineometer type electrode in the anal canal; this patient shows normal reflex inhibition of pelvic floor EMG during straining. (Reproduced with permission from Whitehead et al. [7].)

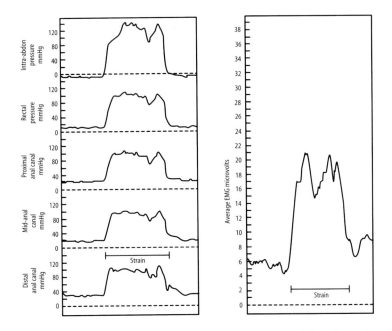

Figure 28.3 Left panel shows paradoxical increases in anal canal pressure during straining to defecate in a patient with pelvic floor dyssynergia. The top channel shows intra-abdominal pressure recorded from a 10 ml air-filled balloon and reflects normal increases in pressure associated with straining. However, the lower four channels all show paradoxical increases in anal canal pressure, which would obstruct defecation, rather than decreases in anal canal pressure, which would permit defecation to occur. The right panel, taken from the same patient, shows that these paradoxical increases in anal canal pressure are accompanied by increases in averaged pelvic floor EMG. (Reproduced with permission from Whitehead et al. [7].)

Leroi and colleagues [54] found a greater incidence of sexual abuse in women with pelvic floor dyssynergia. These authors speculate that following the trauma of sexual abuse, any sensation of rectal fullness may trigger a memory of the original trauma and may lead to an involuntary contraction of the pelvic floor muscles.

Impact on Quality of Life

Patients with symptoms of difficult defecation show significant impairments on the SF-36 scales for bodily pain, role physical (limitations in ability to work or perform usual physical activities), and general health, even when the possible mediating effects of neuroticism (a personality trait associated with a generally pessimistic attitude) are statistically controlled for [16].

Biofeedback Treatment

The earliest behavioral treatment for pelvic floor dyssynergia was simulated defecation: The team of Bleijenberg and Kuijpers [55] described an inpatient program in which water-filled balloons were introduced into the rectum and slowly pulled out while the patient was encouraged to attend to the sensations produced by the balloon and to try to facilitate balloon passage. At other times, these patients had porridge introduced into the rectum to simulate stool, and they practiced defecating this. This approach is used infrequently because it is offensive to some patients and some physicians. Moreover, one study [56] found EMG biofeedback to be more effective than simulated defecation.

The largest series of constipated patients treated with biofeedback was reported by Gilliland and colleagues [57]. In this series of 194 patients, 63% of patients who completed the treatment protocol reported complete success (≥3 unassisted bowel movements per week). If patients were included who discontinued treatment prematurely, 35% had complete success (defined as at least 3 unassisted bowel movements per week and discontinuation of cathartics), and 13% reported partial success (defined as at least one unassisted bowel movement per week with decreased cathartics).

Heymen and colleagues [58] subsequently compared four approaches to the biofeedback treatment of pelvic floor dyssynergia: (1) EMG biofeedback training alone, (2) EMG plus rectal balloon biofeedback training, (3) EMG plus daily use of a home biofeedback trainer, and (4) EMG, balloon biofeedback, and home trainer combined. There were 8–10 subjects in each group. There was a significant increase in the frequency of unassisted bowel movements in groups 1, 2, and 4; and there was a significant decrease in the use of cathartics by groups 1, 2, and 3. There were no significant differences between groups, although the small sample sizes limited the statistical power of between-group comparisons.

Literature Review on the Outcomes of Biofeedback Treatment

We have systematically reviewed all published studies of biofeedback for pelvic floor dyssynergia, which included a total of 40 studies. This literature may be summarized as follows:

1. Sensory training, in which subjects are taught to recognize the sensations associated with normal defecation, has been a part of many treatment protocols. It is accomplished by inflating a balloon in the rectum and slowly pulling it out [55,59], by having the patient attempt to defecate a balloon [60,61], or by having the patient practice defecating oatmeal or psyllium introduced into the rectum as an enema [55]. In the only study which systematically compared biofeedback with and without such sensory training [56], EMG biofeedback alone appeared to be superior. However, further studies are needed.

2. Most studies in the last 10 years have employed pelvic floor EMG instead of anal canal pressure as the basis for biofeedback. Only two studies directly compared the two types of biofeedback [58,62]. Neither found significant differences.

3. Six parallel group studies have compared biofeedback to conventional therapy, and results were mixed. Five of these studies involved children, and it has been suggested that the etiology of pelvic floor dyssynergia may differ for children compared with adults.

   a) Wald and colleagues [50] compared pressure biofeedback to mineral oil in 50 fecally incontinent children, of whom only 18 had pelvic floor dyssynergia. There were no significant differences between treatments, but there was a trend for patients with pelvic floor dyssynergia to do better with biofeedback and for patients without pelvic floor dyssynergia to do better with mineral oil.

   b) Loening-Baucke [63] compared biofeedback (pressure and EMG) to laxatives in 41 children all of whom had pelvic floor dyssynergia. The biofeedback group did significantly better.

c) Van der Plas and colleagues [64] compared biofeedback (pressure and EMG) to laxatives plus scheduled evacuation in 192 constipated children, 40% of whom had pelvic floor dyssynergia. There were no between-group differences.

d) In a second study from the same group, van der Plas and colleagues [51] compared biofeedback plus laxatives to laxatives alone. At the end of training a higher proportion of children treated with biofeedback plus laxatives were categorized as successful (39% versus 19%), but by 12 months, there were no differences between groups.

e) Nolan and co-workers [65] compared EMG biofeedback plus laxatives to laxatives alone in 29 children, all of whom had pelvic floor dyssynergia. There were no between-group differences.

f) Koutsomanis and colleagues [66] compared EMG biofeedback training to defecate a balloon (n = 29) to guided practice of balloon defecation without visual feedback (n = 30). Both groups reported subjective improvement (69% versus 64%) associated with increased frequency of bowel movements and decreased straining. Limitations of this trial were (1) etiology of constipation was mixed, although approximately 75% had pelvic floor dyssynergia; and (2) relatively few training sessions were provided (average of three).

Biofeedback studies for pelvic floor dyssynergia have been reviewed by others [36,37]. These reviews suggest that approximately two-thirds of adult patients with pelvic floor dyssynergia benefit from biofeedback training. However, there are no controlled trials comparing biofeedback to either sham biofeedback or conventional treatment in adults, and there are no data on long-term efficacy, nor on which component of treatment is most effective. Despite these limitations, biofeedback therapy is often regarded as the treatment of choice for this problem [67].

Functional Anorectal Pain

Recently, the Rome criteria for Functional Anorectal Pain have been revised (Rome II) and two distinct anorectal pain disorders have been identified, levator ani syndrome and proctalgia fugax [7]. While the two disorders may coexist, they differ based upon the duration, frequency, and characteristic of the anorectal pain. Other causes of anorectal pain such as ischemia, fissures, inflammatory bowel disease, solitary rectal ulcer, and intramuscular abscess must be excluded.

Levator Ani Syndrome

Levator ani syndrome has been previously referred to as levator spasm, pyriformis syndrome, puborectalis syndrome, chronic proctalgia, and pelvic tension myalgia. The diagnosis of levator ani syndrome requires at least 12 weeks (which need not be consecutive) during the preceding 12 months of chronic or recurrent rectal pain or aching, with episodes lasting 20 minutes or longer, and exclusion of any organic basis for the pain [7,67]. The prevalence of levator ani syndrome is estimated at 6.6% of the general population [2]. More than half of the affected patients are aged 30–60 years, but the prevalence declines after age 45. It appears to be more common in women. Only 29% of affected individuals consult a physician, although there is significant associated disability [2].

The pathophysiological basis for levator ani syndrome has not been established, but two studies [68,69] show that the majority of patients have chronic elevated levels of tension in the striated pelvic floor muscles and that biofeedback training to teach patients to relax these pelvic floor muscles often provides relief of pain. Moreover, a review of the treatment literature suggests that most of the treatments which have been recommended for this disorder are directed at relaxation of tense pelvic floor muscles (see Whitehead et al. 2000 [7] for a review of these uncontrolled treatment studies).

Heymen and colleagues [48] reported that the MMPI profiles of patients with intractable rectal pain show a preoccupation with bodily symptoms and a fear of disease (shown by elevations on scales 1, 2 and 3 of the MMPI). Salzano and colleagues [69] also reported that these patients have psychological test scores showing elevated levels of anxiety.

Proctalgia Fugax

In contrast to levator ani syndrome, proctalgia fugax is defined as sudden, severe pain localized to the anus or lower rectum that lasts from seconds to several minutes with an absence of anorectal pain between episodes [7]. Attacks are typically infrequent, occurring five times a year in 51% of patients. Community prevalence estimates have ranged from 8 to 18% with only 17–20% of these patients reporting symptoms to their physicians. A small subset of individuals experience proctalgia fugax on a frequent basis. Two studies [70,71] suggest that smooth muscle spasm may be the cause of proctalgia fugax.

When comparing proctalgia fugax patients to healthy controls, patients appear to be more perfectionist, anxious and/or hypochondriacal [72].

Biofeedback Treatment for Chronic Anorectal Pain

Research on rectal pain has been hampered by the lack of a consensus on appropriate diagnostic criteria. It appears that most patients enrolled in biofeedback treatment studies have had levator ani syndrome, but patients with proctalgia fugax may have been included in some studies. No controlled, parallel-group studies of treatment outcome are available, but the following uncontrolled studies suggest that biofeedback training to teach relaxation of the pelvic floor may be effective.

Grimaud and colleagues [68] reported a prospective evaluation of 12 patients with chronic rectal pain (patients with proctalgia fugax and coccygodynia were excluded). Patients received both pre- and post-treatment manometric assessments and defecography, and these data were compared with those of 12 healthy control subjects. Prior to treatment, resting anal pressures averaged 67 mmHg for patients compared with 44 mmHg for controls, and 75% of the patients demonstrated pelvic floor dyssynergia when straining to defecate. Biofeedback training consisted of 30-minute sessions in which anal canal pressure was displayed and subjects were instructed to relax. They also practiced relaxation at home, and used the relaxation technique at times when rectal pain occurred. Patients were treated on a weekly basis until they reported being pain free. Thereafter, patients were seen for three follow-up sessions scheduled on a monthly basis followed by sessions scheduled for every 3 months. All subjects were initially able to achieve a pain-free status in an average of eight treatment sessions. Post-treatment manometric assessment revealed a mean resting anal canal pressure of 42 mmHg, which was similar to that of the healthy controls. All but one of the patients who had pelvic floor dyssynergia at pre-treatment, showed anal pressure relaxation at post-treatment. Only one patient reported a relapse of pain. On reassessment, this patient again showed elevated anal canal pressures. During the assessment session, the patient was able to decrease anal canal pressure to the normal range with cueing and he reported that his pain resolved. Although this study lacks a control for attention and other non-specific aspects of treatment, these investigators demonstrated that they could alleviate anorectal pain in an average of 10 sessions with anal canal pressure biofeedback, and the pain reduction appeared to be

associated with a decrease in anal canal resting pressures and a decrease in inappropriate motor responses (pelvic floor dyssynergia) during simulated defecation.

Ger and colleagues [73] reported a retrospective evaluation of 60 consecutive patients diagnosed with chronic intractable rectal pain. Patients met inclusion criteria if they had either frequent episodic pain or pain of a more long-lasting nature. Patients were presented with three treatment options and chose which form of treatment they desired. Thus, subjects entered treatment groups in a non-randomized fashion to either electrogalvanic stimulation (EGS), biofeedback, or steroid caudal block (SCB). Biofeedback was conducted by a certified therapist through six 50-minute sessions. Using an intra-anal EMG sensor, patients were trained to alternately contract and relax anorectal muscles and were instructed to relax pelvic floor muscles when attempting a bowel movement. Patients were instructed to practice Kegel exercises in a series of 20 sphincter contractions and relaxations without feedback five times a day at home. They were evaluated a mean of 15 months after completing treatment. Of the 14 patients initially receiving biofeedback, 14.3% reported complete relief of symptoms (compared with 6.9% for EGS and 0% for SCB) and 28.6% reported acceptable improvement in the frequency and intensity of pain (compared with 31.0% for EGS and 18.2% for SCB). While biofeedback produced the highest success rate, none of the procedures benefited even half of the patients.

This research team also examined retrospectively the records of 86 patients who completed more than one session of intra-anal EMG biofeedback to assess the efficacy of biofeedback and to identify variables which might predict treatment success [74]. All biofeedback was conducted by a trained and experienced biofeedback therapist using intra-anal EMG feedback. There were 34.7% of patients who reported an improvement in symptoms. The major predictor variable for success was whether the patients completed therapy versus terminating biofeedback training prematurely. Age, duration of symptoms, and the presence of paradoxical puborectalis contraction were not predictive of success.

Two studies have used biofeedback based on anal canal pressures rather than EMG activity from the pelvic floor. Heah and colleagues [75] studied 16 patients with levator ani who had an average duration of symptoms of 32 months. Pain ratings decreased from a median of eight before treatment to a median of two after treatment, and the patients reported a significant reduction in the use of non-steroidal anti-inflammatory drugs (NSAIDs). However, pain reduction was not associated with significant reductions in anal canal pressures. In the second study [69], 31 patients with chronic anal pain were treated with pressure biofeedback, and all reported improvements in anal pain. In contrast to the previous study, these authors reported that symptom improvement was associated with significant reductions in anal canal pressures.

To date, no studies have included control groups with random assignment to treatment condition in order to control for placebo effects. Moreover, with the exception of the Heah et al. [75] study, investigators have not distinguished patients with proctalgia fugax from those with levator ani syndrome. Given the different presentation of these disorders, it is reasonable to hypothesize that there may be different pathophysiological mechanisms underlying the disorders (e.g. smooth muscle spasm versus spasm of striated pelvic floor muscles). It is recommended that future research utilize the Rome II consensus criteria in selecting patient groups.

In contrast to fecal incontinence and constipation, less is known about the pathophysiology of functional rectal pain disorders. Without knowing the underlying pathophysiology of the disorder, it is difficult to know what aspect of physiology biofeedback should address. For example, if proctalgia fugax is indeed a disorder produced by spasm of smooth muscles, then biofeedback using intra-anal EMG electrodes, which primarily reflect striated external anal sphincter activity, may not provide useful information to the patient in being able to regulate their pain. With greater understanding of the underlying pathophysiology of the disorders, new biofeedback procedures may be developed to facilitate changes in physiological self-regulation more specific to the disorders.

Presently, the findings of uncontrolled empirical studies suggest that biofeedback may be useful to some patients in managing chronic rectal pain. Biofeedback is not associated with side effects or adverse events that may occur as a result of medications or surgery nor has it been shown to worsen or exacerbate symptoms. Comparisons with other treatment alternatives (i.e., surgery, electrogalvanic stimulation, sacral blockade, analgesic medications) suggest (but do not prove) that biofeedback may be more effective. Given the significant disability associated with functional anorectal pain disorders, further development of biofeedback therapies and alternative treatment modalities is needed. However, future studies should focus on more restrictive and more carefully characterized patient groups (e.g. patients with levator ani syndrome who have elevated anal canal pressure or elevated pelvic floor

EMG), and they should take into account the psychological symptoms that have been found to be associated with chronic rectal pain.

Summary

Biofeedback training is a form of motor skills learning in which the patient practices an activity and learns from their successes and failures how to refine their performance. What is unique about biofeedback training is that electronic devices are used to enhance the amount of sensory information available to patients on the success of their efforts. This is especially useful in situation such as muscle weakness due to partial denervation or chronic muscle tension, where intrinsic sensory feedback is limited.

Biofeedback is considered the treatment of choice for fecal incontinence associated with weak pelvic floor muscles and/or decreased ability to perceive rectal distension. On average 75% of patients are improved, although only about 50% are cured. The appeal of biofeedback for incontinence is that it is completely safe and it is relatively inexpensive compared with surgery, which produces comparable outcomes overall.

For constipation related to pelvic floor dyssynergia, biofeedback is used to teach the patient to relax pelvic floor muscles during defecation, and it has been found to be effective in approximately 67% of cases. However, some studies suggest that it may not be superior to laxative regimens, especially in children. It is therefore recommended only after a trial of osmotic laxatives and patient education.

For chronic rectal pain associated with tense pelvic floor muscles, biofeedback is also reported to be one of the most effective treatments. However, there are too few studies to establish firm indications for treatment or to estimate the proportion of patients likely to benefit.

The success of biofeedback training depends on the skill of the trainer/therapist and varies between centers. Additional research is needed to standardize treatment protocols, to identify predictors of success, and to document efficacy in controlled studies.

Acknowledgment

This work was supported in part by NIDDKD grant RO1 DK50487.

References

1. Nelson R, Norton N, Cautley E, Furner S. Community-based prevalence of anal incontinence. JAMA 1995;274:559–61.
2. Drossman DA, Li Z, Andruzzi E, Temple RD et al. US Householder Survey of functional gastrointestinal disorders. Dig Dis Sci 1993;38:1569–80.
3. Harari D, Gurwitz JH, Avorn J, Bohn R, Minaker KL. Bowel habit in relation to age and gender. Findings from the National Health Interview Survey and clinical implications. Arch Intern Med 1996;156:315–20.
4. Preston DM, Lennard-Jones JE. Anismus in chronic constipation. Dig Dis Sci 1985;30:413–18.
5. Wald A, Caruana BJ, Freimanis MG, Bauman DH, Hinds JP. Contributions of evacuation proctography and anorectal manometry to the evaluation of adults with constipation and defecatory difficulty. Dig Dis Sci 1990;35:481–7.
6. Barnett JL, Raper SE. Anorectal diseases. In: Yamada T, Alpers DH, Owyang C, Powell DW, Silverstein, FE, editors. Textbook of Gastroenterology. New York: JB Lippincott, 1991; 1813–32.
7. Whitehead WE, Wald A, Diamant N, Enck P, Pemberton J, Rao S. Functional disorders of the anus and rectum. In: Drossman DA, Corazziari E, Talley NJ, Thompson WG, Whitehead WE, editors. Rome II: The Functional Gastrointestinal Disorders. Falls Church, VA: Degnon Associates, 2000.
8. Bellman M. Studies on encopresis. Acta Paediatr Scand 1966;56(Supplement 170):1–151.
9. Schaefer CE. Childhood Encopresis ad Enuresis: Causes ad Therapy. New York: Van Nostrand Reinhold, 1979.
10. Kinnunen O. Study of constipation in a geriatric hospital, day hospital, old people's home and at home. Aging 1991;3:161–70.
11. Cheskin LJ, Schuster MM. Fecal incontinence. In: Hazzard WR, Andres R, Bierman EL, Blass JP, editors. Principles of Geriatric Medicine and Gerontology, 2nd edn. New York: McGraw-Hill, 1990; 1143–5.
12. Nelson R, Furner S, Jesudason V. Fecal incontinence in Wisconsin nursing homes: Prevalence and associations. Dis Colon Rectum 1998;41:1226–9.
13. Thomas TM, Egan M, Walgrove A, Meade TW. The prevalence of fecal and double incontinence. Community Md 1984;6:216–20.
14. Huppe D, Enck P, Kruskemper G, May B. Psychosoziale Aspekte der Stuhlinkontinenz, Leber Magen Darm 1992;22:138–42.
15. O'Keefe EA, Talley NJ, Zinsmeister AR, Jacobsen SJ. Bowel disorders impair functional status and quality of life in the elderly: a population-based study .J Gerontol: Series A, Biological Sciences & Medical Sciences 1995;50:M184–9.
16. Burnett C, Whitehead WE, Drossman D. Psychological distress and impaired quality of life in patients with functional anorectal disorders. Gastroenterology 1998;114:A729.
17. Rockwood TH, Churh JM, Fleshman JW et al. FIQL: A quality of life instrument for patients with fecal incontinence. Dis Colon Rectum 2000;43:9–17.
18. Lahr CJ. Evaluation and treatment of incontinence. Practical Gastroenterol 1988:12:27–35.
19. Read NW, Celik AF, Kassinelos P. Constipation and incontinence in the elderly. J Clin Gastroenterol 1995;20:61–70.
20. Whitehead WE, Orr WC, Engel BT, Schuster MM. External anal sphincter response to rectal distention: Learned response or reflex. Psychophysiology 1982;19:57–62.
21. Wald A, Tunuguntla K. Anorectal sensorimotor dysfunction in fecal incontinence and diabetes mellitus. Modification with biofeedback therapy. N Engl J Med 1984;310:1282–7.
22. Whitehead WE, Parker L, Bosmajian L et al. Treatment of fecal incontinence in children with spina bifida: Comparison of biofeedback and behavior modification. Arch Phys Med Rehabil 1986;67:218–24.
23. Sultan AH, Kamm MA, Hudson CN, Thomas JM, Bartram CI. Anal sphincter disruption during vaginal delivery. N Engl J Med 1993;329:1905–11.
24. Whitehead WE, Wald A, Norton NJ. Treatment options for fecal incontinence. Dis Colon Rectum 2001;44:131–42.
25. Whitehead WE, Thompson WG. Motility as a therapeutic modality: Biofeedback. In Schuster MM, editor. Atlas of Gastrointestinal Motility in Health and Disease. Baltimore: Williams & Wilkins, 1993; 300–16.
26. Engel BT, Nikoomanesh P, Schuster MM. Operant conditioning of rectosphincteric responses in the treatment of fecal incontinence. N Engl J Med 1974;290:646–9.
27. Cerulli M, Nikoomanesh P, Schuster MM. Progress in biofeedback conditioning for fecal incontinence. Gastroenterology 1979;76:742–6.
28. Glia A, Gylin M, Akerlund JE et al. Biofeedback training in patients with fecal incontinence. Dis Colon Rectum 1998;41:359–64.
29. Patankar SK, Ferrara A, Larach SW et al. Electromyographic assessment of biofeedback training for fecal incontinence and chronic constipation. Dis Colon Rectum 97;40(8):907–11.
30. Whitehead WE, Burgio K, Engel BT. Biofeedback treatment of fecal incontinence in geriatric patients. J Am Geriatr Soc 1985;33:320–4.
31. Heymen S, Wexner SD, Vickers D, Nogueras J, Weiss EG, Pikarsky A. A prospective randomized trial comparing four biofeedback techniques for patients with fecal incontinence. Int J Colorectal Dis, in press.
32. Miner PB, Donnelly TC, Read NW. Investigation of mode of action of biofeedback in treatent of fecal incontinence. Dig Dis Sci 1990;35:1291–8.
33. Guillemot F, Bouche B, Gower-Rousseau C et al. Biofeedback for the treatment of fecal incontinence. Long-term clinical results. Dis Colon Rectum 1995;38:393–7.
34. Latimer PR, Campbell D, Kasperski J. A component analysis of biofeedback in the treatment of fecal incontinence. Biofeedback Self Regul 1984;9:311–24.
35. Buser WE, Miner PB. Delayed rectal sensation with fecal incontinence. Gastroenterology 1986;91:1186–91.
36. Enck P. Biofeedback training in disordered defecation: A critical review. Dig Dis Sci 1993;38:1953–60.
37. Rao SS, Enck P, Loening-Baucke V. Biofeedback therapy for defecation disorders. Dig Dis Sci 1997;15(Suppl 1):78–92.
38. Stewart WE, Liberman JN, Sandler RS, Woods MS, Stemhagen A, Farup CE. A large US national epidemiological study of constipation. Gastroenterology 1998;114:A44.
39. Surrenti E, Rath DM, Pemberton JH, Camilleri M. Audit of constipation in a tertiary referral gastroenterology practice. Am J Gastroenterol 1995;90:1471–5.
40. Kuijpers HC. Application of the colorectal laboratory in diagnosis and treatment of functional constipation. Dis Colon Rectum 1990;33:35–9.
41. Lestar B, Penninck FM, Kerremans RP. Defecometry: a new method for determining the parameters of rectal evacuation. Dis Colon Rectum 1989;32:179–201.
42. Kuijpers HC, Bleijenberg G. The spastic pelvic floor syndrome. A cause of constipation. Dis Colon Rectum 1985;28:669–72.
43. Kuijpers HC, Bleijenberg G, De Moiree H. The spastic pelvic floor syndrome. Large bowel outlet obstruction caused by pelvic floor dysfunction: a radiological study. Int J Colorectal Dis 1986;1:44–8.

44. Roberts JP, Womack NR, Hallan RI, Thorpe AC, Williams NS. Evidence from dynamic integrated proctography to redefine anismus. Br J Surg 1992;79:1213–15.

45. Duthie GS, Bartolo DCC. Anismus: the cause of constipation? Results of investigation and treatment. World J Surg 1992;16:831–5.

46. Schouten WR, Briel JW, Auwerda JJA et al. Anismus: fact or fiction? Dis Colon Rectum 1997;40:1033–41.

47. Mertz H, Naliboff B, Mayer EA. Symptoms and physiology in severe chronic constipation. Am J Gastroenterol 1999;94:131–8.

48. Heymen S, Wexner SD, Gulledge AD. MMPI assessment of patients with functional bowel disorders. Dis Colon Rectum 1993;36:593–6.

49. Whitehead WE. Illness behaviour. In: Kamm MA, Lennard-Jones JE, editors. Constipation. Petersfield, UK: Wrightson Biomedical Publishing, 1993; 95–100.

50. Wald A, Chandra R, Gabel S, Chiponis D. Evaluation of biofeedback in childhood encopresis. J Pediatr Gastroenterol Nutr 1987;6:554–8.

51. van der Plas RN, Benninga MA, Redekop WK, Taminiau JA, Buller HA. Randomized trial of biofeedback training for encopresis. Arch Dis Child 1996;75:367–74.

52. Keren S, Wagner Y, Heldenbert D, Golan M. Studies of manometric abnormalities of the rectoanal region during defecation in constipated and soiling children: modification through biofeedback therapy. Am J Gastroenterol 1988;83:827–31.

53. Loening-Baucke V. Factors determining outcome in children with chronic constipation and faecal soiling. Gut 1989;30:999–1006.

54. Leroi AM, Berkelmans I, Denis P, Hemond M, Devroede G. Anismus as a marker of sexual abuse. Consequences of abuse on anorectal motility. Dig Dis Sci 1995;40:1411–16.

55. Bleijenberg G, Kuijpers HC. Treatment of the spastic pelvic floor syndrome with biofeedback. Dis Colon Rectum 1987;30:108–11.

56. Bleijenberg G, Kuijpers HC. Biofeedback treatment of constipation: A comparison of two methods. Am J Gastroenterol 1994;89:1021–6.

57. Gilliland R, Heymen S, Altomare DF, Park UC, Vickers D, Wexner SD. Outcome and predictors of success of biofeedback for constipation. Br J Surg 1997;84:1123–6.

58. Heymen S, Wexner SD, Vickers D, Nogueras J, Weiss EG, Pikarsky A. A prospective randomized trial comparing four biofeedback techniques for patients with constipation. Dis Colon Rectum 1999;42:1388–93.

59. Fleshman JW, Dreznik Z, Meyer K et al. Outpatient protocol for biofeedback therapy of pelvic floor outlet obstruction. Dis Colon Rectum 1992;35:1–7.

60. Kawimbe BM, Papachrysostomou M, Binnie NR, Clare N et al. Outlet obstruction constipation (anismus) managed by biofeedback. Gut 1991;32:1175–9.

61. Rao SS, Welcher KD, Pelsing RE. Effects of biofeedback on anorectal function in obstructed defecation. Dig Dis Sci 1997;42:2197–205.

62. Glia A, Glyin M, Gullberg K, Lindberg G. Biofeedback retraining in patients with functional constipation and paradoxical puborectalis contraction. Comparison of anal manometry and sphincter electromyography for feedback. Dis Colon Rectum 1997;40:889–95.

63. Loening-Baucke V. Modulation of abnormal defecation dynamics by biofeedback treatment in chronically constipated children with encopresis. J Pediatr 1990;116:214–22.

64. van der Plas RN, Benninga MA, Buller HA et al. Biofeedback training in treatment of childhood constipation: a randomized controlled study Lancet 1996;348:776–8.

65. Nolan T, Catto-Smith T, Coffey C, Wells J. Randomized controlled trial of biofeedback training in persistent encopresis with anismus. Arch Dis Child 1998;79:131–5.

66. Koutsomanis D, Lennard-Jones JE, Roy AJ, Kamm MA. Controlled randomised trial of visual biofeedback versus muscle training without a visual display for intractable constipation. Gut 1995;37:95–9.

67. Diamant NE, Kamm MA, Wald A, Whitehead WE. AGA technical review on anorectal testing techniques. Gastroenterology 1999;116:735–60.

68. Grimaud JC, Bouvier M, Naudy B, Guien C, Salducci J. Manometric and radiologic investigations and biofeedback treatment of chronic idiopathic anal pain. Dis Colon Rectum 1991;34:690–5.

69. Salzano A, Carbone M, Rossi E et al. [Defecography and treatment of essential anal pain.] [Italian] Radiologia Medica 1999;98:48–52.

70. Rao SSC, Hatfield RA. Paroxysmal anal hyperkinesis: a characteristic feature of proctalgia fugax. Gut 1996;39:609–12.

71. Eckardt 1996.

72. Pilling LF, Swenson WM, Hill JR. The psychologic aspects of proctalgia fugax. Dis Colon Rectum 1972;8:372–376.

73. Ger GC, Wexner SD, Jorge JM et al. Evaluation and treatment of chronic intractable rectal pain – a frustrating endeavor. Dis Colon Rectum 1993;36:139–45.

74. Gilliland R, Heymen JS, Altomare DF, Vickers D, Wexner SD. Biofeedback for intractable rectal pain: outcome and predictors of success. Dis Colon Rectum 1997;40:190–6.

75. Heah SM, Ho YH, Tan M, Leong AF. Biofeedback is effective treatment for levator ani syndrome. Dis Colon Rectum 1997;40:187–9.

6 Surgical Approaches to Urinary and Fecal Incontinence

29 Anterior Colporrhaphy

Shawna L. Johnston and James A. Low

Introduction

Urinary incontinence and pelvic organ prolapse are common. Estimates of prevalence for urinary incontinence in adult females range between 10 and 30% [1]. Though genital prolapse remains one of the most common indications for gynecologic surgery, its prevalence is unknown. Beck [2] has reported prevalence estimates of as high as 50%. Olsen et al. [3] have estimated a lifetime risk (by age 80) for primary surgery for prolapse or urinary incontinence of 11%, with an incidence of re-operation estimated at 29%. Pelvic floor dysfunction, and its surgical management, are thus important health care considerations.

Over 200 different operations have been described for the surgical management of urinary stress incontinence [4]. The earliest surgeries involved repair via the vaginal route, including the anterior colporrhaphy. In the last century, there has been a move away from vaginal procedures because of higher failure rates. Nonetheless, there still remains a place for anterior colporrhaphy, particularly for the management of anterior vaginal wall prolapse alone, without associated urinary incontinence.

Historical Review

In the late nineteenth century, J. Marion Sims [5], considered by many to be the father of urogynecology, described a vaginal procedure for cystocele repair which involved simple excision of a portion of the anterior vaginal wall in an oval or rectangular shape and then closure of the vaginal incision. Numerous modifications then ensued. Kelly [6] published his classic description of anterior colporrhaphy in 1914. The operative technique additionally included dissection between the bladder and vagina

(Figure 29.1), with two or three mattress sutures placed in the vesical wall beneath the bladder neck to reapproximate, or plicate, the torn or relaxed tissues at the urethrovesical junction (Figures 29.2a, 29.2b, and 29.3). Redundant vaginal mucosa, as with the Sims technique, was excised, and the anterior prolapse thus corrected. Kennedy [7] later recommended, along with plication sutures at the bladder

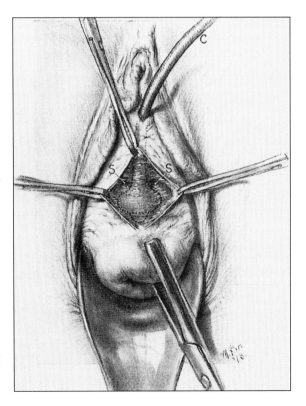

Figure 29.1 Kelly's original drawing showing the location of the vaginal incision, and the surgical dissection between the vagina and bladder. (Reproduced with permission from Kelly and Dumm [6].)

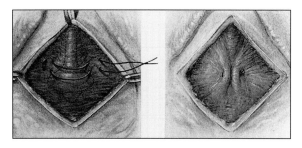

Figure 29.2 **a** Kelly's original drawing depicting placement of the Kelly plication suture at the bladder neck. **b** Kelly plication suture tied. (Reproduced with permission from Kelly and Dumm [6].)

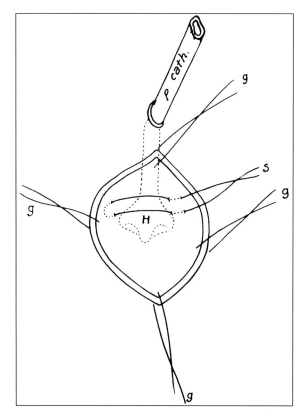

Figure 29.3 Kelly's diagrammatic representation of suture placement. (Reproduced with permission from Kelly and Dumm [6].)

neck, a two-layered plication of the proximal third of the urethra, in the area which he speculated also contained urethral sphincter components.

The goal of surgery suggested by these early authors was to reconstruct and tighten the sphincteric tissue between the bladder and vagina, and thus restore continence. More contemporary thinking, however, has rather focused on bladder neck support and normal abdominal pressure transmission to the urethra, and not on urethral sphincters

in the vaginal wall per se, which probably do not exist.

Modifications to the anterior colporrhaphy have thus been proposed with the intent of correcting bladder neck position and support with increased intra-abdominal pressure. These modifications include the placement of deep lateral sutures into the so-called pubourethral ligaments on either side of the bladder neck (Figure 29.4). Support has also been bolstered in other ways. In 1952, Ingelman-Sundberg [8] reported improved postoperative success after anterior colporrhaphy using suburethral placement of portions of the pubococcygeus muscle. Other variations have added synthetic mesh materials as an extra layer to support the bladder neck and vagina [9,10]. Zacharin proposed using a full-thickness vaginal epithelial graft under the bladder neck to achieve this effect [11].

Surgical Anatomy

Cystocele and its companion urethrocele have been described as herniations or defects in the bladder and urethra. However, these terms do not correctly depict the anatomical abnormalities of prolapse. Cystocele is described more accurately as anterior vaginal prolapse (loss of support of the anterior vagina with resultant loss of support of the bladder). Urethrocele is a condition of urethral hypermobility (loss of support at the bladder neck and urethra).

Support for the anterior vaginal wall is accrued from both midline and lateral connective tissue support. In theory, anterior colporrhaphy would be best suited for prolapse of the anterior vaginal wall from a central defect in support, the so-called distension or pulsion cystourethrocele. For prolapse occurring from a loss of lateral support, either the Burch colposuspension or the paravaginal repair would be best. However, as yet there are no controlled outcome studies comparing these different approaches.

A note should be made regarding terminology. Current concepts regarding the etiology of prolapse involve genetic, biochemical and mechanical alterations in vaginal wall fascia which compromise its integrity and strength. Furthermore, current descriptions of anterior colporrhaphy rely on surgical dissection and plication of vaginal fascia. However, fascia, per se, is characterized histologically by regular arrangements of mainly collagen. It typically covers skeletal muscle, not smooth muscle, and is attached to bone. The collagen in the vaginal walls is mainly perivascular and does not have organized arrangement of fibers. Elastin fibers and adipose tissue are intermingled. It is thus not, by definition, fascia, and its plication cannot thus be expected to invest the same strength as if it were parietal fascia elsewhere in the body. Based on gross and microscopic examination of full-thickness sections of the bladder and vagina from autopsy specimens, Weber and Walters [12] have concluded, "The vagina and bladder are not invested in their own separate layer of adventitia or connective tissue capsule. There is no vaginal fascia."

Whether or not this layer of connective tissue that is dissected and plicated during anterior colporrhaphy is a true fascial layer thus remains debatable. Nonetheless, there is a layer of connective tissue in the vaginal wall, which can usually be readily identified at surgery. Perhaps the inferior long-term surgical results with anterior colporrhaphy reflect the fact that true fascia is not used in the repair. On the other hand, in cases of successful repair, the authors speculate that it is the fibrous scar tissue from surgical dissection that maintains long-term support.

Patient Selection

Proper patient selection for anterior colporrhaphy is crucial. Surgery requires healthy vaginal tissues, and adequate vaginal capacity and depth. Preoperative estrogen replacement may be useful in improving the integrity of postmenopausal vaginal tissues. "Adequate" vaginal capacity has not been well quantified, though the authors suggest that a vagina that easily admits two fingers on digital examination be considered to have adequate capacity.

A patient with a completely asymptomatic cystourethrocele and no incontinence does not require surgery. Furthermore, there is no role for "prophylactic" surgery while the prolapse is small; it may not worsen with time, and may thus never become symptomatic. Repair of an asymptomatic cystourethrocele may result in postoperative debilitating stress incontinence, or, more rarely, detrusor instability or voiding dysfunction.

Patients with a symptomatic cystourethrocele and no urinary incontinence may develop urinary stress incontinence after anterior colporrhaphy. It is not entirely clear why this happens, though one possibility is that a marked cystourethrocele results in kinking or obstruction of an incompetent bladder neck, creating an artificial continence mechanism [13]. When this urethral kinking is corrected at surgery, urethral sphincter incompetence (genuine stress incontinence) is unmasked. This has been referred to as latent or occult genuine stress incontinence. Prevalence predictions of occult genuine

stress incontinence range between 15 and 80% [14,15].

A vaginal pessary used during preoperative urodynamic evaluation is helpful. Patients are fitted with a pessary, and if they remain continent during cystometry, they are assumed to have a competent urethral sphincter. Surgery in this scenario is necessary only to correct the vaginal wall relaxation. On the other hand, patients who become incontinent with a pessary in place during urodynamics are assumed to have occult genuine stress incontinence, with surgery then chosen to address the genuine stress incontinence in addition to the prolapse.

In patients with a symptomatic cystourethrocele and urinary incontinence, urodynamics are necessary to make an accurate and objective preoperative diagnosis. Patients with prolapse who have detrusor instability do not require an operation for relief of incontinence, and thus need surgery only for the correction of the prolapse. If genuine stress incontinence is confirmed, nonsurgical management should initially be offered, particularly in the young patient or in the patient with symptoms of mild severity, prior to considering surgery. Non-surgical management has been reported successful in 60–70% of patients [16]. A vaginal pessary or bladder neck support prosthesis that provides mechanical support to the bladder neck is often helpful. When surgery is necessary, it must address both the genuine stress incontinence and the prolapse.

There is little role for a second anterior colporrhaphy if the first surgery failed to provide significant improvement or cure, particularly for urinary incontinence where failure rates for repeat operation have been estimated to be as high as 70% [17].

Technique

Anterior colporrhaphy with Kelly plication of the bladder neck was originally described in 1911 by Howard Kelly.

The patient is placed in the supine lithotomy position. General or regional anesthesia is used, though the procedure can be performed with local anesthesia and sedation only [4]. The vagina and perineum are prepared and draped in sterile fashion, and a urethral Foley catheter with a 10 ml balloon placed to delineate the position of the bladder neck. The bladder is not drained, with the catheter connected to a spigot; inadvertent cystotomy during the procedure is thus more easily recognized. A preoperative dose of a broad-spectrum

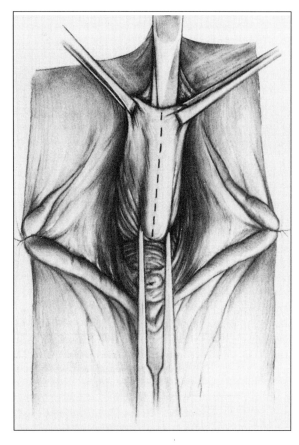

Figure 29.4   A transverse mucosal incision is made near the apex of the vagina. (Reproduced with permission from Thompson JD, Wall LL, Growdon WA, Ridley JH. Urinary stress incontinence. In: Thompson JD, Rock JA, editors. Te Linde's Operative Gynecology, 7th edn, Lippincott, 1992; 887–940.)

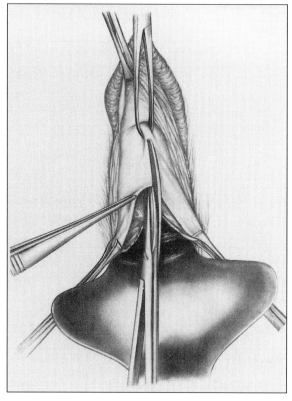

Figure 29.5   Dissection in the avascular plane between the vagina and bladder is performed bluntly by opening and closing the scissors tips. The mucosa is then incised in the midline to within one centimeter of the urethral meatus. (Reproduced with permission from Thompson JD, Wall LL, Growdon WA, Ridley JH. Urinary stress incontinence. In: Thompson JD, Rock JA, editors. Te Linde's Operative Gynecology, 7th edn, Lippincott, 1992; 887–940.)

antibiotic (a third generation cephalosporin) is given as prophylaxis against infection.

A weighted speculum is placed in the vagina. Either saline or a dilute solution of bupivacaine (with epinephrine) is injected submucosally, to decrease bleeding and to facilitate surgical dissection. A small transverse mucosal incision is made near the apex of the vagina (Figure 29.4), and through this the vesicovaginal space entered with the tips of a pair of Metzenbaum scissors. Dissection is then performed bluntly by opening and closing the scissors just beneath the vaginal mucosa (Figure 29.5). The mucosa is incised as dissection continues, along the length of the vaginal wall to within one centimeter of the urethral meatus. The final success of the procedure is likely related to the thoroughness of this dissection and to the wide mobilization of the proximal urethra and the surrounding periurethral tissue at the bladder neck.

The vaginal epithelium along the line of incision is then grasped using arterial clamps, and retracted laterally. Sharp and blunt dissection are used to mobilize connective tissue ("vesicovaginal fascia"), bladder, and urethra away from the overlying epithelium (Figures 29.6 and 29.7). Dissection should be carried out just beneath the mucosa; Thompson [4] speculated that the success of the procedure depends upon the integrity of the fascial layer left attached to the bladder. Dissection in the proper avascular plane is also important, especially in the spaces lateral to the urethrovesical junction where large perivesical vessels are found. Lateral dissection into the space beneath the inferior pubic ramus is necessary bilaterally.

Repair should begin at the urethrovesical junction, which can be identified visually or by palpation of the inflated Foley bulb. The Kelly plication sutures are first placed, using permanent suture (Ethibond 2.0). A tissue bite is taken laterally, in the strong

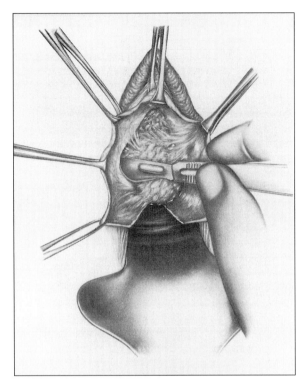

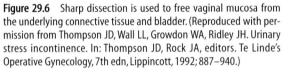

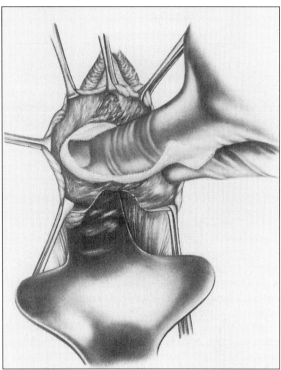

Figure 29.6 Sharp dissection is used to free vaginal mucosa from the underlying connective tissue and bladder. (Reproduced with permission from Thompson JD, Wall LL, Growdon WA, Ridley JH. Urinary stress incontinence. In: Thompson JD, Rock JA, editors. Te Linde's Operative Gynecology, 7th edn, Lippincott, 1992; 887–940.)

Figure 29.7 Blunt dissection with a gauze sponge is also used to mobilize tissues. (Reproduced with permission from Thompson JD, Wall LL, Growdon WA, Ridley JH. Urinary stress incontinence. In: Thompson JD, Rock JA, editors. Te Linde's Operative Gynecology, 7th edn, Lippincott, 1992; 887–940.)

periurethral tissue just under the symphysis pubis, with the suture crossing under the bladder neck before a similar bite is taken in periurethral tissue on the other side (Figure 29.8). When this suture is tied, the periurethral tissue is approximated toward the midline, and the bladder neck moves to a high retropubic position. One to three delayed absorbable sutures are then placed distally, to reduce the posterior component of the cystocele. Occasionally, when the cystocele is very large, a distal purse-string suture is additionally required (Figure 29.9). Care must be taken with these latter sutures to avoid deep tissue bites, as such bites may result in ureteral kinking. Cystoscopy can be performed if there is any suspicion of penetration of permanent suture material through the bladder mucosa.

After the entire cystourethrocele is repaired, excess vaginal mucosa is trimmed bilaterally (Figure 29.10) and the anterior vaginal wall closed with interrupted vertical mattress sutures that include the underlying connective tissue (Figure 29.11). Delayed absorbable suture material (Vicryl 2.0) is used here.

Following completion of the procedure, the urethral Foley catheter is connected to straight drainage, and left in place for 48 hours prior to removal and a trial of voiding. Alternatively, a suprapubic catheter can be placed intraoperatively, in closed fashion, after retrograde filling of the bladder to 500 ml. Suprapubic catheterization has the advantage of allowing spontaneous voiding to occur before final removal without the need for catheter reinsertion (which is often difficult and painful) to measure post-void residual volume. In patients with preoperative urodynamic parameters which suggest voiding difficulty, a suprapubic catheter following anterior repair is advisable. A vaginal pack can be placed for 24 hours, to minimize the chance of postoperative hematoma formation.

Complications

In general, anterior colporrhaphy is well tolerated, with a low incidence of both postoperative pain and

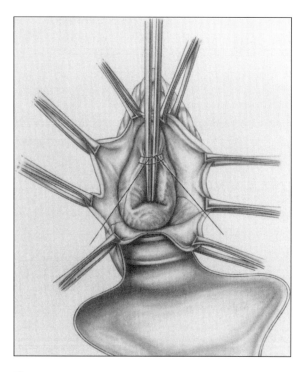
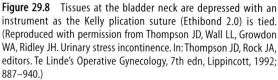

Figure 29.8 Tissues at the bladder neck are depressed with an instrument as the Kelly plication suture (Ethibond 2.0) is tied. (Reproduced with permission from Thompson JD, Wall LL, Growdon WA, Ridley JH. Urinary stress incontinence. In: Thompson JD, Rock JA, editors. Te Linde's Operative Gynecology, 7th edn, Lippincott, 1992; 887–940.)

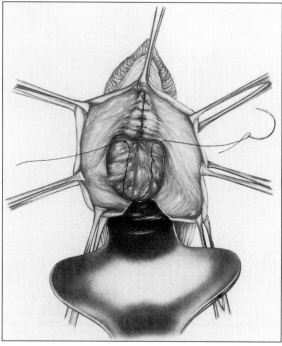

Figure 29.9 Occasionally, a distal purse string suture (Vicryl 2.0) is required to reduce the large posterior component of the cystourethrocele. (Reproduced with permission from Thompson JD, Wall LL, Growdon WA, Ridley JH. Urinary stress incontinence. In: Thompson JD, Rock JA, editors. Te Linde's Operative Gynecology, 7th edn, Lippincott, 1992; 887–940.)

patient morbidity. The operating time required is relatively short. The length of postoperative hospitalization is usually short (2–3 days), with discharge on resumption of normal voiding.

Anterior colporrhaphy is generally a straightforward procedure, but it is not free from complication. Excessive bleeding from periurethral venous plexuses can occur intraoperatively, and can be difficult to manage. Postoperative bleeding can result in hematoma formation, with or without infection, and cellulitis in the vaginal wall can occur. The incidence of each of these complications is unknown.

Accidental cystotomy can occur, particularly in those patients who have had previous vaginal surgery, especially previous anterior colporrhaphy. The site of cystotomy is usually easily identified. If proximity to either ureteric orifice is suspected, cystoscopy (through the cystotomy site if it is small) with intravenous indigo carmine dye should be first performed to identify ureteric efflux. The defect is closed in two layers using delayed absorbable suture. The efficacy of bladder closure can be

assessed intraoperatively using methylene blue dye in saline, instilled retrograde, or intravenous indigo carmine as mentioned above. After cystotomy repair, the bladder is drained for 5–7 days to allow for adequate healing. Ureteric injury can alternatively occur from intravesical suture, particularly during placement of the Kelly plication sutures. The distance between anterior colporrhaphy sutures and ureteric orifices can be as short as 0.9 mm, as reported by Hofmeister [4].

While short-term voiding difficulty is common after anterior colporrhaphy, long-term (greater than 3 months) problems are uncommon. The actual incidence is unknown. Voiding difficulty will occur more often in women with some degree of preoperative voiding dysfunction, as suggested by preoperative urodynamic parameters including elevated post-void residual volume, decreased peak urinary flow rate, and low voiding detrusor pressure (Table 29.1). Treatment of voiding dysfunction in the immediate postoperative weeks is by adequate bladder drainage with a Foley catheter or with intermittent self-catheterization until spontaneous

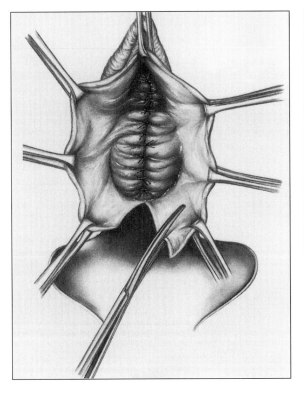

Figure 29.10 Excess vaginal mucosa is trimmed bilaterally. (Reproduced with permission from Thompson JD, Wall LL, Growdon WA, Ridley JH. Urinary stress incontinence. In: Thompson JD, Rock JA, editors. Te Linde's Operative Gynecology, 7th edn, Lippincott, 1992; 887–940.)

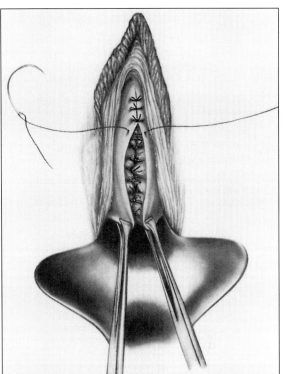

Figure 29.11 The anterior vaginal wall is closed with interrupted sutures (Vicryl 2.0). (Reproduced with permission from Thompson JD, Wall LL, Growdon WA, Ridley JH. Urinary stress incontinence. In: Thompson JD, Rock JA, editors. Te Linde's Operative Gynecology, 7th edn, Lippincott, 1992; 887–940.)

voiding resumes, usually within 6 weeks. Treatment of urinary tract infection is also important, particularly if intermittent catheterization is being used. Long-term voiding difficulty is best managed with clean intermittent self-catheterization.

Tanagho [18] and others [12] have suggested that the surgical dissection around the urethra and bladder neck at anterior colporrhaphy damages the delicate parasympathetic and sympathetic nerves, partially denervating the urethra and detrusor muscle and potentially causing detrusor instability. Stanton and colleagues [19] have disputed this; in 73 patients followed for 2 years after anterior repair, objective assessment with urodynamics (prior to and following surgery) did not show significant increases in the incidence of detrusor instability.

Genuine stress incontinence can occur de novo following anterior repair, presumably from denervation injury to the urethral sphincter. An alternate explanation is overcorrection of the cystocele component of the prolapse, so that there is a loss in the normal posterior urethrovesical angle between the bladder base and bladder neck. This concept is,

however, an old one, now replaced by the concept that de novo postoperative incontinence occurs because latent genuine stress incontinence is unmasked when urethral kinking is surgically corrected.

Additional complications following anterior repair result from decreased vaginal mobility and capacity of the vagina from postoperative scarring. This renders subsequent surgery to correct incontinence more difficult to perform and more likely to fail. Sexual function can also be compromised secondary to dyspareunia. Haase and Skibsted [20] reported significant dyspareunia in 9% of 55 patients undergoing colporrhaphy.

Results

Despite the fact that over 200 operations have been described for the management of genuine stress incontinence, there still remains no clear consensus as to which procedure is the most effective. No one

Table 29.1 Urodynamic parameters of voiding function

Urodynamic parameter	Normal value
Post-void residual volume	Less than 100 ml
Peak voiding flow rate	Greater than 15 ml/s
Voiding detrusor pressure	Greater than 15 cmH$_2$0

operation is capable of curing all patients, so that the physician treating female urinary incontinence needs to have more than one operation in his/her surgical armamentarium.

Procedures for genuine stress incontinence can be broadly categorized into one of three groups based on the method of bladder neck suspension. The first group includes the anterior colporrhaphy, along with its many modifications. The second group comprises the needle suspension procedures (e.g., Raz, Stamey, Pereyra), and the third the retropubic urethropexies, including the Burch and more recently popularized paravaginal repair of Cullen Richardson [21].

Comparison of surgical results in the treatment of genuine stress incontinence has been difficult for many reasons. Most reports are descriptive, retrospective, and uncontrolled, with small numbers. They are thus open to bias and confounding. In general, these studies lack both subjective and objective criteria for assessing surgical outcome. Surgical success and cure are variably defined, and sometimes not defined at all. Objective preoperative urodynamic evaluation is often not performed, with a resultant failure to identify coexistent detrusor instability, or low urethral closure pressure, the latter thought to be important in determining surgical success or failure [22,24]. Additional related patient factors are often not reported, including patient age, body weight, and the presence or absence of associated pelvic floor neuropathy. Finally, the duration and adequacy of patient follow-up differs dramatically between studies.

Marked variability in success rates for anterior colporrhaphy for the treatment of incontinence have been thus been reported. Excellent objective results 2 years following surgical repair have been reported by Beck and McCormick [23]; in their series of 33 patients, primary anterior colporrhaphy was curative in 91% of patients. The authors cited their use of permanent suture material for Kelly plication as a contributing factor to their good surgical outcome. These results have not, however, been reproduced by other investigators. Low [24] noted objective cure or improvement in only 65% of patients after anterior colporrhaphy, with surgical failure in 35%. Weil et al. [25] reported subjective cure at 6 months in 77% of 30 patients on whom anterior repair was performed,

though with objective assessment via urodynamics demonstrating cure in only 57% of the same population. Though the aim of anterior colporrhaphy is to improve pressure transmission to the urethra, a decrease in mean urethral closure pressure was seen following colporrhaphy, secondary to denervation and devascularization of urethral sphincter components during surgical dissection as suggested by the authors. van Geelan et al. [26] documented objective cure in 45% in 56 patients 1–2 years following primary anterior repair. An even lower objective cure rate of 36%, only 3–6 months after surgery, was reported by Stanton and Cardozo [27].

Only a handful of studies addressing surgical outcome for genuine stress incontinence have been conducted in a prospective, randomized and controlled fashion. Bergman and Elia [28] reported comparative long-term results for three procedures, the Kelly plication, modified Pereyra needle suspension, and Burch urethropexy. All surgeries were primary, and all 127 subjects were randomly assigned one of the three procedures. Follow-up was conducted at 1 and 5 years using both subjective and objective (urodynamic) criteria. For anterior colporrhaphy with Kelly plication, objective cure at 1 year was 63%, dropping to a dismal 37% at 5 years. Cure with the needle suspension occurred in 65% (1 year) and 43% (5 years), and for the Burch procedure in 89% (1 year) and 82% (5 years). More recent studies have reported similarly poor comparative results for the anterior repair. In a randomized study of 81 women with primary genuine stress incontinence, Liapis and colleagues [29] noted objective cure in 57% of those who had undergone anterior repair, in contrast to objective cure in 88% of those who had undergone Burch urethropexy. Kammerer-Doak et al. [30] randomly assigned 35 patients to undergo anterior colporrhaphy or Burch colposuspension; objective cure was demonstrated in 89 and 31% respectively at 1 year. In this study, there was no increase in perioperative morbidity and length of hospital stay between groups, disputing the often cited advantages of the vaginal approach.

Studies evaluating outcome for anterior colporrhaphy for anterior wall prolapse alone (without incontinence) are scarce, and flawed as are those evaluating surgical outcome for incontinence. Reasonable success with the procedure has been reported in the limited studies available, with recurrent cystocele formation reported in 3–33% of patients [31,32]. Prolapse itself, whether primary or recurrent, has not yet, however, been described in objective terms, making outcome measures difficult to assess. The International Continence Society has recently developed a standardized scoring system to address this problem [33].

Conclusions

Anterior colporrhaphy with Kelly plication of the bladder neck has been performed for more than 100 years. It is, in general, a straightforward procedure which affords few serious risks and complications, and offers low patient morbidity. It may well have a role for the surgical correction of the cystourethrocele without associated urinary incontinence, but it is not an operation for the management of genuine stress incontinence. Objective cure rates for incontinence have been repeatedly reported to be inferior to other procedures, particularly the Burch retropubic colposuspension. Long-term cure rates are especially disappointing. Anterior colporrhaphy for the management of genuine stress incontinence should be avoided, unless patient factors like advanced age or surgical frailty seriously compromise the choice of surgery. It remains then in current standard practice an operation only to correct prolapse.

References

1. Mallet VT, Bump RC. The epidemiology of female pelvic floor dysfunction. Curr Opin Obstet Gynecol 1994;6:308–12.
2. Beck RP. Pelvic relaxational prolapse. In: Kase NG, Weingold AB, editors. Principles and Practice of Clinical Gynecology. New York: John Wiley & Sons, 1983; 677–85.
3. Olsen AL, Smith VJ, Bergstrom JO, Colling JC, Clark AL. Epidemiology of surgically managed pelvic organ prolapse and urinary incontinence. Obstet Gynecol 1997;89:501–6.
4. Thompson JD, Wall LL, Growdon WA, Ridley JH. Urinary stress incontinence. In: Thompson JD, Rock JA, editors. Te Linde's Operative Gynecology, 7th edn. Philadelphia: Lippincott, 1992; 887–940.
5. Sims JM. Clinical notes on uterine surgery. London Obstet Trans 1866;7:228.
6. Kelly HA, Dumm WM. Urinary incontinence in women, without manifest injury to the bladder. Surg Gynecol Obstet 1914;18: 444–50.
7. Kennedy WT. Incontinence of urine in the female, the urethral sphincter mechanism, damage of function, and restoration of control. Am J Obstet Gynecol 1937;34:576–89.
8. Ingelman-Sundberg A. Urinary incontinence in women excluding fistulas. Acta Obstet Gynecol Scand 1952;31:266.
9. Friedman EA, Meltzer RN. Collagen mesh prosthesis for repair of endopelvic fascial defect. Am J Obstet Gynecol 1970;106:430–3.
10. Moore J, Armstrong JT, Willis SH. The use of tantalum mesh in cystocele with critical report of ten cases. Am J Obstet Gynecol 1955;69:1127–35.
11. Zacharin RF. Free full-thickness vaginal epithelium graft in correction of recurrent genital prolapse. Aust NZ J Obstet Gynaecol 1992;32:146–8.
12. Weber AM, Walters MD. Anterior vaginal prolapse: Review of anatomy and techniques of surgical repair. Obstet Gynecol 1997;89:311–18.
13. Richardson DA, Bent AE, Ostergard DR. The effect of uterovaginal prolapse on urethral pressure dynamics. Am J Obstet Gynecol 1983;146:901–5.
14. Versi E, Lyell DJ, Griffiths DJ. Videourodynamic diagnosis of occult genuine stress incontinence in patients with anterior vaginal wall relaxation. J Soc Gynecol Invest 1998;5:327–30.
15. Bhatia NN, Bergman A. Pessary test in women with urinary incontinence. Obstet Gynecol 1985;65:220–6.
16. Bo K, Hagen RH, Kvarstein B, Jorgensen J, Larsen S. Pelvic floor muscle exercise for the treatment of female stress urinary incontinence. III. Effects of two different degrees of pelvic floor muscle exercise. Neurourol Urodyn 1990;9:489–502.
17. Warrell D. Anterior Repair. In: Stanton SL, Tanagho EA, editors. Surgery of Female Incontinence, 2nd edn. Berlin, Heidelberg: Springer-Verlag, 1986; 77–85.
18. Tanagho EA. Colpocystourethropexy: The way we do it. J Urol 1976;116:751–3.
19. Stanton SL, Norton C, Cardozo LD. Clinical and urodynamic effects of anterior colporrhaphy and vaginal hysterectomy for prolapse with and without incontinence. Br J Obstet Gynaecol 1982;89:459–63.
20. Haase P, Skibsted L. Influence of operations for stress incontinence and/or genital descensus on sexual life. Acta Obstet Gynecol Scand 1988;67:659–61.
21. Richardson AC, Edmonds PB, Williams NL. Treatment of stress urinary incontinence due to the paravaginal fascial defect. Obstet Gynecol 1981;57:357–62.
22. Sand PK, Bowen LW, Panganiban R, Ostergard DW. The low pressure urethra as a factor in failed retropubic urethropexy. Obstet Gynecol 1987;69:399–402.
23. Beck RP, McCormick S. Treatment of urinary stress incontinence with anterior colporrhaphy. Obstet Gynecol 1982;59:269–74.
24. Low JA. Management of anatomic urinary incontinence by vaginal repair. Am J Obstet Gynecol 1967;97:308–15.
25. Weil A, Reyes H, Bischoff P, Rottenberg RD, Krauer F. Modifications of the urethral rest and stress profiles after different types of surgery for urinary stress incontinence. Br J Obstet Gynaecol 1984;91:46–55.
26. Van Geelan JM, Theeuwes AGM, Eskes TKAB, Martin CB. The clinical and urodynamic effects of anterior vaginal repair and Burch colposuspension. Am J Obstet Gynecol 1988;159:137–44.
27. Stanton SL, Cardozo LD. A comparison of vaginal and suprapubic surgery in the correction of incontinence due to urethral sphincter incompetence. Br J Urol 1979;51:497–9.
28. Bergman A, Elia G. Three surgical procedures for genuine stress incontinence: Five-year follow-up of a prospective randomized study. Am J Obstet Gynecol 1995;173:66–71.
29. Liapis A, Pyrgiotis E, Kontoravdis A, Louridas C, Zourlas PA. Genuine stress incontinence: prospective randomized comparison of two operative methods. Eur J Obstet Gynecol Reprod Biol 1996;64:69–72.
30. Kammerer-Doak DN, Dorin MH, Rogers RG, Cousin MO. A randomized trial of Burch retropubic urethropexy and anterior colporrhaphy for stress urinary incontinence. Obstet Gynecol 1999;93:75–8.
31. Kohli N, Sze EHM, Roat TWR, Karram MM. Incidence of recurrent cystocele after anterior colporrhaphy with and without concomitant transvaginal needle suspension. Am J Obstet Gynecol 1996;175:1476–82.
32. Porges RF, Smilen SW. Long-term analysis of the surgical management of pelvic support defects. Am J Obstet Gynecol 1994;171:1518–28.
33. Bump RC, Mattiason A, Bo K, Brubaker L, DeLancey JDL, Klarskov P, Shull BL, Smith ARB. The standardization of terminology of female pelvic organ prolapse and pelvic floor dysfunction. Am J Obstet Gynecol 1996;175:10–17.

30 Buttress Procedures and Tension-free Slings for the Treatment of Prolapse and Stress Incontinence

Corrine F.I. Jabs, Harold P. Drutz and Ian Currie

Introduction

There is incredible diversity in the number of procedures that have been developed for the treatment of stress incontinence in women. This fact alone tells us that there is no perfect operation which is suitable for all patients and which has no risk of recurrence of symptoms. Most of the procedures for stress incontinence can be grouped under the headings of anterior repairs, needle suspensions, retropubic urethropexies and slings. Within each of these groups there are variations in technique between centers and individual surgeons. These standard procedures are discussed in the appropriate chapters of this text. This chapter will discuss examples of other surgical procedures that cannot be included in the previously mentioned groups and fall under a classification which includes significant modifications of the anterior repair and non-anchored slings.

Anterior repair with plication of the fascia lying between the vaginal mucosa, urethra and bladder base with removal of excess vaginal mucosa has been used for decades for the treatment of stress incontinence and prolapse of the anterior vaginal wall. It is a low morbidity procedure with a relatively low risk of complications, short period of hospitalization and quick recovery. Unfortunately the long-term success for the treatment of stress incontinence is low, with objective cure rates at 1 year approximately 65–70% which drop to 37% at 5 years [1].

A few surgeons may have higher success rates with anterior repair when care is taken to take deep bites of tissue in the fascia incorporating the area described as the pubourethral ligament located superior and lateral to the urethra [2]. The mechanism of improved continence after anterior repair is similar to that of retropubic urethropexies. The transmission of abdominal pressure to the proximal urethra is improved in successful cases although the enhancement of transmission is less prominent and less consistent in women undergoing anterior repair for the treatment of stress incontinence than in those undergoing retropubic urethropexy [3]. Several modifications of the anterior repair attempt to provide an increase in suburethral resistance and compression of the urethra only at the time of straining to enhance pressure transmission.

Anterior repair remains the most commonly used procedure for the treatment of prolapse of the anterior vaginal wall. Unfortunately the recurrence rate following anterior repair is high. Following vaginal repair of stage III or IV prolapse, Bump [4] found recurrent stage II anterior wall descent at 6-month follow-up in 36% of patients. The use of needle suspension in addition to anterior repair has been shown to increase the risk of recurrence [4,5], possibly by producing an iatrogenic paravaginal defect by separating the periurethral attachments to the pubic bone and lateral pelvic sidewall. The use of mesh has been introduced to try to increase the strength and longevity of the anterior repair. Permanent synthetic mesh reinforces the fascial repair and increases formation of scar tissue, which may reduce the risk of recurrent cystocele. Several techniques for the use of mesh have been described.

Modifications Not Using Mesh

Vaginal Paravaginal Repair for Prolapse

The paravaginal repair was designed as a treatment for cystourethrocele caused by anterior vaginal wall lateral defects in which the lateral sulcus of the vagina had separated from the arcus tendineus fasciae pelvis (white line). Shull in 1994 published his series of 62 vaginal paravaginal repairs in conjunction with repair of other pelvic support defects [6]. His dissection opened the retropubic space bilaterally through the anterior vaginal incision. Sutures were placed through the white line/obturator fascia, periurethral pubocervical fascia and vaginal epithelium to recreate anterior support for the lateral aspects of the vagina. All patients had repair of support defect in other sites (including central cystocele plication) and 69% had previous pelvic surgery. At a median of 1.6 years of follow-up, 4 (7%) of the women had recurrent cystocele larger than grade 1.

Randomized comparison of abdominal paravaginal repair and retropubic urethropexy for stress incontinence has shown paravaginal repair to be inferior to retropubic urethropexy with objective cure of only 61% [7]. The vaginal paravaginal repair is technically challenging and may not be possible in women with a narrow subpubic arch [6]. Vaginal paravaginal repair would likely not have higher success than the easier abdominal approach, and is not recommended for the treatment of stress incontinence.

Tuck Procedure for Stress Incontinence

Petros and Ulmsten experimented with a minor vaginal procedure to tighten the suburethral vaginal wall in an attempt to treat stress incontinence with minimal morbidity [8]. The rationalization for the procedure was based on their integral theory of female urinary incontinence which theorized that urinary incontinence resulted from inadequate or excessive tension in the vaginal wall affecting the surrounding muscles and nerves [9]. Their tuck procedure involved removal of ellipses of vaginal mucosa on either side of the urethra (but not beyond the bladder neck) measuring approximately 1 cm in length and 0.3–0.5 cm in width. The success rate at 1 year was only 47% and the technique was not recommended as an isolated procedure.

Suburethral Duplication of the Vaginal Wall for Stress Incontinence

The principle of Lazarevski's modification of the anterior repair involves the creation of a trapezoidal duplication of the anterior vaginal wall under the proximal urethra and bladder neck [10]. A standard cystocele plication is performed followed by suburethral plication of the vaginal mucosa (Figure 30.1). This vaginal plication does not use the urethral,

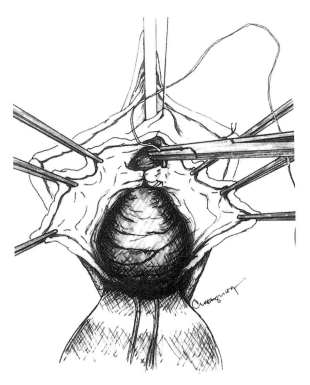

Figure 30.1   Three layers of suture grasp 10 mm, 12–13 mm and 15 mm of tissue on the left and right sides of the vaginal wall producing a duplication of the vaginal wall which does not include peri-urethrovesical tissues. (Reproduced with permission from Lazarevski MB. Suburethral duplication of the vaginal wall – an original operation for urinary stress incontinence in women. Int Urogynecol J Pelvic Floor Dysfunct 1995;6:73–7; Figure 3.)

vesical or periurethral tissue as in the Kelly or Kennedy procedures but sutures the vaginal wall together to act as a bar to support the bladder neck (Figure 30.2). One-year follow-up of patients undergoing the Lazarevski procedure for the treatment of stress incontinence had a cure rate of 93.3%. There were no cases of de novo detrusor instability and a very low incidence of voiding disorder. Following removal of the catheter on postoperative day 3, further catheterization was required in only 3.1% of patients. This procedure does not produce compression of the urethra at rest or during micturition but provides a small but sufficient compressive force of the urethra during increases in intra-abdominal pressure to improve continence.

Modifications Using Mesh

The variety of materials and the number of different attachment points available for suburethral slings

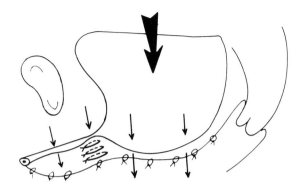

Figure 30.2 Schematic view of the urethrovesical pressure relationships with the suburethral duplication procedure. The suburethral trapezoidal wedge of the vaginal wall underlies the proximal urethra. (Reproduced with permission from Lazarevski MB. Suburethral duplication of the vaginal wall-an original operation for urinary stress incontinence in women. Int Urogynecol J Pelvic Floor Dysfunct 1995;6:73–7; Figure 5.)

have led to multiple procedure modifications to support the bladder neck for the treatment of stress incontinence. The approach for placement of the sling may be abdominal, vaginal or both. This chapter will be limited to suburethral slings that do not have a solid upper attachment point but simply act as a suburethral buttress.

The materials used for slings include autologous, heterologous and artificial materials.

Significant concerns with the use of synthetic mesh material include the risk of infection, erosion and fistula formation. The American Urologic Association clinical guidelines compare the use of autologous and synthetic materials in the use of slings and found these complications to be higher when synthetic materials were used [11]. Erosion, fistula and sinus formation occurred in 3.4% of cases using synthetic materials and 0.9% of cases using autologous material (rectus fascia and fascia lata) [11].

There are several considerations that make synthetic materials more acceptable and useful for buttress procedures. Buttress procedures are generally under no or low tension, making erosion into the urethra unusual. With buttress procedures there is no abdominal incision to allow the harvesting of rectus fascia. Synthetic materials allow the use of larger pieces that can be cut to the exact size required by the dissection and the woman's anatomy and distribute pressure to a larger surface area. Synthetic materials are now available with an open weave pattern which allows the ingrowth of native tissue to increase the strength of the repair and reduce abscess formation. Conservative surgical management of vaginal sling erosion with excision

of exposed mesh and granulation tissue with two-layer closure of the vaginal defect is generally successful [12].

To reduce the risk of vaginal mesh erosion it is recommended to avoid excessive excision of vaginal mucosa and to use a tension-free vaginal closure. The use of mesh material that has pores large enough to allow the entry of immunologically active cells and ingrowth of tissue can possibly reduce the risk of infection and sinus formation. The use of permanent monofilament suture material is recommended for anchoring of the mesh to tissue, and permanent braided suture should be avoided. Most authors also use perioperative prophylactic antibiotics.

Dyspareunia is also a concern but sexual function is only now starting to be documented in prolapse and incontinence literature and there is little evidence to determine the effect of the use of mesh.

Mesh Procedures Used Primarily to Treat Prolapse

Modified anterior repair with needle suspension of the periurethral fascia and vaginal mucosa has been described along with the use of dissolvable polyglycolic acid mesh [13]. Plicating sutures were tied over a crumpled ball of polyglycolic acid mesh that was used simply to reduce the herniation of the cystocele defect and was not sutured into place.

Several authors have described reinforcement of the anterior wall repair with permanent mesh. Typically a piece of mesh is laid over the plicating stitches of an anterior repair and lies beneath the vaginal mucosa.

Flood published a series of 142 patients in which a piece of Marlex mesh approximately 4 cm by 1 cm was placed at the bladder neck [14]. The mesh was laid over the plicating stitches of the anterior repair with the ends extending into periurethral "tunnels" that had been dissected through the urogenital diaphragm into the retropubic space (Figure 30.3). Sutures were placed only to prevent the mesh from shifting position from the bladder neck and the mesh was essentially without tension (Figure 30.4). The mesh was fixed beneath the bladder neck with four "stay" sutures, two paraurethrally and two over the base of the bladder. In this group with mean follow-up of 3.2 years, there were no cases of anterior wall descent to the level of the hymen, although 5.7% had symptomatic recurrent rectocele and/or vault descent. Of the 30 patients with preoperative demonstrable stress incontinence, 74% were cured. Only one patient of the 142 studied developed de

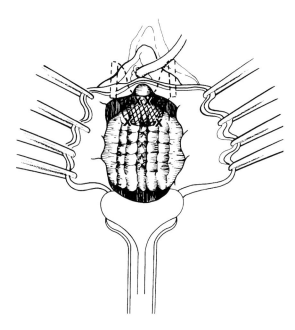

Figure 30.3 Mesh position in relation to the pelvis and bladder neck. (Reproduced with permission from Flood CG, Drutz HP, Waja L. Anterior colporrhaphy reinforced with Marlex mesh for the treatment of cystoceles. Int Urogynecol J Pelvic Floor Dysfunct 1998; 9:200–4; Figure 4.)

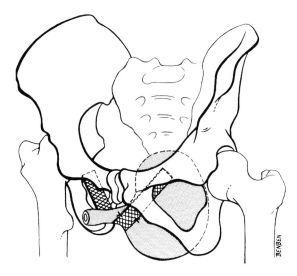

Figure 30.4 Marlex mesh is placed under the bladder neck and into the retropubic space and secured. (Reproduced with permission from Flood CG, Drutz HP, Waja L. Anterior colporrhaphy reinforced with Marlex mesh for the treatment of cystoceles. Int Urogynecol J Pelvic Floor Dysfunct 1998; 9:200–4; Figure 5.)

novo stress incontinence and no patient developed de novo detrusor instability. The rate of vaginal mesh erosion was 2%, with no case of erosion into

the bladder or urethra. Erosions were treated successfully with excision of the exposed mesh and reapproximation of the vaginal edges. The main author of this technique has now modified the shape of the mesh to include a jacket-shaped portion in the center that is wider to support the upper portion of the cystocele, with similar results. Currently Drutz is prospectively evaluating the effect of combining the above procedure with the Lazarevski procedure to see if even better success rates can be obtained in women with cystocele, overt and latent stress incontinence [15].

Nicita has described a similar procedure using a relatively large piece of polypropylene mesh laid over the cystocele extending from the bladder neck to the cervix/vault with lateral wings sutured to the arcus tendineus fasciae pelvis [16]. Results were similar to Flood's report of the Drutz procedure. With median 13.9-month follow-up of 44 patients there was no recurrence of cystocele and only 1 patient with vaginal mesh erosion (in a case where tension on the vaginal incision was known to be high). Migliari also describes using a large piece of mixed absorbable/non-absorbable fiber mesh over the fascial plicating sutures of an anterior repair with the most distal portion of the mesh fixed in a similar fashion to a needle suspension procedure [17].

Tension-free Slings (TVT): Mesh Procedure Used Primarily for Stress Incontinence

The tension-free vaginal tape (TVT) is a suburethral sling which shows promise as a low morbidity, day-surgery treatment for stress incontinence [18]. The TVT procedure has been designed to correct the tension of the pubourethral ligament and is placed at the mid-urethra, unlike most other stress incontinence procedures that elevate the bladder neck. The TVT is attached to disposable introducer needles that are inserted on either side of the urethra through a central vaginal incision with minimal lateral dissection (Figure 30.5). The needle is directed upward behind the posterior aspect of the pubic bone to exit through the abdominal wall just above and lateral to the pubic symphysis (Figure 30.6). A rigid catheter guide is used to move the urethra laterally to allow safe passage of the needle. Cystoscopy is performed with each needle in place to ensure the bladder has not been perforated. The sling material is Prolene tape covered in a removable plastic sheath which allows smooth passage through tissue and also reduces contamination of the tape upon passage through the vagina.

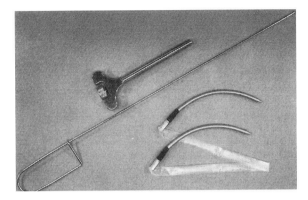

Figure 30.5 Tension-free vaginal tape instruments. (Reproduced with permission from Ulmsten U, Johnson P, Rezapour M. A three-year follow up of tension free vaginal tape for surgical treatment of female stress urinary incontinence. Br J Obstet Gynaecol 1999; 106:345–50; Figure 1.)

The procedure is performed with local anaesthetic plus intravenous sedation or spinal anaesthetic. The patient is asked to cough with a full bladder and the sling is tightened only to the point of allowing drops of urine to escape. Following removal of the plastic sleeves, tissue friction holds the sling in place with no other attachment or suturing of the sling required. This has likely contributed to the low rate of urinary retention with this procedure. Ninety percent of women were able to urinate spontaneously the day of surgery, 10% require short-term intermittent catheterization [19]. Most patients are discharged the same day or the next day.

In the series published, the effectiveness of the TVT as primary surgical treatment is similar to that of retropubic urethropexies with 85% objective cure and 11% improvement at 3-year follow-up [18–22]. Randomized clinical trials of TVT versus open retropubic urethropexy are currently underway. As the TVT is placed at the level of the mid-urethra, there is no alteration of the anatomy of the proximal vaginal wall; therefore this procedure is not useful for the treatment of prolapse. In trials published to date, prolapse has been an exclusion criterion. The possibility of using this procedure in addition to other vaginal procedures for prolapse has yet to be explored in the literature.

Summary

There are numerous procedures designed for the treatment of stress incontinence and prolapse. Buttress procedures that are modifications of the anterior repair may be appropriate in many cases to improve the treatment of stress incontinence or reduce the recurrence of anterior wall prolapse. The novel use of mesh can assist in these goals and several procedures have been developed for these purposes.

The various buttress procedures we have described in this chapter need to be compared in a

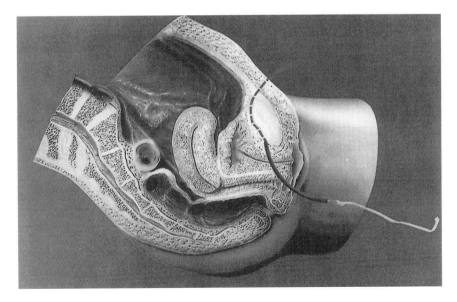

Figure 30.6 Schematic illustration of insertion of the TVT needle. Directly after the needle tip has perforated the urogenital diaphragm and entered the retropubic space, it is brought up to the abdominal incision in close contact with back of the pubic bone. (Reproduced with permission from Ulmsten U, Johnson P, Rezapour M. A three-year follow up of tension free vaginal tape for surgical treatment of female stress urinary incontinence. Br J Obstet Gynaecol 1999; 106:345–50; Figure 2.)

well-designed randomized control trial before evidence-based conclusions are drawn.

References

1. Black NA, Downs SH. The effectiveness of surgery for stress incontinence in women: A systematic review. Br J Urol 1996;78:497–510.
2. Beck RP, McCormick S, Nordstrom L. A 25-year experience with 519 anterior colporrhaphy procedures. Obstet Gynecol 1991;78(6):1011–18.
3. van Geelen JM, Theeuvew AG, Eskes TK, Martin CB Jr. The clinical and urodynamic effects of anterior vaginal repair and Burch colposuspension. Am J Obstet Gynecol 1988;159(1):137–44.
4. Bump RC, Hurt WG, Theofrastous JP, Addision WA, Fantl JA, Wyman JF, McClish DK. Randomized prospective comparison of needle colposuspension versus endopelvic fascia plication for potential stress incontinence prophylaxis in women undergoing vaginal reconstruction for stage III or IV pelvic organ prolapse. Am J Obstet Gynecol 1996;175:326–35.
5. Kohli N, Sze EHM, Roat TW, Karram MM. Incidence of recurrent cystocele after anterior colporrhaphy with and without concomitant transvaginal needle suspension. Am J Obstet Gynecol 1996;175:1476–82.
6. Shull BL, Benn SJ, Kuehl TJ. Surgical management of prolapse of the anterior vaginal segment: an analysis of support defects, operative morbidity, and anatomical outcome. Am J Obstet Gynecol 1994;171(6):1429–36.
7. Colombo M, Milani R, Vitobello D, Maggioni A. A randomized comparison of Burch colposuspension and abdominal paravaginal defect repair for female stress urinary incontinence. Am J Obstet Gynecol 1996;175(1):78–84.
8. Petros PEP, Ulmsten UI. The tuck procedure: a simplified vaginal repair for treatment of female urinary incontinence. Acta Obstet Gynecol Scand 1990;69 (suppl 153):41–2.
9. Petros PEP, Ulmsten UI. An integral theory of female urinary incontinence. Acta Obstet Gynecol Scand 1990;69(suppl 153):7–31.
10. Lazarevski MB. Suburethral duplication of the vaginal wall – An original operation for urinary stress incontinence in women. Int Urogynecol J Pelvic Floor Dysfunct 1995;6:73–9.
11. Leach GE, Dmochowski RR, Appell RA, Blaivas JG, Hadley HR, Luber KM et al. Female stress urinary incontinence clinical guidelines panel summary report on surgical management of female stress urinary incontinence. J Urol 1997;158:875–80.
12. Myers DL, LaSala CA. Conservative surgical management of Mersilene mesh suburethral sling erosion. Am J Obstet Gynecol 1998;179(6 Pt 1):1424–8.
13. Safir MH, Gousse A, Rovner ES, Ginsberg DA, Raz S. 4-defect repair of grade 4 cystocele. J Urol 1999; 161:587–94.
14. Flood CG, Drutz HP, Waja L. Anterior colporrhaphy reinforced with Marlex mesh for the treatment of cystoceles. Int Urogynecol J Pelvic Floor Dysfunct 1998;9:200–4.
15. Smith KM, Al-Badr AH, Drutz HP. Suburethral buttress with Marlex mesh with or without Lazarevski procedure for treatment of cystocele, overt and latent stress incontinence: A cohort study (submitted).
16. Nicita G. A new operation for genitourinary prolapse. J Urol 1998;160:741–5.
17. Migliari R, Usai E. Treatment results using a mixed fiber mesh in patients with grade IV cystocele. J Urol 1999;161:1255–8.
18. Ulmsten U, Henriksson L, Johnson P, Varhos G. An ambulatory surgical procedure under local anesthetic for treatment of female urinary incontinence. Int Urogynecol J Pelvic Floor Dysfunct 1996;7(2):81–5.
19. Ulmsten U, Johnson P, Rezapour M. A three-year follow up of tension free vaginal tape for surgical treatment of female stress urinary incontinence. Br J Obstet Gynaecol 1999;106:345–50.
20. Falconer C, Ekman-Orderberg G, Malmstrom A, Ulmsten U. Clnical outcome and changes in connective tissue metabolism after intravaginal slingplasty in stress incontinent women. Int Urogynecol J Pelvic Floor Dysfunct 1996;7(3):133–7.
21. Ulmsten U, Falconer C, Johnson P, Jomaa M, 6Lanner L, Nilsson CG, Olsson I. A multicenter study of tension-free vaginal tape (TVT) for surgical treatment of stress urinary incontinence. Int Urogynecol J Pelvic Floor Dysfunct 1998;9(4):210–13.
22. Ulmsten U, Petros P. Intravaginal slingplasty (IVS): an ambulatory surgical procedure for the treatment of female urinary incontinence. Scand J Urol Nephrol 1995;29:75–82.

31 Endoscopic Suspensions

Sender Herschorn and Lesley K. Carr

Introduction

The first reports of surgical management of stress incontinence from the early part of the twentieth century recommended a vaginal approach with plication of the periurethral tissue to narrow the urethral lumen and elevate the bladder neck [1]. By the 1940s, concepts regarding etiology changed and procedures to address lateral support defects were published. Retropubic suspensions [2] or slings [3] followed in an attempt to improve efficacy and durability. To achieve elevation as in the retropubic suspension with reduced morbidity Pereyra introduced the vaginal needle suspension in 1959 [4]. There have been many subsequent modifications with regard to the extent of dissection, location of sutures, method of fixation, and types of ligature carrier. The most widely adopted procedures, the modified Pereyra [5], Stamey [6], Raz [7], and Gittes [8] procedures, will be discussed below.

While initial reports with relatively short-term follow-up showed success rates equivalent to retropubic suspensions, with less postoperative morbidity, longer-term outcomes have been worse [9–11]. A review of published studies by the American Urological Association Female Stress Urinary Incontinence Clinical Guidelines Panel [12] showed a significantly lower cure (dry) rate beyond 4 years with transvaginal suspensions (67%) compared to retropubic suspensions (84%) or slings (83%). The review panel still considered transvaginal suspensions to be a good option for the appropriate women with stress incontinence, those with smaller volume incontinence, less intrinsic urethral sphincter deficiency, and those who are willing to accept worse long-term benefit in favor of lower immediate morbidity.

Recently, however, with the introduction of newer procedures that have addressed the inherent deficiencies of the endoscopic suspensions, the outcome appears to have improved. The newer modifications will also be discussed in this chapter.

Pre- and Intraoperative Management

Vaginal suspensions are routinely performed under general or regional anesthesia. Local anesthesia with sedation has recently been advocated for newer minimally invasive techniques [13]. Antibiotic prophylaxis is commonly employed, although there are no specific data supporting its use. Patients are positioned in dorsal lithotomy with Trendelenburg to optimize visibility and lower the chance of bowel injury with needle or suprapubic catheter passage. A weighted vaginal speculum, or Simms retractor, and pinning of the labia with sutures or a Scott retractor to spread the vaginal introitus, improve access. A Foley catheter is inserted to allow identification of the bladder neck by palpation and to decompress the bladder to allow safe passage of the ligature carrier. With the vaginal incision, injection of sterile saline into the mucosa facilitates the development of the submucosal plane. Hematuria from the Foley catheter should alert one to suture penetration of the bladder (usually laterally, near the bladder neck). Stamey [6] first introduced the idea of intraoperative cystoscopy to check suture placement and elevation and ruling out bladder or urethral injury. This gave origin to the term endoscopic suspension. A vaginal packing may be left at the end of the procedure depending on the amount of bleeding encountered. Postoperative bladder drainage is with either a urethral Foley or suprapubic catheter. A urethral catheter avoids potential complications of blind insertion of a suprapubic catheter. However, with prolonged retention, the women must master intermittent catheterization in the face of adjacent surgical swelling and pain. Care must be taken with percutaneous insertion of a suprapubic catheter, especially if there is a history of previous lower abdominal surgery or radiation. The bladder must be very distended with the patient in exaggerated Trendelenburg to minimize the risk of bowel penetration.

Surgical Techniques

Modified Pereyra

Pereyra's original description involved a T-shaped vaginal incision with minimal periurethral dissection and no penetration into the retropubic space [4]. A single needle stylet and absorbable suture were used to suspend the periurethral tissue over the rectus fascia. The needle stylet was delivered into the vagina through a single midline lower abdominal incision.

Subsequently, Pereyra modified the procedure by incorporating bladder neck plication but still using absorbable suture. He reported a 94% cure rate with one-year follow-up in 210 patients [5].

Stamey Needle Bladder Neck Suspension

Stamey's modifications to the transvaginal suspension incorporated three different aspects [6]. Endoscopy was an adjunct to ensure sutures were placed at the bladder neck. Non-absorbable sutures were used with Dacron tube vaginal pledgets to buttress both sides of the urethra and prevent suspensory suture pull-through on the vaginal side. He also designed a single-pronged blunt-tipped needle (Stamey needle) that is still commonly used in many versions of transvaginal suspensions. The procedure involved two lateral suprapubic incisions and a suprapubic catheter was inserted for bladder drainage. The procedure is shown in Figure 31.1.

Many large published series have documented success in 72–91% of cases [10,14]. Success tends to lessen with longer follow-up [10] and in younger patients [15]. Erosion of the Dacron pledgets has also been reported at up to 3 years after surgery [16].

Gittes Bladder Neck Suspension

Gittes and Loughlin [8] described a no-incision pubovaginal suspension. Two lateral suprapubic stab

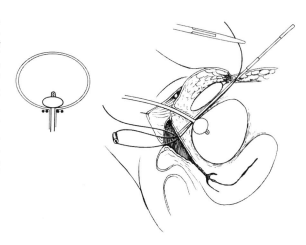

Figure 31.1   Stamey endoscopic suspension. The Stamey needle has been passed the first time to withdraw one end of the suture through the abdominal incision. It is passed for the second time on the ipsilateral side. The other end of the suture has been passed through a small piece of Dacron and then through the eye of the needle, which is withdrawn for the second time. The procedure is repeated on the other side, resulting in two suspension sutures with Dacron bolsters at the level of the bladder. Cystoscopy is done to verify suture position and urethral and bladder integrity. (From Raz S, Stothers L, Chopra A. Vaginal reconstructive surgery for incontinence and prolapse. In: Walsh PC, Retik AB, Vaughan Jr ED, Wein AJ, editors. Campbell's Urology, 7th edn. Philadelphia, WB Saunders Company, 1998; 1059–94, with permission.)

incisions are made and the Stamey needle is passed twice on each side from over the rectus fascia through the vaginal wall at the bladder neck (guided by the Foley balloon) to retrieve the ends of a no. 2 polypropylene stitch. A Mayo needle is used to take helical bites of vaginal mucosa prior to delivering the second end of the stitch to the abdominal wall. The sutures are tied over the rectus fascia without tension. Gittes postulated that the vaginal suspension sutures under slight traction will cut through the vaginal wall and become buried in scar, creating an "autologous pledget". A suprapubic catheter was also used.

Although favorable short-term results were published [8,17,18], the no-incision technique has the poorest reported long-term outcome of endoscopic suspensions. Kondo and co-workers compared their experience with 382 patients undergoing a Stamey or Gittes suspension with a mean follow-up of more than 5 years in both groups [10]. The Kaplan–Meier cumulative continence rates were 71.5% for the Stamey at 14 years and 37.0% for the Gittes at 6 years postoperatively (p < 0.0001). Elkabir and Mee [9] found a similarly low cure rate of 38.5% at 2 years with the Gittes technique.

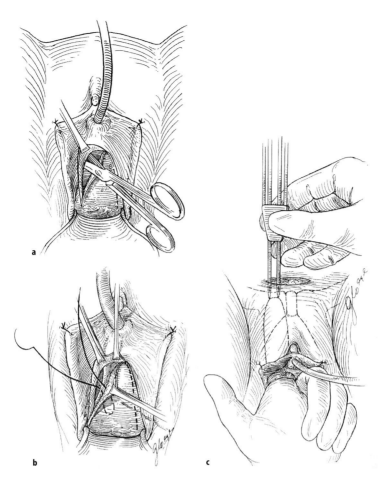

Figure 31.2 Raz bladder neck suspension. **a** Inverted U-shaped incision is made in the anterior vaginal wall with the base of the U at a point midway between the bladder neck and the urethral meatus. The vaginal wall is dissected off the surface of the periurethral fascia. The retropubic space is entered by detaching the endopelvic fascia from the arcus tendineus. **b** A no. 1 polypropylene suture is placed to include the endopelvic fascia and pubocervical fascia which underlies the vaginal wall. A similar suture is placed on the opposite side. **c** A midline transverse incision is made just above the pubis and carried down to the rectus fascia. The double-prong suture carrier is placed through the rectus fascia and muscle and the tips are palpated with the index finger in the retropubic space. The suture carrier is guided down and out through the vaginal incision. The sutures are placed into the needle holes and guided back up through the rectus fascia. Cystoscopy is carried out. The vaginal incision is closed and the sutures are tied suprapubically. The vagina is packed and the suprapubic incision is closed. (From Raz S. Female Genitourinary Dysfunction and Reconstruction. Philadelphia: WB Saunders Company, 1996, with permission.)

Raz Procedures for Stress Incontinence

In 1981, Raz [7] reported a modification of the Pereyra procedure (Figure 31.2). The technique employed an inverted U-shaped vaginal incision to improve access. It also was the first to enter the retropubic space sharply via the vaginal route by detaching the periurethral connective tissue and endopelvic fascia from the arcus tendineus and pelvic sidewall. Opening the retropubic space facilitates blind passage of the ligature carrier from the abdomen to the vaginal incision by allowing finger guidance, permitting urethrolysis if required, and allowing placement of helical sutures into the abdominal and vaginal sides of the periurethral connective tissue, which results in a more secure purchase of tissue. Another subsequent modification was the double-pronged ligature carrier that is passed twice via a midline suprapubic incision to retrieve the no. 1 non-absorbable suture. A suprapubic catheter was also utilized.

Early results with 15-month follow-up reported by Raz [19] showed a 92% success rate. Severity of incontinence was found to be a negative predictor for outcome. Other groups have confirmed good early results and low morbidity with Raz's modified Pereyra procedure [20]. However, there are more reports of poor long-term results from this version of the Raz procedure [11,21–23]. Masson and Govier [11] showed that of 135 patients with a mean follow-up of more than 4 years, only 14% were dry and 53% continued to wear pads.

Raz Vaginal Wall Sling

In 1989, Raz et al. reported a new vaginal technique to treat stress incontinence due to intrinsic sphincter dysfunction [24]. A rectangular flap of vagina was buried at the bladder neck and suspended by non-absorbable sutures at each corner by passage of a ligature carrier. In 1992, they reported on 54 patients with this procedure, showing a success rate of 94% after a mean follow-up of 24 months [25]. Other investigators confirmed similar short-term success and low morbidity [26].

Subsequently, Raz and co-workers modified the procedure in that the vaginal flap was no longer buried. The current technique is based on the importance of the mid-urethral mechanism to prevent incontinence. The surgical goals of the anterior vaginal wall "sling" were (1) to provide elastic support to the mid-urethra and bladder neck and (2) to create a strong hammock of vaginal wall and underlying tissues, which provides a backboard against which the urethra can be compressed with increases in intra-abdominal pressure [27]. It is applicable to patients with any type of stress incontinence.

Two oblique incisions are made in the anterior vaginal wall extending from the level of the mid-urethra to 3 cm beyond the level of the bladder neck. The incisions are 1 cm medial to the folded lateral margin of the anterior vaginal wall. The same dissection to enter the retropubic space is then carried out as above. The proximal (bladder neck) sutures are placed in the same fashion as the modified Pereyra stitches using no. 1 non-absorbable suture with the addition of several helical passes under the vaginal epithelium capturing further periurethral and perivesical tissue. The distal (mid-urethral) sutures are then placed again using no. 1 non-absorbable suture. To facilitate multiple helical passes with a good purchase of periurethral tissue in this location, Russian forceps are opened widely in the retropubic space with gentle downward traction maintaining the forceps parallel to the ground. After this deep tissue is taken, several helical bites of anterior periurethral fascia underlying the vaginal epithelium are taken at the mid-urethra level. Care must be taken to avoid urethral perforation by maintaining the needle parallel to the vagina. The identical sutures are then placed on the contralateral side.

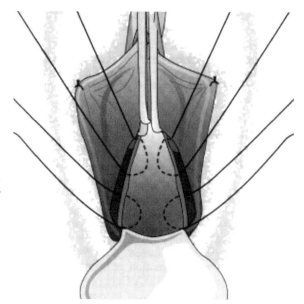

Figure 31.3 Illustration of the two pairs of no. 1 polypropylene sutures which create a hammock of support after being transferred to the retropubic space by the suture carrier. (From Raz S, Stothers L, Chopra A. Vaginal reconstructive surgery for incontinence and prolapse. In: Walsh PC, Retik AB, Vaughan Jr ED, Wein AJ, editors. Campbell's Urology, 7th edn. Philadelphia: WB Saunders Company, 1998; 1059–94, with permission.)

These four sutures suspend a rectangle of support ("sling") for the bladder neck and mid-urethra (Figure 31.3). The double-pronged ligature carrier is then passed in the same fashion as the Raz procedure through a midline suprapubic incision. It must be passed four times to transfer the sutures, which are then tied over the immobile portion of the rectus fascia. The vaginal incisions are closed using running, locking 2-0 delayed absorbable suture. Cystoscopy is used to rule out bladder or urethral penetration.

Early results in 160 women with incontinence due to either sphincteric deficiency or hypermobility who underwent the Raz vaginal wall sling, with a median follow-up of 17 months, showed 152 to be cured of stress incontinence [27]. Longer-term results and comparative trials are awaited.

Tension-free Vaginal Tape Procedure

Another technique focusing on the mid-urethral continence mechanism, is the tension-free vaginal tape procedure (TVT). Early attempts to place a fine mesh "sling" around the urethra showed 90% success at a mean follow-up of 16 months. However, a rejection rate approaching 10% was found using Gore-tex and Mersilene tapes [28]. Revisions in this

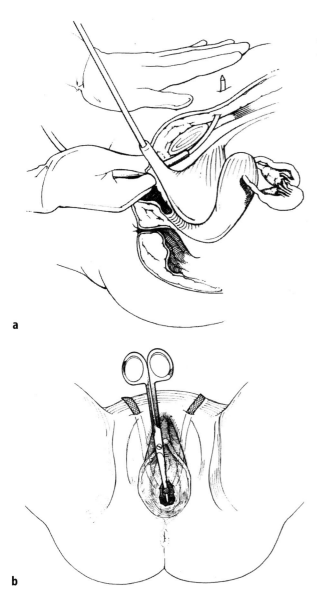

a

b

Figure 31.4 **a** Tension-free vaginal tape placement. Passage of the curved trocar through the endopelvic fascia, retropubic space, and abdominal wall. **b** Tension adjustment using Mayo scissors as a spacer. (From Carlin BI, Klutke JJ, Klutke CG. The tension-free vaginal tape procedure for the treatment of stress incontinence in the female patient. Urology 2000; 56(Supplement 6A):28–31, with permission.)

early methodology, including the use of loose weave polypropylene mesh, have led to the current technique (Figure 31.4). The TVT does not seem to abolish urethral hypermobility as assessed by pre- and postoperative Q-tip tests [29]. Additionally, Lo and co-workers [30] in a study using ultrasound

and urodynamics postulated that urinary continence after surgery is most probably achieved by creating a dynamic mid-urethral knee angulation by which the urethra is closed, i.e. kinked at stress.

Procedure

A neuroleptic or regional anesthetic with pre-procedure antibiotic coverage is recommended. The patient is placed in dorsal lithotomy and a urethral Foley catheter (18F) is inserted to drain the bladder. Then 60–80 ml of dilute local anesthetic with epinephrine is injected into the abdominal skin above the pubis and downwards along the back of the pubic bone to the space of Retzius. Two abdominal skin incisions of 1 cm are made, one on each side of the midline, just above the symphysis, approximately 5 cm apart. Further local anesthetic is then injected transvaginally into the periurethral area extending up to the retropubic space. A midline 1.5 cm long incision is made starting 1 cm from the external urethral meatus. Two small lateral periurethral spaces are created, not entering the retropubic space. The TVT rigid catheter guide is inserted into the Foley catheter. The purpose of the guide is to move the bladder and urethra away from where the tip of the needle passes into the retropubic space. Using the handle with the pre-loaded needles, the surgeon inserts the tip of the needle into the paraurethral space on the right side of the urethra (catheter guide pushed to the right to displace the bladder to the left). The endopelvic fascia is perforated and the tip of the needle is brought up to and through the abdominal incision by hugging the back of the pubic bone. Cystoscopy is performed to rule out bladder perforation. The procedure is then repeated on the left side. When the sling is placed in a U shape around the mid-urethra, the patient is asked to cough with a full bladder and the tension of the tape is adjusted just to the point of abolishing leakage. Tension on the tape is avoided. The plastic sheaths are then removed. The abdominal ends are cut flush with the skin and are not sutured in place. Friction from the coarse weave of the mesh holds the tape in place. The skin and vaginal incisions are then closed. The bladder is drained or a Foley is inserted for postoperative drainage.

Results

Until recently, most published series of TVT were for primary repairs. In a multicenter trial Ulmsten and colleagues [13] showed a 91% cure rate in 131 patients with a minimum one-year follow-up. Mean operative time was 28 minutes and all procedures were performed under local anesthetic with 90% as outpatients. Three-year follow-up in

50 consecutive women showed an 86% cure rate with no mesh rejection or permanent retention [31]. Wang and Lo [32] found a subjective cure rate of 87% in 70 women using the same technique. Epidural anesthesia was used and mean hospital stay was 3 days. Three bladder perforations occurred but healed with conservative management.

Recent reports include patients with previously failed surgery. Haab and co-workers from France described 16 patients with previous retropubic or vaginal suspension undergoing successful TVT [33]. In their series of 62 women followed over a median of 16.2 months, 87% were cured and 9.6% improved. No erosion or infection occurred. In a recent study of 67 women with previous failed surgery, Azam and colleagues from Britain [34] reported that at 12 months 54 women (81%) were cured, 4 (6%) were significantly improved and 9 (13%) were no better. No serious morbidity was noted after the procedure. A similarly good outcome, after a mean of 4 years, was reported by Rezapour and Ulmsten in 34 women with previously failed surgical procedures [35].

Longer-term data were published by Nilsson and co-workers [36]. The median follow-up time was 56 months with a range of 48 to 70 months. In their study of 90 patients 5 could not be evaluated physically. Seventy-two (84.7%) of the 85 patients who were fully evaluated were both objectively and subjectively completely cured. Another 9 patients (10.6%) were significantly improved and 4 (4.7%) were regarded as failures. No long-term morbidity was seen. Finally, Ward and colleagues have undertaken a multicenter randomized clinical trial of TVT versus colposuspension in Britain [37]. At 6 months 103 (66%) out of 170 TVT patients and 90 (71%) out of colposuspension patients reported a subjective cure of stress incontinence. The CMG (cystometrogram) cure rates were both higher at 89% and 85% respectively. The incontinence outcomes were similar but mean blood loss, analgesia requirement, and hospital stays were significantly less in the TVT group. Bladder perforation occurred in 15 (9%) of the TVT group and 3 (2%) of the colposuspension group. The patients are to be followed for at least 2 years.

Complications include bladder perforation (0–10%). It is treated by repositioning the needle and continuing Foley catheter drainage for 1–2 days postoperatively. Voiding difficulty may occur in fewer than 5% [38]. If persistent, tape adjustment may be necessary. Potential and rare severe complications may require surgical exploration and include retropubic hematoma and bleeding (<1%) [38–40] and bowel perforation [41]. Obturator nerve injury may occur as

well [31,38,42]. Other problems, which are rarely mentioned, may include prosthesis erosion and infection.

In an effort to reduce the rate of bladder perforation and potential bleeding, thought to be associated with introducing the tape through the vaginal route, a device that pulls the tape in via an abdominally introduced system has been released. No data are yet published.

Bone Anchoring Techniques

Most transvaginal suspensions for stress incontinence fix the suspensory sutures over the anterior rectus fascia. Some investigators have postulated that since the rectus fascia is mobile this motion leads to shearing forces that may lead to pull-through of the suspensory suture at the vaginal end (Figure 31.5). Others feel that stitches placed laterally in this region lead to nerve entrapment and prolonged postoperative pain. In an effort to combat these theoretical problems, various bone anchoring systems have been developed and marketed, including the In-Tac, and Vesica, systems.

The In-Tac, bone anchor system was first described by Nativ in 1997 [43]. Nickel/titanium alloy bone anchors threaded with no 1 non-absorbable sutures are inserted transvaginally via a spring-loader multi-use inserter. Initial experience of 50 women with type I or II stress incontinence showed a one-year cure rate of 82%. Transient dyspareunia occurred in 6% [43]. El-Toukhy et al. used a similar surgical technique in 30 women, reporting a one-year subjective cure rate of 80%. Dyspareunia due to the vaginal polypropylene stitches occurred in 23%, requiring successful revision in all [44]. Braided non-absorbable suture is now used to avoid this complication. There are no reports of anchor infection after transvaginal insertion to date [45].

The Vesica, system uses a drill to place screws into the pubic symphysis via a suprapubic incision [46,47]. Non-absorbable no. 1 polybutester suture is preloaded into the screws and is then passed via a suture passer into the vagina to suspend the bladder neck. Appell and co-workers in a report on percutaneous bladder neck stabilization using the Vesica, system showed a 94% cure rate at 1 year in 71 women [48]. The results of Schultheiss and co-workers were not as good. Of 37 patients with maximum follow-up of 18 months, 43% were dry and 24% were significantly improved. Furthermore, 25% of patients reported prolonged pelvic pain. Surgical removal of the anchors was necessary in two patients for bacterial infection and painful granuloma [49]. Tebyani and co-workers also reported disappointing results, with cure in 5% and improvement in 12% of 42 patients with mean

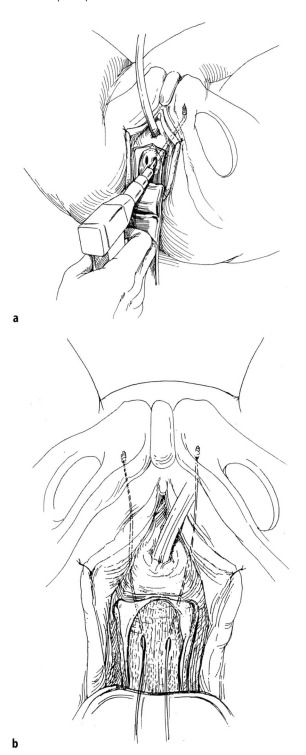

a

b

Figure 31.5 **a** Placement of transvaginal bone anchor insertion tool. Vaginal incision was inverted U-shape. **b** Transvaginal bone anchor placement. Note suture fixation to anchors on undersurface of pubis. (From Winters JC, Scarpero HM, Appell RA: Use of bone anchors in female urology. Urology 2000; 56 (Supplement 6A):15–22, with permission.)

follow-up of 29 months. Recurrent hyper-mobility, shown by urodynamics, was the most common cause for recurrent stress incontinence with 2 women showing bone anchor migration. Surgical debridement of osteomyelitis was required in another woman [50]. Bernier and Zimmern [51] reported difficulties in removing painful bone anchors which required wedge excision of the pubis.

The issue of bone anchor infections was addressed in a review by Rackley and co-workers [45]. They reported that prevalence of suprapubic bone anchors was 6 cases in 698 procedures (0.86%). For transvaginal bone anchor procedures no infectious cases were reported in the combined series of 314 procedures. The overall prevalence is 0.6% and since it so low there was no significant difference between the techniques.

While bone anchoring offers an alternative for suture stabilization, there is insufficient evidence at present to suggest that they are superior to traditional needle suspensions in the short or long term. With their increased cost compared to traditional methods of rectus fascia anchoring, cost-effectiveness will also have to be addressed.

Complications of Endoscopic Suspensions

Intraoperative Complications

The most commonly encountered intraoperative complications are bleeding, suture passage through the bladder, or laceration of the bladder or urethra during dissection. Bleeding from vaginal veins may be brisk, but can usually be controlled by electrocautery or absorbable stitches. Bleeding from retropubic dissection may be more problematic and is often a result of dissection too far laterally into the obturator fossa. Temporary vaginal packing along with digital compression can slow bleeding. Suture ligatures may be required. Vaginal closure with packing may tamponade bleeding that is not too brisk or flowing freely into the retropubic space. Rarely, an abdominal exploration may be required to control bleeding. Transfusion requirement for endoscopic suspensions is estimated at 1% [12].

When hematuria is identified after passage of a ligature carrier, bladder puncture is likely. Cystoscopy should be done and the suture removed. It is usually on the lateral side, near the bladder neck. Removal and replacement of the stitch along with catheter bladder decompression for 48 hours are generally sufficient. Finally, if dissection leads to urethral or bladder laceration, this should be repaired using multilayer absorbable suture closure and consideration given to longer-term bladder drainage.

Postoperative Complications

Postoperative complications from stress incontinence surgery are not unique to transvaginal suspension techniques. Many result from an increased urethral resistance or relative obstruction and as such are felt to be more common following sling type procedures [12]. The most commonly encountered postoperative complication is urinary retention. This persists beyond 2 weeks in 5–8% [9,10,12,52]. Permanent retention is a rare complication and may not be predicted by preoperative urodynamics. De novo instability symptoms or worsening of pre-existing instability symptoms such as frequency, urgency, and urge incontinence are estimated to occur in 4–16% [10,12,19,22]. For some patients this is quite problematic and may not respond to anticholinergics. Both retention and de novo instability symptoms, if from obstruction, may respond to urethrolysis [53,54]. Cutting the suspensory sutures beyond the initial postoperative period is not generally effective. Other complications that are less frequent but well recognized include: persistent pelvic pain or dyspareunia in 5% [9,19], pelvic prolapse including enterocele, rectocele, or cystocele in 6% [19], and death 0.05% [12].

Conclusions

In general, the long-term success of transvaginal endoscopic suspensions is not as good as open retropubic repairs or sling procedures. Of the transvaginal suspensions, the Gittes no-incision procedure appears to be the least durable. However, the morbidity associated with transvaginal suspensions for stress incontinence is lower than that with open retropubic or sling surgery.

With the introduction of a synthetic mesh prosthesis to support the mid-urethra the results of endoscopic suspension improved. Long-term and comparative trials are in progress. There is still some concern over short- and long-term morbidity, although increasing experience and modifications in the design over time will settle these issues. Bone anchor techniques have also been shown to be safe but still require long-term reporting of outcomes to justify their cost.

References

1. Kelly HA, Dumm WM. Urinary incontinence in women without manifest injury to the bladder. Surg Gynecol Obstet 1914;8:444–50.
2. Marshall VF, Marchetti AA, Krantz KE. The correction of stress incontinence by simple vesicourethral suspension. Surg Gynecol Obstet 1949;88:509–18.
3. Aldridge AH. Transplantation of fascia for relief of urinary stress incontinence. Am J Obstet Gynecol 1942;44:398–411.
4. Pereyra AJ. A simplified surgical procedure for the correction of stress incontinence in women. West J Surg Obstet Gynecol 1959;67:223–6.
5. Pereyra AJ, Lebherz TB. Combined urethrovesical suspension and vaginourethroplasty for correction of urinary stress incontinence. Obstet Gynecol 1967;30:537–46.
6. Stamey TA. Endoscopic suspension of the vesical neck for urinary incontinence. Surg Gynecol Obstet 1973;136:547–54.
7. Raz S. Modified bladder neck suspension for female stress incontinence. Urology 1981;17:82–5.
8. Gittes RF, Loughlin KR. No-incision pubovaginal suspension for stress incontinence. J Urol 1987;138:568–70.
9. Elkabir JJ, Mee AD. Long-term evaluation of the Gittes procedure for urinary stress incontinence. J Urol 1998;159:1203–5.
10. Kondo A, Kato K, Gotoh M, Narushima M, Saito M. The Stamey and Gittes procedures: Long-term followup in relation to incontinence types and patient age. J Urol 1998;160:756–8.
11. Masson DB, Govier FE. Modified Pereyra bladder neck suspension in patients with intrinsic sphincter deficiency and bladder neck hypermobility: Patient satisfaction with a mean follow-up of 4 years. Urology 2000;55:217–22.
12. Leach GE, Dmochowski RR, Appell RA, Blaivas JG, Hadley HR, Luber KM, Mostwin JL, O'Donnell PD, Roehrborn CG. Female stress urinary incontinence clinical guidelines panel summary report on surgical management of female stress urinary incontinence. J Urol 1997;158:875–80.
13. Ulmsten U, Falconer C, Johnson P, Jomaa M, Lanner L, Nilsson CG, Olsson I. A multicenter study of tension-free vaginal tape (TVT) for surgical treatment of stress urinary incontinence. Int Urogynecol J 1998;9:210–13.
14. Stamey TA. Endoscopic suspension of the vesical neck for urinary incontinence in females. Ann Surg 1980;192:465–71.
15. Hilton P, Mayne CJ. The Stamey endoscopic bladder neck suspension. A clinical and urodynamic investigation, including actuarial follow-up over four years. Br J Obstet Gynaecol 1991;91:1141–9.
16. Bihrle W 3d, Tarantino AF. Complications of retropubic bladder neck suspension. Urology 1990;35:213–14.
17. Kil PJ, Hoekstra JW, van der Meijden AP, Smans AJ, Theeuwes AG, Schreinemachers LM. Transvaginal ultrasonography and urodynamic evaluation after suspension operations: Comparison among the Gittes, Stamey and Burch suspensions. J Urol 1991;146:132–6.
18. Conquy S, Zerbib M, Younes E. Retrospective comparative study of three surgical procedures in the treatment of urinary stress incontinence in women: Apropos of 119 patients treated from 1985 to 1990. J Urol (Paris) 1993;99:16–19.
19. Raz S, Sussman EM, Erickson DB, Bregg KJ, Nitti VW. The Raz bladder neck suspension: Results in 206 patients. J Urol 1992;148:845–50.
20. Golomb J, Goldwasser B, Mashiach S. Raz bladder neck suspension in women younger than sixty-five years compared

with elderly women: Three years' experience. Urology 1994;43:40–3.

21. Korman IU, Sirls LT, Kirkemo AK. Success rate of modified Pereyra bladder neck suspension determined by outcomes analysis. J Urol 1994;152:1453–7.
22. Trockman BA, Leach GE, Hamilton J, Sakamoto M, Santiago L, Zimmern PE. Modified Pereyra bladder neck suspension: 10-year mean followup using outcomes analysis in 125 patients. J Urol 1995;154:1841–7.
23. Das S. Comparative outcome analysis of laparoscopic colpo-suspension, abdominal colposuspension and vaginal needle suspension for female urinary incontinence. J Urol 1998;160:368–71.
24. Raz S, Siegel AL, Short JL, Synder JA. Vaginal wall sling. J Urol 1989;141:43.
25. Juma S, Little NA, Raz S. Vaginal wall sling: four years later. Urology 1992;39:424–8.
26. Couillard DR, Deckard-Janatpour KA, Stone AR. The vaginal wall sling: a compressive suspension procedure for recurrent incontinence in elderly patients. Urology 1994;43:203–8.
27. Raz S, Stothers L, Young GPH, Shrot J, Marks B, Chopra A, Wahle GR. Vaginal wall sling for anatomical incontinence and intrinsic sphincter dysfunction: Efficacy and outcome analysis. J Urol 1996;156:166–70.
28. Ulmsten U, Petros P. Intravaginal slingplasty. An ambulatory surgical procedure for treatment of female urinary inconti-nence. Scand J Urol Nephrol 1995;29:75–82.
29. Klutke JJ, Carlin BI, Klutke CG. The tension-free vaginal tape procedure: correction of stress incontinence with minimal alteration in proximal urethral mobility. Urology 2000;55:512–14.
30. Lo TS, Wang AC, Horng SG, Liang CC, Soong YK. Ultrasonographic and urodynamic evaluation after tension free vagina tape procedure (TVT). Acta Obstet Gynecol Scand 2001;80:65–70.
31. Ulmsten U, Johnson P, Rezapour M. A three-year follow up of tension free vaginal tape for surgical treatment of female stress urinary incontinence. Br J Obstet Gynaecol 1999;106:345–50.
32. Wang AC, Lo TS. Tension-free vaginal tape: A minimally invasive solution to stress urinary incontinence in women. J Reprod Med 1998;43:429–34.
33. Haab F, Sananes S, Amarenco G, Ciofu C, Uzan S, Gattengno B, Thibault P. Results of the tension-free vaginal tape proce-dure for the treatment of type II stress urinary incontinence at a minimum followup of 1 year. J Urol 2001;165:159–62.
34. Azam U, Frazer MI, Kozman EL, Ward K, Hilton P, Rane A. The tension-free vaginal tape procedure in women with previous failed stress incontinence surgery. J Urol 2001;166:554–6.
35. Rezapour M, Ulmsten U. Tension-free vaginal tape (tvt) in women with recurrent stress urinary incontinence – a long-term follow up. Int Urogynecol J 2001;12:S9–S11.
36. Nilsson CG, Kuuva N, Falconer C, Rezapour M, Ulmsten U. Long-term results of the tension-free vaginal tape (TVT) procedure for surgical treatment of female stress urinary incontinence. Int Urogynecol J 2001;12:S5–S8.

37. Ward K, Hilton P, Browning J. A randomized trial of colpo-suspension and tension free vaginal tape (TVT) for primary genuine stress incontinence. (Abstract). Neurourol Urodyn 2000;19:386–8.
38. Meschia M, Pifarotti P, Bernasconi F, Guercio E, Maffiolini M, Magatti F, Spreafico L. Symposium: Tension-Free Vaginal Tape: Analysis of outcomes and complications in 404 stress incontinent women. Int Urogynecol J 2001;12:S24–S27.
39. Vierhout ME. Severe hemorrhage complicating tension-free vaginal tape (tvt): a case report. Int Urogynecol J 2001;12:139–40.
40. Zilbert AW, Farrell SA. Case report: External iliac artery laceration during tension-free vaginal tape procedure. Int Urogynecol J 2001;12:141–3.
41. Brink DM. Bowel injury following insertion of tension-free vaginal tape [letter]. S African Med J 2000;90:450, 452.
42. Moran PA, Ward KL, Johnson D, Smirni WE, Hilton P, Bibby J. Tension-free vaginal tape for primary genuine stress incontinence: a two-centre follow-up study. BJU Int 2000;86:39–42.
43. Nativ O, Levine S, Madjar S, Issaq E, Moskovitz B, Beyar M. Incisionless per vaginal bone anchor cystourethropexy for the treatment of female stress incontinence: Experience with the first 50 patients. J Urol 1997;158:1742–4.
44. El-Toukhy TAA, Tolba MA, Davies AE. Assessment of a new bone anchor system for the treatment of female genuine stress incontinence. BJU Int 1999;84:780–4.
45. Rackley RR, Abdelmalak JB, Madjar S, Yanilmaz A, Appell RA, Tchetgen MB. Bone anchor infections in female pelvic reconstructive procedures: a literature review of series and case reports. J Urol 2001;165:1975–8.
46. Leach GE. Bone fixation technique for transvaginal needle suspension. Urology 1988;31:388–90.
47. Leach GE, Appell R. Percutaneous bladder neck suspension. Urol Clin North Am 1996;23:511–16.
48. Appell RA, Rackley RR, Dmochowski RR. Vesica percuta-neous bladder neck stabilization. J Endourol 1996;10:221–5.
49. Schultheiss D, Hofner K, Oelke M, Grunewald V, Jonas U. Does bone anchor fixation improve the outcome of percuta-neous bladder neck suspension in female stress urinary incontinence? Br J Urol 1998;82:192–5.
50. Tebyani N, Patel H, Yamaguchi R, Aboseif SR. Percutaneous needle bladder neck suspension for the treatment of stress urinary incontinence in women: long term results. J Urol 2000;163:1510–12.
51. Bernier PA, Zimmern PE. Bone anchor removal after bladder neck suspension. Br J Urol 1998;82:302–3.
52. Tamussino KF, Zivkovic F, Pieber D, Moser F, Haas J, Ralph G. Five-year results after anti-incontinence opera-tions. Am J Obstet Gynecol 1999;181:1347–52.
53. Nitti VW, Raz S. Obstruction following anti-incontinence procedures: diagnosis and treatment with transvaginal ure-throlysis. J Urol 1994;152:93–8.
54. Carr LK, Webster GD. Voiding dysfunction following incon-tinence surgery: diagnosis and treatment with retropubic or vaginal urethrolysis. J Urol 1997;157:821–3.

32 Retropubic Urethropexies

David H.L. Wilkie

Genuine stress incontinence is a common condition, particularly in multiparous patients, and frequently results in a request for surgical correction. Vaginal and abdominal procedures have been described in the literature over the last 100 years but it is only within the last 20 to 25 that choice of surgery has been influenced by evidence-based medicine. Initially, anterior colporrhaphy was the gynecological procedure of choice, following which an abdominal procedure could correct the shortcomings of the former. Marshall et al. [1] described a simple retropubic suspension that could be performed either as a primary or secondary operation to support the bladder neck. This transformed the prognosis for women with stress incontinence as consistently high cure rates began to be appreciated. Burch [2] later reported his colposuspension with virtually the same success rate but with reduced complications.

Despite the long history, these two procedures remain the most commonly chosen in North America for primary and recurrent stress incontinence. This chapter will focus on anatomical and physiological changes in the pelvis, on the indications for surgery, and will review the surgical techniques to correct the bladder neck defect. The chapter will review clinical results and complications of retropubic urethropexy.

Diagnosis

Genuine stress incontinence (GSI) is a diagnosis that applies to loss of urine coincident with a rise of intra-abdominal pressure in the absence of detrusor activity [3]. The urethral sphincter is incompetent at this time, owing to failure of pressure transmission, to intrinsic sphincter deficiency or to a combination of both. These concepts have replaced the earlier impression that the posterior urethrovesical angle was critical to maintaining continence. Instead, it is the failure of support to the proximal urethra at the time of increased abdominal pressure that occurs in the majority of patients with GSI. When this is combined with a lack of intrinsic muscular tone, GSI may be quite severe.

Etiology

Vaginal parity is most commonly implicated in the pelvic floor changes that result in GSI. Dilation of the pelvic floor and birth canal with vaginal delivery may result in disruption of levator ani attachments and trauma to the pudendal nerve. Denervation and subsequent reinnervation of the pelvic floor leave the urethra less able to match the contraction effort of other abdominal muscle groups [4]. The pelvic floor and urethrovesical junction then descend at times of effort. For a fraction of a second, the pressure in the proximal urethra is exceeded by the pressure in the bladder and urine escapes. This is compounded if the intrinsic muscles of the urethra are compromised by such changes as denervation, devascularization and scarring from previous lacerations or surgery. Other factors play a role in the occurrence and severity of GSI and these include obesity, chronic obstructive lung disease, severity of work or recreation related activities, aging changes and estrogen deficiency [5].

Therapeutic Options

Therapy for GSI is directed to improving pelvic floor pressure transmission to the proximal urethra and/or to improving intrinsic sphincter tone.

Conservative options include weight reduction, discontinuation of smoking, pelvic floor exercises to improve levator tone, vaginal prostheses to support the bladder neck (tampon, incontinence pessary), drug manipulation (estrogen, alpha-agonists, discontinuation of alpha-blockers) and surgery. The conservative treatment for pelvic floor disorders is described in an earlier section of this book. Similarly, vaginal repair and endoscopic needle suspensions have been described but shortcomings or complications of these techniques limit their use in the modern treatment of GSI. Retropubic surgery for GSI is now preferred for uncomplicated patients who have demonstrated a significant failure of pressure transmission to the proximal urethra.

In 1949, a retropubic urethrovesical suspension for treatment of GSI was described by Marshall, Marchetti and Krantz [1]. Although this seemed a somewhat radical procedure for supporting the proximal urethra, it became accepted as a surgical choice because of the recognized failure of vaginal repair. In 1961, Burch [2] described a different form of retropubic support using Cooper's ligament instead of the symphysis pubis. Over time, the procedures became increasingly popular as improved operative and anesthesia techniques reduced the morbidity of retropubic surgery. Studies now have confirmed a definite superiority of retropubic support surgery over vaginal repair [6,7].

Indications for Surgery

Patients who are chosen for retropubic repair should have attempted the conservative treatments described above. In particular, they should have optimized their surgical suitability (weight and smoking reduction) so as to reduce postoperative risks of thromboembolism, pneumonia and surgical infections. Weight and chest symptoms also play a role in the long-term outcome of surgery such that failure to control these factors probably reduces the overall cure rate.

The diagnosis of GSI must be secure. This involves the history of loss of urine promptly at the time of sudden movement or coughing. Ideally, other symptoms such as irritative bladder complaints and voiding dysfunction are absent. With a half speculum retracting the posterior vagina, the patient strains and obvious descent of the bladder neck is usually present. If a lubricated Q-tip swab is placed in the urethra, a deflexion of more than 30 degrees from resting position indicates urethral hypermobility and is called a positive Q-tip test [8]. Coughing may reveal stress incontinence, though this is frequently absent while supine. The patient is

then examined standing with urine in the bladder and, if necessary, with the perineal and posterior vaginal tissues retracted by the observer's hand. Coughing will usually demonstrate stress incontinence in this situation. Further confirmation would involve the patient performing a "pad test" in which she attends with a comfortably full bladder and proceeds through a standardized set of activities while wearing a pre-weighed perineal pad [9]. The pad is inspected and weighed afterwards to confirm urinary loss during these activities. Urodynamic testing is recommended if the diagnosis has not yet been otherwise confirmed or if there are conflicting symptoms involving urgency and voiding dysfunction. This is particularly true if previous bladder neck surgery has been performed [10].

When the patient proceeds to retropubic surgery, the consent should include a full description of the nature of the surgery, how it is performed, length of stay in hospital, convalescent period at home and activity restriction. Potential complications should be reviewed including a discussion of the success and failure rate of the technique. The rest of this chapter will focus on these issues.

Surgical Technique

The Marshall–Marchetti–Krantz procedure (MMK) involves retropubic dissection and exposure of the catheterized proximal urethra. The surgeon's vaginal finger elevates the anterior vagina and the structure is elevated into view. Either absorbable or non-absorbable sutures are then placed into the upper wall of the vagina adjacent to the urethra and through the lateral wall of the urethra. These are located up to the level of the urethrovesical junction. Care is taken to avoid going into the lumen of the urethra or bladder. The sutures are brought through the symphysis pubis and tied. This has the effect of placing the urethra immediately behind the symphysis in the midline (Figure 32.1). Seen laterally, the urethrovesical junction now makes an acute angle behind the symphysis pubis. The catheter is left per urethra or it may be inserted suprapubically.

The Burch colposuspension also involves retropubic dissection down to the bladder and urethrovesical junction. The proximal urethra and vagina are identified during the course of dissection. With the bladder catheterized, the catheter bulb can be palpated and this helps to identify the urethrovesical junction. The operator's vaginal finger elevates the vagina on either side of bladder neck. Urethral and bladder tissue are gently retracted medially to expose a safe area of paravaginal tissue

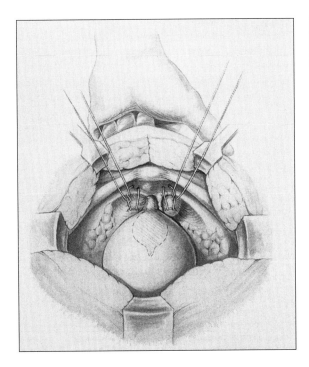

Figure 32.1 Marshall–Marchetti–Krantz Procedure (From Walters MD, Karram MM (1993) In: Clinical Urogynecology. Mosby Year-Book Inc., p 200, with permission.)

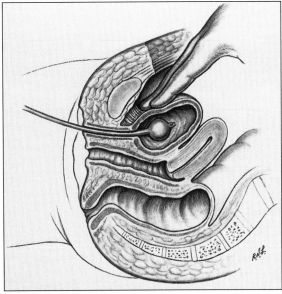

Figure 32.2 Burch procedure – retropubic dissection between symphysis and bladder (From Stanton SL, Tanagho EL (1986) In: Surgery of Female Incontinence. Springer-Verlag, p 99, with permission.)

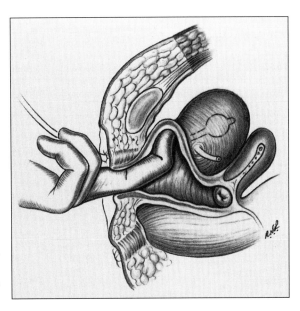

Figure 32.3 Burch procedure – digital elevation of paravaginal tissue adjacent to bladder neck. (From Stanton SL, Tanagho EL (1986) In: Surgery of Female Incontinence. Springer-Verlag, p 99, with permission.)

(Figures 32.2–32.5). Absorbable or non-absorbable suture is then passed through this paravaginal tissue and ideally does not penetrate the vagina. These sutures are brought through ipsilateral Cooper's ligaments and held. A check for urethral and bladder integrity is appropriate and different techniques are used. In the course of dissection, the operator identifies the "roll-back" of the urethrovesical junction just medial to the area of suture placement. By visualizing a clear sulcus between vagina and adjacent urethrovesical junction, paravaginal tissue can be safely sutured. Methylene blue can be instilled per catheter to check that sutures have not actually penetrated the bladder itself. Many practitioners cystoscope their patients at this point. This has the advantage of excluding bladder pathology and penetrating sutures. Ureteric function is confirmed by visualizing efflux of urine from each orifice. With a cystoscope at the bladder neck, satisfactory support will be visualized at the time of gentle traction on the sutures.

The patient is recatheterized. The sutures are then gently tied in a manner that simply takes up the "slack" of bladder neck hypermobility. In this manner, the Burch colposuspension would be more appropriately described as urethral stabilization. The support given by the paravaginal tissue under the proximal urethra acts as a stabilizing point and permits more effective compression of the bladder neck at the instant of increased abdominal pressure.

The bladder is left catheterized, either per urethra or by the suprapubic route. The advantage of the latter is that the patient may begin attempts at voiding the day after surgery with the catheter clamped. The catheter, however, provides a release mechanism for the patient who has postoperative voiding difficulty. Selected patients do quite well

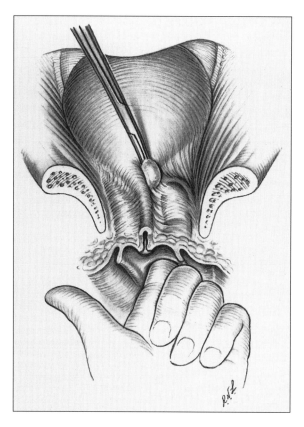

Figure 32.4 Burch procedure – bladder neck is mobilized medially and shows "Roll-back" sulcus. (From Stanton SL, Tanagho EL (1986) In: Surgery of Female Incontinence. Springer-Verlag, p 99, with permission.)

with a simple urethral catheter that is removed from one to two days after surgery. It is quite uncommon to have postoperative voiding delay if the supportive sutures are under minimal tension.

Outcome of Surgery

When offering patients surgery for stress incontinence it is essential that they know the likelihood of success and failure of the procedure that is chosen and also the potential for complications. It was recognized several generations ago that vaginal repair for stress incontinence had a high failure rate and the earlier attitude to incontinent women was to "try first from below and then go from above". The development of retropubic surgery came as a response to the obvious deficiency of vaginal surgery for incontinence. Surgeons began to offer retropubic support as primary surgery for GSI. Early reports of success rates were optimistic but objectivity was limited by lack of standardized ways of assessing outcome. These have gradually been refined, particularly with the advent of urodynamic

testing, "pad testing" and more recently still, the use of quality of life assessment tools [11]. Studies of the MMK and Burch colposuspension have shown consistently high success rates when measured subjectively (patient denies incontinence) and objectively (patient is observed to be dry with a full bladder during stress provocation).

In Bergman and Elia's classic randomized control study [6], patients who underwent anterior colporrhaphy, modified Pereyra needle suspension and Burch colposuspension were followed for 2 and 5 years. The anterior repair distinguished itself early with a poor outcome. By 5 years there was no significant difference between anterior repair and needle suspension with cure rates between 37 and 43% respectively. The Burch colposuspension produced objective cure in 82%. Similar results were reported by Kammerer-Doak et al. in 1999 [7]. Columbo et al. [12] reported a comparison in 1994 between Burch colposuspension and MMK. Subjective and objective cure rates were not significantly different, with 92 and 80% for the Burch colposuspension and 85 and 65% for the MMK. There was longer hospital stay and catheter requirement in the MMK patients. Their conclusion was that both provided a high cure rate but that the Burch colposuspension was preferable. A 10- to 20-year review of the Burch colposuspension was reported by Alcalay et al. [13]. Patients who underwent Burch colposuspension either as a primary or secondary procedure were followed and a 69% objective cure rate was found between the 10- and

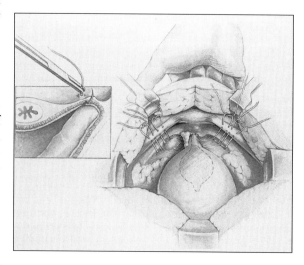

Figure 32.5 Burch procedure – sutures are placed through paravaginal tissue and then Cooper's ligament. They are tied with minimal tension, stabilizing the proximal urethra. (From Walters MD, Karram MM (1993) In: Clinical Urogynecology, Mosby Year-Book Inc., p 199, with permission.)

20-year interval. Factors adversely affecting the cure were previous bladder neck surgery, obesity, difficult dissection and development of postoperative detrusor instability.

Complications

Perioperative complications are uncommon following retropubic surgery. However, severe hemorrhage has been reported to occur occasionally, typically in patients undergoing repeat retropubic procedures [14]. Serious infection at the operative site is also very uncommon and it is rare to have to remove sutures after the fact. Transvesical and transurethral sutures have been identified occasionally; these typically present with symptoms of bladder irritation and persistence of stress incontinence. Damage to viscera is uncommon and typically involves laceration of the bladder at the time of repeat retropubic dissection. Nerve injuries, though rare, can be particularly worrisome when lateral cutaneous nerves are compressed or cut, giving paresthesia to the anterior thigh. Femoral nerve injury may result in significant weakness in the anterior thigh. The proposed mechanism here is of compression by the retractor or by abnormal leg positioning for the procedure with subinguinal compression. The long-term issues include de novo detrusor instability, development of a fistula, osteitis pubis, voiding dysfunction, pelvic pain and genital prolapse. Detrusor instability can occur in 3–25% of women who undergo Burch colposuspension [15]. Luckily most of these patients have transient symptoms and only a small portion require treatment. Patients with preoperative detrusor instability should be warned that their urgency symptoms may persist despite satisfactory bladder neck support. Voiding difficulty with slow stream is common after retropubic surgery for incontinence but retention is rare. A patient known to void by Valsalva preoperatively should be instructed to let detrusor effort alone empty the bladder. Gentle traction on the supporting sutures reduces postoperative voiding delay. Urogenital fistulas are also uncommon. However, Mainprize and Drutz [16] reported 7 fistulas in 2712 MMK procedures. Osteitis pubis has been one of the most worrisome complications of the MMK and occurs approximately in 2.5% of patients. The etiology is unknown and it is an intense inflammatory response to sutures in the symphysis pubis associated with the MMK. The disability experienced by these patients has impressed incontinence surgeons to the extent that the Burch procedure is increasingly preferred to the MMK. Occasionally, post colposuspension pain has been reported and has required release of one or more of the supporting sutures if physiotherapy is not successful.

In the original description of the Burch colposuspension, postoperative enterocele formation was found to occur in 7.6% of patients [1]. Other authors have noted this to be less common but it is still a concern when operating on a patient who has pelvic floor relaxation and stress incontinence. The shift of the mid-anterior vagina behind the symphysis may allow for the descent of a mobile retroverted uterus or early enterocele. Hysterectomy or Moscowitz enterocele closure has been recommended if patients are thought to be at risk. No randomized control trial has been performed to evaluate the benefit of concomitant enterocele closure at the time of Burch colposuspension.

Summary

In the straightforward patient with a hypermobile bladder neck and stress incontinence, the intrinsic sphincter mechanism is usually relatively normal. Because of this, retropubic urethropexy, particularly the Burch colposuspension, has become the gold standard for surgical treatment of GSI. It is against this procedure that other operations must be compared and this follow-up should extend beyond 10 years [13]. The Burch colposuspension has been clearly shown to be effective and to have a low complication rate in properly selected patients. The open procedure can be performed in a surgical day care setting with appropriate multimodality analgesia techniques (Wilkie D, Gofton E (1999), submitted for publication). Postoperative narcotic pain requirements are minimal and patients can expect to return to normal activities at approximately 2 weeks postoperatively. The Burch colposuspension is an easily taught technique and all graduates of gynecology residencies should be familiar and comfortable with this operation.

References

1. Marshall VF, Marchetti AA, Krantz KE. The correction of stress incontinence by simple vesicourethral suspension. Surg Gynecol Obstet 1949;88:509–18.
2. Burch JC. Urethrovaginal fixation to Cooper's ligament for correction of stress incontinence, cystocele and prolapse. Am J Obstet Gynecol 1961;100:764–74.
3. Bates P, Bradley WE, Glen E, Griffiths D, Melchoir H, Rowan D et al. The standardization of terminology of lower urinary tract function. J Urol 1979;121:551–4.
4. Smith ARB, Hosker GL, Warrell DW. The role of partial denervation of the pelvic floor in the aetiology of genitourinary

prolapse and stress incontinence of urine: a neurophysiological study. Br J Obstet Gynaecol 1989;96:24–8.

5. Walters M. Epidemiology and social impact of urinary incontinence. In: Clinical Urogynecology. St Louis: Mosby Year-Book, 1993.

6. Bergman A, Elia G. Three surgical procedures for genuine stress incontinence: five year follow-up of a prospective randomized study. Am J Obstet Gynecol 1995;173(1):66–71.

7. Kammerer-Doak DN, Dorin MH, Rogers RG, Cousin MO. A randomized trial of Burch retropubic urethropexy and anterior colporrhaphy for stress urinary incontinence. Obstet Gynecol 1999;93(1):75–8.

8. Karram MM, Bhatia NN. The Q-tip test: standardization of the technique and its interpretation in women with urinary incontinence. Obstet Gynecol 1988;71(6, Pt 1):807–11.

9. International Continence Society. Quantification of urine loss. In: Fifth Report on the Standardization of Terminology. Aachen, West Germany: International Continence Society, 1983.

10. Drutz HP, Farrell SA, Mainprize TL, Wilkie D. Guidelines for the evaluation of genuine stress incontinence prior to primary surgery. In: Society of Obstetricians and Gynaecologists of Canada Clinical Practice Guidelines Policy Statement 1997;60:1–9.

11. Robinson D, Pearce KF, Preisser JS, Dugan E, Suggs PK, Cohen SJ. Relationship between patient reports of urinary incontinence symptoms and quality of life measures. Obstet Gynecol 1998;91(2):224–8.

12. Columbo M, Scalambrino S, Maggioni A, Milani R. Burch colposuspension versus modified Marshall-Marshetti-Krantz urethropexy for primary genuine stress incontinence: a prospective randomized clinical trial. Am J Obstet Gynecol 1994;171(6):1573–9.

13. Alcalay M, Monga A, Stanton SL. Burch colposuspension a 10–20 year follow-up. Br J Obstet Gynaecol 1995;102(2):740–5.

14. Nygaard IE, Kreder KJ. Complications of incontinence surgery. Int Urogynecol J 1994;5:353–60.

15. Cornella JL. Long term complications of retropubic urethropexy: review and clinical opinion. In: Quarterly Report, American Urogynecologic Society 1997;15(1):1–4.

16. Mainprize TC, Drutz HP. The Marshall-Marchetti-Kranz procedure: a critical review. Obstet Gynecol Surv 1988;43(12):724–9.

33 Slings

Jane A. Schulz and J. Edwin Morgan

Background

Throughout the past century, hundreds of different surgical procedures have been described for the management of stress urinary incontinence. However, the sling procedure, despite its many variations, has maintained a constant presence in both the urologic and urogynecologic communities.

Three European physicians pioneered sling procedures in the early 1900s. Goebell first suggested transplantation of the pyramidalis muscle in 1910 [1]. This was followed by Frangheim who, in 1914, recommended using the pyramidalis or strips of rectus muscle as a suburethral sling by attaching the muscle to overlying fascia [2]. In 1917, Stoeckel suggested combining the techniques of Goebell and Frangheim and adding plication of the vesical neck [3].

Throughout the twentieth century there have been many variations of sling procedures described in the literature. In 1907, Giordano suggested the use of gracilis muscle by wrapping it around the urethra [4]. Shortly thereafter, in 1911, Souier described the use of levator ani muscles by placing them between the vagina and urethra [5], and, in 1923, Thompson recommended the use of strips of rectus muscle, surrounded by fascia, to be passed in front of the pubic bones and around the urethra [6]. The Aldridge sling was introduced in 1942 [7], and then in 1968 Chasser Moir introduced the gauze hammock operation [8] as a modification of the original Aldridge technique.

Over time, there has been recognition that retropubic procedures provide better long-term success rates than vaginal procedures. Until the 1990s, sling procedures were usually used after other incontinence procedures had failed. However, a sling procedure is now indicated if intrinsic sphincter deficiency, with or without bladder neck hypermobility, is diagnosed preoperatively, regardless of whether the patient has had a previous incontinence operation [9]. Since many women have some intrinsic sphincter deficiency, this has led to a trend to do primary sling procedures in all patients [10]. There is also literature and widespread opinion that incontinence secondary to hypermobility should be treated with a sling if other comorbidities, such as obesity, chronic chest conditions, or other repetitive strenuous activity, predispose the patient to a higher risk of postoperative failure [11,12].

Indications

The most common indication for a sling is type III stress urinary incontinence or intrinsic sphincter deficiency. Slings are used in those patients who have low urethral closure pressures that require a more compressive or obstructive procedure than a standard suspension procedure, such as a Burch or a Marshall–Marchetti–Krantz retropubic urethropexy. There is a spectrum of stress urinary incontinence; some women have pure hypermobility, some women have pure intrinsic sphincter deficiency (often with the classic leadpipe or pipestem urethra), but many women have some component of both. Although slings have traditionally been used after previous failed continence surgery, there is a role for primary slings in certain patients. The three main options available for the management of intrinsic sphincter deficiency are slings, injectable bulking agents, and the artificial sphincter. Of these, the sling is the most desirable as long as the patient can tolerate the procedure medically. We currently have no ideal urethral bulking agent and the long-term success of this procedure is quite poor (30–40% still dry at 5-year follow-up [13]). Artificial sphincters carry a risk of infection and malfunction and are a much more morbid procedure than the sling.

Intrinsic sphincter deficiency has a multifactorial etiology; these factors lead to decreased urethral integrity, which affects the ability of the submucosal and muscular layers to coapt and compress the urethral lumen. Etiologic factors are related to devascularization, denervation, or trauma and may include: neurologic injury from childbirth or other neurologic conditions (myelodysplasia, sacral agenesis, T12 spinal cord injury); previous radiation exposure; previous surgery; connective tissue abnormalities; catheter trauma; and menopausal hormone loss. Certain women, who have severe urinary leakage and positive cough test supine, are more likely to have intrinsic sphincter deficiency [14] and benefit from a primary sling procedure. Other patients that will benefit more from a sling than a retropubic urethropexy include those with a funneled bladder neck on imaging, obesity, chronic chest conditions, and those that perform extreme physical activity [15]. Slings can be used in any age group of patients as long as the patient or caregiver has the ability to do clean intermittent catheterization afterwards if needed.

Certain patients may request a sling with a goal to complete retention and long-term clean intermittent catheterization. This is often a desirable procedure in patients with neurogenic disease, who may develop urethral erosions related to Foley bulb expulsion, rather than resorting to bladder neck closure which has risk of fistulizing or causing chronic problems with leakage.

The goal of the sling operation is to restore sufficient outlet resistance to the damaged urethra to prevent urine loss with stress maneuvers, while preventing urethral obstruction. In addition to facilitating urethral coaptation and increasing intrinsic urethral closure pressure, slings provide some bladder neck suspension to increase the transmission of intra-abdominal pressure to the urethra. Therefore, the sling procedure is not only adequate for patients with pure intrinsic sphincter deficiency, but will also correct hypermobility in those that have a mix of type II and III incontinence.

As with all pelvic floor repairs, correction of any prolapse or concomitant pelvic pathology should be addressed in addition to the incontinence

Investigations Prior to a Sling

As with all patient assessment, a full history and physical examination should be completed. Particular attention should be paid to genitourinary symptomatology, the severity of the incontinence, previous surgery, previous radiation, and history of neurologic injury. Physical examination should include a general examination, a neurologic assessment, examination of all pelvic floor compartments for prolapse, and assessment of any other pelvic pathology.

Urinalysis, uroflowmetry, and post-void residual are easily performed in a clinic setting and the latter two are good screening tools for voiding dysfunction. Patients with prolonged intermittent uroflow patterns and high residuals are potential risks for voiding problems after any surgical procedure for incontinence. If urodynamic assessment confirms preoperative voiding dysfunction the patient must be counseled that this could become much worse with a sling; a patient of this type should also learn clean intermittent catheterization preoperatively [16].

Prior to a sling patients should have video urodynamics, or multichannel urodynamics and some imaging of the bladder neck. An assessment of urethral resistance should also be performed with either a Valsalva leak point pressure (VLPP) or maximal urethral closure pressure (MUCP). Diagnosis of intrinsic sphincter deficiency involves assessment of many factors on clinical history and physical examination but also includes assessment of bladder neck mobility and either a VLPP less than 60 cmH$_2$O, or an MUCP less than 20 cmH$_2$O [17]. There have been studies looking at the correlation of low MUCP and low VLPP and the results are somewhat discrepant. Nager et al. showed good correlation between low MUCP and low VLPP [18]; however, Peschers et al. showed poor correlation [19]. Regardless of the controversies, a measure of urethral resistance should be performed preoperatively; the urologic community tends to use VLPP and the gynecologic community uses MUCP. Concerns exist about reproducibility of Valsalva effort, but this is a more dynamic representation of the incontinence event. Many feel that a funneled bladder neck on cystogram or on video urodynamics is also an indication for a sling [20,21]; however, some controversy exists in this area.

Urodynamics are also useful to check for detrusor instability, to assess voiding function and bladder compliance. The Society of Obstetricians and Gynecologists of Canada has developed guidelines for the assessment of patients prior to primary and secondary continence surgery [22,23]. Both recommend the use of urodynamics studies; the use of urethral pressure studies is recommended prior to secondary surgery, but many authors feel it is advisable prior to any sling procedure. Throughout the years there has been controversy about the role of urodynamic testing as a diagnostic tool, and regarding how relevant it is in the final decision-making process [24]. However, a recent review by Abrams et al. of over 5000 women still concludes with the recommendation that urodynamics assessment be performed prior to incontinence surgery [25]. This was reinforced by the group at Duke University who concluded that the predictive value of stress symptoms alone was not high enough to serve as the basis for surgical management [26].

When assessing patients with intrinsic sphincter deficiency, the physician must be aware that any complaint of urinary frequency may be related to altered voiding habits to keep the bladder empty and avoid leakage, and not due to detrusor instability. When performing urodynamic studies on patients with intrinsic sphincter deficiency, it may be difficult to assess bladder capacity because of the ease of urinary leakage. A Foley catheter in place with gentle traction on the bulb to prevent bypassing may be useful during assessment of capacity, and also to allow sufficient bladder filling to demonstrate any detrusor instability or abnormal bladder compliance.

Cystoscopic evaluation of the lower urinary tract should definitely be performed in any patient who has had prior continence surgery and in those with irritative voiding symptoms. The role of cystoscopy for the evaluation of patient with primary stress urinary incontinence is controversial; however, it can play a role in assessment of the bladder neck.

Types of Sling

There are many described techniques and materials used for slings. In this chapter, we will overview the most commonly used procedures and materials. The tension-free vaginal tape is a new procedure that has many properties of the traditional sling; this will be discussed in a separate chapter.

Fascial Slings

The first fascial sling was described in 1933 by Price, who used fascia lata in a woman with sacral agenesis and urinary incontinence, and fixed the sling to the rectus muscles [27]. In the 1940s both Millen and Aldridge described the use of paired strips of rectus fascia to form a sling. Millen looped the fascial strips around the urethra and tied them above, whereas Aldridge sutured the strips of fascia below the urethra.

Modifications of this pubovaginal sling technique continue to be commonly used in practice today. An incision is made in the vaginal mucosa from the mid-urethra to the bladder neck; the bladder is then dissected off the anterior vaginal mucosa.

Alternatively, an inverted U-shape incision can be made to expose the urethra and bladder neck. If available, a Lone Star retractor may be useful to retract the edges of the vaginal mucosa. The fascial strip is placed under the bladder neck and passed through the space of Retzius behind the pubic rami. Depending on the operator's preferred technique, the sling can be sutured directly to Cooper's ligament, or can be brought through and tied over the top of the rectus fascia. Preference is often given to securing the sling to the rectus fascia to allow for a more dynamic result; when the patient increases their intra-abdominal pressure the sling responds by tightening and providing posterior urethral support and preventing urinary leakage. Some authors describe attachment of the sling to the pubic tubercle, but this carries a higher risk of osteitis pubis and osteomyelitis [28,29]. The sling can be secured vaginally to the fascial tissues with a 2-0 or 3-0 Vicryl or Dexon suture to prevent movement or rolling of the sling and to allow the sling tension to maintain an even distribution. Once the sling has been placed, cystourethroscopy should be performed to rule out bladder injury; certain authors also describe the use of indigo carmine dye to ensure ureteric patency.

A few options are available for the acquisition of fascial material. The first decision is whether to use autologous or cadaveric fascia. Autologous fascia can be obtained from the anterior rectus sheath or from the fascia lata of the leg. It is a good choice with minimal associated morbidity and few concerns about tissue infection, rejection, or erosion [30]. With the emergence of more tissue banks, cadaveric fascia has become a more popular option as it reduces the morbidity of autologous fascial harvest. However, caution must be taken in the choice of banked fascia; there have been reports of rapid tissue breakdown and failure of incontinence and prolapse repair with some cadaveric fascia [31–33]. The suspicion is that the specimens that failed may have been over-irradiated during processing leading to tissue breakdown and failure. Another concern with cadaveric fascia use is the risk, although low, of infection transmission.

When harvesting a rectus fascial strip, either a 15 cm by 2 cm strip can be completely detached and used to pass from the vagina to the space of Retzius, or the central portion of the strip can be left attached and the two ends of the fascia tunneled from the abdomen to the vagina and wrapped below the bladder neck.

Fascia lata has the advantage of being uniformly strong regardless of age or medical condition. One study showed triple the tensile strength in fascia lata compared to rectus sheath [34]. Fascia lata may also be the autologous material of choice in patients that have had previous abdominal surgery and have significant scarring in the suprapubic area. It has the advantage of allowing a smaller abdominal incision for securing the sling, and therefore, a lower risk of creation of hernia or postoperative pain, which may occur in the larger rectus fascial harvest incision. The main disadvantages of using fascia lata are the need to reposition the patient and the need for an additional leg incision. When using fascia lata, a strip of 20–25 cm length and 2 cm width can be easily harvested through two small incisions in the lateral thigh; some physicians use a fascial stripper tool to aid in harvest, but this is not necessary. Caution must be taken to avoid injury to the common peroneal nerve near the lateral femoral condyle. The fascial defect can be repaired with figure-of-eight absorbable sutures, a drain placed, and a pressure dressing applied.

Synthetic Slings

The morbidity associated with fascial harvest may be avoided with the use of artificial materials. A continuous piece of material may be used for the body and arms of the sling, or a patch of synthetic material may be used with arms of non-absorbable suture. The advantages of using synthetic material are that it is cheap (especially when compared to cadaveric fascia), readily available, and there is no dependence on previous surgical scars, body habitus, or experience in harvesting the graft. Since the synthetic strips can be prepared in advance, this theoretically decreases operative time; also, patients should have decreased postoperative pain and risk of hernia formation. The disadvantages are that the use of any foreign substance is accompanied by increased risks of infection and erosion. However, overall risks of erosion are now likely to be less with the trend towards tension-free slings.

Polyethylene terephthalate (Mersilene, Ethicon) mesh was one of the first used in 1966 by Ridley. He described use of a Mersilene ribbon in 17 patients, but noted serious complications in 18%, including mesh erosion, graft infection, and urinary retention [35].

Sling Techniques

Abdominal Approach

This technique is not used very commonly; it should be reserved for patients in whom the lithotomy position is contraindicated (perhaps due to significant limitation of hip mobility), in the rare circumstance where a decision is made intraoperatively to do a sling, or where concomitant proce-

dures dictate the need to have the patient supine. However, in our experience, with the use of new hydraulic stirrups that allow easy repositioning, there should be very few contraindications to the lithotomy position.

With the abdominal approach the retropubic space is opened, and a tunnel is created under the proximal urethra at the bladder neck with sharp and blunt dissection without making a vaginal incision. The sling is then passed under the bladder neck and brought up to Cooper's ligament or the rectus fascia. There may be significant scarring due to previous surgery in the area; it may be necessary to open the bladder to aid in the dissection under the bladder neck. With this technique, there is a risk of placing the sling too distally, thereby increasing the risk of obstruction.

Abdomino-vaginal Approach

This method is quite common and allows for concomitant vaginal and abdominal repairs if required. We use this method in our unit with rectus fascia and have found it to be very successful with comparable cure and improvement rates to other series of slings. This method facilitates accurate perforation of the arms of the sling and placement of the sling under the bladder neck by using a combined technique of dissection into the retropubic space and vaginal dissection. Advantages include improved exposure both vaginally at the bladder neck, and in the space of Retzius to decrease the amount of retropubic dissection required (Figure 33.1).

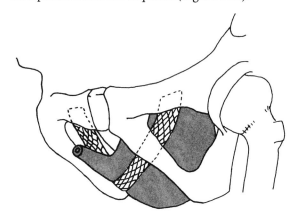

Figure 33.1 Combined abdomino-vaginal Marlex sling procedure. This is a two-team operation in which the surgeon passes the Marlex mesh through tunnels created in the urogenital diaphragm into the space of Retzius, where it is sutured to Cooper's ligament. (Reproduced with permission from Drutz HP, Buckspan M Flax S, Mackie L (1990) Clinical and urodynamic re-evaluation of combined abdomino-vaginal Marlex sling operations for recurrent stress urinary incontinence. International Urogynecology Journal and Pelvic Floor Dysfunction 1:71; Figure 1.)

Vaginal Approach

A vaginal incision is used to place the sling under the bladder neck. Using a finger or instrument, dissection is carried up into the retropubic space; the sling is passed up blindly using a needle passer or a packing forcep. Only a small abdominal incision is then required to secure the sling to the rectus fascia. This method also has the advantage of decreasing the dissection required in the retropubic space; however, there is an increased risk of bladder or urethral injury due to the blind passage of the sling.

Vaginal Wall Sling

The final technique that has been described in the urologic literature is the vaginal wall sling. This involves making two parallel incisions in the vaginal mucosa just lateral to the urethra. Bites of fascia are then taken, also incorporating a portion of the rectangular vaginal wall overlying the urethra centrally. The remainder of the technique is similar to the vaginal approach, with the pairs of permanent sutures on each side then being passed blindly up ipsilaterally to the small suprapubic incision and secured to the rectus fascia. The features of this technique are more comparable to needle suspension techniques and will not be discussed further here.

Adjusting Sling Tension

There is no useful way to measure sling tension intraoperatively that has prognostic value in terms of either achieving continence or preventing long-term clean intermittent catheterization. Many techniques have been tried and described to attempt to secure correct sling tension intraoperatively but none have proven consistent, or predictive of postoperative outcome.

Techniques that have been described include the use of urethral pressure profilometry in the operating room. However, since slings only seem to increase functional urethral length and not maximal urethral closure pressure, the measurement of maximal urethral closure pressures intraoperatively is not helpful and has been found to have no predictive value [15,36]. Endoscopic assessment of the bladder neck may also be performed to ensure easy passage of the cystoscope (no obstruction), and to ensure adequate urethral coaptation, but again this has no predictive value. With the more recent use of more regional (spinal) anesthesia, the patient can be cough tested with 300–500 ml fluid in the bladder, and sling tension adjusted such that there is no leak or just a drop of leakage. However, there is some muscle weakness associated with use of the spinal anesthesia; also, it is difficult for many patients to cough adequately in the modified lithotomy position. In general, we are trying to create a backrest for the urethra, re-creating some of the lost intrinsic sphincter pressure. Putting the sling under no tension, and secured under the bladder neck for an even distribution of support, are reasonable general guidelines.

Postoperative Care

Postoperative care is similar for any continence procedure, but varies between centers. Some physicians routinely teach patients to perform intermittent self-catheterization preoperatively, thereby preparing patients for this in the event of postoperative voiding dysfunction. In this instance the patient has a Foley catheter indwelling for 24 to 48 hours postoperatively, which is then removed for a voiding trial. If patients have voiding difficulty after a sling, they should be encouraged to try to void every 4 hours and then catheterize for residuals or if unable to void. Other institutions routinely use suprapubic catheter drainage, which can then remain in place for up to 6 weeks with postoperative voiding dysfunction. During their trial voids, if patients void more than 100 ml with residuals less than 100 ml on two consecutive occasions post-void residual assessments can be discontinued and the suprapubic catheter removed.

Routine use of postoperative antibiotics should only be considered if synthetic material has been used for the sling. In the event of prolonged time in the modified lithotomy position, the use of prophylactic subcutaneous heparin is advisable. If used, vaginal packing may be removed on the first postoperative day.

Success Rates of Slings

Success rates of all types of slings (Table 33.1) are relatively similar with reported objective cure rates of 61-100% and subjective cure rates of 73-93% [37]. Cure rates tend to be higher for primary slings than for secondary procedures [38]. A review by the American Urological Association reported an overall subjective cure rate of 82% [39]; this was in keeping with a previous meta-analysis that revealed an objective cure rate of 85.3% and a subjective cure rate of 82.4% [40].

Table 33.1 Sling success rates

Author	Material used	n	Follow-up	Objective cure (%)
Stanton et al. [41]	Silastic	30	1–2 years	83
Horbach et al. [42]	Gortex	17	3 months	85
Weinberger and Ostergard [43]	Gortex	108	38 months	61
Young et al. [44]	Mersilene	110	13 months	93
Morgan et al. [12]	Marlex	208	5 years	77.4
Amaye-Obu and Drutz [38]	Marlex	92	1–12 years	66-69
McGuire and Lytton [36]	Autologous rectus fascia	52	2–3 years	80
Carr et al. [45]	Autologous rectus fascia	96	22 months	90
Chaikin et al. [46]	Autologous rectus fascia	251	Over 1 year	92[a]
McLennan et al. [47]	Autologous fascia lata	62	No data	87
Handa et al. [48]	Cadaveric fascia lata	16	6–12 months	79
Jarvis and Fowlie [49]	Porcine dermis	50	21 months	78

[a] Subjective cure.

Complications of Slings

Failure

Slings performed for recurrent stress urinary incontinence certainly have a lower success rate than those performed primarily. In general, any repeat surgical procedure for stress urinary incontinence has a lower success rate than when performed primarily [38]. One recent article showed a higher rate of objective failure after a pubovaginal sling in women who were preoperative Valsalva voiders [50]. Any failure should be approached as a new case of urinary incontinence. A thorough history and physical examination should be completed with multichannel urodynamics. Since prior surgery has occurred, a cystoscopy should also be performed. Recurrent stress urinary incontinence will occur in 10-15% patients, but many cases of perceived sling failure are related to detrusor overactivity.

Voiding Dysfunction

Many studies have attempted to examine factors predisposing to postoperative voiding dysfunction following incontinence surgery. Slings are associated with the highest rate of voiding dysfunction with rates reported between 2 and 16%. Preoperative Valsalva voiders with prolonged or intermittent uroflow curves and reduced maximal flow rate are at risk of prolonged postoperative voiding dysfunction [47]. In women at risk of postoperative voiding problems, the risk must be explained in detail, including the risk of prolonged postoperative catheterization and the potential need for long-term clean intermittent catheterization in 1.5–7.8% [51].

Many physicians will insist on this "at risk" group of women learning intermittent catheterization preoperatively.

Bladder Perforation

This is a more common complication in women having secondary surgery for recurrent stress urinary incontinence. It will often occur close to the bladder neck near the sites of previous suture placement. The risk of bladder perforation is approximately 10%; it may be higher in patients that have had multiple prior retropubic surgeries [52]. If bladder perforation does occur, the laceration should be repaired and continuous catheter drainage implemented for 7 days. A cystogram can then be completed and, if normal, the catheter removed and trial void attempted.

Pain

Wound pain is most likely to occur in patients with large abdominal incisions for fascial harvest. The risk for development of incisional hernia is also greatest in this group. Wound pain may be related to nerve entrapment, hematoma, or a hernia. Patients often complain of a mild tugging sensation at the site of sling attachment abdominally; this usually resolves with time. Any wound pain should be assessed; in the event of suspected nerve entrapment, these patients may respond to local steroid or local anesthetic injection.

Detrusor Instability

Persistent urgency incontinence has been reported in 3–31% patients after a sling. De novo detrusor instability has been reported in 10–40% women [36,53,54]. Certainly, higher rates of de novo detrusor instability are often reported with more extensive dissection; therefore, with some of the newer, less extensive procedures, a decrease in this complication may become apparent. Some de novo detrusor instability is likely related to bladder outlet obstruction. Patients should be cautioned that a response to anticholinergics preoperatively might not persist after surgery. Symptoms of persistent urgency and urge incontinence can be quite debilitating and are the most common reason for perceived sling failure; severe cases may require takedown of the sling or augmentation cystoplasty.

Sling Erosion/Migration

Sling erosions are usually due to uneven compression of the urethra, too much tension on the sling, or technical error, such as unrecognized bladder perforation. Erosions are seen more commonly with synthetic slings with an erosion rate of 1–4% [55]; this may involve erosion into the vagina, bladder or urethra. With some of the bone anchor slings, there have been reports of migration and pull out of the metal anchors [56]. There has been one report of fascia lata erosion into the urethra [57]. Erosion can be prevented by avoiding any tension on the sling and by using a wide strip of sling material secured in place to allow even distribution of sling tension over the bladder neck and proximal urethra.

Infection

Wound and urinary tract infections are the most common infectious complications of slings. A preoperative antibiotic dose administered one hour before surgery will reduce the risk of infection [58]. Infectious complications are more of a concern with the use of synthetic mesh owing to the potential risk of chronic infection and the need to remove the sling if there is no response to antibiotics. If a sling does have to be removed, there is approximately a 25% risk of recurrent stress urinary incontinence [59].

Other Complications

Vaginal inclusion cysts are another potential complication that usually do not cause significant morbidity [60]. If they are troublesome they may be excised.

Conclusions

There are multiple descriptions of different sling techniques. However, regardless of technique or material used, the success rates are relatively similar. With the emergence now of tension-free techniques this should reduce the rate of some of the more troublesome complications such as voiding dysfunction and de novo detrusor instability.

References

1. Goebell RG. Zur operativen Behandlung der Incontinenz der männlichen Harnröhre (About the surgical procedure for the treatment of incontinence of the urethra in men). Z Gynäk Urol 1910;2:187.
2. Frangheim P. Zur operativen Behandlung der Incontinenz (About the surgical treatment of incontinence). Zentral Verhandl d. Deutsch. Geseusch Chir 1914;43:149.
3. Stoeckel W. Über die Verwändung der Musculi Pyramidalis bei der opeutinen Behandlung der Incontinentia Urinae (About the use of the musculi pyramidalis for the surgical treatment of urinary incontinence). Allgemeine Gynäkologie und Urologie 1917;41:11.
4. Giordano D. Twentieth Congress Franc de Chir 1907;506.
5. Souier JB. Med Rec 1911;79:868.
6. Thompson R. Br J Dis Child 1923;20:116.
7. Aldridge AH. Transplantation of fascia for relief of urinary stress incontinence. Am J Obstet Gynecol 1942;44:398–411.
8. Chasser Moir J. The gauze-hammock operation (a modified Aldridge sling procedure). J Obstet Gynaecol Br Commonw 1968;75:1–9.
9. Rovner ES, Ginsberg DA, Raz S. Female stress urinary incontinence clinical guidelines panel summary report on surgical management of female stress urinary incontinence. J Urol 1997;158 (3 part 1):875-80.
10. Appell RA. Argument for sling surgery to replace bladder neck suspension for stress urinary incontinence. Urology 2000;56(3):360–3.
11. Cespedes RD, Cross CA, McGuire EJ. Pubovaginal fascial slings. Techniques in Urology 1997;3(4):195–201.
12. Morgan JE, Farrow GA, Stewart FE. The Marlex sling operation for the treatment of recurrent urinary stress incontinence: a 16 year review. Obstet Gynecol 1985;151:224–6.
13. Gorton E, Stanton SL, Monga A, Wiskind AK, Lentz GM, Bland DR. Periurethral collagen injection: a long-term followup study. BJU 1999;84(9):966–71.
14. Hsu TH, Rackley RR, Appell RA. The supine stress test: a simple method to detect intrinsic urethral sphincter dysfunction. J Urol 1999;162(2):460–3.
15. McGuire EJ, Gormley EA. Abdominal fascial slings. In: Raz S, editor. Female Urology, 2nd edn. Philadelphia, PA: WB Saunders, 1996; 369–75.
16. Weinberger MW, Ostergard DR. Postoperative catheterization, urinary retention, and permanent voiding dysfunction after polytetrafluroethylene suburethral sling placement. Obstet Gynecol 1996;87(1):50–4.
17. Bump RC, Coates KW, Cundiff GW, Harris RL, Weidner AC. Diagnosing intrinsic sphincter deficiency: comparing urethral closure pressure, urethral axis, and valsalva leak point pressures. Am J Obstet Gynecol 1997;177(2):303–10.

18. Nager CW, Schulz JA, Wise B, Monga A, Stanton SL. Comparison of water maximal urethral closure pressure and valsalva leak point pressure with each other and with measures of urinary incontinence severity. Abstract from proceedings of the International Continence Society, Jerusalem, Sept 1998, pp 79–80.
19. Peschers UM, Jundt K, Dimpfl T. Differences between cough and valsalva leak-point pressure in stress incontinence women. Neurourol Urodyn 2000;19(6):677–81.
20. Olesen KP, Walter S. Bladder base insufficiency. Radiological, urodynamic, and clinical aspects. Acta Obstet Gynecol Scand 1978;57(5):463–8.
21. English SF, Amundsen CL, McGuire EJ. Bladder neck competency at rest in women with incontinence. J Urol 1999;161(2):578–80.
22. Drutz HP, Farrell SA, Mainprize TC. Guidelines for the evaluation of genuine stress incontinence prior to primary surgery. Society of Obstetricians and Gynecologists of Canada (SOGC) Policy Statement No. 60, May 1997.
23. Drutz HP, Farrell SA, Lemieux MC, Mainprize TC, Wilkie DHL. Guidelines for the evaluation and treatment of urinary incontinence following pelvic floor or incontinence surgery. SOGC Policy Statement No. 74, July 1998.
24. Weber AM, Walters MD. Cost-effectiveness of urodynamics testing before surgery for women with pelvic organ prolapse and stress urinary incontinence. Am J Obstet Gynecol 2000;183(6):1338–46.
25. James M, Jackson S, Shepherd A, Abrams P. Pure stress leakage symptomatology: is it safe to discount detrusor instability? Br J Obstet Gynecol 1999;106(12):1255–8.
26. Weidner AC, Myers ER, Visco AG, Cundiff GW, Bump RC. Which women with stress incontinence require urodynamic evaluation? Am J Obstet Gynecol 2001;184(2):20–7.
27. Price PB. Plastic operations for incontinence of urine and faeces. Arch Surg 1933;26:1043–8.
28. Fitzgerald MP, Gitelis S, Brubaker L. Pubic osteomyelitis and granuloma after bone anchor placement. Int Urogynecol J Pelvic Floor Dysfunct 1999;10(5):346–8.
29. Kane L, Chung T, Lawrie H, Iskaros J. The pubofascial anchor sling procedure for recurrent genuine urinary stress incontinence. BJU Int 1999;83(9):1010–14.
30. Fitzgerald MP, Mollenhauer J, Brubaker L. The fate of rectus fascia suburethral slings. Am J Obstet Gynecol 2000;183(4):964–6.
31. Fitzgerald MP, Mollenhauer J, Bitterman P, Brubaker L. Functional failure of fascia lata allografts. Am J Obstet Gynecol 1999;181(6): 1339–44 (discussion 1344–6).
32. Fitzgerald MP, Mollenhauer J, Brubaker L. Failure of allograft suburethral slings. BJU Int 1999;84(7):785–8.
33. Carbone JM, Kavaler E, Hu JC, Raz S. Pubovaginal sling using cadaveric fascia and bone anchors: disappointing early results. J Urol 2001;165(5):1605–11.
34. Crawford JS. Nature of fascia lata and its fate after implantation. Am J Ophthalmol 1969;67:900.
35. Ridley JH. Appraisal of the Goebell–Stoeckel sling procedure. Am J Obstet Gynecol 1996;95:714-21.
36. McGuire EJ, Lytton B. Pubovaginal sling for stress incontinence. J Urol 1978;119:82–4.
37. Bidmead J, Cardozo L. Sling techniques in the treatment of genuine stress incontinence. Br J Obstet Gynecol 2000;107(2):147–56.
38. Amaye-Obu FA, Drutz HP. Surgical management of recurrent stress urinary incontinence: A 12 year experience. Am J Obstet Gynecol 1999;181(6):1296-307.
39. Leach G, Dmochowski R, Appell R et al. Female stress urinary incontinence clinical guidelines panel summary on surgical management of stress urinary incontinence. J Urol 1997;158:875–80.
40. Jarvis GJ. Surgery for genuine stress incontinence. Br J Obstet Gynecol 1994;101:371-4.
41. Stanton SL, Brindley GS, Holmes DM. Silastic sling for urethral sphincter incompetence in women. Br J Obstet Gynecol 1985;92:747–50.
42. Horbach NS, Blanco JS, Ostergard DR. A suburethral sling procedure with PTFE for the treatment of genuine stress incontinence in patients with low urethral closure pressure. Obstet Gynecol 1988;71:648–52.
43. Weinberger M, Ostergard D. Long-term clinical and urodynamic evaluation of the polyterafluoroethylene suburethral sling for treatment of genuine stress incontinence. Obstet Gynecol 1995;86:92–6.
44. Young SB, Rosenblatt PL, Pingeton DM, Howard A, Baker SP. The Mersilene mesh suburethral sling: a clinical and urodynamic evaluation. Am J Obstet Gynecol 1995;173:1719–26.
45. Carr L, Walsh P, Abraham V, Webster G. Favorable outcome of pubovaginal slings for geriatric women with stress incontinence. J Urol 1997;157:125–8.
46. Chaikin D, Rosenthal J, Blaivas G. Pubovaginal fascial slings for all types of stress urinary incontinence: long term analysis. J Urol 1998;160:1312–16.
47. McLennan MT, Melick CF, Bent AE. Clinical and urodynamic predictors of delayed voiding after fascia lata suburethral sling. Obstet Gynecol 1998;92:608–12.
48. Handa V, Jensen J, Germain M, Ostergard D. Banked human fascia lata for the suburethral sling procedure: a preliminary report. Obstet Gynecol 1996;88:1045–9.
49. Jarvis GJ, Fowlie A. A clinical and urodynamic assessment of the porcine dermis bladder sling in the treatment of genuine stress incontinence. Br J Obstet Gynaecol 1985;92:1189–91.
50. Iglesia CB, Shott S, Fenner DE, Brubaker L. Effect of pre-operative voiding mechanism on success rate of autologous rectus fascia suburethral sling procedure. Obstet Gynecol 1998;91(4) 577–81.
51. Ghonheim G, Shaaban A. Sub-urethral slings for the treatment of stress urinary incontinence. Int Urogynecol J 1994;5:228–39.
52. Ascher-Walsh CJ, DeMarco E, Bloomgarden A, Blanco JS. Initial experience with a bone-anchored sling for stress urinary incontinence. Obstet Gynecol 2000;95(4 suppl 1):S2.
53. Hom D, Desautel MG, Lumerman JH, Feraren RE, Badlani GH. Pubovaginal sling using polypropylene mesh and Vesica bone anchors. Urology 1998;51(5):708–13.
54. Cross CA, Cespedes RD, McGuire EJ. Our experience with pubovaginal slings in patients with stress urinary incontinence. J Urol 1998;159(4):1195–8.
55. Clemens JQ, DeLancey JO, Faerber GJ, Westney OL, McGuire EJ. Urinary tract erosions after synthetic pubovaginal slings: diagnosis and management strategy. Urology 2000;56(4):589–94.
56. Winters JC, Scarpero HM, Appell RA. Use of bone anchors in female urology. Urology 2000;56(suppl 1):15–22.
57. Beck RP, Grove D, Arnusch D, Harvey J. Recurrent stress urinary incontinence treated by the fascia lata sling procedure. Am J Obstet Gynecol 1974;120:613.
58. Giuliani B, Periti E, Mecacci F. Antimicrobial prophylaxis in obstetric and gynecologic surgery. J Chemother 1999;11(6):577–80.
59. Goldman HB, Rackley RR, Appell RA. The efficacy of urethrolysis without re-suspension for iatrogenic urethral obstruction. J Urol 1999;161(1):196–8.
60. Baldwin DD, Hadley HR. Epithelial inclusion cyst formation after free vaginal wall sling procedure for stress urinary incontinence. J Urol 1997;157(3):952.

34 Artificial Sphincters

Sender Herschorn and Martine Jolivet-Tremblay

Introduction

Surgical treatment of female urinary incontinence has progressed considerably in the past 20 years and most patients who qualify for treatment will not require an artificial urinary sphincter (AUS). While in males it is the procedure of choice for post-radical prostatectomy stress incontinence [1], in females controversy exists regarding the indications as many patients, even those with severe incontinence following multiple surgeries, can be managed successfully with surgery that does not involve implantation of a mechanical prosthesis. However, it does have a place and this chapter will outline the historical aspects, clinical evaluation and indications, the surgical procedure, results and complications of its use in females.

History of the Device and Current Design

In the past thirty years, several prostheses to control incontinence have been developed primarily for male patients. In 1974, Scott and co-workers [2] reported the first one designed for implantation around the bladder neck in female patients. The work was done in collaboration with American Medical Systems. The first device, the 721, consisted of an inflatable cuff, inflate and deflate pumps with a reservoir between the two of them and was controlled by unidirectional valves. The "V4" valve controlled the pressure. The reservoir was placed just outside the peritoneal cavity below the rectus muscles. The intra-abdominal pressure was supposed to be transmitted to the device during exercise, coughing or Valsalva. Hydrodynamic pressure

forced the cuff to stay closed with the additional pressure transmitted to it during exercise maneuvers. The main problem with this system was the defect in the V4 valve. The excessive pressure transmitted to the cuff also led to urethral or bladder neck erosion.

Following the 721, the 761 was modified with an extra balloon between the cuff and the deflate pump to control the given amount of pressure in the system. The principal problem with this AUS was the larger number of components and malfunctioning of the different components. The device was then simplified and redesigned with fewer components [3].

In 1978, at the VIIth International Congress of Nephrology the new simpler device, the 742, was introduced. It had a pressure-regulating balloon, with preset elasticity that controlled cuff pressure and closure and one deflate pump. There was also a choice of balloon pressures. After the patient deflated the cuff it automatically closed or reinflated as the balloon pressure forced fluid back into the cuff through a resistor. This is the mechanism of the current AUS. Additional modifications were made for facilitating implantation and included miniaturization of the resistor and valves and production changes to the silicone components (balloon, cuff, and pump) by dip-coating technology [3].

In 1982, with the AMS 800, two new elements were incorporated into the device to diminish complications. First, the control, or resistor, and the deflate pump were joined into one piece. Second, the deactivation button, permitting delayed activation without additional surgery, and control by either the urologist or the patient, was incorporated into the pump. The cuff was also modified into a belt design and the overall material was also strengthened [3].

In 1987, the introduction of a narrow-backed cuff design improved the transmission of the pressure to the urethra to decrease possible erosion [4,5].

The AMS 800 is the sphincter device that has generally withstood the test of time. The only new modifications in the 10 past years were coordinated tubing colors in the components to assist in implantation and reinforcement of the tubing insertion into the pump. A photograph of the current device is shown in Figure 34.1. The device works by maintaining a predetermined pressure to close the urethra. The pressures are determined by the specific implanted balloon and are 51–60, 61–70, and 71–80 cmH$_2$O and are selected by the surgeon at implantation. When the patient wants to void she compresses the pump to transfer fluid from the cuff into the balloon (Figure 34.2). The balloon then causes the fluid to return to the cuff, thereby recompressing the urethra. Reinflation of a collapsed cuff takes about 3 minutes. This gives the patient a long enough time for voiding or intermittent catheterization.

Indications and Contraindications

The AUS is an alternative treatment for intrinsic sphincter deficiency or even sphincteric absence

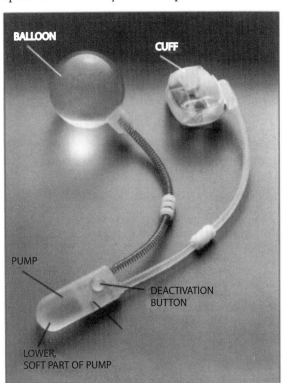

Figure 34.1 AMS Sphincter 800™ urinary prosthesis. (Courtesy of American Medical Systems, Inc., Minnetonka, Minnesota; www.visitAMS.com.)

[6]. There are many reports of its use in patients after previous unsuccessful surgery and the results will be presented below [3,7–17]. These reports also had patients who had not had previous surgery. In general, females with hypermobility-related incontinence are treated satisfactorily with suspension procedures [6]. The AUS can be used for patients with sphincter deficiency, without adverse risk factors enumerated below, and who are felt not to be candidates for sling procedures. Additionally patients who are at high risk for retention after a sling and who are prepared to have a prosthetic device to facilitate voiding may also be candidates.

The AUS has been used in conjunction with augmentation enterocystoplasty when sphincteric resistance is too low [18,19], as well as in continent urinary diversion [20]. It has been used extensively in the pediatric age group with congenital anomalies such as myelomeningocele, sacral dysgenesis [21,22] and exstrophy/epispadias complex [23].

The AUS can also be used in patients with neuropathic sphincteric dysfunction, a stable bladder, and a low-pressure storage system. Intermittent catheterization may safely be used for bladder emptying if necessary [24]. A major concern is the pediatric neurologic patient with myelodysplasia who develops poor bladder compliance after AUS insertion. If uncontrolled this may lead to hydronephrosis and renal deterioration [22], underscoring the need for close follow-up and treatment. Upper tract deterioration has not been reported in the non-neurologic patient with overactive bladder dysfunction but adjunctive pharmacologic control of the dysfunction with anticholinergics may be necessary. Patients with low-volume hyperreflexia or instability are not good candidates for implantation unless the bladder dysfunction can be controlled pharmacologically or surgically with augmentation since the bladder pressure may override the sphincter pressure.

Prior radiotherapy is also a risk factor since cuff erosion may occur in the devascularized tissues [25]. Active urinary infection, stone disease, recurrent bladder tumors requiring frequent instrumentation, vesicoureteral reflux may be relative contraindications. Urethral diverticula and urethrovesicovaginal fistulas must be treated prior to insertion.

Since the AUS requires patient compliance and manual dexterity to operate it, various types of cognitive and physical impairments may preclude insertion.

Since 1972, more than 52 000 patients have AUS implants worldwide and of these 19% have been female [26].

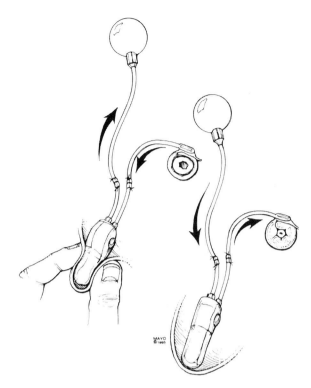

Figure 34.2 Functioning of the AMS 800 artificial sphincter. Pressure on the pump transfers fluid out of the cuff to the pressure balloon to allow voiding. The cuff then fills passively by pressure from the balloon. (From Barrett DM, Licht MR. Implantation of the artificial genitourinary sphincter in men and women. In: Walsh PC, Retik AB, Vaughan Jr ED, Wein AJ, editors. Campbell's Urology, 7th edn. Philadelphia: WB Saunders Company, 1998; 1121–34.)

Patient Evaluation and Selection

The primary goal of the urologic work-up is to eliminate patients who, if they undergo implantation of an artificial urinary sphincter, are at high risk of device complication, failure, or deterioration of the upper urinary tract.

The recommended evaluation includes basic assessment with history, physical examination, and urine culture as in other patients with urinary incontinence [27]. Manual dexterity and cognitive function should also be assessed. Since these patients almost always have complex problems, additional testing with cystoscopy and urodynamic studies is warranted. Visual inspection of the urethral mucosa by cystoscopy is important to assess integrity and vascularity, especially with a history of previous surgery or radiation [6]. Videourodynamic studies are particularly helpful. Pressure/flow studies may be of some predictive value for postoperative voiding function. Imaging of the upper urinary tract may also be neces-

sary, especially if there are congenital anomalies, vesicoureteral reflux, fistulas, or neurologic disease.

Patients with clinically significant detrusor instability or hyperreflexia demonstrated on urodynamics should be treated prior to implantation of the AUS with pharmacologic agents. Other options may include nerve blocks or even sacral neuromodulation. If it is impossible to abolish the detrusor uninhibited contractions, augmentation enterocystoplasty may be an option, especially in the presence of neurologic disease. The augmentation may be done prior to or at the same time as AUS insertion [18,19].

Patients with inability to void are also candidates but must be taught intermittent catheterization before the procedure.

A most important aspect during the evaluation is to assess the patient's motivation. She must be aware of the different therapies, the risks, complications and the possible consequences of the AUS. Unique to the AUS is the possibility of device malfunction, infection and erosion that may necessitate removal or revision at any time during the patient's life. The patient must be willing to accept this.

Preoperative Management

The major goal is to reduce the risk of infection as it may lead to removal of the device. The urine has to be free of bacteria with appropriate antibiotic treatment before the surgery. Skin infections and open sores are also a risk factor and should be treated prior to AUS insertion. *Staphylococcus epidermidis* is responsible for 35–80% of all genitourinary prosthesis infection [28,29], and Gram-negative organisms are responsible for the rest. The reason that prosthesis infection has to be resisted is that the surface bacteria produce and live in a biofilm that is resistant to antibiotic treatment [30]. This almost always necessitates surgical removal of the prosthesis. Infection prevention strategy is therefore a key point.

Patients are admitted on the day of surgery. Some centers recommend an antiseptic shower on the night before surgery [6]. One hour before induction of the anesthesia, broad-spectrum intravenous antibiotics such as gentamicin and cephalosporin are given to achieve high concentration at the time of surgery. Shaving of the pubic and genital areas is done in the operating room after induction to reduce possible colonization of small nicks and scratches. The patient is positioned in low lithotomy to ensure simultaneous vaginal and abdominal access. Skin and mucosal preparation of the vagina should be done with an organic iodide soap and solution for 10–15 minutes

[3]. The bladder is catheterized after the patient is draped in order for the surgeon to access the catheter during the procedure if necessary.

Surgical Technique

The AUS can be implanted through an abdominal or vaginal approach.

With the abdominal approach, the retropubic space is usually entered through a lower midline or Pfannenstiel incision. The rectus muscles are separated and dissection is done towards the pubis to separate the bladder from the symphysis and to identify the anterior vaginal wall on both sides of the bladder neck and urethra. With previous retropubic surgery the area may be densely scarred. Dissection is done sharply with Metzenbaum scissors, using the symphysis as the landmark. The fluid volume in the bladder can be varied to facili-

tate dissection. The peritoneal cavity should be avoided but if violated can easily be repaired. After the bladder, urethra, and anterior vaginal wall are separated from the pubis, a ring retractor is deployed to optimize exposure.

The next part involves cuff insertion. The bladder neck region can be palpated just below the Foley balloon. Bilateral incisions are made in the endopelvic fascia (Figure 34.3). A plane is created between the urethra and anterior vaginal wall with a right-angled clamp. Vaginal veins may bleed at the site of entry into the endopelvic fascia and may require suture ligatures. One must be careful not to penetrate the bladder, urethra, or vaginal wall. Inadvertent penetration of the urinary tract can be demonstrated with irrigation of the Foley catheter. Methylene blue may be helpful but it tends to stain the tissues. Penetration of the vaginal mucosa can usually be palpated, or irrigation fluid can be seen emanating from the vagina. The holes should be repaired with absorbable suture. Once the space is

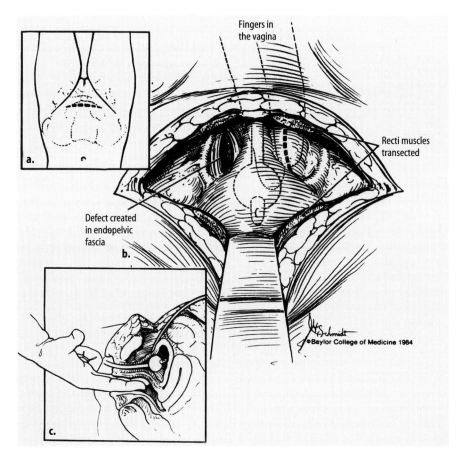

Figure 34.3   Abdominal approach for artificial sphincter implantation. The plane between the urethra and vagina is carefully dissected with a right-angled clamp while the surgeon keeps his/her fingers in the vagina. (From Scott FB. The use of the artificial sphincter in the treatment of urinary incontinence in the female patient. Urol Clin North Am 1985;12:305–15.)

created the cuff size should be selected by insertion of the cuff sizer. The cuff is placed around the bladder neck and fastened together. If difficulty is encountered at any time, the bladder may be opened to ensure proper position of the cuff.

The space for the pump in the labium majorum is then created. A subcutaneous tunnel is then made from the abdominal incision down to the lowermost aspect of the labium and enlarged with either a Hegar dilator or urethral sound. The pump is then inserted. Right-handed patients usually need the pump placed on the right side.

The balloon is then inserted into the retropubic space and the cuff and balloon tubes are brought through the rectus muscle into the subcutaneous area on the same side as the pump. The balloon is then filled with 22 ml of saline or an appropriate concentration of radiographic contrast and the connections are made between the cuff and balloon tubes and pump. The device can then be deactivated by emptying the pump, waiting until it partially refills, and then pressing the deactivation button. A Jackson–Pratt drain is optional and the incision is closed. Care must be taken not to damage the tubes during the closure.

With the vaginal approach [10,11], an inverted U-shaped incision is made in the anterior vaginal wall, with the apex halfway between the bladder neck and meatus. The retropubic space is entered bilaterally at the level of the bladder neck and blind dissection is carried around the bladder neck ante-riorly. Cystoscopy can be done to check the site. The cuff is inserted and snapped in place after sizing. The reservoir placed into the retropubic space through a separate small transverse incision through which the cuff tubing, placed in from below, is accessed. The labial pouch for the pump is created and the pump is inserted; 22 ml of saline or contrast are placed into the balloon and the connections are made. The device is also deactivated as above and the incisions are closed.

During the procedure the components are placed into a basin with antibiotic solution and the wounds are irrigated with a similar solution. Although there are no data showing efficacy, the antibiotic irrigation may minimize operating room acquired bacterial contamination of the device. The device must also be handled carefully with avoidance of any sharp objects coming into contact with it.

The patient is catheterized with a Foley for a few days postoperatively.

Postoperative Care and Follow-up

The patient is usually hospitalized for 2–3 days. Intravenous antibiotics may be administered and

then changed to oral. The Foley catheter can be removed after the first day and the bladder checked for emptying with a bladder scan. The patient is instructed on how to gently pull the pump down in the labium to keep it in position. The Jackson–Pratt drain, if placed, can be removed on the first postoperative day.

The patient is discharged from hospital with oral cephalosporin, for 1–2 weeks. Restriction of activity is similar to other abdominal or vaginal procedures. Incontinence is expected until the device is activated. The patient is instructed to watch for any symptoms and signs of wound or urinary infection. She is also given instructions about obtaining a Medic-Alert bracelet.

Early follow-up visits may be necessary. After 6–8 weeks, if there is no more swelling or tenderness in the labia, the surgeon activates the device by squeezing the pump firmly until the fluid is forced out of it. The patient is then instructed how to cycle the device and should demonstrate her ability to do it (Figure 34.4). She is given additional printed instructions. Patients on intermittent catheterization are taught to open the device prior to catheterization. Patients who are at high risk for erosion are taught how to deactivate the device at night time. Subsequent visits are arranged.

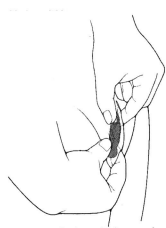

Squeeze and release the lower, soft part of the pump several times.

Figure 34.4 Patient instructions on cycling the device. (Courtesy of American Medical Systems, Inc., Minnetonka, Minnesota; www.visitAMS.com.)

Complications

Complications may occur as a result of the surgery or anesthesia in general but those specific to the AUS will be discussed.

Perforation

When intraoperative bladder, urethral or vaginal perforations occur, they should be closed immediately with absorbable suture. Usually the AUS can proceed but if a satisfactory closure is not assured the procedure may have to be abandoned.

Hematoma

Bleeding and hematoma formation can occur in the anterior vaginal wall, the labia majora, or subcutaneous tissue after blunt dissection. Usually it resolves without any further complication and no drainage is necessary.

Urinary Retention

Occasionally patients will have difficulty voiding after the Foley is removed. This may be from periurethral swelling and usually subsides. However, deactivation and emptying of the cuff should be verified by repeating the deactivation procedure. Retention after activation may be from inadvertent deactivation by the patient. If the device has not been deactivated, cystoscopy should be done to make sure that cuff erosion has not occurred. If there is no erosion then bladder function may have changed and should be checked with urodynamic studies.

Infection

As mentioned above, device infection may have to be treated with removal of the whole device because of inability of antibiotics to eradicate the bacteria. The overall infection rate for genitourinary implants is 1–3% [28,29,31]. Early infection may be from intraoperative bacterial contamination and later acquired infection may be from the urinary tract but can also be from an indolent organism acquired early on. The clinical presentation may range from swelling over the pump to purulent infections with fever, chills, abscess formation and drainage from the prosthesis to the skin. The infection may also result from unrecognized urethral cuff erosion. Treatment usually involves removal of the whole device, as the infection tends to travel along its entire surface. The device may be reimplanted after

3–6 months if the AUS is still considered to be appropriate treatment for the patient's incontinence.

Cuff Erosion

Cuff erosion can occur at any time, but is most common 3–4 months after implantation [6]. Symptoms and signs may range from minor with minimal urethral bleeding to major with infection, abscess formation, and retention. Early erosion, before activation, may be from unrecognized intraoperative urethral injury. Later erosion, after 3–4 months, may be from infection or loss of urethral integrity with a relatively too high a balloon pressure. Cystoscopy should be done to confirm the erosion and then surgical treatment is mandated. If there is no infection, the cuff alone can be removed and the tubing capped for subsequent connection to another implanted cuff. A Foley catheter can be left indwelling for 3–6 weeks and urethral healing confirmed cystoscopically. If there is associated infection, the whole device should be removed. Reimplantation can take place after 3–6 months.

Recurrent or Persistent Incontinence

Incontinence following implantation of an AUS can result principally from (a) alteration in bladder function, (b) urethral atrophy, (c) mechanical failure of the device [1]. Rarely, a fistula may have resulted from an unrecognized intraoperative injury [6].

Alteration in Bladder Function
This has been reported in patients with neurogenic bladder dysfunction, especially in children [22]. These changes include, de novo uninhibited detrusor contractions, decrease in bladder compliance, and the development of a high-pressure system, causing incontinence, hydronephrosis and ultimately renal failure. There has never been a published report of hydronephrosis following implantation of an artificial sphincter for incontinence after prostatectomy or non-neurologic disease [32]. However, the bladder dysfunction will have to be treated appropriately as required.

Urethral Atrophy
This may occur at the cuff site and is reported in the literature in 3–9.3% of patients [4,33–35]. Treatment involves changing the cuff to a smaller size or replacing the balloon with a higher pressure model.

Mechanical Failure
This includes perforation of one of the components of the AUS with loss of fluid volume with or without

leaking of tissue fluid and organic debris into the system. This causes the cuff not to close. Other mechanical problems are tubing kinks and disconnections. The incidence of these complications varies widely and ranges from 0% [4] to 52.5% [35] in the series with the longest follow-up. In this latter study, the cuff seemed to be the most vulnerable part of the system (22 cuff failures in 18 patients, most of them occurring during the first 2 or 3 years following implantation), followed by pump failure (six times in 4 patients). The revision rate for reported female series is outlined in the results below.

Diagnosis and Management of Sphincter Failure

The diagnostic evaluation of incontinence after the placement of the AUS is important for management of these patients. Several diagnostic and management algorithms have been proposed, some relatively simple, others more complex [1,36]. A simplified scheme is shown in Figure 34.5.

Physical examination should exclude infection at the site of the cuff or the labial pump. Difficulty

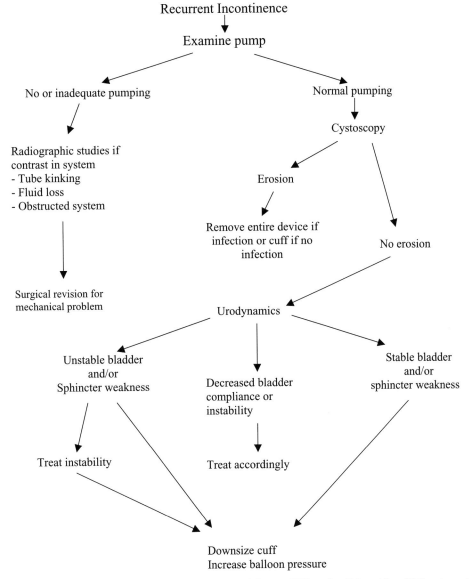

Figure 34.5 Algorithm for the investigation and treatment if incontinence following AUS insertion. (Adapted from [1] Herschorn et al. Surgical treatment of urinary incontinence in men. In: Abrams P, Khoury S, Wein A, editors. Incontinence. Plymouth: Health Publications Ltd, 1999; 691–729.)

Table 34.1 Results of artificial sphincter insertion in women

Author	No. of patients	Complications	Revisions and reasons	Outcome
Scott [3]	139	4 infections (3%) 5 erosions (4%)	11 removed (8%)	84% success (dry and improved)
Light and Scott [7]	39	1 infection (3%) 3 erosions (7%)	21 revisions in 14 patients (36%) (11 cuff malfunctions)	87% dry 5% improved
Donovan et al. [8]	31	9 erosions (29%) 1 infection (3%)		68% continent
Diokno et al. [9]	32	1 dehiscence (3%) 1 pelvic abscess (3%)	7 revisions (22%) (4 cuff malfunctions)	91% dry 3% improved
Abbassian [10]	4	0		100% dry
Appell [11]	34	0	3 revisions (0.9%)	100% dry
Parulkar and Barrett [12]	24	4 erosions and infections (17%)	12 revisions (50%)	17 good (71%) 3 fair (12.5%)
Duncan et al. [13]	29	8 erosions (28%) 1 infection (3.5%)	1 revision (3.4%)	52% continent
Webster et al. [14]	25	1 postoperative death (4%)	4 revisions (16%)	92% dry 8% improved
Hadley et al. [15]	18	2 erosions (11%)		89% dry
Stone et al. [16]	54	4 lost to follow-up 3 erosions (6%) 2 unable to use (4%)	11 revisions (20%)	84% dry 12% improved
Costa et al. [17]	207	51 operative injuries (25%) 12 erosions (6%) 2 hernias (1%)	6 revisions (3%)	81% dry 7% improved

compressing the pump suggests tube kinking, fluid loss or an obstructed system. If the pump cycles normally, urodynamic studies may demonstrate changes in bladder behavior as described above. If the system was filled with radiographic contrast, plain X-ray of the abdomen or pelvis may show fluid loss. Cystoscopy will show a cuff erosion and cystourethrography could demonstrate a urethral diverticulum at the site of a previous cuff erosion [1]. Management is outlined in the algorithm.

Results

As with many other surgical procedures there is no standardization of assessing and reporting of treatment outcomes. Cure usually refers to "dry" or nearly "dry" and improvement indicates "social continence with pads". Table 34.1 shows the reported success rates along with complications in a total of 636

patients from a number of series of incontinent female patients.

Success rates range from 52 to 100% with most in the 80–90% range. The erosion rate ranges from 7% to 29% and the revision rate for mechanical malfunctions range from 8% to 50%. The longer series have higher revision rates.

Since the AUS is a mechanical device and subject to deterioration over time, a higher revision rate with longer follow-up is expected. One can then look at the durability over time. Klijn and co-workers [37] found it useful to consider patients with "primary adequate function" (PAF) when no revision is necessary to achieve continence separately from those with "additional procedure-assisted adequate function" (APA-AF), where one or more revisions are necessary to obtain favorable outcome. Applying Kaplan–Meier curves to this concept showed that in their series the median time to failure for the PAF group was 48 months, the mean time to the first failure following the initial implant was 14 months (range: 0–48 months). In the

APA-AF group at 72 months, the median time to definite failure could not yet be established while the mean time to a second failure after a revision was 15 months (range: 0–61 months).

Conclusion

The AUS has proved to be a safe and reliable treatment for sphincteric incompetence. The device has undergone considerable modification and design improvements since it was introduced in the early 1970s, but very little has changed in the past 10 years. Although most female patients with stress incontinence can be treated satisfactorily with suspension or sling procedures there are still some patients who will benefit from the AUS. Success rates compare favorably with other procedures but there have not been any comparison trials. In assessing results, in contrast to other procedures, there is a predictable revision rate that has to be mentioned in the discussion with the patient, and factored into the overall cost.

References

1. Herschorn S, Boccon-Gibod L, Bosch JLHR et al. Surgical treatment of urinary incontinence in men. In: Abrams P, Khoury S, Wein A, editors. Incontinence. Plymouth: Health Publications, 1999; 691–729.
2. Scott FB, Bradley WE, Timm GW. Treatment of urinary incontinence by an implantable prosthetic urinary sphincter. J Urol 1974;112:75–80.
3. Scott FB. The use of the artificial sphincter in the treatment of urinary incontinence in the female patient. Urol Clin North Am 1985;12:305–15.
4. Light JK, Reynolds JC. Impact of the new cuff design on reliability of the AS 800 artificial urinary sphincter. J Urol 1992;147:609–11.
5. Leo ME, Barrett DM. Success of the narrow-backed cuff design of the AMS 800 artificial urinary sphincter. Analysis of 144 patients. J Urol 1993;150:1412–14.
6. Barrett DM, Licht MR. Implantation of the artificial genitourinary sphincter in men and women. In: Walsh PC, Retik AB, Vaughan Jr ED, Wein AJ, editors. Campbell's Urology, 7th edn. Philadelphia: WB Saunders, 1121–34; 1998.
7. Light JK, Scott FB. Management of urinary incontinence in women with the artificial urinary sphincter. J Urol 1985;134:476–8.
8. Donovan MG, Barrett DM, Furlow WL. Use of the artificial sphincter in the management of severe in females. Surg Gynecol Obstet 1985;161:17–20.
9. Diokno AC, Hollander HB, Anderson TP. Artificial urinary sphincter for recurrent female urinary incontinence: Indications and results. J Urol 1987:138:778–80.
10. Abbassian A. A new operation for insertion of the artificial urinary sphincter. J Urol 1988;140:512–13.
11. Appell RA. Techniques and results in the implantation of the artificial urinary sphincter in women with type III stress incontinence by a vaginal approach. Neurourol Urodyn 1988:7:613–18.
12. Parulkar BG, Barrett DM. Application of the AS 800 artificial sphincter for intractable urinary incontinence in females. Surg Gynecol Obstet 1990;171:131–8.
13. Duncan HJ, Nurse DE, Mundy AR. Role of the artificial urinary sphincter in the treatment of stress incontinence in women. Br J Urol 1992;69:141–3.
14. Webster GD, Perez LM, Khoury JM et al. Management of type III stress urinary incontinence using artificial urinary sphincter. Urology 1992;39:499–503.
15. Hadley RA, Loisides P, Dickinson M. Long-term follow-up (2–5 years) of transvaginally placed artificial urinary sphincters by an experienced surgeon. J Urol 1995;Part 2 153:432A, abstract 816.
16. Stone KT, Diokno AC, Mitchell BA. Just how effective is the AMS 800 artificial urinary sphincter? Results of long-term follow-up in females. J Urol 1995;Part2 153:433A, abstract 817.
17. Costa P, Motte N, Rabut B, Thuret R, Ben Naoum K, Wagner L. The use of an artificial sphincter in women with type III incontinence and a negative Marshall test. J Urol 2001;165:1172–6.
18. Light JK, Lapin S, Vohra S. Combined use of bowel and the artificial urinary sphincter in reconstruction of the lower urinary tract: Infectious complications. J Urol 1995;153:331–3.
19. Strawbridge LR, Kramer SA, Castillo OA, Barrett DM. Augmentation cystoplasty and the artificial genitourinary sphincter. J Urol 1989: 142:297–301.
20. Mitrofanoff P, Bonnet O, Annoot MP et al. Continent urinary diversion using an artificial urinary sphincter. Br J Urol 1992;70:26–9.
21. Gonzalez R, Koleilat N, Austin C, Sidi AA. The artificial sphincter AS 800 in congenital urinary incontinence. J Urol 1989;142:512–15.
22. Bosco PJ, Bauer SB, Colodny AH et al. The long-term results of artificial sphincters in children. J Urol 1991;146:396–9.
23. Decter RM, Roth DR, Fishman IJ et al. Use of the AS 800 device in exstrophy and epispadias. J Urol 1988;140:1202–3.
24. Barrett DM, Furlow WL. Incontinence, intermittent catheterization and the artificial genitourinary sphincter. J Urol 1984;132:268–9.
25. Wang Y, Hadley HR. Experiences with the artificial urinary sphincter in the irradiated patient. J Urol 1992;147:612–13.
26. Data on file. American Medical Systems Inc., Minnetonka, Minnesota, USA.
27. Fantl JA, Newman DK, Colling J et al. Urinary Incontinence in Adults: Acute and Chronic Management. Clinical Practice Guideline No. 2, 1996 Update. Rockville, MD: U.S. Department of Health and Human Services. Public Health Service, Agency for Health Care Policy and Research. AHCPR Publication No. 96-0682. March 1996.
28. Carson CC III. Infections in genitourinary prostheses. Urol Clin North Am 1989;16:139–47.
29. Blum MD. Infections of genitourinary prostheses. Infect Dis Clin North Am 1989;259–74.
30. Nickel JC, Heaton J, Morales A, Costerton JW. Bacterial biofilm in persistent penile prosthesis-associated infection. J Urol 1986;135:586–8.
31. Radomski SB, Herschorn S. Risk factors associated with penile prosthesis infection. J Urol 1992;147:383–5.
32. Montague DK, Angermeier KW. Postprostatectomy urinary incontinence: the case of artificial urinary sphincter implantation (Editorial). Urology 2000;55:2–4.
33. Fishman IJ, Shabsigh R, Scott FB. Experience with the artificial urinary sphincter model AS800 in 148 patients. J Urol 1989;141:307–10.
34. Montague DK. The artificial urinary sphincter (AS 800): Experience in 166 consecutive patients. J Urol 1992;147:380–2.

35. Fulford SC, Sutton C, Bales G, Hickling M, Stephenson TP. The fate of the "modern" artificial sphincter with a follow-up of more than 10 years. Br J Urol 1997;79:713–16.

36. Furlow WF, Barrett DM. Recurrent or persistent urinary incontinence in patients with the artificial urinary sphincter. Diagnostic considerations and management. J Urol 1985;133:792–5.

37. Klijn AJ, Hop WC, Mickisch G, Schroder FH, Bosch JL. The artificial urinary sphincter in men incontinent after radical prostatectomy: 5 year actuarial adequate function rates. Br J Urol 1998;82:530–3.

35 Minimal Access Surgery in the Management of Genuine Stress Incontinence

Kevin M. Smith and Rose C. Kung

Introduction

Genuine stress incontinence (GSI) is a common condition in women. Prevalence studies underestimate the magnitude of the problem, but typically the rates are said to be between 10% and 20% of women, regardless of age [1]. The treatment options for GSI are discussed in detail elsewhere in this volume, but can basically be divided into conservative therapies (Kegel exercises, hormone replacement, biofeedback and α-agonists), periurethral injections and surgical treatments. Surgical procedures, reported since 1906, were either vaginal repairs as advocated by Kelly and Kennedy or urethral sling procedures, as pioneered by Goebel [2]. In the 1940s, Marshall and Marchetti [3] developed a retropubic approach that was later modified by Burch in 1961 [4]. More recently, an alternative theory on pelvic relaxation [5] has led to the surgical repair of defects in the pubo-cervical fascia (paravaginal repair) in the treatment of vaginal prolapse and GSI.

The evolution of the surgical approach for the correction of GSI has focused on devising a minimally invasive technique to place the proximal urethra in a high retropubic position, which avoids a large abdominal incision with its incumbent morbidity. Advances in imaging and instrument design over the last 15 years have enabled surgeons to perform procedures under endoscopic vision rather than through conventional open wounds, and retropubic colposuspension, urethral sling procedures and paravaginal repairs can now be included in the list of procedures that can be performed laparoscopically. It should be remembered that laparoscopic procedures are not new operations, but merely a different way of accessing the surgical field.

The aim of this chapter is to outline some of the described laparoscopic approaches for the treatment of GSI and to review the evidence in the literature for the efficacy of these approaches.

Laparoscopic Retropubic Colposuspension

Despite more than 100 different surgical techniques for the treatment of GSI in the literature, the Burch colposuspension has endured as one of the most successful [6]. The only two randomized trials comparing "open" Burch colposuspension with two other procedures for the treatment of GSI (modified Pereyra and anterior repair) report the Burch to have the highest long-term cure rates (87%) [7,8]. It is not, therefore, surprising that laparoscopic approaches to this operation have been devised. The technique of performing an "open" Burch colposuspension is far from standardized. The number, placement and type of suture, as well as the tension placed on the sutures, varies from surgeon to surgeon. The same is true for the Burch procedure performed laparoscopically. Vancaille and Schuessler first described a laparoscopic approach to bladder neck suspension in 1991 [9]. Since then, other investigators have described transperitoneal and extraperitoneal approaches to the space of Retzius as well as a laparoscopic approach to the Stamey procedure. Also, different types of suture material, including mesh and staples [10,11], have been described.

Transperitoneal Technique

The majority of the laparoscopic Burch procedures performed at Women's College Hospital, Toronto, is by a transperitoneal method described by

Kung et al. [12]. The patient is placed in the Lloyd-Davies position and is cleaned, draped and catheterized using a Foley catheter with a 30 ml balloon. A Veress needle is inserted through an umbilical incision. After adequate insufflation with a high flow carbon dioxide (CO_2) insufflator, a 10 mm reusable cannula is inserted infra-umbilically and an operating laparoscope introduced. Accessory cannulae are inserted in the right and left lower quadrants, lateral to the inferior epigastric vessels, and an additional 5 mm cannula is placed in the right upper quadrant, lateral to the rectus muscle, at approximately the level of the umbilicus. A transverse incision is made in the abdominal peritoneum, approximately 5–6 cm above the symphysis pubis, between the obliterated umbilical vessels, using either a coherent CO_2 laser or unipolar scissors. The anterior peritoneum is dissected from the anterior abdominal wall and the space of Retzius is exposed with a combination of sharp and blunt dissection. Cooper's ligaments are identified and the fatty tissue along the ligaments and the paravaginal fascia is removed. A blunt grasper and suction-irrigator are used to dissect the bladder medially from the paravaginal fascia, with the aid of an assistant's finger inserted into the vagina at the level of the urethrovesical junction, as delineated by the catheter balloon. Permanent sutures of 0 polypropylene are placed in a figure-of-eight fashion through the paravaginal fascia, lateral to the urethrovesical junction. Two sutures are placed on each side and secured to Cooper's ligament. The knots are tied extracorporeally and slid into position using a knot pusher. Cystoscopy is then performed to ensure that no suture material has been inadvertently placed through the bladder wall, and that both ureters are patent. A suprapubic catheter is inserted under direct laparoscopic and cystoscopic vision. The peritoneum is then closed using a 2-0 polydioxanone suture. Fascial incisions are then closed with polyglactin and skin incisions with 3-0 Monocril sutures.

Extraperitoneal Technique

This approach is of use principally on patients without previous abdominal surgery. The patient is placed supine in the Lloyd-Davies position and the abdomen, upper thighs and perineal area, including the vaginal vault, are prepared and draped. A small, open laparoscopic, para-umbilical incision is made, and blunt dissection is performed down to the anterior rectus sheath. The rectus fascia is incised just lateral to the midline. The rectus muscle is identified and deflected laterally and a finger inserted to begin blunt dissection anterior to the posterior rectus

fascia. A balloon dissector can then be placed against the posterior rectus sheath and tunneled inferiorly down to the symphysis pubis. It can then be inflated to a volume of approximately one liter to bluntly develop the space of Retzius. The laparoscope provides visualization during dissection from within the balloon. Once the pubic tubercle and Cooper's ligaments have been identified and adequate space has been created for insertion of bilateral lower ports, the balloon is deflated, removed, and replaced with a Hasson-type, blunt-tip laparoscopic port. Carbon dioxide insufflation of the retropubic space is then performed to a pressure of 10–15 mmHg. Lower ports can then be inserted bilaterally under direct vision and the operation completed in the same manner as described previously when using a transperitoneal approach.

Variations on this technique have been described, including insertion of the balloon dissector through a suprapubic incision [13] or an incision in the midline, midway between the symphysis pubis and the umbilicus [14]. Also, home-made balloon dissectors have been described, using a rubber glove [15] or a finger cut from a glove [14] tied over a Foley catheter. Polascik et al. [13] also describe the creation of a tense pneumo-retroperitoneum using a Veress needle inserted suprapubically before insertion of the balloon dissector. Other authors have described the use of hernia mesh and staples to elevate the urethra [11], while Das and Palmer [15] secured the sutures elevating the urethra to bone anchors sited in holes drilled into the pubic ramus 4 cm from the midline. It should be remembered, however, that regardless of these variations in surgical approach, the objective of the operation remains the same as that of an "open" Burch procedure: the surgical placement of the proximal urethra in a retropubic position.

Success of Laparoscopic Colposuspension

Two of the problems in assessing the efficacy of incontinence procedures, both open and laparoscopic, are the lack of prospective, randomized, controlled trials and a lack of standardization of the procedures. This makes it difficult to compare case series. A MEDLINE search back to 1990 revealed only one prospective, randomized study [16]. This showed that the "open" colposuspension was significantly more effective than the laparoscopic approach (p = 0.03), with a cure rate of only 60% at 36 months in the laparoscopic group. The main criticisms of this study are that the author, at the time the series was performed, was a novice laparoscopist and that an absorbable suture was used. It should be remembered that there are individual studies looking at open colposuspension which report disappointing intermediate-term results [17,18], and yet meta-analysis of all the studies on open colposuspension gives an acceptable success rate [6].

Five non-randomized, comparative studies found no difference in cure rate between the open and laparoscopic approach (Table 35.1). Sixteen observational case series were found (Table 35.2). A total of 922 patients were included in all these papers with

an overall "cure" rate of 91% (Table 35.3). It has been shown that previous incontinence surgery militates against the success of a colposuspension [19]. In most of the papers reviewed, it was not apparent whether the patients had undergone previous incontinence surgery. Therefore, although it is not ideal, it was necessary to combine the results from patients undergoing their first surgical procedure for stress incontinence with those undergoing recurrent surgery.

Table 35.1 Summary of prospective randomized (PR) and retrospective comparative (RC) studies

Study	Year	Study type	Procedure	n	Follow-up (months)	Outcome measurement	Cure rate (%)	p	95% CI
Burton GA [16]	1994	PR	OL	30	12	O	97	<0.005	
				30	12	O	73		83–100
Polascik TJ et al. [13]	1995	RC	O	10	35.6	S	70	NS	35–93
			L	12	20.8	S	83		52–98
Ross JW [45]	1995	RC	O	30	12	O	93	NS	78–99
			L	32	12	O	94		79–99
Das S, Palmer JK [15]	1995	RC	O	10	10	S	100		69–100
			L	10	10	S	90		56–100
			Raz	10	10	S	100		69–100
McDougall EM et al. [14]	1995	RC	L	19	3	O	82		57–96
			Raz	23	3	O	95		75–100
Kung RC et al. [12]	1996	RC	L	31	14.4	O	97		94–100
			O	31	32.4	O	90		87–100

L, laparoscopic; O, "Open"; S, subjective; O, objective.

Table 35.2 Summary of observational clinical series

Study	Year	Study type	n	Technique	Follow-up (months)	Outcome measurement	Cure rate (%)	95% CI
Saidi MH et al. [46]	1998	P	70	E/S	15.9	S	91	84–98
Ross JW [23]	1998	P	48	T/S	30–41	S+O	89	80–98
Pelosi MA et al. [47]	1998	?	63	?	24	?	90	82–98
Foote AJ, Lam A [48]	1997	R	10		3	S	100	
Papasakelariou C et al. [49]	1997	P	32	T/S	(24)	S	91	81–100
O'Shea RT et al. [50]	1996	R	58	28 E/S				
				30 T/S	6–33	?	98	94–100
Flax S [24]	1996	R	47	E/S	2–15	S	73	57–85
Radomski SB and Herschorn S [51]	1996	R	46	T+E/S	12–26			
					Av 17.3	S	85	69–95
Lobel PW and Sand PK [52]	1996	R	35	?/S	Av 30	S	68.6	51–83
Cooper MJW et al. [22]	1996	R	113	T+E/S	1–28			
					Av 108	S	87	80–93
Langebrekke A et al. [53]	1995	R	8	E/S	3	S+O	88	47–100
Lam AM et al. [21]	1995	P	16	T/S	1.5–9	S	100	77–100
von Theobald P et al. [10]	1995	?	37	E/M+St	18–42			
					Av 24.9	S	86	53–84
Liu CY [54]	1993	R	58	T/S	6–22	S+O	95	85–99
Liu CY and Peak W [55]	1993	R	107	T/S	3–27	S+O	97	89–99
Ou C-S et al. [11]	1993	R	40	T/M+St	Av 6	S	100	91–100

P, prospective; E, extraperitoneal; T, transperitoneal; Su, sutures; St, staples; M, mesh.

Table 35.3 Showing the cure rate of laparoscopic Burch procedure as taken from the literature review summarized in Tables 35.1 and 35.2

	n	Cured n (%)	95% CI
Subjective assessment	589	519 (88)	85–91
Objective assessment	333	318 (96)	94–98
Total	922	837 (91)	89–93

It is important to define precisely what is meant by "success" in an anti-incontinence operation. If the patient is no longer incontinent, this may be considered a successful outcome. However, numerous studies have already observed that results assessed subjectively by the patient give a greater cure rate for incontinence than do those studies that use some form of objective measure [20]. While subjective assessment of cure may be satisfactory in clinical practice, it is clearly unsatisfactory, for the above reason, in the scientific assessment of a procedure. An objective method of assessment is taken to be cure assessed by urodynamic testing, for example a pad test, a cystometrogram, or clinically by a cough stress test with a full bladder. Only 333 of the 922 patients had been assessed objectively and in this group the cure rate was 96% (Table 35.3). This compares favorably with the outcomes of other incontinence procedures (Table 35.4) as calculated from the results reported in papers gleaned in a comprehensive literature review by Jarvis in 1994 [6].

The length of follow-up for reported cases of incontinence surgery is also important. It has been shown that cure of incontinence following colposuspension is time dependent [19]. Unfortunately there is no standardization in the literature of the way in which length of follow-up is reported, and the

Table 35.4 Comparison of the success rate of laparoscopic Burch procedure as determined from the literature review summarized in Tables 35.1 and 35.2, with the success rates of other incontinence procedures as reported in a literature review by Jarvis [6]

Procedure	Subjective cure n (%)	Objective cure n (%)
Laparoscopic colposuspension	589 (88)	333 (96)
"Open" colposuspension	1726 (90)	2300 (84)
MMK	6827 (93)	443 (89)
Sling procedure	1712 (82)	720 (85)
Bladder buttress	1481 (81)	490 (72)
Injectables	319 (56)	133 (60)

MMK, Marshall–Marchetti–Krantz.
Adapted from Jarvis [6].

follow-up periods reported for the cases of laparoscopic retropubic colposuspension reviewed varied from three months to 50 months. Most cases have quite a short follow-up period, as the authors were reporting their initial experiences with the procedure. Studies showing the long-term results of laparoscopic colposuspension are lacking, but the technique was initially described only a few years ago, and we are only just reaching the time when case series with 5-year follow-up can be anticipated.

Intraoperative and Postoperative Complications of Laparoscopic Colposuspension

When considering the results of surgery for benign disease, it is important to consider the complications or consequences of the procedure. The incidence of adverse events during or following the reported cases of laparoscopic colposuspension is low. The most frequently reported was bladder injury. Some of the complications reported are peculiar to laparoscopic surgery, such as injury to the inferior epigastric artery [21,22] and Richter's hernia [23]. Others, for example bladder injury, sutures in the bladder [24], ureteric injury [25] and vesicocutaneous fistula [22], could also be sustained during an open colposuspension. Postoperative voiding disorders and de novo detrusor instability, which occur respectively in a mean of 12.5% and 9.6% of patients undergoing open colposuspension [6], have also been reported following laparoscopic colposuspension, but it is not possible to calculate an incidence. To date there have been no reports on injury to intra-abdominal organs, peritonitis or intraoperative or postoperative deaths.

Duration of Surgery, Hospital Stay and Cost of Laparoscopic Colposuspension

As the cost of health care has come under increasingly rigorous scrutiny, the duration of surgical procedures, particularly laparoscopic procedures which are being touted as an alternative to conventional surgery, has become an issue of concern. Figure 35.1 shows the mean duration of laparoscopic colposuspension reported by different groups. The time varies from 35 to 196 minutes. The duration of an operation depends not only on the nature of the operation, but on the surgeon and whether or not the surgeon is training a junior. It is accepted that there is a learning curve for any procedure, particularly for laparoscopic surgery, and most of the cases presented in the literature to date are the initial experiences of different units with the technique. The operation times presented may not, therefore, be a true representation of the duration of surgery in experienced hands. It is estimated that about 35 procedures should be performed before the operation time stabilizes at around 60 minutes [26]. It is generally accepted, however, that laparoscopic procedures take longer than open procedures. This is certainly borne out by the three studies that made a direct comparison (Figure 35.2). This increased duration of surgery is an issue to be considered if it results in prolonged waiting lists.

It is often said that a decreased hospital stay following laparoscopic surgery offsets the overall cost of a longer duration of surgery. Indeed, numerous studies have reported significantly shorter length of hospitalization following laparoscopic colposuspension [12,13,15,23,24,27] compared with open colposuspension. However, these results are not based on appropriately designed, randomized studies. MacKenzie [28] illustrated, in patients recovering from hysterectomy, that preoperative information given to the patients has a major influence on the time for recovery. The apparent rapid recovery following laparoscopic surgery may, at least in part, be produced by the patient's and physician's expectations. The Sheffield cholecystectomy study [29] showed that when patients were blinded to the method of gall bladder removal, their recovery rates were the same for open and laparoscopic techniques. Ideally a similar study is required to assess whether there is any difference in immediate postoperative recovery from colposuspension when the patients and the attendant nursing staff do not know by which technique the operation was performed.

Although laparoscopy has been reported to be more cost-effective than laparotomy in the surgical treatment of ectopic pregnancy [30], the cost-effectiveness of laparoscopy in other areas of gynecology, such as hysterectomy, has been controversial [31,32]. Data from the general surgical literature support laparoscopy as a cost-effective alternative to the traditional abdominal approach for procedures such as cholecystectomy and appendicectomy [33–35]. It is difficult to compare evaluations of cost from different hospitals, because the expenses incurred are unique to a particular institution. Also the costing structure of hospitals varies in different countries. It is important, also, to take into account the success rate of the operation. A particular operation may be cheap to perform, but if it has a low success rate the economy is false. This brings into account the definition of "success" of a procedure and over what time period it should be evaluated; a complex issue which is far from standardized.

Kohli et al. [27] performed a non-randomized, retrospective cost analysis comparing open colposuspension with laparoscopic colposuspension, and found the operating room charges to be higher for the laparoscopic approach, but the postoperative hospitalization charges to be significantly lower. Overall, however, the total cost of the laparoscopic approach was significantly higher for the laparoscopic group. This study assumes comparable cure rates and was based on hospital charges to the patient and not on actual costs to the hospital. Kung et al. [12] performed an extremely rigorous, retrospective, cost-effectiveness analysis of laparoscopic versus abdominal colposuspension. They performed the analysis from the point of view of the Ministry

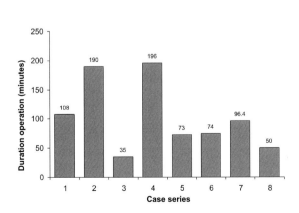

Figure 35.1 Average duration of laparoscopic Burch procedure reported in different case series. 1, Cooper et al. [22]; 2, Lobel and Sand [52]; 3, von Theobald et al. [10]; 4, Radomski and Herschorn [51]; 5, Liu [54]; 6, Liu and Peak [55]; 7, Flax [24]; 8, Lam et al. [21].

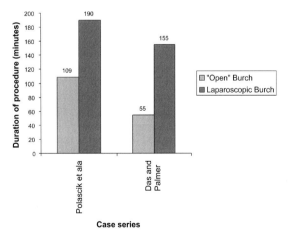

Figure 35.2 Duration of open Burch compared to laparoscopic Burch as reported in comparative studies (Polascik et al. [13], Das and Palmer [15]).

of Health (Canada) and the cost of professional fees (physicians, nurses, nursing assistants), investigations, drugs, capital equipment, disposable equipment, length of hospital stay and indirect hospital costs (overhead expenses, heating, pharmacy, housekeeping etc.) were all taken into account. They found that the laparoscopic approach was more cost-effective than the abdominal, principally due to decreased postoperative hospitalization. A criticism of this study is that it included patients in the open group who underwent multiple concurrent procedures, which may have accounted for a lengthier postoperative stay.

Discussion

Laparoscopic colposuspension has gained widespread use despite the fact that a thorough assessment of the success rate and cost of the procedure has not been performed so far. The available information would suggest an acceptable short-term success rate, but longer-term success of the procedure has yet to be evaluated. There does not seem to be a significant difference in the intermediate complication rate between open and laparoscopic colposuspension. Laparoscopy provides better visualization of the space of Retzius, less postoperative pain, less postoperative voiding dysfunction, shorter hospital stay and earlier return to work [13–15,23]. However, these observations are not documented on the basis of appropriately designed, randomized, controlled trials. It is also postulated that early mobilization of the patient may carry a risk of suspension rupture because of weak scarification [36]. There is obviously a need for randomized, prospective study of laparoscopic colposuspension in terms of efficacy and cost. The procedure was originally described only in 1991 [9], so hopefully over the next few years one can anticipate at least some case series reporting follow-up at five years or more.

Sling Procedure

Sling procedures have been used for many years in the treatment of GSI, usually in patients with failed primary procedures, low urethral closure pressures, poorly mobile or drainpipe urethras (intrinsic sphincter deficiency). Many different approaches to the sling procedure have been described and are outlined elsewhere in this textbook. As an "open" procedure it is generally regarded as one of the largest surgical interventions for incontinence, but it is one of the most successful. The success rate

of the procedure, as reported in Jarvis's meta-analysis [6] is 93.9% when performed as a primary procedure and 86.1% when performed for recurrent incontinence. This makes it the most effective operation in the urogynecologist's repertoire for treating stress incontinence.

Nearly 30 years ago, Morgan [37] described a combined abdominal and vaginal, two-team approach using a polypropylene mesh. The vaginal surgeon dissects out and completely mobilizes the bladder neck. A para-urethral tunnel can then be created on each side, to the level of the pubocervical fascia. The abdominal surgeon dissects down into the space of Retzius to expose the pubocervical fascia on each side of the bladder neck, similar to the approach used when performing a colposuspension. The vaginal surgeon can then pass a pre-cut sling, in this case made of polypropylene, up into the para-urethral tunnels and through the pubocervical fascia (urogenital diaphragm) into the space of Retzius. The abdominal surgeon then secures the ends of the mesh to Cooper's ligament on each side. The advantage of this two-team, combined approach is that the sling is passed through the urogenital diaphragm under the direct vision of the abdominal surgeon, so minimizing the risk of vascular or bladder trauma that may occur when the sling is passed blindly into the space of Retzius.

Recently, Kung et al. [38] published the preliminary results of the first one hundred cases of the same procedure performed using a laparoscopic approach to the abdominal part of the operation. Both extraperitoneal and transperitoneal approaches were used. The mean follow-up was 1.5 years and the overall success rate, assessed objectively, was 95%, which compares favorably with the open procedure. The mean duration of surgery was 70 minutes and the average hospital stay was 1.5 days. Complications included small bowel perforation (1%), inadvertent cystotomy (3%), erosion of the mesh (3%) and postoperative voiding dysfunction (3%). Postoperative voiding dysfunction occurs in an average of 10.4% (range 2–20%) of patients undergoing open sling procedures [6], so in this respect, the laparoscopic approach seems preferable. This may be because it is more difficult to put too much tension on the sling through the laparoscope. When a postoperative wound infection rate of 12% (range 4.7–48%) [6] following open slings is considered, the laparoscopic approach seems alluring. Interestingly, Kreder and Winfield [39] described a similar laparoscopic sling technique, but failed to show any benefits to the patients in terms of decreased cost or convalescence compared with the open vaginal sling.

Blander et al. [40] report on 24 cases using a similar technique to Kung et al. [38], but using a stapling device to fix the mesh rather than a suture. The mean follow-up was 29 months and the cure rate, assessed subjectively, was 80%. There was also a 25% de novo incidence of urgency and urge incontinence following the procedure. This is a recognized complication of incontinence surgery and sling procedures in particular. Jarvis [6] reports an incidence of 16.6% (range 4–29%) following conventional open surgery. Blander and colleagues [40] felt that the use of the stapling device would reduce the operating time. However, the mean duration of surgery, 69 minutes, is similar to that reported by Kung et al. [38], highlighting the fact that duration of surgery depends not only on the nature of the operation, but also the individual surgeon and also other factors like the training of juniors.

Pelosi and Pelosi [41] utilized the concept of improved visualization to decrease inadvertent injury associated with blind manipulations within the space of Retzius and described a single, suprapubic puncture technique, with transperitoneal laparoscopic dissection of the bladder neck to define the areas of periurethral fascial perforation and anterior abdominal wall fixation of the sling.

Paravaginal Repair

A new theory of vaginal support was proposed by Richardson in 1976 [5]. He contends that the support of the anterior vaginal wall, bladder and urethra is dependent on the inherent strength of the pubocervical fascia and its peripheral attachment to the pelvic sidewalls. The anterior vaginal fornix and its underlying pubocervical fascia are attached to the sidewall at the arcus tendineus fascia pelvis, or the white line, overlying the obturator internus muscle. It is postulated that a proximal break in this lateral attachment may result in a cysto-urethrocele, whereas a distal break, in the area of the bladder neck, may result in bladder neck hypermobility with associated stress urinary incontinence. Often, both entities coexist and present as prolapse *and* incontinence.

The idea of repairing defects in the endopelvic fascia to restore urinary continence is not new. In 1961, Burch [4] described the placement of three sutures of number 2 chromic catgut "from the perivaginal fascia to the iliopectineal line and fascia over the levator muscle" in seven patients. However, he believed that the ileopectineal line did not hold the suture well and changed the placement of these sutures to Cooper's ligament. Richardson et al. [42], in 1981, described a similar method of repairing the defects in the paravaginal fascia as a treatment of

stress urinary incontinence. This extraperitoneal technique involves mobilization of the bladder edge medially to expose the endopelvic fascia and its attachment to the lateral pelvic sidewalls. A suture is then passed through the full thickness of the fascial margin next to the bladder neck and carried laterally through the fascial covering of the levator muscle at the level of the ileopectineal line. This first suture is placed far enough posteriorly on the pelvic sidewall to reposition the urethra back into the pelvis so that the external meatus lies at the level of the anterior surface of the pubic bone. Up to three sutures are then placed anterior to this key stitch and three posterior to it, to reattach the endopelvic fascia to the pelvic sidewall. The procedure may be repeated on the contralateral side if necessary. In his initial series of 233 patients, a complete cure of stress incontinence was reported in 80% of the patients after a minimum of two years' follow up (range 2–8 years) and "satisfactory" bladder function in 95.3%. More recently, the same investigator reported a laparoscopic approach to this procedure [43] while Miklos and Kohli [44] describe a laparoscopic approach to a combined colposuspension and paravaginal repair. The procedure is quite new and, as yet, objective reports on its efficacy are lacking.

Conclusions

Technological innovations in instrumentation, illumination and imaging over the last few years have opened up an exciting new approach to surgery. The advantages of laparoscopic surgery have been demonstrated in the field of general surgery [33–35] and in certain aspects of gynecological practice [29,30]. Surgical procedures for stress incontinence would seem to lend themselves perfectly to a laparoscopic approach and, indeed, most of the few case series that have been published reviewing laparoscopic colposuspension report a good short- and intermediate-term success rate. The value of this information is diluted by the fact that the surgical technique is far from standardized, the laparoscopic experience of the different investigators is variable and the follow-up assessments are often inadequate. Ultimately, to evaluate these procedures properly, a multicenter, randomized, controlled trial is required which standardizes the indication for surgery, the approach employed, the materials used and which measures postoperative complications. Objective assessments of the outcomes for at least a 5-year period will need to be performed.

References

1. Mohide EA. The prevalence and scope of urinary incontinence. Clin Geriatr Med 1986;2(4):639–55.

2. Kohorn EI. The surgery of stress incontinence. Obstet Gynecol Clin North Am 1989;16(4):841–52.

3. Marshall VF, Marchetti AA, Krantz KE. The correction of stress incontinence by simple vesicourethral suspension. Surg Gynecol Obstet 1949;88:509.

4. Burch JC. Urethrovaginal fixation to Cooper's ligament for correction of stress incontinence, cystocoele and prolapse. Am J Obstet Gynecol 1961;81:281.

5. Richardson AC, Lyons JB, Williams NL. A new look at pelvic relaxation. Am J Obstet Gynecol 1976;126:568.

6. Jarvis GJ. Surgery for genuine stress incontinence. Br J Obstet Gynaecol 1995;101:397

7. Bergman A, Ballard CA, Koonings PP. Comparison of three different surgical procedures for genuine stress incontinence: Prospective randomized study. Am J Obstet Gynecol 1989;160(5):1102–6.

8. Bergman A, Koonings PP, Ballard CA. Primary stress urinary incontinence and pelvic relaxation: Prospective randomized comparison of three different operations. Am J Obstet Gynecol 1989;161(1):97–101.

9. Vancaille TG, Schuessler W. Laparoscopic bladder neck suspension. J Laparoendoscop Surg 1991;3:169–73.

10. von Theobald P, Guillaumin D, Levy G. Laparoscopic preperitoneal colposuspension for stress incontinence in women. Technique and results of 37 procedures. Surg Endosc 1995;9(11):1189–92.

11. Ou C-S, Presthus J, Beadle E. Laparoscopic bladder neck suspension using hernia mesh and surgical staples. J Laparoendosc Surg 1993;3:563–6.

12. Kung RC, Lie K, Lee P et al. The cost effectiveness of laparoscopic versus abdominal Burch procedures in women with urinary stress incontinence. J Am Assoc Gynecol Laparosc 1996;3(4):537–44.

13. Polascik TJ, Moore RG, Rosenberg MT et al. Comparison of laparoscopic and open retropubic urethropexy for treatment of stress urinary incontinence. Urology 1995;45:647–52.

14. McDougall EM, Klutke CG, Carnell T. Comparison of transvaginal versus laparoscopic bladder neck suspension for stress urinary incontinence. Urology 1995;45:641–9.

15. Das S, Palmer JK. Laparoscopic colposuspension. J Urol 1995;154:1119–21.

16. Burton GA. A randomised comparison of laparoscopic and open colposuspension. Neurourol Urodyn 1994;13:497–8.

17. Galloway NTM, Davies N, Stephenson TP. The complications of colposuspension. Br J Urol 1987;60:122–4.

18. Eriksen BC, Hagen B, Eik-Nes SH et al. Long-tern effectiveness of the Burch colposuspension. Acta Obstet Gynaecol Scand 1990;69:45–50.

19. Alcalay M, Monga A, Stanton S. Burch colposuspension: a 10–20 year follow up. Br J Obstet Gynaecol 1995;102:740–5.

20. Mundy AR. A trial comparing the Stamey bladder neck suspension with colposuspension for the treatment of stress incontinence. Br J Urol 1983;55, 687–90.

21. Lam AM, Jenkins GJ, Hyslop RS. Laparoscopic Burch colposuspension for stress incontinence: preliminary results. Med J Aust 1995;2;162(1):18–21.

22. Cooper MJW, Cario G, Lam A et al. A review of the results in a series of 113 laparoscopic colposuspensions. Aust NZ J Obstet Gynaecol 1996;36:44–8.

23. Ross JW. Multichannel urodynamic evaluation of laparoscopic Burch colposuspension for genuine stress incontinence. Obstet Gynecol 1998;91(1):55–9.

24. Flax S. The gasless laparoscopic Burch bladder neck suspension: Early experience. J Urol 1996;156:1105–7.

25. Aslan P, Woo HH. Ureteric injury following laparoscopic colposuspension. Br J Obstet Gynaecol 1997;104:266–8.

26. Lose G. Laparoscopic Burch colposuspension. Acta Obstet Gynecol Scand Suppl 1998;168; 77:29–33.

27. Kohli N, Jacobs PA, Sze EH et al. Open compared with laparoscopic approach to Burch colposuspension: a cost analysis. Obstet Gynecol 1997;90(3):411–15.

28. MacKenzie IZ. Reducing hospital stay after abdominal hysterectomy. Br J Obstet Gynaecol 1996;103:175–8.

29. Majeed AW, Troy G, Nicholl JP et al. Randomised, prospective, single-blind comparison of laparoscopic versus small-incision cholecystectomy. Lancet 1996;347:989–94.

30. Gray DT, Thorburn J, Lundorff P et al. A cost-effectiveness study of a randomised trial of laparoscopy versus laparotomy for ectopic pregnancy. Lancet 1995;345:1139–43.

31. Nezhat C, Bess O, Admon D et al. Hospital cost comparison between abdominal, vaginal and laparoscopically-assisted vaginal hysterectomy. Obstet Gynecol 1994;83:713–16.

32. Messina MJ, Garavaglia MM, Walsh RT et al. Laparoscopically-assisted vaginal hysterectomy: Cost analysis and review of initial experience in a community hospital. J Am Osteopath Assoc 1995;95:31–6.

33. Bass EB, Pitt HA, Lillemoe KD. Cost-effectiveness of laparoscopic cholecystectomy versus open cholecystectomy. Am J Surg 1993;165:466–71.

34. Fisher KS, Reddick EJ, Olsen DO. Laparoscopic cholecystectomy: Cost analysis. Surg Laparosc Endosc 1991;1:77–81..

35. Martin LC, Puente I, Sosa JL et al. Open versus laparoscopic appendicectomy. A prospective, randomised comparison. Ann Surg 1995;222:256–61.

36. Korram MM. Laparoscopic colposuspension operation. J Gynecol Surg 1995;10:205–6.

37. Morgan JE. A sling operation, using Marlex polypropylene mesh, for the treatment of recurrent stress incontinence. Am J Obstet Gynecol 1970;106:369–77.

38. Kung R, Lie KI, Morgan JE et al. Laparoscopic Two-team sling for Urinary Stress Incontinence. J Am Assoc Gynecol Laparosc 1996;3(4, Supplement):S23.

39. Kreder KJ, Winfield HN. Laparoscopic urethral sling for the treatment of intrinsic sphincter deficiency. J Endourol 1996;10(3):255–7.

40. Blander DS, Carpiniello VL, Harryhill JF et al. Extraperitoneal laparoscopic urethropexy with Marlex mesh. Urology 1999;53(5):985–9.

41. Pelosi MA 3rd, Pelosi MA. Laparoscopically-assisted pubo-vaginal sling procedure for the treatment of stress urinary incontinence. J Am Assoc Gynecol Laparosc 1996;3(4):593–600.

42. Richardson AC, Edmonds PB, Williams NL. Treatment of stress urinary incontinence due to paravaginal fascial defect. Obstet Gynecol 1981;57(3):357–62.

43. Richardson AC, Saye WB, Miklos JR. Repairing paravaginal defects laparoscopically. Contemp Obstet Gynecol 1997;42:130.

44. Miklos JR, Kohli N. "Paravaginal Plus" Burch Procedure. A laparoscopic approach. J Pelvic Surg 1998;4(6):297–302.

45. Ross JW. Laparoscopic Burch repair compared to laparoscopic Burch for cure of urinary stress incontinence. Int Urogynecol J 1995;6:323–8.

46. Saidi MH, Sadler RK, Saidi JA. Extraperitoneal laparoscopic colposuspension for genuine urinary stress incontinence. J Am Assoc Gynecol Laparosc 1998;5(3):247–52.

47. Pelosi MA, Papasakelariou C, Pelosi MA 3rd. Laparoscopic colposuspension with a transvaginal illuminator. J Am Assoc Gynecol Laparosc 1998;5(2):179–82.

48. Foote AJ, Lam A. Laparoscopic colposuspension in women with previously failed anti-incontinence surgery. J Obstet Gynaecol Res 1997;23(3):313–17.
49. Papasakelariou C, Papasakelariou B. Laparoscopic bladder neck suspension. J Am Assoc Gynecol Laparosc 1997;4(2):185–9.
50. O'Shea RT, Seman E, Taylor J. Laparoscopic Burch Colposuspension for Urinary Stress Incontinence. J Am Assoc Gynecol Laparosc 1996;3(4, Supplement):S36.
51. Radomski SB, Herschorn S. Laparoscopic bladder neck suspension: Early results. J Urol 1996;155:515–18.
52. Lobel PW, Sand PK. Long-term results of laparoscopic Burch colposuspension. Neurourol Urodyn 1996;15:398–9.
53. Langebrekke A, Dahlstrom B, Eraker R et al. The laparoscopic Burch procedure. A preliminary report. Acta Obstet Gynecol Scand 1995;74(2):153–5.
54. Liu CY. Laparoscopic retropubic colposuspension (Burch procedure). A review of 58 cases. J Reprod Med 1993;38(7):526–30.
55. Liu CY, Peak W. Laparoscopic retropubic colposuspension (Burch Procedure). J Am Assoc Gynecol Laparosc 1993;1:31–4.

36 Bulking Agents

Sender Herschorn and Patricia Lee

Introduction

Murless, in 1938, first reported on injection of sodium morrhuate around the urethra [1], and since then various materials have been injected for urinary incontinence as an alternative to surgery. Quackels [2] reported paraffin wax in 1955 and Sachse [3] used sclerosing agents in 1963. The initial results were poor and significant complications such as pulmonary emboli and urethral sloughing were seen. Polytetrafluoroethylene (Teflon) paste was first introduced by Berg [4] and then popularized by Politano [5] in the 1970s. Shortliffe et al. [6] published the first report on glutaraldehyde cross-linked collagen and more recently autologous fat injection [7] has been described. Newer agents, such as silicone microparticles [8] and injectable microballoons, have also been reported [9].

Despite a tremendous growth in interest recently in injectable agents, there have been few published prospective randomized trials comparing different agents or injectables to other treatments for SUI. Outcome measures have not been standardized. This chapter will summarize the properties, published results, and complications of the various agents as well as examine some of the controversies.

Mechanism of Action of Injectables

It is generally agreed that these agents improve intrinsic sphincter function. Collagen injections have been reported [10,11] to augment urethral mucosa, improve coaptation and intrinsic sphincter function as evidenced by an increase in post-treatment abdominal leak pressure [12–14]. Initial inves-tigators with collagen [15,16] postulated obstruction as a mechanism of action, but Monga et al. [11] showed that successfully treated patients have an increased area and pressure transmission ratio in the first quarter of the urethra. They suggested that placement of the injectable at the bladder neck or proximal urethra prevents bladder neck opening under stress. Proper placement of the injectable, possibly just below the bladder neck, rather than actual quantity [17] of the agent improves intrinsic sphincter deficiency (ISD).

The ideal injectable agent [18] should be easily injectable and conserve its volume over time. If unsuccessful it should not interfere with subsequent surgical intervention. It should also be biocompatible, non-antigenic, non-carcinogenic and non-migratory. To date, no substance has met all of these requirements.

Patient Selection

Patients with ISD and normal detrusor function are candidates for injectable agents [19]. McGuire et al. [20] identified these patients with the use of abdominal leak pressures to measure the strength of the intrinsic sphincter. Low leak pressures (<65 cm water) correlate well with type III videourodynamic findings, i.e. a poorly functioning bladder neck and proximal urethra (ISD), and higher leak pressures correlated with types I or II hypermobility.

The presence of ISD is the primary indication for the use of injectable agents in patients with stress incontinence [10]. Since ISD can coexist with hypermobility [21], injectables have been administered to patients with hypermobility, to improve the ISD component of their incontinence. Furthermore, elderly women with hypermobility, who are poor operative risks, have also been injected [22].

Injection Techniques

The materials can be administered under local anesthesia with cystoscopic control as an outpatient procedure. Both the *periurethral* and *transurethral* methods are done to implant the agent within the urethral wall, preferably into the submucosa or lamina propria. It is thought that the implant should be positioned at the bladder neck or proximal urethra. Different sites can be chosen such as 3 and 9 o'clock or 4 and 8 o'clock positions. The needle size depends on the viscosity of the injectable. Pre- and postoperative antibiotics are usually administered. The technique of injection is seen in Figures 36.1 and 36.2.

With the periurethral approach, perimeatal blebs are raised with 1% or 2% lidocaine at the 3 and 9 or 4 and 8 o'clock positions approximately 3 to 4 mm lateral to the urethral meatus. A 20F urethroscope with a 30° telescope is inserted into the urethra after instillation of topical urethral lidocaine. The periurethral needle is introduced and advanced parallel to endoscope sheath until its position can be seen cystoscopically just below the bladder neck within the mucosa. Care must be taken to prevent the needle from getting to close to or entering the urethral lumen as rupture of the mucosa and extravasation will occur. Rocking the needle will confirm the position of the tip. If penetration of the mucosa occurs the needle should be removed and reposi-

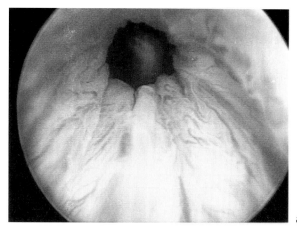

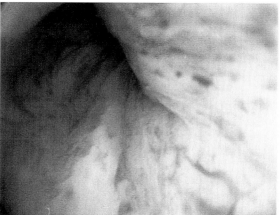

Figure 36.2 **a** Cystoscopic view of the open bladder neck region prior to injection. **b** Collagen has been injected via the periurethral route on the patient's left side. Note the intraluminal bulking effect of the agent.

tioned. The substance is injected either uni-laterally or bilaterally to create the appearance of "prostatic" lobes. The patient is asked to cough or strain in the supine and then upright position. If leakage still occurs more agent may be given. If no leakage is seen the procedure may be terminated. The patient then voids and can be discharged. Acute retention can be treated by insertion of a fine 8F catheter.

The implant can also be injected transurethrally through the cystoscope with specially designed needles. Teflon, silicone microparticles, and fat, due to their high viscosity, may require the use of injection guns.

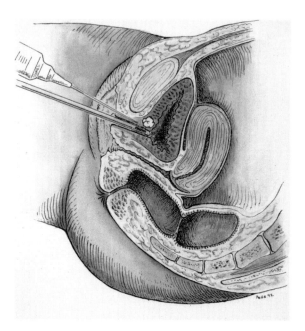

Figure 36.1   Periurethral collagen injection. The 20F cystoscope with a 30 degree lens is positioned in the urethra while the while the substance is injected into the bladder neck region.

Collagen

Glutaraldehyde cross-linked collagen or Gax-collagen is a highly purified suspension of bovine collagen in normal saline containing at least 95%

type I collagen and 1–5% type III collagen [23]. This cross-linking makes the Gax-collagen resistant to the fibroblast-secreted collagenase. As a result of this, the Gax-collagen is only very slightly resorbed. The implant causes no inflammatory reaction or granuloma formation and is colonized by host fibro-blasts and blood vessels. It is not known to migrate. However, it does degrade over time and is replaced by host collagen, to explain its persistence [23].

Since 2–5% of patients [24] are sensitized to collagen through dietary exposure, all patients must undergo a skin test into the volar aspect of the forearm 30 days prior to treatment. Positive responders should be excluded.

Collagen Results

Numerous reports of its efficacy, safety, ease of administration, and relative lack of morbidity have appeared since the first description of collagen injections for urinary incontinence. Our original report, with short-term follow-up of 6 months [12], showed a cured and improved rate of 90.3%. With longer follow-up the success rate decreased, but there were still long-term cures. Table 36.1 lists various reported series.

Persistence of the implant itself has been demonstrated with magnetic resonance imaging of the urethra at intervals of up to 22 months after injection although the measured volume was less than that injected [25]. Early results are generally good with success rates of 72–100% (Table 36.1). Maintenance of good results in the long term may be from durability of the initial procedure itself or from reinjections with additional collagen. It is important for authors to differentiate the durability of the original procedure(s) from reinjections or top-ups by reporting the follow-up period starting from after the last injection.

Longer-term results, of more than 1 to 2 years, vary from 57%, cure and improved [17], to 94% [33]. Most patients need 1–2 treatment sessions with means of 5.6 to 15 cm^3 of collagen. Since patients are treated at different times and durations of follow-up vary, the Kaplan–Meier curve can be useful to display the persistence of a good result. In our series [30], the probability of remaining dry was 72% at 1 year, 57% at 2 years, and 45% at 3 years (Figure 36.3). Winters and Appell [13] also reported a similar 50% rate of complete continence in the multicenter trial after 2 years. Additional administration of collagen usually resulted in restoration of continence and this has to be factored into the reporting.

Berman and Kreder [34] analyzed the cost-effectiveness of collagen versus sling cystourethropexy for type III incontinence. They concluded that surgery was more cost-effective than collagen.

The use of collagen for patients with hypermobility has been reported. Moore et al. [29] included patients with both type I and type III abnormalities. Faerber [22] treated elderly patients with type I abnormality. In the report by McGuire and Appell [10], the results at more than one year in women with ISD were similar to those in women with hypermobility, although there were far more women with ISD. However, Appell [19] subsequently reported that these patients with hypermobility all required bladder neck surgery within 2 years. Monga et al. [11] included patients with hypermobility and found that cure rates were not reduced for women with up to 2.5 cm of movement. In our series of 181 patients there was no significant difference in outcome in patients with or without hypermobility [30].

Collagen Complications

Treatment-related morbidity has been minimal. Urinary retention ranges from 1 to 21% [12,13,19] and can be managed with intermittent catheterization or short-term Foley. Urinary tract infection occurs in 1–25% [12,13,19]. Extravasation resolves quickly with flushing away of the dilute collagen suspension and sealing over of the small needle site. Hematuria can occur in 2% of patients [19]. Other rare complications include periurethral abscess formation [35].

Other complications include de novo instability, seen in 11 of 28 elderly women (39%) treated by Khullar et al. [17]. Stothers et al. reported de novo urgency with urgency incontinence in 43 of

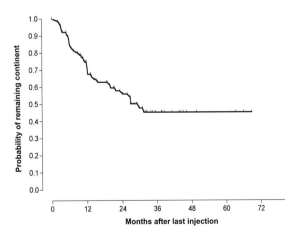

Figure 36.3 Durability: Kaplan–Meier curve showing durability of cure of incontinence after the last collagen injection in 78 patients [30].

Female Pelvic Medicine and Reconstructive Pelvic Surgery

Table 36.1 Comparison of collagen parameters and results

Study	No. patients	Type of incontinence	Follow-up (months)	No. patients dry (%)	No. patients improved (%)	No. patients failed (%)
Stricker and Haylen [26]	50	ISD	Mean:11 Range:1–21	21 (42)	20 (40)	7 (14)
Kieswetter et al. [27]	16	Not specified	9	7 (44)	7 (44)	2 (12)
Eckford and Abrams [15]	25	Not specified	3	16 (64)	4 (16)	5 (20)
O'Connell et al. [28]	44	42 with ISD	1–2 (longest 7)	20 (45)	8 (18)	16 (37)
Moore et al. [29]	11	2 hypermobile Types I and III	2	1 (9)	7 (63)	2 (18)
Winters and Appell [13]	50	ISD	>12	48 (96) dry or socially continent		2 (4)
McGuire and Appell [10]	17	Mobile	>12	8 (47)	3 (17)	6 (35)
Faerber [22]	137	ISD	>12	63 (46)	47 (34)	29 (19)
	12	Type I	10.3 (Range 3–24)	10 (83)	2 (17)	0
Monga et al. [11]	60	Some hypermobile	3 (n = 59) 12 (n = 54) 24 (n = 29)	27 (46) 22 (40) 14 (48)	24 (40) 20 (37) 6 (20)	
Richardson et al. [14]	42	ISD	46 (10–66 after 1st injection)	17 (40)	18 (43)	7 (17)
Herschorn et al. [30]	181	Type I:54 Type II:67 Type III:60	Mean:22 (Range 4–69)	42 (23)	94 (52)	45 (25)
Smith et al. [31]	94	Type III	>=24 (n = 62) >=36 (n = 25)	27 (43.5) 13 (52)	29 (46.8) 8 (32)	6 (9.7) 4 (16)
Khullar et al. [17]	21	Not specified	Median:14	36 (38.3)	27 (28.7)	31 (33)
Swami et al. [32]	107	Some hypermobile	24 (minimum)	10 (48)	2 (9)	9 (43)
Cross et al. [33]	103	Type III (Range 6–36)	24 (minimum) Median:18	27 (25) Substantially improved 103 (74)	43 (40) 29 (20)	37 (35) 7 (6)

Table 36.2 Teflon results for female stress incontinence

Study	No. patients	Follow-up (months)	Patients dry (%)	Patients improved (%)	Patients failed (%)
Politano et al. [42]	51	6	26 (51)	10 (20)	15 (29)
Lim et al. [43]	28	–	6 (21)	9 (33)	13 (46)
Schulman et al. [44]	56	3	39 (70)	9 (16)	8 (14)
Deane et al. [45]	28	3–24	9 (32)	8 (28)	11 (40)
Beckingham et al. [46]	26	36	2 (7)	7 (27)	17 (66)
Harrison et al. [47]	36	61	4 (11)	8 (22)	24 (67)
Lotenfoe et al. [48]	21	11	8 (38)	4 (19)	9 (43)
Lopez et al. [49]	74	31	41 (56)	15 (20)	18 (24)
Vesey et al. [50]	36	9 (3–36)	20 (56)	4 (11)	12 (33)
Herschorn and Glazer [41]	46	12	14 (31)	19 (41)	13 (28)

337 patients (12.9%), 21% of whom did not respond to anticholinergics [36].

Another rare complication is a reaction in the previously negative skin test site following a urethral collagen injection [24]. This occurred in 3 patients (1.9%) and was associated with arthralgias in 2. This reaction has been reported before in the dermatologic literature [37] and two negative pretreatment skin test have been suggested to prevent it. The potential for hypersensitivity reactions is present since antibody production is stimulated by collagen injection [38].

Polytetrafluoroethylene Paste (PTFE, Teflon, Urethrin)

Polytetrafluoroethylene paste (Teflon) is composed of equal parts Teflon paste and glycerin with polysorbate 20 [39]. Teflon is a resin polymer with a very high molecular weight, high viscosity and composed of small particles (40 mm in diameter). It is inert, stable, and does not induce an allergic response. However, it does cause a local inflammatory response with histiocytes phagocytizing the particles and coalescing to form foreign body giant cells and a granuloma. There is also fibrous tissue ingrowth that adds to the bulk formed by the Teflon. Owing to the small particle size, Malizia et al. [40] also showed distant migration of Teflon particles to pelvic nodes, lung, brain, and kidneys of experimental animals.

Teflon paste has been used to treat urinary incontinence since 1964, but it was not reported until 1975 by Berg [4]. Since that time, numerous reports relating to its use in treating incontinence have appeared in the literature. Although not approved in the United States, Teflon has been approved in Canada and in other countries.

It may be injected via the periurethral route and volumes of up to 10–20 ml are reported. The procedure is done under local or spinal anesthesia and repeats may be done after 6 months. We have modified the procedure by injecting small amounts (2.5 ml) via the periurethral approach under local anesthetic [41]. Heating the Teflon reduces its viscosity and allows injection without a gun.

Teflon Results

Table 36.2 lists various series. There are wide-ranging outcomes with longer-term series showing poorer results (33–76% cure and improved) than those of short-term series (57–86%).

Teflon Complications

Since relatively large volumes of Teflon have been injected with the patient under general anesthetic, the incidence of urinary retention at 25% [42] is higher than that of collagen. Irritative voiding symptoms have also been seen transiently in 20% [44]. Urinary infection is rare at 2% [43]. Perineal discomfort may occur in 5% [42] and transient fever in 10–15% of patients. Perforation and extravasation can occur and, if recognized at the time of injection, the Teflon should be removed,.

Although Teflon particles can migrate [40], only one case of clinical significance has been reported in the literature in humans. Claes et al. [51] described a woman previously treated with large volumes of periurethral Teflon for urinary incontinence who later presented with lymphocytic alveolitis and fever. Light microscopy showed Teflon particles in the lungs. She was treated successfully with steroids. Mittleman and Marraccini [52] reported an incidental finding of postmortem interstitial pulmonary granulomas in a previously

Table 36.3   Results of autologous fat injection

Study	No. patients	Follow-up (months)	No. patients dry (%)	No. patients improved (%)	No. patients failed (%)
Cervigni and Panei [7]	14	9.7	8 (57)	4 (29)	2 (14)
Santarosa and Blaivas [61]	12	11	7 (58)		5 (42)
Trockman and Leach [59]	32	6	4 (12)	14 (44)	14 (44)
Haab et al. [62]	45	7	6 (13)	13 (29)	26 (58)
Su et al. [60]	26	Mean; 17.4 (range 12–30)	13 (50)	4 (15)	9 (35)
Palma et al. [63]	30	12	1 injection: 4/13 (34) 2 injections: 11/17 (67)		

asymptomatic man who had received Teflon. Kiilhoma et al. [53] reported 3 complications out of 22 women, a sterile periurethral abscess, a urethral diverticulum, and a urethral granuloma, which all required surgical intervention. In another case, the material migrated into the bulbar corpus spongiosum causing perineal pain for 3 months necessitating medication for pain relief [54].

Although neoplastic transformation was hypothesized [40], there has never been a clinical occurrence reported. Furthermore, in a long-term rat study, Dewan et al. [55] demonstrated no increase in tumor risk and no tumors found at the injection site.

Despite the potential for complications with Teflon the actual rate of reported problems is low.

Autologous Fat

Autologous fat has been used for aesthetic and defect reconstruction since the 1980s [56]. Although fat is biocompatible and readily available, 50–90% of the transferred adipose tissue graft may not survive [57]. Graft survival depends on minimal handling, low suction pressure during liposuction, and the use of large bore needles. Smaller grafts survive better than larger ones [58].

The procedure involves harvesting abdominal wall fat by liposuction either under local [59] or general anesthesia [60]. The injection is usually carried out via the periurethral route with a 16- or 18-gauge needle. Post procedure care may involve intermittent catheterization or even a suprapubic tube [60].

Autologous Fat Results

A number of reports of urethral fat injections have been published and appear in Table 36.3. Most of the series report short-term results with success apparently lower than that of other injectables, apart from the study of Su et al. [60] with a follow-up of more than 12 months. Palma et al. [63] showed that repeat injections improved the cure rate from 31% to 64%. Haab et al. [62] reported a comparative study with collagen. After a mean of 7 months 13% of the women with fat injection were cured versus 24% of the women with collagen injections. The subjective improvement rate was also higher with the collagen.

Autologous Fat Complications

Reported complications are similar to other injectables with urinary infection, retention, hematuria, and extravasation. Additional problems with donor site, the abdominal wall, such as pain, hematomas, and infection, may also be seen. Other noteworthy complications are urethral pseudolipoma [64] and fat embolism [35,65].

Silicone Microimplants

Silicone microimplants [8] are solid polydimethylsiloxane (silicone rubber) particles suspended in a non-silicone carrier gel that is absorbed by the reticuloendothelial system and excreted unchanged in the urine. Since 99% of the particles are between 100 mm and 450 mm in diameter, the likelihood of migration is low. Henly et al. [66] demonstrated distant migration of small particles, less than 70 mm, but no migration of particles greater than 100 mm in diameter. Although there was a typical histiocytic and giant cell reaction within the injection site, there was no granuloma formation in response to the larger particles. Since the substance is quite viscous it must be injected with an injection gun and a 16-gauge tip transurethral needle.

Silicone Microimplant Results

Hariss et al. [8] reported on 40 patients followed for a minimum of 3 years at which time 16 (40%) were dry, 7 (18%) were improved, and 17 (42%) failed. Twelve of the 16 required one injection and four needed two injections to become dry. Sheriff et al. [67] reported an overall success of 48% in 34 patients after unsuccessful stress incontinence surgery and Koelbl et al. [68] reported a 60% success rate in 32 women after 12 months but noted a time-dependent decrease in success. Radley et al. reported a success rate of 61% (19.6% cured and 41.1% improved) in 60 women after a mean of 19 months [69].

Silicone Microimplant Complications

Self-limited side effects of hematuria, dysuria, frequency, and retention have been reported in a minority of patients. The lack of a granulomatous reaction and migration of the large silicone particles may provide some benefit over Teflon although long-term data are not yet available. Despite the laboratory and clinical evidence of safety with the large particles, concerns still exist about the small silicone particle migration and long-term tissue response to the injection [57].

Implantable Microballoons

In order to obviate the degradation and movement of injectable materials Atala and co-workers [70] developed a self-detachable implantable balloon system. The balloon is a silicone elastomer with a check valve that prevents escape of the solution that is injected at the time of implant. The filling solution is a biocompatible cross-linked hydrogel that maintains its volume within the silicone shell. The balloons are inserted into the submucosal area, usually periurethrally, with cystoscopic control.

Pycha et al. [9] reported that 8 (42%) of 19 women were dry and 7 (36.8%) were improved after a mean of 14.4 months. The patients with hypermobility had a poor outcome. Rare complications included bladder instability and balloon extrusion.

Conclusions

Considerable progress has been made since the introduction of collagen injections. Injectable agents are used for buttressing the ISD component of the incontinence but patients with concomitant hypermobility may benefit as well. They have also been administered to elderly patients who are not surgical candidates. However, there are still a number of areas in which further study is needed.

Durability is a concern. Although long-term successes have been reported with collagen and Teflon the results of both deteriorate over time. Similarly autologous fat and silicone microimplants yield poorer long-term than short-term results. Comparisons of injectables and injectables to surgery have been done to a limited degree and prospective studies have yet to be reported. Despite the ease of the technique and the attractiveness to patients of an outpatient procedure that can be repeated if necessary, the cost-effectiveness of injectable agents relative to other treatments, such as newer minimally invasive surgical procedures, still has to be addressed.

Safety of the material is also a concern. All of the injectables have excellent safety profiles, although the risk of migration and granuloma formation with Teflon has prevented its widespread use. Rare but serious complications have also been reported with collagen and autologous fat. The long-term risks of silicone microparticles and balloons are unknown. Newer agents, such as carbon beads and calcium hydroxylapatite crystals [71], which are not yet widely available, also appear to be safe. Longer-term and comparative studies may settle these issues.

References

1. Murless BC. The injection treatment of stress incontinence. J Obstet Gynaecol Br Emp 1938;45:67–73.
2. Quackels R. Deux incontinences après adénectomie guéries par injection de paraffine dans la périnée. Acta Urol Belg 1955;23:259–62.
3. Sachse H. Treatment of urinary incontinence with sclerosing solutions. Indications, results, complications. Urol Int 1963;15:225–44.
4. Berg S. Polytef augmentation urethroplasty. Correction of surgically incurable urinary incontinence by injection technique. Arch Surg 1973;107:379–81.
5. Politano VA, Small MP, Harper JM, Lynne CM. Peri-urethral Teflon injection for urinary incontinence. J Urol 1974;111:180–3.
6. Shortliffe LMD, Freiha FS, Kessler R, Stamey TA, Constantinou CE. Treatment of urinary incontinence by the periurethral implantation of glutaraldehyde cross-linked collagen. J Urol 1989;141:538–41.
7. Cervigni M, Panei M. Periurethral autologous fat injection for type III stress urinary incontinence. J Urol 1993;149 (Part 2):403A.
8. Harriss DR, Iacovou JW, Lemberger RJ. Peri-urethral silicone microimplants (Macroplastique7) for the treatment of genuine stress incontinence. Br J Urol 1996;78:722–8.
9. Pycha A, Klingler CH, Haitel A, Heinz-Peer G, Marberger M. Implantable microballoons: An attractive alternative in the

management of intrinsic sphincter deficiency. Eur Urol 1998;33:469–75.

10. McGuire EJ, Appell R. Transurethral collagen injection for urinary incontinence. Urology 1994;43:413–15.

11. Monga AK, Robinson D, Stanton SL. Periurethral collagen injections for genuine stress incontinence. Br J Urol 1995;76:156–60.

12. Herschorn S, Radomski SB, Steele DJ. Early experience with intraurethral collagen injections for urinary incontinence. J Urol 1992;148:1797–800.

13. Winters JC, Appell R. Periurethral injection of collagen in the treatment of intrinsic sphincter deficiency in the female patient. Urol Clin North Am 1995;22:673–8.

14. Richardson TD, Kennelly MJ, Faerber GJ. Endoscopic injection of glutaraldehyde cross-linked collagen for the treatment of intrinsic deficiency in women. Urology 1995;46:378–81.

15. Eckford SD, Abrams P. Para-urethral collagen implantation for female stress incontinence. Br J Urol 1991;68:586–9.

16. Appell RA. New developments: Injectables for urethral incompetence in women. Int Urogynecol J 1990;1:117–19.

17. Khullar V, Cardozo LD, Abbott D, Anders K. GAX collagen in the treatment of urinary incontinence in elderly women: a two year follow up. Br J Obstet Gynaecol 1997;104: 96–9.

18. Kershen RT, Atala A. New advances in injectable therapies for the treatment of incontinence and vesicoureteral reflux. Urol Clin North Am 1999;26:81–94.

19. Appell RA. Periurethral injection therapy. In: Walsh PC, Retik AB, Vaughan Jr ED, Wein AJ, editors. Campbell's Urology, 7th edn. Philadelphia: WB Saunders, 1998; 1109–20.

20. McGuire EJ, Fitzpatrick CC, Wan J, Bloom D, Sanvordenker J, Ritchey M, Gormley EA. Clinical assessment of urethral sphincter function. J Urol 1993;150:1452–4.

21. Raz S, Little N, Juma S. Female Urology. In: Walsh PC, Retik AB, Stamey TA, Vaughan ED, editors. Campbell's Urology, 6th edn. Philadelphia: WB Saunders, 1992;2782–2828.

22. Faerber GJ. Endoscopic collagen injection therapy in elderly women with type I stress urinary incontinence. J Urol 1996;155:512–14.

23. Remacle M, Bertrand B, Eloy P, Marbaix E. The use of injectable collagen to correct velopharyngeal insufficiency. Laryngoscope 1990;100:269.

24. Stothers L, Goldenberg SL. Delayed hypersensitivity and systemic arthralgia following transurethral collagen injection for stress urinary incontinence. J Urol 1998;159: 1507–9.

25. Carr LK, Herschorn S, Leonhardt C. Magnetic resonance imaging of intraurethral collagen injected for stress urinary incontinence. J Urol 1996;155:1253–5.

26. Stricker P, Haylen B. Injectable collagen for type III female stress incontinence: the first 50 Australian patients. Med J Australia 1993;158:89–91.

27. Kieswetter H, Fischer M, Wöber L, Flamm J: Endoscopic implantation of collagen (GAX) for the treatment of urinary incontinence. Br J Urol 1992;69:22–5.

28. O'Connell HE, McGuire EJ, Aboseif S, Usui A. Transurethral collagen therapy in women. J Urol 1995;154:1463–5.

29. Moore KN, Chetner MP, Metcalfe JB, Griffiths DJ. Periurethral implantation of glutaraldehyde cross-linked collagen (contigen7) in women with type I or type III stress incontinence: quantitative outcome measures. Br J Urol 1995;75:359–63.

30. Herschorn S, Radomski SB. Collagen injections for genuine stress urinary incontinence: Patient selection and durability. Int Urogynecol J 1997;8:18–24.

31. Smith DN, Appell RA, Winters JC, Rackley RR. Collagen injection therapy for female intrinsic sphincteric deficiency. J Urol 1997;157:1275–8.

32. Swami S, Batista JE, Abrams P. Collagen for female genuine stress incontinence after a minimum 2-year follow-up. Br J Urol 1997;80:757–61.

33. Cross CA, English SF, Cespedes RD, McGuire, EJ. A followup on transurethral collagen injection therapy for urinary incontinence. J Urol 1998;159:106–8.

34. Berman CJ, Kreder KJ. Comparative cost analysis of collagen injection and fascia lata sling cystourethropexy for the treatment of type III incontinence in women. J Urol 1997;157:122–4.

35. Sweat SW, Lightner DJ. Complications of sterile abscess formation and pulmonary embolism following periurethral bulking agents. J Urol 1999;161:93–6.

36. Stothers L, Goldenberg SL, Leone EF. Complications of periurethral collagen injection for stress urinary incontinence. J Urol 1998;159:806–7.

37. Elson ML. The role of skin testing in the use of collagen injectable materials. J Derml Surg Oncol 1986;15:301.

38. McClelland M, DeLustro F. Evaluation of antibody class in response to bovine collagen treatment in patients with urinary incontinence. J Urol 1996;155:2068–73.

39. Diagnostic and Therapeutic Technology Assessment (DATTA). Use of Teflon preparations for urinary incontinence and vesicoureteral reflux. JAMA 1993;269:2975–80.

40. Malizia AA, Reiman HM, Myers RP, Sande JR, Barham SS, Benson RC, Dewanjee MK, Utz WJ. Migration and granulomatous reaction after periurethral injection of Polytef (Teflon). JAMA 1983;251: 3277–81.

41. Herschorn S, Glazer AA. Early experience with small volume periurethral teflon for female stress urinary incontinence. J Urol 2000;163:1838–42.

42. Politano VA. Periurethral polytetrafluoroethylene injection for urinary incontinence. J Urol 1982;127:439–442.

43. Lim, KB, Ball AJ, Feneley RCL. Periurethral teflon injection: A simple treatment for urinary incontinence. Br J Urol 1983;55:208–10.

44. Schulman CC, Simon J, Wespes E et al. Endoscopic injections of teflon to treat urinary incontinence in women. Br Med J 1984;288:192.

45. Deane AM, English P, Hehir M, Williams JP, Worth PHL. Teflon injection in stress incontinence. Br J Urol 1985;57:78–80.

46. Beckingham IJ, Wemyss-Holden G, Lawrence WT. Long-term follow-up of women treated with perurethral Teflon injections for stress incontinence. Br J Urol 1992;69:580–3.

47. Harrison SC, Brown C, O'Boyle PJ. Periurethral Teflon for stress urinary incontinence: medium-term results. Br J Urol 1993;71:25–7.

48. Lotenfoe R, O'Kelly JK, Helal M, Lockhart JL. Periurethral polytetrafluoroethylene paste injection in incontinent female subjects: surgical indications and improved surgical technique. J Urol 1993;149:279–82.

49. Lopez AE, Padron OF, Patsias G, Politano VA. Transurethral polytetrafluoroethylene injection in female patients with urinary incontinence. J Urol 1993;150:856–8.

50. Vesey SG, Rivett A, O'Boyle PJ. Teflon injection in female stress incontinence. Effect on urethral pressue profile and flow rate. Br J Urol 1988;62:39–41.

51. Claes H, Stroobants D, van Meerbeek J et al. Pulmonary migration following periurethral polytetrafluoroethylene injection for urinary incontinence. J Urol 1989;142:821–2.

52. Mittleman RE, Marraccini JV. Pulmonary teflon granulomas following periurethral teflon injection for urinary incontinence. Arch Pathol Lab Med 1983;107:611–12.

53. Kiilhoma, PJ, Chancellor MB, Makinen J, Hirsch IH, Klemi PJ. Complications of teflon injection for stress urinary incontinence. Neurourol Urodyn 1993;12:131–7.

54. Stanisic TH, Jennings CE, Miller JI. Polytetrafluoroethylene injection for post-prostatectomy incontinence: experience with 20 patients during 3 years. J Urol 1991;146:1575–7.

55. Dewan PA, Owen AJ, Byard RW. Long-term histologic response to subcutaneously injected Polytef and Bioplastique in a rat model. Br J Urol 1995;76:161–4.

56. Billings E, May JW. Historical review and present status of free fat graft autotransplantation in plastic and reconstructive surgery. Plast Reconstr Surg 1989;83:368–81.

57. Horl HW, Feller AM, Bieuner E. Technique for liposuction fat re-implantation and long-term evaluation by magnetic resonance imaging. Ann Plast Surg 1991;26:248–58.

58. Bircoll M, Novack BH. Autologous fat transplantation employing liposuction techniques. Ann Plast Surg 1987;18:327–9.

59. Trockman BA, Leach GE. Surgical treatment of intrinsic urethral dysfunction: injectables (fat). Urol Clin North Am 1995;22:665–71.

60. Su T-H, Wang K-G, Hsu C-Y et al. Periurethral fat injection in the treatment of recurrent genuine stress incontinence. J Urol 1998;159:411–14.

61. Santarosa RP, Blaivas JG. Periurethral injection of autologous fat for the treatment of sphincteric incontinence. J Urol 1994;151:607–11.

62. Haab F, Zimmern PE, Leach GE. Urinary stress incontinence due to intrinsic sphincteric deficiency: experience with fat and collagen periurethral injections. J Urol 1997;157:1283–6.

63. Palma PC, Riccetto CL, Herrmann V, Netto NR Jr. Repeat lipoinjections for stress urinary incontinence. J Endourol 1997;11:67–70.

64. Palma PC, Riccetto CL, Netto Jr NR. Urethral pseudolipoma: a complication of periurethral lipo-injection for stress urinary incontinence in a woman. J Urol 1996;155:646.

65. Currie I, Drutz HP, Beck J, Oxorn D. Adipose tissue and lipid droplet embolism following periurethral injection of autologous fat – case report and review of the literature. Int Urogynecol J 1997;8(6):377–80.

66. Henly DR, Barrett DM, Weiland TL, O'Connor MK, Malizia AA, Wein AJ. Particulate silicone for use in periurethral injections: local tissue effects and search for migration. J Urol 1995;153: 2039–43.

67. Sherriff MKM, Foley S, McFarlane J, Nauth-Misir R, Shah PJR. Endoscopic correction of intractable stress incontinence with silicone micro-implants. Eur Urol 1997;32:284–8.

68. Koelbl H, Saz V, Doerfler D, Haeusler G, Sam C, Hanzal E. Transurethral injection of silicone microimplants for intrinsic sphincter deficiency. Obstet Gynecol 1998;92: 332–6.

69. Radley SC, Chapple CR, Mitsogiannis IC, Glass KS. Transurethral implantation of Macroplastique® for the treatment of female stress urinary incontinence secondary to urethral sphincter deficiency. Eur Urol 2001;39:383–9.

70. Yoo JJ, Magliochetti M, Atala A. Detachable self-sealing membrane system for the endoscopic treatment of incontinence. J Urol 1997;158: 1045–8.

71. Mayer R, Lightfoot M, Jung I. Preliminary evaluation of calcium hydroxylapatite as a transurethral bulking agent for stress urinary incontinence. Urology 2001;57:434–8.

37 Fecal Incontinence; Rectal Prolapse

Martin Friedlich and Marcus J. Burnstein

Fecal incontinence can be a devastating problem with major social implications. The prevalence of fecal incontinence is 0.5–1.5% in the general population, and if soiling is included, the prevalence reaches approximately 5% [1,2]. Fecal incontinence is much more common in women: the incidence in 45-year-old women is eight times higher than in men of a similar age, and 6–10% of women experience urgency and incontinence after vaginal delivery. Studies using endoanal ultrasound have shown that one-third of women have occult injury of the anal sphincter after vaginal delivery [3,4]. These occult obstetrical injuries may cause immediate problems or may predispose to incontinence later in life, as menopause and aging add their effects.

Table 37.1 Classification of the etiology of fecal incontinence

Altered stool consistency: diarrheal states
irritable bowel syndrome
inflammatory bowel disease
laxative abuse
infectious diarrhea
Inadequate reservoir capacity or compliance
proctitis
absent rectal reservoir (sphincter-saving resection)
overflow incontinence
Abnormal sphincter mechanism
anatomic sphincter defect (obstetic injury, anorectal surgery)
pelvic floor and sphincter denervation
congenital abnormalities
miscellaneous (aging, rectal prolapse)

Mechanisms of Continence

Fecal continence is maintained through multiple, interrelated mechanisms and disturbances to any of these may be associated with diminished continence (Table 37.1) [5,6]. The involuntary, smooth muscle internal anal sphincter has intrinsic tone and is responsible for 50–85% of resting anal pressure. The remainder of the resting anal tone is provided by the external sphincter and the hemorrhoidal cushions [7]. The external sphincter contributes to resting tone as a result of a reflex arc between stretch receptors in the sphincter and pelvic floor muscles and the cauda equina [8]. The external anal sphincter and levator ani muscles are comprised predominantly of type I, fatigue-resistant, skeletal muscle fibers, making them suitable for tonic activity [9]. The external sphincter and pelvic floor are innervated by the pudendal nerves and the inferior rectal nerves.

The internal anal sphincter transiently relaxes in response to rectal distension, the so-called rectoanal inhibitory reflex. This reflex permits rectal contents to be assessed or "sampled" by the rich sensory nerve endings of the upper anal canal. Anal sensation and sampling are important in fine control and allow discrimination between solid, liquid, and gas within the rectum [10]. Defective anal sensation and sampling may contribute to fecal incontinence.

Aging significantly affects continence and physiologic tests reveal decreasing resting tone and deteriorating pudendal nerve function with increasing age [11].

Disruption of the internal anal sphincter primarily results in passive fecal incontinence – loss of stool without awareness or warning. External anal sphincter dysfunction results in urgency incontinence because of the patient's inability to squeeze [12].

Incontinence Following Childbirth

Diminished continence after childbirth is a significant problem: in one survey of women who delivered vaginally without sustaining a clinically obvious tear, 5% were found to have fecal incontinence if loss of flatus was included [13]; in another survey, 4% described the new development of significant fecal incontinence after delivery [14].

The etiology of fecal incontinence after childbirth is sphincter disruption, nerve injury, or both [15]. The vast majority of these women have structural damage to one or both sphincters. In a prospective study, Sultan et al. demonstrated sphincter defects by endoanal ultrasound in 35% of primiparous women, and this increased to 80% following a forceps delivery [16,17]. Women with sphincter defects had lower anal pressure than those without and all the women with symptoms had sonographic sphincter defects. There was no correlation between pudendal nerve function, as measured by pudendal nerve terminal motor latency, and the development of fecal incontinence [16]. Pudendal nerve terminal motor latency was prolonged in 16% of women after vaginal delivery but only one-third of these remained prolonged at 6 months [18]. Others have found that the damage persists [19]. Changes in pudendal nerve function were associated with a heavier infant and a prolonged second stage. The degree to which pudendal nerve injury contributes to incontinence after childbirth is arguable. Recent work with endoanal ultrasonography strongly supports the concept that disruption of the sphincter is the dominant mechanism. Isolated pudendal neuropathy appears to be rare [20].

Between 0.5 and 1% of women delivering vaginally sustain a third-degree tear defined as a perineal laceration involving the anal sphincter, with or without involvement of the anal mucosa. Risk factors for third-degree tears are forceps, primiparous delivery, large infant (greater than 4 kg), occipitoposterior presentation and a prolonged second stage of labour [19,20]. Despite primary repair of the laceration in the delivery suite, there is a high incidence of residual structural damage and diminished continence. Incontinence after a third-degree tear occurs in 7–20%, and if urgency is included, 47% of patients with third-degree tears have control problems [20].

The role of episiotomy is controversial. Episiotomy certainly does not provide complete protection against third-degree tears [21]. In a randomized controlled trial, midline episiotomy was associated with a higher risk of sphincter injury

than mediolateral episiotomy [22]. Instrumental vaginal delivery has been found to be an independent variable associated with the development of fecal incontinence [16]. Forceps appear to be associated with more severe perineal and occult sphincter trauma than the vacuum extractor [4,17,23].

Impaired anal sensation has been demonstrated in women after vaginal delivery compared to controls or women delivered by cesarean section, but this effect appears to be transient, and at 6 months there was no difference between groups [24].

Management

Management of the patient with fecal incontinence is determined by the severity of the problem, and whether the sphincter is anatomically disrupted or intact (Figure 37.1) [6]. It is important to determine the degree to which fecal incontinence is interfering with the patient's quality of life and restricting their professional, social, and sexual activity. The need for pads, changes of underwear, and the frequency of incontinence episodes for solids and liquids are good indicators of the severity of the problem. Scoring systems allow a more objective assessment of function and facilitate comparison before and after treatment, as well as comparisons between different treatments [5] (Table 37.2).

The severity of fecal incontinence is the major determinant of the therapeutic approach: the less

Table 37.2 Continence grading system

Type of continence	never	rarely	frequency sometimes	usually	always
Solid	0	1	2	3	4
Liquid	0	1	2	3	4
Gas	0	1	2	3	4
Wears pad	0	1	2	3	4
Lifestyle alteration	0	1	2	3	4

0 = perfect.
20 = complete incontinence.
Never = 0 (never).
Rarely = < 1/month
Sometimes = < 1/week, ≥ 1/month.
Usually = < 1/day, ≥ 1/week.
Always = ≥ 1/day.
The continence score is determined by adding points from the above table, which takes into account the type and frequency of incontinence and the extent to which it alters the patient's life.

From Jorg JMM, Wexner SD. Etiology and management of faecal incontinence. Dis Colon Rectum 1993;36:77–97 (with permission).

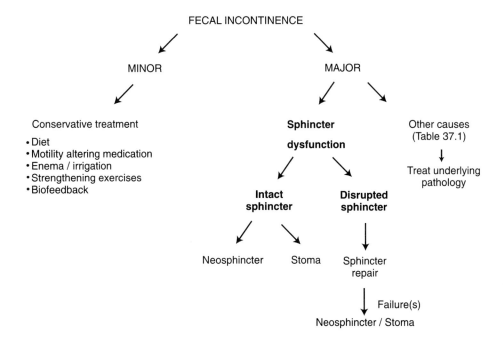

Figure 37.1 Treament of fecal incontinence

severe the incontinence the less aggressive the thera-peutic response. A good surgical rule is never try to fix flatus incontinence. If the problem with dimin-ished continence is not accompanied by lifestyle alterations or restrictions in daily activities, a non-operative approach is best. Minor degrees of inconti-nence are common in elderly multiparous women, and the great majority of these patients are success-fully managed with a conservative approach. Conservative treatment principles include increasing stool consistency though diet and anti-diarrhoeal medications, pelvic floor strengthening exercises, and biofeedback. Loperamide has a constipating effect, increases internal anal sphincter tone, and is well tolerated [25]. "Planned" bowel movements with the use of enemas or irrigation techniques may also prove helpful. In biofeedback, the voluntary activity of the external anal sphincter is displayed to the patient with either a manometric or electromyo-graphic technique. The patient receives feedback on sphincter response and encouragement is given to improve the response. Biofeedback can improve both external anal sphincter contraction and rectal sensa-tion. Complete recovery or significant reduction in incontinence episodes has been reported in two-thirds of patients. The success of biofeedback has been correlated more with improved sensation than sphincter strengthening. Patient selection is based on patient motivation and the preservation of some rectal sensation and voluntary sphincter contraction [5]. The impact of biofeedback may be transient [26,27]. Perineal strengthening exercises have not been well evaluated, but their impact appears to be modest [5].

The presence of a major sphincter disruption can generally be determined by careful history and physical examination. A detailed obstetrical history is essential. Physical examination, including sigmoi-doscopy, provides information regarding resting tone, squeeze pressure, the integrity of the sphinc-ter, anorectal sensation, and rectal compliance. Rectal prolapse should be ruled out, especially in older patients, and this may necessitate examination with the patient in a squatting position. This diag-nosis must be considered even when the patient is not complaining of protrusion. Structural assess-ment by endoanal ultrasound and physiologic assessment by anal manometry and pudendal nerve terminal motor latency are useful adjuncts. Endosonography is able to characterize internal and external sphincter structural damage and help guide treatment selection [28]. Prolonged pudendal nerve terminal motor latency predicts a poor result from operative repair of a disrupted sphincter. Normal pudendal nerve terminal latency does not exclude nerve damage [8].

Patients with severe incontinence and a single or dominant defect in the external anal sphincter should undergo operative repair. Overlapping anterior sphincteroplasty achieves continence for solids and liquids in 70–80% of patients [5,28,29] (Figure 37.2). The scar tissue at the site of sphincter

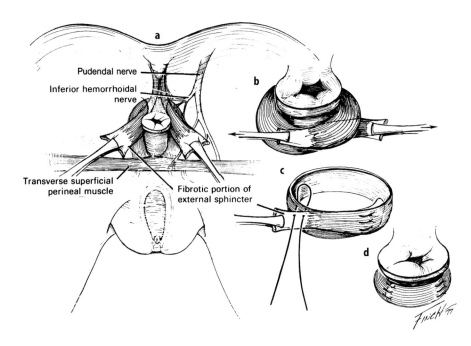

Figure 37.2 Sphincteroplasty. **a**, The divided sphincter is mobilized with preservation of scar tissue **b, c, d**, The fibro, muscular ends are overlapped and mattress sutures placed. (SM Goldberg, PH Gordon, A Nivatvongs. *Essentials of Anorectal Surgery*, 1st edn. Philadelphia, JB Lippincott, 1980.)

disruption is divided. The fibromuscular ends are mobilized and overlapped to re-establish a ring of sphincter muscle. The operation is done under mechanical and antibiotic bowel preparation, and stool softeners are given in the early postoperative period. A temporary diverting stoma is not needed. In women who are able to cope with their symptoms, it may be prudent to postpone operative repair until childbearing is complete. If symptoms are unmanageable, repair should be undertaken and cesarean section should be recommended for future deliveries. Anorectal function is not affected by elective cesarean section [4,19].

For patients who fail to improve after sphincter reconstruction, for those with weak but intact sphincters, or for those with complex sphincter injuries, the treatment is much less clear [20]. The options are continued conservative treatment, a stoma, or a neosphincter procedure, either the artificial anal sphincter device or a skeletal muscle transposition. Parks postanal repair, which involves posterior dissection in the intersphincteric plane and plication of the puborectalis and external sphincter muscles, has been used in the treatment of fecal incontinence due to intact but weak sphincters. The results have generally been poor and the procedure has become increasingly uncommon [30–32].

Early results with the artificial anal sphincter device are promising [33–35]. The artificial anal sphincter is a modification of the artificial urinary sphincter (Figure 37.3). It comprises three Silastic components: an inflatable cuff, a pressure regulating balloon, and a control pump. The cuff is implanted around the anus, the control pump in the scrotum or labia majora, and the balloon in the space of Retzius. Silastic tubing connects the three components, and the system is filled with fluid. The cuff distends with fluid, occludes the anal canal and provides continence. When the patient has the urge to defecate, the control pump is compressed several times and fluid is displaced from the cuff to the

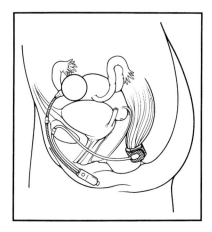

Figure 37.3 Artificial bowel sphincter. (Courtesy of American Medical Systems, Inc., Minnetonka, Minnesota, USA)

balloon. The cuff deflates and defecation can occur. Fluid returns to the cuff over the next 7–10 minutes. Continence to solids and liquids is reported in 70–90% of patients, continence for flatus in approximately 50%. Infectious complications and mechanical problems occur in 33% of patients and explantation because of complications or poor function has been reported in a similar percentage. Data on long-term function and morbidity are not available. A protecting stoma is not routinely used.

The greatest experience with muscle transposition involves wrapping the gracilis muscle around the anus. Dynamic graciloplasty involves electrical stimulation of the transposed muscle via a pacemaker [36] (Figure 37.4). Low frequency electrical stimulation generates tonic contraction and promotes conversion of the skeletal muscle fibers from fatigue prone, type II fibers to fatigue resistant, type I fibers. Continence to solids and liquids has been achieved in 60–78% following dynamic graciloplasty [36–39]. Technical, infectious and functional complications are common but can often be treated [38].

There is one report of the application of sacral nerve stimulation in which improvement in sphincter pressures and continence is described in three patients [40]. The place of the two neosphincter procedures and of sacral nerve stimulation in the management of fecal incontinence is in evolution.

Conclusion

Sphincter injury is common following vaginal delivery. When a single defect is associated with significant fecal incontinence, an overlapping sphincter repair achieves satisfactory results in the majority of patients. When the sphincter muscles are weak but intact, when only the internal sphincter is disrupted, or when there are multiple defects in both sphincters, the therapeutic approach is not clear. Some patients may achieve a satisfactory level of continence with bowel management and biofeedback. For the rest, the neosphincters represent an exciting new alternative to colostomy.

Rectal Prolapse

Rectal prolapse is a circumferential full-thickness intussusception of the rectum in which the lead point of the intussusception descends through the anal canal to appear on the outside. Rectal prolapse primarily affects elderly women. It is a miserable condition, usually associated with fecal incontinence, and frequently associated with constipation and disordered defecation. Patients can rarely cope with the symptoms and operative repair of rectal

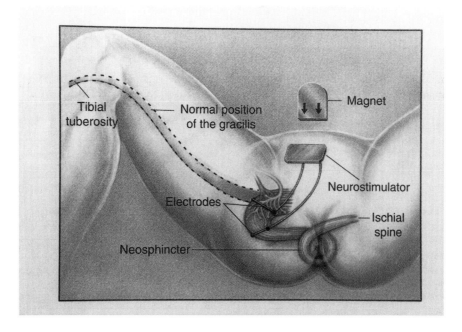

Figure 37.4 Dynamic gracilplasty. From Baeten CG, Geerdes BP, Adang EM, Heineman E, Konsten J, Engel GL, Kester AS, Spaans F, SOeters PB. Anal dynamic graciloplasty in the treatment of intractable faecal incontinence. N Engl J Med 1995;332(24):1600–1605, with permission. © 1995 Massachusetts Medical Society. All rights reserved.

prolapse is almost always indicated. Unfortunately, repairing the prolapse often fails to alleviate the associated symptoms. The best way to repair rectal prolapse remains one of the most difficult and contentious issues in colorectal surgery.

Etiology and Pathogenesis

It is well accepted that rectal prolapse is an intussusception of the rectum, with the lead point 6–8 cm above the pelvic floor [41] (Figure 37.5). The primary cause of the intussusception remains uncertain and the many anatomic defects seen in association with rectal prolapse may all be secondary phenomena. The five most consistent anatomic abnormalities are: (1) diastasis of the levator muscles, (2) a deep cul-de-sac, (3) a redundant rectosigmoid colon, (4) a patulous anus, and (5) loss of the normal "horizontal" position of the

rectum within the sacral hollow [42]. Other frequent features are pudendal neuropathy, uterine prolapse, cystocele, rectocele, enterocele, and perineal descent. Combined rectal and genitourinary prolapse is common but sequential rather than synchronous occurrence is the rule, with descent of the genitourinary system usually preceding rectal prolapse [43]. The gastrointestinal and genitourinary findings in patients with rectal prolapse indicate a diffuse loss of support within the pelvis. Whether this is primarily an abnormality of nerves, pelvic floor muscles, or the endopelvic fascia is not clear. Neither parity nor obstetrical injury appears to play a significant role in the etiology of rectal prolapse [42].

Clinical Features

Women predominate in a ratio of 6 to 1. The incidence of rectal prolapse in women begins to rise in

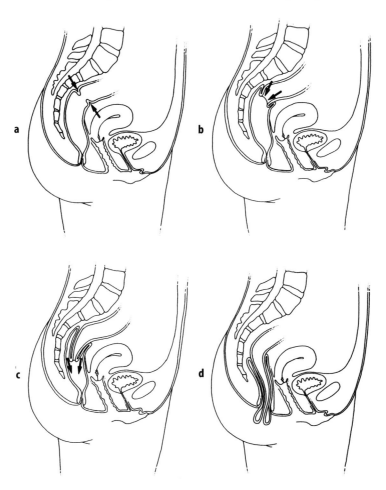

Figure 37.5 Rectal prolapse progressing from internal intussusception (a–c) to complete procidentia (d). From Gordon PH, Nivatvongs A. Principles and Practice of Surgery for the Colon, Rectum and Anus. Quality Medical Publishing, INc., St. Louis, Missouri, 1992, with permission.

the fifth decade, and peaks in the seventh decade. The incidence in men has an even age distribution [42]. Patients complain not only of tissue protrusion but also of fecal incontinence, mucus discharge, constipation, difficult or incomplete evacuation, bleeding, and discomfort. The functional symptoms, especially fecal incontinence and discharge, often predominate, and the history of protrusion may need to be specifically sought. The mass may protrude only at defecation, or may protrude with slight exertion, or even by assuming an upright posture. Manual reduction of the prolapse is usually required. Urinary incontinence and symptoms of gynecologic prolapse may also be present.

Physical findings include a patulous lax anus which may gape open with separation of the buttocks. Straining demonstrates perineal descent followed by the appearance of concentric mucosal folds. The mucosa may be erythematous or even ulcerated. Bidigital palpation of the prolapse reveals the double wall of an intussusception. An enterocele may be felt anteriorly. Cystocele, uterine prolapse, and rectocele may coexist. If rectal prolapse is suspected but not confirmed on routine examination, it is essential to accompany the patient to the toilet, where the patient can strain in a squatting position and more readily demonstrate the prolapse. Sigmoidoscopy may reveal erythema and edema, especially on the anterior rectal wall between 6–10 cm.

Prolapsing internal hemorrhoids may share some symptoms with rectal prolapse, but these two clinical conditions can be distinguished on physical examination. Prolapsing internal hemorrhoids are characterized by radial mucosal folds and a normal or high tone sphincter on digital examination, in contrast to the concentric mucosal folds and low tone sphincter of rectal prolapse [42,44].

Investigation

Other pathology in the colon and rectum should be excluded by colonoscopy or by a combination of sigmoidoscopy and barium enema. Defecography may be indicated when the diagnosis cannot be confirmed by physical examination. The need for additional work-up is controversial. It has been suggested that the operative treatment of rectal prolapse can be tailored to the associated pathophysiology and that each patient should therefore be evaluated with respect to colonic transit (marker study), anal sphincter function (anal manometry, pudendal nerve terminal motor latency), and rectal function (balloon expulsion testing, defecography, and tests of rectal compliance and sensation) [45]. Although there are few data to support this, a selec-

tive approach to physiologic testing may be appropriate, as determined by the clinical setting and the dominant symptoms.

Treatment

Many operations have been described, and there is no consensus regarding which is best. It is becoming increasingly accepted that no single operation is best in all circumstances. In selecting the best procedure for an individual patient, the surgeon must consider the general health and age of the patient, the morbidity, mortality and recurrence rates for the operation, and the effect of the operation on concomitant symptoms like fecal incontinence, constipation, and ineffective emptying. It is important to recognize that, regardless of the operative approach taken, correction of the prolapse is not equivalent to symptom control: fecal incontinence, constipation, mucus discharge, and tenesmus may persist despite operative control of the prolapse [46]. The following is a simplified and subjective overview of the treatment of rectal prolapse.

The main operative approaches to rectal prolapse are abdominal and perineal. In general, the abdominal operations have lower rates of recurrence than the perineal operations, but are associated with greater morbidity. The complications of abdominal operations are related to laparotomy, rectal mobilization, and colorectal resection, including bleeding from presacral veins, infection, bowel obstruction, and particularly in male patients, sexual dysfunction secondary to pelvic autonomic nerve injury. The morbidity of abdominal operations may be reduced by a laparoscopic approach. The common abdominal operations have all been performed laparoscopically with efficacy and safety [47–50].

The true incidence of constipation and fecal incontinence in patients with rectal prolapse and the real impact of the various operations on these symptoms are extremely difficult to establish. This is the result of inconsistent definitions for incontinence and constipation and inconsistent preoperative and postoperative documentation of these symptoms. Interpreting the data is made more difficult by the many minor modifications of the same operation performed by different surgeons.

Constipation is seen in about one-third to one-half of patients with rectal prolapse. After abdominal repairs, an increase in the incidence of constipation and evacuation problems can be expected, up to double the preoperative rate. An exception to this may be abdominal repairs that include colonic resection, where an improvement in bowel function seems more likely, especially with more extensive resections. The impact of perineal operations on constipation and ineffective rectal emptying is unpredictable – symptoms are equally likely to improve, deteriorate, or not change.

Fecal incontinence is reported in up to 100% of patients with rectal prolapse. Incontinence may be due to repeated stretching of the sphincter by the prolapsing rectum, or to pudendal neuropathy secondary to chronic perineal descent. Alternatively, incontinence and prolapse may both be manifestations of the same underlying neuromuscular deficiency. Following abdominal operations, continence improves in about half the patients by 6–12 months. Better results are reported for perineal operations that include plication of the levator muscles. The mechanism for improved continence following abdominal operations is not certain. Improvement may be related to removal of the source of persistent rectoanal inhibition or to the prolapse no longer holding the anus open [51]. An improvement in fecal continence cannot be reliably predicted preoperatively. However, patients with worse incontinence and worse function on physiologic tests appear less likely to benefit from repair. Worsening of fecal incontinence may occur in up to 5% [42,44,52]. Residual fecal incontinence after successful prolapse repair is extremely problematic. Biofeedback and bowel management with constipating medications, dietary modification, and enemas, may be beneficial. Parks postanal repair, a plication of the puborectalis and external anal sphincter, has been used in this setting with mixed results. A reliable salvage procedure for persistent fecal incontinence has not yet been described [42,52].

Problems of genitourinary prolapse may predate rectal prolapse and have usually already been dealt with by the gynecologist. Rarely, synchronous operations involving the urogynecologist and colorectal surgeon are performed to address coexistent rectal procidentia and prolapse of the genitourinary system [43].

Abdominal operations

The medically fit patient has conventionally been treated by an abdominal approach. The popular abdominal operations incorporate fixation of the mobilized rectum to the presacral fascia, with or without resection.

Rectopexy

The rectum is fully mobilized and as the rectum is retracted in a cephalad direction, the lateral liga-

ments of the rectum (or lateral rectal tissues) are fixed with sutures to the presacral fascia. The degree to which the rectum should be mobilized anteriorly and laterally is controversial, but there is complete agreement that full posterior mobilization to the tip of the coccyx is important in reducing recurrence. This is a simple procedure with a recurrence rate in the range of 5% in most series. The mobilized rectum may be anchored to the presacral fascia with the use of a prosthetic mesh which partially encircles the rectum (Figure 37.6). Different absorbable and non-absorbable materials and configurations have been used. A partial wrap, leaving the anterior quarter to half of the rectal circumference free, prevents obstruction. Anchoring the mesh to the presacral fascia 1 cm off the midline decreases the risk of injuring presacral veins. The peritoneum is closed over the mesh to avoid adhesion of small bowel loops. The recurrence rate with the mesh approach is also very low, less than 5% in many large series [42,44,52].

Rectopexy is associated with improved continence in approximately half. Constipation is inconsistently affected, but most authors have described worsening constipation and often severely disturbed rectal emptying following rectopexy. The tendency for constipation to persist or worsen following rectopexy, especially with prosthetic mesh, has led some to avoid this operation when constipation is present [51].

Resection

The resectional procedures are combination rectopexy–resection, anterior resection, and low anterior resection. When resection of the redundant sigmoid colon is added to rectopexy, prosthetic mesh is avoided because of the risk of infection. The colonic resection is extended proximally to eliminate the redundant colon. Recurrence is in the range of 5–10%. Resection-rectopexy may improve constipation and the likelihood of improvement is loosely related to the extent of resection. At the University of Minnesota, constipation was improved in 2/9 patients when sigmoidectomy was added to rectopexy and in 4/6 patients when subtotal colectomy was added [52,53]. Incontinence was improved in approximately one-third of the patients and was worsened in a similar number. Resection should be applied cautiously when incontinence is prominent because of the risk of diarrhoea [11]. At the Mayo Clinic, anterior resection with complete rectal mobilization achieved rates of recurrence of 6% at 5 years and 12% at 10 years [54]. Extending the resection below the peritoneal reflection increased morbidity without decreasing the recurrence rate.

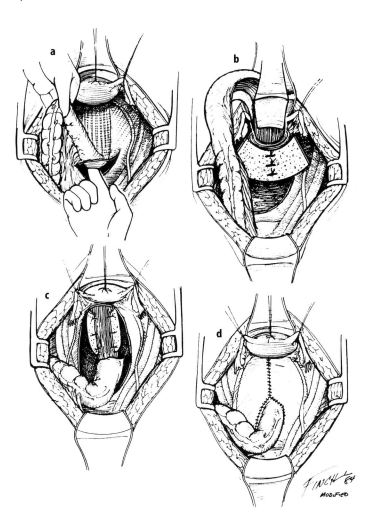

Figure 37.6 Rectopexy with prosthetic mesh. **a** The rectum is mobilized posteriorly to the tip of the coccyx. **b**, **c** A strip of mesh is anchored to the presacral fascia, partially wrapped around the rectum, and sutured to the rectal wall. **d** The pelvic peritoneum is closed over the mesh. (From Madoff RD, Watss JD, Rothenberger DA, Goldberg SM. Rectal prolapse: treatment. In: Henry MM, Swash M, editors. Coloproctology and the Pelvic Floor, 2nd edition. Butterworth-Heinemann Ltd, Toronto, 1992, pp 321–350, with permission.)

Perineal Approaches

The principal attraction of the perineal operations is that they are well tolerated by the elderly, often frail patients most commonly affected by this condition. Laparotomy is avoided and the perineal operations can be performed under regional or local anesthesia. Perineal procedures are especially attractive where there has been previous pelvic surgery. The convention of reserving the perineal approach for high risk patients has been challenged in recent years in the wake of improving results with these operations. The main perineal operations are the perineal proctosigmoidectomy and the Delorme procedure. As with the abdominal operations, full mechanical and antibiotic bowel preparation is used. The patient may be placed in lithotomy or prone jackknife position.

Delorme Procedure (Figure 37.7)

In this operation, the mucosa is circumferentially stripped off the underlying muscle from 1.5 cm proximal to the dentate line to the tip of the prolapsed rectum; the mucosal tube is dissected until resistance is encountered. A submucosal injection of 1:200,000 epinephrine solution facilitates the dissection. The denuded rectal wall is longitudinally plicated with a series of absorbable sutures, the mucosal tube is excised, and the mucosa is reapproximated. Morbidity and mortality are consistently very low. Recurrence rates range from 5 to

408

Female Pelvic Medicine and Reconstructive Pelvic Surgery

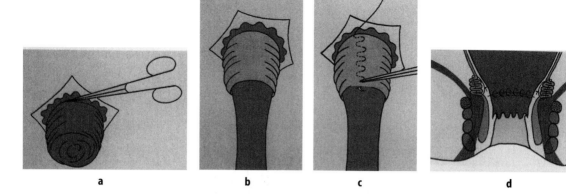

Figure 37.7 Delorme procedure. **a, b** Mucosectomy is begun 1.5 cm proximal to the dentate line and continued until there is resistance. **c, d** The muscle coat is plicated and mucosa re-approximated. (From Gordon PH, Nivatvongs A. Principles and Practice of Surgery for the Colon, Rectum and Anus. Quality Medical Publishing, Inc., St. Louis, Missouri, 1992, with permission.)

27%. Improved continence can be expected in 36–83% and worse continence in 0–3% [52,55–57].

Perineal Proctosigmoidectomy (Figures 37.8 and 37.9)

With the rectum prolapsed, a circumferential incision 2 cm proximal to the dentate line is deepened through the full thickness of the bowel wall. The peritoneum is opened and the rectosigmoid is mobilized until the redundant bowel cannot be pulled down any further. Anterior and posterior plication of the levator muscles may be added at this point. About 2 cm distal to the anus the inner tube of the rectosigmoid is transected along with its mesentery. An anastomosis is performed 1–2 cm proximal to the dentate line. Morbidity and mortality are low, but infectious complications and bleeding rates appear to be higher than with the Delorme procedure. Recurrence rates range from 0 to 60% with most recent reviews reporting recurrence rates of 5 to 10%. The concomitant levatorplasty has been reported to have a significant impact on continence with several authors indicating improved continence in 90% and full continence in two-thirds of patients [52,58–61].

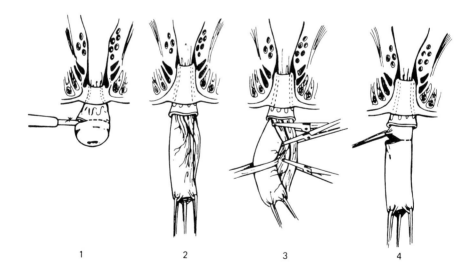

Figure 37.8 Perineal proctosigmoiddectomy. 1, Beginning of incision 2–3 cm proximal to the dentate line (when stapling devices are used, the bowel should be transected 1 cm longer). 2, Unfolding of the prolapse. 3, Mesenteric division. 4, Division of the inner cylinder of the intrussusception. (From Madoff RD, Watss JD, Rothenberger DA, Goldberg SM. Rectal prolapse: treatment. In: Henry MM, Swash M, editors. Coloproctology and the Pelvic Floor, 2nd edition. Butterworth-Heinemann Ltd, Toronto, 1992, pp 321–350, with permission.)

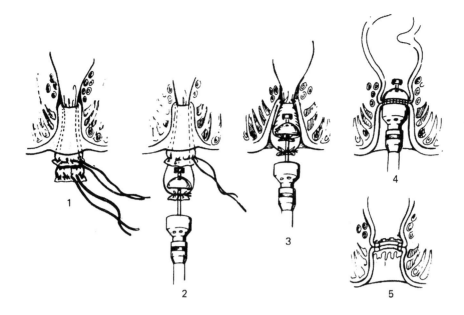

Figure 37.9 Perineal proctosigmoidectomy–continued. 1, Placement of purse-string sutures. 2, Proximal purse-string secured around anvil. 3, Distal purse-string secured. 4, Closure of instrument. 5, Completed anastomosis. (From Madoff RD, Watss JD, Rothenberger DA, Goldberg SM. Rectal prolapse: treatment. In: Henry MM, Swash M, editors. Coloproctology and the Pelvic Floor, 2nd edition. Butterworth-Heinemann Ltd, Toronto, 1992, pp 321–350, with permission.)

Anal Encirclement

Encircling the anus with mesh, Silastic tubing, or suture is not recommended because of the high complication rate, in particular the high rate of fecal impaction and related problems of bowel function. Infectious complications and erosion of the foreign body are also encountered. The advantage of technical simplicity has not been sufficient to sustain this operation, which has been supplanted by the more technically demanding Delorme procedure and perineal proctosigmoidectomy, both of which can be performed in even the most frail of patients.

Internal Intussusception

Defecography may demonstrate rectal intussusception in which the lead point remains above the pelvic floor, so-called internal intussusception or "occult" rectal prolapse. Although this may represent an early stage of rectal prolapse, it is not clear that internal intussusception eventually progresses to true procidentia [42,45]. In fact, a degree of rectal intussusception may be seen on defecography in a variety of pelvic floor disorders, as well as in normal controls [62].

Patients found to have internal intussusception have usually presented with symptoms of obstructed defecation. Straining, self-digitation, pain, mucus, bleeding, and incontinence are often present. Sigmoidoscopy may reveal the changes of solitary rectal ulcer syndrome, most commonly at 6–10 cm on the anterior wall. These changes include mucosal edema, hyperemia, solitary or multiple shallow ulcers, or heaped up polypoid mucosa resembling a neoplasm. The histopathology is characterized by a lamina propria expanded with collagen, fibroblasts, and smooth muscle cells. The smooth muscle cells pass upwards from the muscularis mucosa at right angles to the longitudinal axis. Colitis cystica profunda is a form of the condition in which dilated glands are displaced in the submucosa where they may be mistaken for carcinoma [63]. The changes of solitary rectal ulcer syndrome may also be encountered in association with true rectal prolapse, but are more commonly seen in association with internal intussusception [45,63].

The treatment of internal intussusception, with or without associated solitary rectal ulcer syndrome, is directed at the underlying defecation disorder [63,64]. Dietary modification, avoidance of straining, and biofeedback "retraining" of the defecation mechanism, benefit most patients. Operative correction of internal intussusception, by either rectopexy or resection, is not recommended. When solitary rectal ulcer syndrome is accompanied by true procidentia, as it is in about one-third of patients, abdominal repair of the prolapse is indicated. Ulcer healing can be expected, but as in all patients with rectal prolapse, symptomatic improvement is much less certain [52,63].

Conclusion

Our understanding of rectal prolapse is incomplete and our treatment is imperfect. Abdominal operations have demonstrated the ability to reliably correct prolapse, but troublesome constipation, evacuation disturbance, and incontinence often persist or worsen. Perineal repairs are well tolerated, but the reported experience in terms of recurrence and residual fecal incontinence is diverse. Recent reports are encouraging and perineal operations are becoming more widely applied. Our challenges are to gain a better understanding of the pathophysiology of rectal prolapse, to develop operations which better address the concomitant functional disturbances, and to learn how better to select patients for the various operations.

References

1. Drossman DA, Sander RS, Broome CM, McKee DC. Urgency and faecal soiling in people with bowel dysfunction. Dig Dis Sci 1986;31:1221–5.
2. Enck P, Bielefeld TK, Rathman W et al. Epidemiology of faecal incontinence in selected patient groups. Int J Colorect Dis 1991;6:143–6.
3. Henry NM. Pathogenesis and management of faecal incontinence in the adult. Gastroenterol Clin North Am 1987;16:35–45.
4. Sultan AH, Kamm MA. Faecal incontinence after childbirth. Br J Obstet Gynaecol Sept 1997;104:979–82.
5. Jorge JMM, Wexner SD. Etiology and management of faecal incontinence. Dis Colon Rectum 1993;36:77–97.
6. Burnstein MJ. Constipation and faecal incontinence: is surgery necessary? Canadian Journal of CME, Mar 1997;49–57.
7. Read NW, Sun WM. Anal manometry. In: Henry MM, Swash M, editors. Coloproctology and the Pelvic Floor, 2nd edn. Toronto: Butterworth-Heinemann, 1992;119–45.
8. Swash M, Snooks SJ. Motor nerve conduction studies of the pelvic floor innervation. In: Henry MM, Swash M, editors. Coloproctology and the Pelvic Floor, 2nd edn. Toronto: Butterworth-Heinemann, 1992;196–206.
9. Swash M. Histopathology of pelvic floor muscles in pelvic floor disorder. In: Henry MM, Swash M, editors. Coloproctology and the Pelvic Floor, 2nd edn. Toronto: Butterworth-Heinemann, 1992;173–83.
10. Miller R, Bartolo DC, Cewero F, Mortensen NJ. Anorectal sampling: a comparison of normal and incontinent patients. Br J Surg 1988;75:44–7.
11. Jameson JS, Chia YW, Kamm MA, Speakman CT, Chye YH, Henry MM. Effect of age, sex and parity on anorectal function. Br J Surg 1994;81:1689–92.
12. Gee AS, Durdey P. Urge incontinence of faeces is a marker of severe external anal sphincter dysfunction. Br J Surg 1995;82:1179–82.
13. Ryhammer AM, Beck KM, Laurberg S. Multiple vaginal deliveries increase the risk of permanent incontinence of flatus and urine in normal premenopausal women. Dis Colon Rectum 1995;38:1206–9.
14. MacArthur C, Bick DE, Keighley MRB. Fecal incontinence after childbirth. Br J Obstet Gynaecol 1997;104:46–50.
15. Snooks SJ, Henry MM, Swash M. Faecal incontinence due to external anal sphincter division in childbirth is associated with damage to the innervation of the pelvic floor musculature: a double pathology. Br J Obstet Gynaecol 1985;92:824–8.
16. Sultan AH, Kamm MA, Hudson CN, Thomas JM, Bartram CI. Anal sphincter disruption during vaginal delivery. N Engl J Med 1993;329:1905–11.
17. Sultan AH, Kamm MA, Bartram CL, Hudson CN. Third degree obstetric anal sphincter tears: Risk factors and outcome of primary repair. BMJ 1994;308:887–91.
18. Sultan AH, Kamm MA, Hudson CN. Pudendal nerve damage during labour: prospective study before and after childbirth. Br J Obstet Gynaecol 1994;101:22–8.
19. Snooks SJ, Swash M, Mathers SE, Henry MM. Effect of vaginal delivery on the pelvic floor: a 5 year follow-up. Br J Surg 1990;77:1358–60.
20. Vaisey CJ, Kamm MA, Nicholls RJ. Recent advances in the surgical treatment of faecal incontinence. Br J Surg 1998;85:596–603.
21. Cook TA, Mortenson NJMC. Management of faecal incontinence following obstetrical injury. Br J Surg 1998;85:293–8.
22. Coats PM, Chan KK, Wilkins M, Beard RJ. A comparison between midline and nediolateral episiotomies. Br J Obstet Gynaecol 1980;87:408–12.
23. Johanson RB, Rice C, Doyle M et al. A randomized prospective study comparing the new vacuum extractor policy with forceps delivery. Br J Obstet Gynaecol 1993;100:524–30.
24. Cornes H, Bartolo DC, Stirrat GM. Changes in anal canal sensation after childbirth. Br J Surg 1991;78:74–7.
25. Hallgren T, Fasth S, Delbro DS, Nordgren S, Oresland T, Hulten L. Loperamide improves anal sphincter function and continence after restorative proctocolectomy. Dig Dis Sci 1994;39(12):2612–18.
26. Glia A, Gylin M, Akerlund JE, Lindors U, Lindberg G. Biofeedback training in patients with fecal incontinence. Dis Colon Rectum 1998;41(3):359–64.
27. Guillemot F, Bouche B, Gower-Rousseau C, Chartier M, Wolschies E, Lamblin MD, Haebonnier E, Cortot A. Biofeedback for the treatment of fecal incontinence. Long term clinical results. Dis Colon Rectum 1995;38(4):393–7.
28. Engel AF, Kamm MA, Sultan AH, Bartram CI, Nichols RJ. Anterior anal sphincter repair for patients with obstetric trauma. Br J Surg 1994;81:1231–4.
29. Briel JW, deBoer LM, Hop WC, Schouten WR. Clinical outcome of anterior overlapping external anal sphincter repair with internal anal sphincter imbrication. Dis Colon Rectum 1998;41(2):209–14.
30. Engel AF, van Baal SJ, Brummelkamp WH. Late results of postanal repair for idiopathic faecal incontinence. Eur J Surg 1994;160:637–40.
31. Jameson JS, Speakman CT, Danzi A, Chia YW, Henry MM. Audit of postanal repair in the treatment of faecal incontinence. Dis Colon Rectum 1994;37:369–72.
32. Rieger NA, Sarre RG, Saccone GT, Hunter A, Toouli J. Postanal repair for faecal incontinence: long-term follow up. Aust NZ J Surg 1997;67(8):566–70.
33. Lehur PA, Michot F, Denis P, Grise P, Leborgne J, Teniere P, Buzelin JM. Results of artificial sphincter in severe anal

incontinence. Report of 14 consecutive implantations. Dis Colon Rectum 1996;39(12):1352–5.

34. Wong WD, Jensen LL, Bartolo DC, Rothenberger DA. Artificial anal sphincter. Dis Colon Rectum 1996;39(12):1345–51.

35. Vaizey CJ, Kamm MA, Bartram CI, Halligan S, Nichols RJ. Clinical, physiological, and radiological study of an new purpose-designed artificial bowel sphincter. Lancet 1998;352(9122):105–9.

36. Baeten CG, Geerdes BP, Adang EM, Heineman E, Konsten J, Engel GL, Kester AS, Spaans F, Soeters PB. Anal dynamic graciloplasty in the treatment of intractable faecal incontinence. N Engl J Med 1995;332(24):1600–5.

37. Adang EM, Engel GL, Rutten FF, Geerdes BP, Baeten CG. Cost-effectiveness of dynamic graciloplasty in patients with fecal incontinence. Dis Colon Rectum 1998;41(6):725–33.

38. Geerdes BP, Heineman E, Konsten J, Soeters PB, Baeten CG. Dynamic graciloplasty. Complications and management. Dis Colon Rectum 1996;39(8):912–17.

39. Wexner SD, Gonzalez-Padron A, Teoh TA, Mon HK. The stimulated gracilis neosphincter for fecal incontinence: a new use for an old concept. Plast Reconstr Surg 1996;98(4):693–9.

40. Matzel KE, Stadelmeir U, Hohenfelner M, Gall FP. Electrical stimulation of sacral spinal nerves for treatment of faecal incontinence. Lancet 1995;346:1124–7.

41. Broden B, Snellman B. Procidentia of the rectum studies with cinedefecography: a contribution to the discussion of causative mechanism. Dis Colon Rectum 1968;11:330–47.

42. Gordon PH, Nivatvongs A. Principles and Practice of Surgery for the Colon, Rectum and anus. MO: Quality Medical Publishing, St Louis, 1992.

43. Sullivan ES, Strasburg CO, Sandoz IL, Tarnasky JW, Longaker CJ. Repair of total pelvic prolapse: an overview. In: Schrock T, editor. Perspectives in Colon and Rectal Surgery. MO: Quality Medical Publishing, St Louis, 1990;3(1):119–31.

44. Corman ML. Colon and Rectal Surgery, 3rd edn. Philadelphia, PA: JB Lippincott, 1993.

45. Keighley M. Rectal prolapse: clinical features and pathophysiology. In: Henry MM, Swash M, editors. Coloproctology and the Pelvic Floor, 2nd edn. Toronto: Butterworth-Heinemann, 1992;316–21.

46. Eu KW, Seow-Choen F. Functional problems in adult rectal prolapse and controversies in surgical treatment. Br J Surg 1997;84(7):904–11.

47. Kwok SP, Carey DP, Lau WY, Li AK. Laparoscopic rectopexy. Dis Colon Rectum 1994;37(9):947–8.

48. Ballantyne GH, Laparoscopicaly assisted anterior resection for rectal prolapse. Surg Laparosc Endosc 1992;2(3):230–6.

49. Stevenson AR, Sits RW, Lumley JW. Laparoscopic-assisted resection-rectopexy for rectal prolapse; early and medium follow-up. Dis Colon Rectum 1998;41(1):46–54.

50. Graf W, Stefansson T, Arvidsson D, Pahlman L. Laparoscopic suture rectopexy. Dis Colon Rectum 1995;38(2):211–12.

51. Farouk F, Duthie GS, Bartolo DC, MacGregor AB. Restoration of continence following rectopexy for rectal prolapse and recovery of the internal anal sphincter electromyogram. Br J Surg 1992;79:439–40.

52. Madoff RD, Watts JD, Rothenberger DA, Goldberg SM. Rectal prolapse: treatment. In: Henry MM, Swash M, editors. Coloproctology and the Pelvic Floor, 2nd edn. Toronto: Butterworth-Heinemann, 1992:321–50.

53. Tjandra JJ, Fazio VW, Church JM, Milsom JW, Oakley JR. Lavery IC. Ripstein procedure is an effective treatment for rectal prolapse without constipation. Dis Colon Rectum 1993;36(5):501–7.

54. Madoff RD, Williams JG, Wong WD, Rotenberger DA, Goldberg SM. Long term functional results of colon resection and retopexy for overt rectal prolapse. Am J Gastroenterol 1992;87:101–4.

55. Schlinkert RT, Beart RW Jr, Wolff BG, Pemberton JH. Anterior resection for complete rectal prolapse. Dis Colon Rectum 1985;28:409–12.

56. Kling KM, Rongione AJ, Evans B, McFadden DW. The Delorme procedure: a useful operation for complicated rectal prolapse in the elderly. Am Surg 1996;62(10):857–60.

57. Lechaux JP, Lechaux D, Perez M. Results of Delorme's procedure for rectal prolapse. Advantages of a modified technique. Dis Colon Rectum 1995;38(3):301–7.

58. Agachan F, Pfeifer J, Joo JS, Nogueras JJ, Weiss EG, Wexner SD. Results of perineal procedures for the treatment of rectal prolapse. Am Surg 1997;63(1):9–12.

59. Williams JG, Rothenberger DA, Madoff RD, Goldberg SM. Treatment of rectal prolapse in the elderly by perineal rectosigmoidectomy. Dis Colon Rectum 1992;35(9):830–4.

60. Ramanujan PS, Venkatesh KS, Fietz MJ. Perineal excision of rectal procidentia in elderly high-risk patients. A ten year experience. Dis Colon Rectum 1994;37(10):1027–30.

61. Prasad ML, Pearl RK, Abcarian H et al. Perineal proctectomy, posterior rectopexy, and postanal levator repair for the treatment of rectal prolapse. Dis Colon Rectum 1986;29:547–52.

62. Shorvon PJ, McHugh S, Diamant NE et al. Defaecography is normal volunteers: results and implications. Gut 1989;30:1737–49.

63. Lubowski DZ. Solitary rectal ulcer syndrome: pathophysiology and treatment. In: Henry MM, Swash M, editors. Coloproctology and the Pelvic Floor, 2nd edn. Toronto: Butterworth-Heinemann, 1992;305–15.

64. Park UC, Choi SK, Piccicrillo MF, Verzaro R, Wexner SB. Patterns of anismus and the relation to biofeedback therapy. Dis Colon Rectum 1996;39:768–73.

38 Paravaginal Repairs

Scott A. Farrell and Constance Ling

Introduction

Writing in the Journal of the American Medical Association in June 1909, George R. White said "Ahlfelt states that the only problem in plastic gynaecology left unsolved by the gynaecologist of the past century is that of a permanent cure of a cystocele" [1]. He went on to propose that "The reason for failure seems to be that the normal support of the bladder has not been sought for and restored but instead an irrational removal of part of the anterior vaginal wall has been resorted to, which could result in disappointment and failure". By means of cadaver dissection, White investigated the pelvic structures inherent to the support of the anterior vaginal wall. As a consequence of his investigations, he devised a vaginal approach to correction of the cystocele which involved the attachment of the vaginal sulci to a condensation of fascia overlying the pelvic muscles which he referred to as the "white line of pelvic fascia". Despite the fact that White reported a very high cure rate for cystocele using his new surgical procedure, it was not widely adopted by gynecologic surgeons.

More than 50 years later, A. Cullen Richardson, following the same process of cadaver dissection, developed an abdominal procedure which he termed the paravaginal defect repair [2]. Richardson described four distinct defects in the anterior vaginal wall support and proposed that surgical correction of the prolapse should be directed to the specific defect or defects involved. He went on to report the successful use of the abdominal paravaginal defect repair in 233 patients complaining of combinations of pelvic prolapse and stress urinary incontinence [3]. Benson [4], Baden et al. [5] and Farrell and Ling [6] have described modifications of White's procedure for the vaginal paravaginal defect repair.

Although it is now 90 years since George R. White first called our attention to the problem of recurrent cystocele, its solution remains elusive. Weber and Walters, in a recent review article on cystocele repair, pointed out the deficiencies in the literature on the subject of anterior repair and emphasized the need for prospective studies comparing traditional anterior colporrhaphy with paravaginal repair [7]. The traditional gynecologic approach to a combination of cystocele and urinary incontinence was to do an anterior colporrhaphy. It has now been accepted that the retropubic urethropexy procedure is the best surgical treatment of a primary case of genuine stress incontinence. While it is highly effective at correcting genuine stress incontinence, the retropubic procedure is associated with a significant rate of postoperative pelvic prolapse, particularly in patients who had significant anterior vaginal wall prolapse prior to the procedure [8]. It has been recommended that the retropubic procedures be combined with an abdominal paravaginal repair in these circumstances [9].

While the abdominal approach permits correction of both stress incontinence and the paravaginal defect, it does not allow correction of a central anterior vaginal wall defect. The vaginal approach to paravaginal repair, on the other hand, allows correction of both the paravaginal and the central defects of the anterior vaginal wall. Unfortunately, it is a technically more challenging procedure and, in patients with stress incontinence, must be combined with a vaginal incontinence procedure such as a needle suspension which is less effective than the retropubic procedures [10]. Combination of the vaginal paravaginal repair with either a suburethral sling procedure [11] or tension-free vaginal tape

(TVT) procedure [12], both procedures with high incontinence cure rates, might achieve the best long-term cure of combined anterior wall prolapse and stress incontinence.

Anatomy of the Anterior Vaginal Wall Support

A review of the anatomic basis of the paravaginal defect is critical to an understanding of the rationale for the paravaginal defect repair. DeLancey has described three levels for vaginal support [13]. Level 1 consists of the endopelvic fascial attachments to the upper vagina which arise from a broad area of the upper pelvic bowl and converge as condensations of fibromuscular tissue which we commonly recognize as the uterosacral and cardinal ligaments. At level 2, the mid-portion of the vagina, the vaginal sidewalls come into close approximation with the pelvic sidewall where they derive their support from a lateral attachment to the fascia overlying the levator ani and obturator internus muscles. This lateral attachment occurs along a condensation of fascia referred to as the arcus tendineus fascia pelvis (ATFP), which extends from the ischial spines along the pelvic sidewalls to attach to the back side of the symphysis pubis (Figure 38.1). At this level, the anterior vaginal wall can be viewed as forming a triangular sheet of tissue. The base of this triangle is formed laterally by the cardinal ligaments attached to the ischial spines and more medially by the attachments of the anterior vaginal wall to the

cervix. Extending cranially from the cervix, the uterosacral ligaments attach to the sacrum and provide a continuation of support to the base of this triangle. The sides of this triangle are attached to the ATFP. Below, lies the anterior vaginal wall and above, rests the bladder. It is at this level of attachment that the paravaginal defect occurs. Level 3 corresponds to a short region of the vagina extending from the introitus to 2–3 cm above the hymenal ring, an area where the vagina is firmly attached to surrounding structures.

Richardson, focusing on level 2, described four types of defects (Figure 38.2). The lateral defect is a consequence of the detachment, on one or both sides, of the vaginal fornices from the ATFP. This defect usually results in a mild to moderate cystocele with associated loss of support of the urethrovesical junction and as a consequence, stress urinary incontinence. The transverse defect results from the detachment of the base of the triangular anterior vaginal wall from the cervix in the midline. This defect results in a large pulsion-type cystocele. Because these patients have intact support of the urethrovesical junction they do not experience stress incontinence. The midline defect results from stretching and tearing of the central anterior vaginal wall [7]. As Weber and Walters have clearly demonstrated by performing autopsy dissections of the bladder and vagina, there is no actual fascia in the anterior vaginal wall. The vaginal wall consists of mucosa, muscularis, and adventitia. The central defect, therefore, results from stretching and degeneration of these tissues. Finally, the distal defect results from a detachment of the apex of the trian-

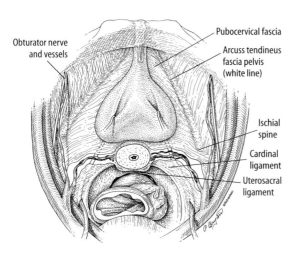
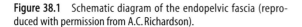

Figure 38.1   Schematic diagram of the endopelvic fascia (reproduced with permission from A.C. Richardson).

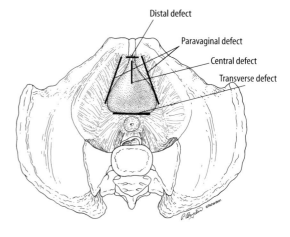

Figure 38.2   Four locations of anterior vaginal wall support defects (reproduced with permission from A.C. Richardson).

gular anterior vaginal wall from the back of the symphysis pubis. This defect is usually a consequence of damage to the pubourethral ligaments and results in a telescoping of the urethra out under the symphysis pubis.

Diagnosis of the Paravaginal Defect

While more objective and precise means of measuring the support defects in the pelvic compartments have been proposed and accepted [14], a standardized approach to diagnosing the paravaginal defect has not been developed. The cornerstone of diagnosis is the pelvic examination. With the patient in the dorsolithotomy position and the bottom half of a Graves speculum retracting the posterior vaginal wall, the patient is asked to perform Valsalva's maneuver. A tongue depressor or ring forceps is placed in the vaginal fornices and the vagina is elevated to the ischial spine, about the level of the inferior margin of the symphysis pubis. If the cystocele is eliminated by uni- or bilateral vaginal fornix support, the defect is diagnosed as a paravaginal defect. This traction-type cystocele is characterized by preservation of the vaginal rugae. If the cystocele persists despite adequate support of the vaginal fornices, it is caused by a central defect. This is a pulsion cystocele, characterized by a vaginal wall which, having lost the healthy rugae, presents as a smooth surface. In patients where elevation of the vaginal fornices reduces the size of the cystocele but does not eliminate it, a combination of paravaginal and central support defects is diagnosed. A combination of two or more of the above defects was rarely encountered in Richardson's experience. In his original report, 66% of patients had lateral attachment defects alone. Of this group, 75% had a unilateral defect (most commonly on the right side) and 25% had a bilateral defect.

The Surgical Procedure

The Abdominal Approach

The abdominal approach to the paravaginal repair can be performed in isolation or in combination with an abdominal hysterectomy and/or a Burch procedure. In the patient who has an indication for hysterectomy (dysfunctional uterine bleeding, or grade 1 to grade 2 uterine prolapse), a cystocele due to a paravaginal defect and genuine stress incontinence, the above-mentioned combined

procedure will correct the problems. The abdominal approach does not permit correction of a central defect.

The abdominal paravaginal repair is begun when the abdomen is opened by means of Pfannenstiel's incision. The rectus muscles are carefully separated in the midline down to the symphysis pubis and dissected off the underlying parietal peritoneum. The palmar surface of the index finger is placed against the posterior aspect of the symphysis pubis on one side and gently swept along the inner surface of the superior pubic ramus to break the attachments of the transversalis fascia to the superior pubic ramus. The obturator vessels and nerves are identified as they pass into the button-hole-shaped obturator foramen, which can be palpated below the superior pubic ramus. The dissection is continued more proximally and inferiorly to separate the bladder from the pelvic sidewalls, down to the level of the ATFP. The arcus should be visualized along its entire length from its attachment to the posterior aspect of the symphysis pubis, running inferiorly and laterally to its attachment at the ischial spine (Figure 38.3).

The non-dominant surgical hand is placed in the vagina and locates the urethrovesical junction (Figure 38.4). The first, or key, suture is placed through the pubocervical fascia approximately 1–2 cm lateral to the urethrovesical junction beneath the prominent veins which course parallel along the vaginal margins. The needle is passed through the tissue from medial to lateral and, before the needle is removed, posterior traction is placed on these tissues pulling them toward the ischial spine (Figure 38.5). The vaginal hand palpates to determine when the external urethral meatus is drawn beneath the middle of the lower

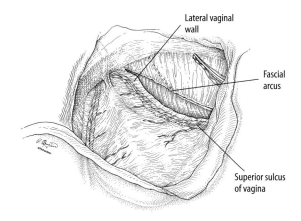

Figure 38.3 The paravaginal defect (reproduced with permission from A.C. Richardson).

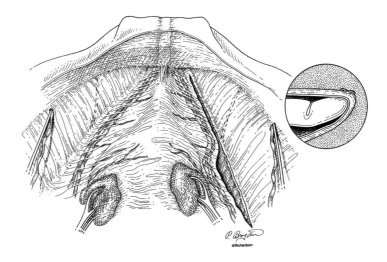

Figure 38.4   Elevation of the right vaginal fornix with the vaginal hand (reproduced with permission from A.C. Richardson).

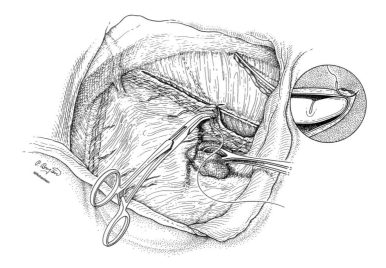

Figure 38.5   Placement of the "key" suture (reproduced with permission from A.C. Richardson).

edge of the symphysis pubis. The needle is then passed through the point on the ATFP adjacent to where the traction has brought it. Additional stitches are placed through the pubocervical fascia and the ATFP at 1 cm intervals both distal and proximal to the key stitch, reattaching the vagina to its original pelvic sidewall fascial support (Figure 38.6). Once all the stitches are placed on one side, they are tied.

It is recommended that the procedure be done on the right side first (the most common location of the paravaginal defect). Silicone-coated Dacron on a gastrointestinal needle is used to do the suturing (Davis and Geck 3.0 Tycron on a T-5 needle). The procedure is then repeated on the left side. Drains were rarely used by Richardson, and an indwelling urethral catheter is not used during or after the procedure. Placement of a transurethral catheter may be useful to help to identify the urethrovesical junction for less experienced surgeons. The course of the ureter as it enters the base of the bladder, although medial to the elevated vaginal fornix, is close to the point of placement of the most cranial stitch. The ureter can often be palpated between vaginal and abdominal fingers and thereby intentionally retracted medially away from the suture site.

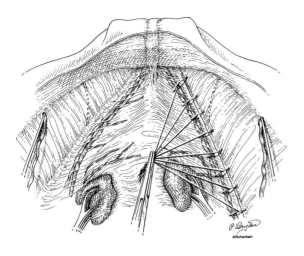

Figure 38.6 Paravaginal repair completed on the right side (reproduced with permission from A.C. Richardson).

Shull employed a modification of this technique in which the sutures were tied as they were placed in order to achieve better hemostasis [15]. The first stitch was placed immediately caudal to the ischial spine. Starting with the most dependent point of the ATFP ensures that any blood will track downward and not obscure the location of subsequent suture placement. He placed his key stitch through the arcus tendineus fascia pelvis and after tying it, further anchored it to Cooper's ligament. Shull routinely inserted a suprapubic catheter and started a postoperative clamping protocol on the first postoperative day. The following modification of the surgical technique is used when combining the paravaginal repair with an abdominal hysterectomy and Burch procedure. The abdominal hysterectomy (often combined with McCall's culdoplasty) is completed first. Only two to three stitches are placed bilaterally on the cranial end of the ATFP. A Tanagho modification of the Burch procedure provides support of the caudal anterior vaginal wall.

The Vaginal Approach

With the patient draped in the dorsolithotomy position, a Foley catheter is inserted into the bladder to permit continuous bladder drainage and to facilitate identification of the urethrovesical junction. Two sets of marker sutures are placed through the anterior vaginal epithelium using a standard absorbable suture. The first set of sutures marks the level of the urethrovesical junction and the second set of sutures is placed bilaterally at the highest points of the vaginal apices (Figure 38.7).

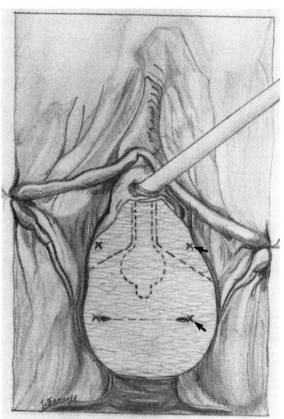

Figure 38.7 Placement of the marker sutures for the vaginal paravaginal repair. Upper arrow: suture marking the urethrovesical junction. Lower arrow: suture marking the vaginal vault. Reprinted with permission from the Society of Obstetricians and Gynaecologists of Canada (S Farrell The Paravaginal Defect Repair, *SGOC journal*).

A standard anterior colporrhaphy is performed using an inverted T-shaped incision of the vaginal epithelium. The ATFP can be palpated as a scallop-shaped ridge of fascia running from the ischial spine up to the pubic symphysis. The paravaginal space should be opened up completely so that a finger can be swept from behind the symphysis pubis along the pelvic sidewall down to the ischial spine. In opening this space the operator is separating the bladder from its attachment to the underlying vagina. This part of the procedure does not, as has been suggested, create an artificial paravaginal defect. The operating table is rotated so that its head swings away from the side of the pelvis on which the repair will be done. This maneuver puts the surgeon at an angle of approximately 30 to 40 degrees to the pelvic sidewall, permitting better visualization of the pelvic sidewall structures. A Briesky–Navaratil retractor is used anteriorly to retract the bladder medially. A Heaney retractor is placed laterally with its tip just above the insertion of the ATFP into the ischial spine. A

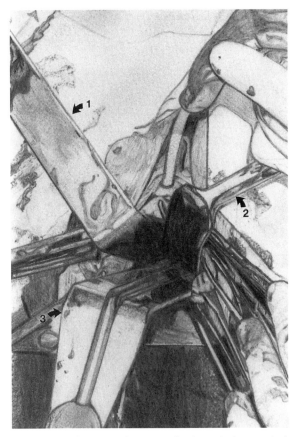

Figure 38.8 Placement of retractors for the vaginal paravaginal repair. 1, Heaney retractor tip over the ischial spine. 2, Briesky–Navaratil retractor retracts bladder medially. 3, Opus fiberoptic retractor illuminates pelvic sidewall. Reprinted with permission from the Society of Obstetricians and Gynaecologists of Canada (S Farrell. The Paravaginal Defect Repair, *SGOC journal*).

fibreroptic retractor is placed inferiorly to expand and illuminate the operative space (Figure 38.8).

Figure 38.9 illustrates the vertical orientation of the ATFP when a patient is in the lithotomy position. Because of this orientation, each suture is both caudal and superior to the previous suture. The first suture of 2.0 silicon-coated Dacron (DuPont, Wilmington, DE) on a T-5 gastrointestinal needle (Davis and Geck, Danbury, CT) is passed using an extra long needle driver from bottom to top through the ATFP approximately 1 cm from its insertion into the ischial spine. The needle is retrieved and with the needle still attached, both ends of the suture are grasped with a hemostat marked with a single piece of autoclavable tape to identify it as suture number one. The suture is then placed in the most lateral teeth of a currycomb held by the contralateral assistant (Figure 38.10). This currycomb is made of solid cast aluminum and measures 10 cm in length by 5 cm in height (Cavalier Equestrian, Stratford, Ontario, Canada). The teeth are blunt and spaced about 2 mm apart. Subsequent

sutures are placed approximately 1 cm apart along the ATFP until the last suture is placed approximately 2 cm from the attachment of the ATFP to the back of the symphysis pubis. Up to five sutures are placed. The sutures held by marked hemostats are placed in the teeth of the currycomb so that hemostat number one is most lateral and number five most medial.

The first currycomb is passed from the contralateral assistant to the ipsilateral assistant. Suture number one, now the most medial suture in the comb, is used to pick up the vesicovaginal muscularis and the underside of the vaginal epithelium corresponding with the marker stitch which was placed at the apex of the vaginal fornix. The needle is driven in a cephalad-to-caudal direction through the vesicovaginal muscularis and in a caudal-to-cephalad direction through the underside of the vaginal epithelium. Care is taken to avoid perforation of the surface of the vaginal epithelium by the needle. The needle is cut off and the two ends of the suture are grasped with the number one hemostat and placed through the most lateral teeth of a second currycomb held by the contralateral assistant (Figure 38.11). In placing the suture, care must be taken to avoid picking up the vaginal epithelium too close to the midline. If this happens, it will be difficult to achieve the midline closure of the vaginal epithelium that completes the procedure. The second suture is placed through the vesicovaginal muscularis and the vaginal mucosa approximately 1 cm above the first suture, the needle is cut off and the ends are grasped with the number two hemostat. This suture is placed more medially in the second currycomb. The fourth suture is usually placed at the level of the marker suture lateral to the urethrovesical junction. When all the sutures have been placed, they are tied in reverse order. Suture number five is tied first, approximating the most caudal portion of the vaginal fornix with the ATFP immediately behind the symphysis pubis. As each suture is tied and cut, the vaginal fornix is elevated and reduced further until it lies along the entire length of the ATFP. The procedure is repeated on the opposite side.

Once the paravaginal defect has been repaired, the degree of central defect will be apparent. The procedure is completed in the standard fashion described for an anterior colporrhaphy [16]. If a vaginal hysterectomy is required, it is completed to the point of placing the Heaney sutures before beginning the paravaginal defect repair. When an incontinence-correcting procedure is required, we use a suburethral sling procedure. These procedures, completed before the paravaginal repair, will correct the caudal anterior vaginal wall defect. After these procedures, only two or three sutures on each side are necessary to correct the paravaginal defect.

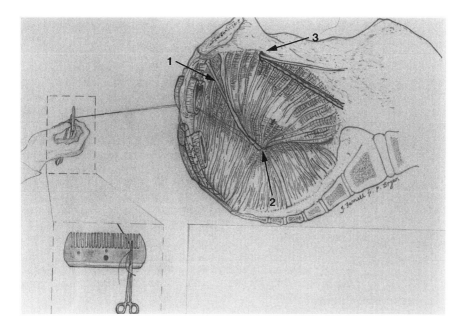

Figure 38.9 Placement of the first suture through the arcus tendineus fascia pelvis and retraction with the currycomb. 1, Arcus tendineus fasciae pelvis. 2, Ischial spine. 3, Obturator canal. Reprinted with permission from the American College of Obstetricians and Gynecologists (Farrell SA, Ling C. Currycombs for the vaginal paravaginal defect repair. *Obstet Gynecol.* 1997 Nov; 90(5): 845–7.)

Indications for the Paravaginal Repair

The paravaginal repair procedure is designed to correct a defect of the lateral attachment of the anterior vaginal wall to the pelvic sidewall. George R. White first devised this procedure to treat cystocele. Cullen Richardson devised an abdominal approach

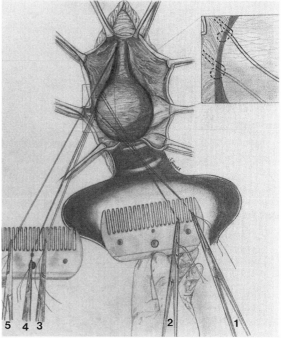

Figure 38.11 Both currycombs retracting the sutures. Inset shows the placement of the sutures through the vesicovaginal tissue and vaginal epithelium. Reprinted with permission from the American College of Obstetricians and Gynecologists (Farrell SA, Ling C. Currycombs for the vaginal paravaginal defect repair. *Obstet Gynecol.* 1997 Nov; 90(5): 845–7.)

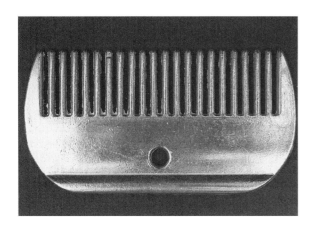

Figure 38.10 Currycomb. Reprinted with permission from the American College of Obstetricians and Gynecologists (Farrell SA, Ling C. Currycombs for the vaginal paravaginal defect repair. *Obstet Gynecol.* 1997 Nov; 90(5): 845–7.)

to the paravaginal repair and used it to treat a combination of cystocele and genuine stress incontinence. Recent evidence suggests that the abdominal approach is an inferior procedure for treating genuine stress incontinence when compared to the Burch retropubic urethropexy [9]. On the other hand, the Burch retropubic urethropexy, although a very effective treatment for genuine stress incontinence, has been associated with a high incidence of postoperative pelvic prolapse problems, particularly in patients who had a large cystocele at the time of their original surgery. A combination of the Burch procedure and the abdominal paravaginal repair may be proven to be superior to either procedure done alone by curing stress incontinence and preventing subsequent prolapse problems.

The vaginal paravaginal repair permits correction of both the paravaginal and central defects which can contribute to a cystocele. In patients with stress incontinence due to intrinsic urethral sphincter deficiency the vaginal paravaginal repair could be combined with a sling procedure. Patients with prolapse associated with stress incontinence due to an extrinsic support defect of the urethra may be treated with a combination of the vaginal paravaginal repair and TVT procedure.

Results of Surgery

The Abdominal Paravaginal Repair

In his first article Richardson reported the results of 60 patients who had stress incontinence and paravaginal defect who underwent abdominal paravaginal repair surgery [2]. At 3–48 months follow-up, he reported satisfactory to excellent results in 55 (92%) of patients, improvement in 3 (5%) and failure in 2 (3%). In 1981 Richardson reported on the results of 233 abdominal paravaginal repair procedures performed in two centers [3]. All patients complained of genuine stress incontinence and, by examination, were found to have paravaginal defects resulting in cystocele. Patients with detrusor instability were excluded from the study group. The group was divided into two subgroups based upon the location in which their surgery took place. Fifty-three percent of group 1 patients were found to have a unilateral paravaginal defect and underwent a unilateral repair. Group 1 patients were managed without catheterization unless necessitated by postoperative voiding difficulties. Group 2 patients all underwent bilateral paravaginal repairs and had indwelling transurethral

catheters during and after the surgery. Follow-up ranged from 2 to 8 years. Eighty-eight percent of the patients were cured (no stress incontinence) and a further 7% experienced only slight urinary incontinence and were satisfied with the results. The author's success rate was 95%. Minimal postoperative voiding difficulties were encountered in group 1 where 18% of the patients required one or more postoperative catheterizations. All patients were voiding well when discharged from hospital. The mean postoperative stay was 5 days and there were no cases of postoperative unstable bladder. The anatomic results paralleled the functional results. Of the 10 failures, 4 were thought to be due to surgical technique and 2 to misdiagnosis of the original support defect. Two patients developed a central defect one year postoperatively, one patient with unilateral repair developed a defect on the other side, and one patient had a true recurrence of their cystocele after one year.

Shull reported the results on 149 patients who underwent his modification of the abdominal paravaginal repair [15]. All patients were found by preoperative evaluation to have paravaginal defects and 11% of the patients had concomitant midline defects. All patients had genuine stress incontinence. Sixteen percent of the patients had mixed incontinence. Twelve percent of these patients had undergone one or more failed surgical procedures for urinary incontinence in the past. Shull modified Richardson's approach by taking the additional step of suspending the sutures supporting the urethrovesical junction from Cooper's ligament. All patients were managed by the insertion of a suprapubic catheter postoperatively.

The mean postoperative hospital stay was 6.2 days and the mean duration of postoperative catheterization was 4 days. Postoperative success rates for cystocele repair and cure of stress incontinence were 95% and 97%, respectively. Duration of follow-up was not clearly specified. Follow-up after the first year was 98%, but by 4 years it was down to 49%. Twenty-one patients experienced postoperative complications: urinary tract infection 16 patients; wound infection 3 patients; and pulmonary embolism 2 patients. Six percent of patients experienced a subsequent vaginal prolapse to a point halfway between the ischial spines and the hymenal ring and 9 patients experienced symptoms of detrusor instability.

Baden and Walker reported a series of 369 patients who underwent a variety of surgical procedures which included both abdominal and vaginal paravaginal defect repair [5]. They reported their results based upon the preoperative rate of incontinence and severity of urethrocele. Patients with a preoperative grade 2 stress incontinence (loss of urine requiring change of underwear) achieved a cure rate of 87%. The cure rate decreased to 66% in patients with preoperative grade 4 stress incontinence (requiring the use of absorbent products at all times). Excluding patients with grade 1 stress incontinence, the abdominal paravaginal repair had a higher success rate of 87% compared to the vaginal paravaginal repair with which patients achieved a 77% cure rate. Since the majority of the vaginal procedures were performed early in their study period, the authors attributed this difference in success rates to the learning curve associated with the surgical procedure. There were a few postoperative complications, the most common being febrile morbidity. The mean hospital stay was 6.3 days and the mean duration of postoperative catheterization was one day.

Colombo et al. published the only randomized comparison of the abdominal paravaginal repair with the Burch retropubic urethropexy for the treatment of genuine stress incontinence [9]. Patients with detrusor instability or who had undergone previous surgery were excluded. This study was terminated after recruitment of only 36 patients because of the obvious difference in the effectiveness of the two surgical procedures. Both the subjective and objective cure rates of incontinence with the Burch procedure were significantly better than those with the paravaginal repair (100% versus 72% and 100% versus 61%, respectively). These authors concluded that the poor results achieved with the paravaginal repair were due to the fact that hypermobility of the urethrovesical junction was not corrected by this procedure. They concluded that the paravaginal repair should not be recommended for the treatment of stress incontinence and added that a combination of the abdominal paravaginal repair with a Burch procedure might be the best treatment for the combination of cystocele and stress incontinence.

Table 38.1 summarizes the results of abdominal paravaginal repair.

The Vaginal Paravaginal Repair

The evidence concerning the efficacy of the vaginal approach to the paravaginal repair is scant. Several small studies were published in the abstract form. Caputo and Benson conducted a study comparing the vaginal paravaginal repair with and without placement of mesh beneath the anterior vaginal mucosa [17]. The group that underwent a standard vaginal paravaginal repair had a failure rate of 34% at 9 months follow-up, compared to an 8.3% failure rate for those treated with the addition of mesh. In a previously mentioned report by Baden and Walker, 47 patients were treated using the vaginal paravaginal repair. The cure rate for urinary incontinence was 77% in this group. There was no mention of the cure rate for cystocele.

In 1994, Shull et al. published the results of the vaginal paravaginal repair on 62 patients [18]; 87% of the patients had a grade 3 to 4 cystocele preoperatively. Sixty-nine percent of patients had previous pelvic operations. At the time of reporting, 56 patients had been followed for a mean of 1.6 years (range 0.1–5.6 years). The rate of successful cure of cystocele was 73%. Amongst the recurrences, 73% (11 patients) had grade 1 defects, 13% (2 patients) had grade 2 defects and 13% (2 patients) had grade 3 defects. Seven patients experienced perioperative morbidity, none of which was directly related to the paravaginal repair. Shull concluded that the vaginal approach to the paravaginal repair was safe and effective and the preferable technique in patients requiring repair of other pelvic floor defects.

In a preliminary report published by Farrell and Ling, 27 patients underwent the vaginal paravaginal

Table 38.1   Cure rates following abdominal paravaginal repair

Author	No. of patients	Cure rates				
		Cystocele		SUI		
		No.	%	No.	%	
Richardson et al. [3]	233	203	95	203	95	
Shull and Baden [15]	149	141	95	145	97	
Baden and Walker [5]	93	NR	NR	81	87	
Pohl and Wall [22]	11	NR	NR	5	45	
Colombo et al. [9]:						
Burch	18	NR	NR	18	100	
APR	18	NR	NR	11	61	

SUI, stress urinary incontinence; NR, not reported; APR, abdominal paravaginal repair.

Table 38.2 Cure rates following vaginal paravaginal repair

Author	No. of patients	Cure rates Cystocele		SUI	
		No.	%	No.	%
Caputo and Benson [17]	50	33	66	NR	NR
Baden and Walker [5]	47	NR	NR	36	77
Farrell and Ling [6]	27	22	80	NA	NA

SUI, stress urinary incontinence; NR, not reported; NA, not applicable.

Table 38.3 Postoperative complication rates following paravaginal repair

Author	No. of patients	Mean hospital stay (days)	Duration postoperative catheterization (days)	UTI	DI	Pelvic prolapse
Shull and Baden [15]	149	6.2	4	11%	NR	10%
Richardson et al. [3]	233	5	5	NR	EX	4%
Baden and Walker [5]	369	6.3	1	NR	NR	1%
Farrell and Ling [6]	27	5	NR	15	0	20%

UTI, urinary tract infection; NR, not reported; DI, detrusor instability; EX, excluded from study group.

repair for cystocele [6]. Preoperatively, 52% of patients had a grade 2 cystocele and 26% had a grade 3 cystocele. The mean follow-up was 8 months. The cystocele cure rate was 80%. Table 38.2 summarizes the results of vaginal paravaginal repair. Table 38.3 summarizes postoperative complications.

Conclusions

George Ball in his remarks concerning the paravaginal repair said that "The paravaginal repair is the best addition to my surgical skills since I finished residency..." [15]. More research is necessary before the appropriate place of the paravaginal repair in our surgical armamentarium can be determined. The paravaginal repair is an attractive surgical procedure because it addresses the paravaginal support defect of the anterior vaginal wall. Evidence would suggest that this defect contributes to more than 50% of cystoceles. The vaginal approach to the paravaginal repair permits simultaneous repair of both the paravaginal and central defects of the cystocele. As such, it takes us a step closer to achieving an effective cure of the cystocele. As Weber and Walters point out in their review of the anterior repair, until a prospective randomized study comparing anterior colporrhaphy to paravaginal repair is conducted, there is no conclusive evidence to show that one procedure is superior to the other [7]. This study remains to be done.

In the work done by Colombo et al., the abdominal paravaginal repair proved to be significantly inferior to the Burch retropubic urethropexy for the treatment of genuine stress incontinence [9]. The high incidence of postoperative genital prolapse following the Burch procedure which was reported by Wiskind et al. may provide us with an indication for the abdominal paravaginal repair. In Wiskind's study, the only identifiable risk factor for subsequent genital prolapse was the presence of a large cystocele at the time of the original surgery [8]. Combining the abdominal paravaginal repair with the Burch procedure may reduce the incidence of subsequent pelvic organ prolapse. Additional pelvic surgery in the form of an internal anterior repair and McCall's culdoplasty has been shown to be beneficial [19]. The theoretical indications for the abdominal paravaginal repair remain to be proven by clinical studies.

At present, the diagnosis of paravaginal repair is made on a clinical basis. Ostrzenski et al. recently reported the use of ultrasound as a means of diagnosing unilateral and bilateral paravaginal defects. This approach to diagnosis is certainly promising, although further work is necessary to determine its accuracy [20].

Future investigation should focus on the effectiveness of the paravaginal defect repair at achieving long-lasting correction of the cystocele. A recent study by Flood et al. describing the use of mesh to reinforce support of the bladder neck at the time of anterior repair found a low incidence of recurrent cystocele with a mean follow-up of 3 years [21]. Until a prospective, randomized study comparing the various surgical options is conducted, there will be no conclusive evidence to support the purported advantage of the paravaginal defect repair over the traditional anterior colporrhaphy.

References

1. White GR. Cystocele. A radical cure by suturing lateral sulci of vagina to white line of pelvic fascia. JAMA 1909;80(21):1707–10.
2. Richardson AC, Lyon JB, Williams NL. A new look at pelvic relaxation. Am J Obstet Gynecol 1976;126:568–73.
3. Richardson AC, Edmonds PB, Williams NL. Treatment of stress urinary incontinence due to paravaginal fascial defect. Obstet Gynecol 1981;57:357–62.
4. Benson JT. Vaginal approach to cystocele repair. In: Benson JT, editor. Female pelvic floor disorders. New York: WW Norton and Company, 1992; 289–94.
5. Baden WF, Walker J. Urinary stress incontinence: evolution of paravaginal repair. The Female Patient 1987;12:89–105.
6. Farrell SA, Ling C. Currycombs for the vaginal paravaginal defect repair. Obstet Gynecol 1997;90:845–7.
7. Weber AM, Walters MD. Anterior vaginal prolapse: Review of anatomy and techniques of surgical repair. Obstet Gynecol 1997;89:311–18.
8. Wiskind AK, Creighton SM, Stanton SL. The incidence of genital prolapse after the Burch colposuspension. Am J Obstet Gynecol 1992;167:399–405.
9. Colombo M, Milani R, Vitobello D, Maggioni A. A randomized comparison of the Burch colposuspension and abdominal paravaginal defect repair for female stress incontinence. Am J Obstet Gynecol 1996;175:78–84.
10. Bergman A, Ballard CA, Koonings PP. Comparison of three different surgical procedures for genuine stress incontinence; prospective randomized study. Am J Obstet Gynecol 1989;160:1102–6.
11. Black NA, Downs SH. The effectiveness of surgery for stress incontinence in women: a systematic review. Br J Urol 1996;78:497–510.
12. Ulmsten U, Falconer C, Johnson P, Jomaq M, Lannér L, Nilsson CG, Olsson I. A multi center study of tension-free vaginal tape (TVT) for surgical treatment of stress urinary incontinence. Int Urogynecol J 1998;9:210–13.
13. DeLancey JOL, Richardson AC. Anatomy of genital support. In: Benson JT, editor. Female Pelvic Floor Disorders. New York: WW Norton and Company, 1992; 19–26.
14. Bump RC, Mattiasson A, Bo K, Brubaker LP, Delancey JO, Klarskov P, Shull BL, Smith AR. The standardization of terminology of female pelvic organ prolapse and pelvic floor dysfunction. Am J Obstet Gynecol 1996;175:10–17.
15. Shull BL, Baden WF. A six year experience with paravaginal defect repair for stress urinary incontinence. Am J Obstet Gynecol 1989;160:1432–40.
16. Thompson JD. Anterior colporrhaphy for repair of cystourethrocele. In: Thompson JD, Rock JA, editors. Telinde's Operative Gynecology, 8th edn. Philadelphia: Lippincott, 1997: 980–95.
17. Caputo RM, Benson JT. Vaginal paravaginal repair with mesh placement for cystocele (Abstract 31). Int Urogynecol J 1993;4:394.
18. Shull BL, Benn SJ, Kuehl TJ. Surgical management of prolapse of the anterior vaginal segment: An analysis of support defects, operative morbidity and anatomic outcome. Am J Obstet Gynecol 1994;171:1429–39.
19. Drutz HP, Baker KR, Lemieux M-C. Retropubic colpourethropexy with transabdominal anterior and/or posterior repair for the treatment of genuine stress urinary incontinence and genital prolapse. Int Urogynecol J 1991;2:201–7.
20. Ostrzenski A, Osborne NG, Ostrzenska K. Method for diagnosing paravaginal defects using contrast ultrasonographic technique. J Ultrasound Med 1997;16:673–7.
21. Flood CG, Drutz HP, Waja L. Anterior colporrhaphy reinforced with Marlex mesh for the treatment of cystoceles. Int Urogynecol J 1998;9:200–4.
22. Pohl JF, Wall LL. Paravaginal defect repair for recurrent urinary incontinence (Abstract 2). Int Urogynecol J 1992;3:263.

7 Surgery for Disorders of Pelvic Support

39 Sacrospinous Vault Suspension and Abdominal Colposacropexy

Bunan Alnaif, Harold P. Drutz and Mohamed H. Baghdadi

Owing to advances in medicine and health care, women are enjoying longer life expectancy. The average North American woman will probably live one-third to one-half of her life after menopause. Menopausal women are not only living longer but also enjoying better quality of life; they are remaining active physically, mentally, socially and sexually. With advancing age, the prevalence of urinary incontinence and genital prolapse increases. Because women expect to be in the best shape possible, they are demanding help with these problems. With the advent of hormone replacement therapy, sexual stimulants made from herbs and medications such as sildenfil (Viagra), and cosmetic and reconstructive surgeries, many women are remaining sexually active well beyond menopause. Advances in anesthesia, pharmacology and support technology have allowed many of the previously so-called surgically unfit patients to undergo surgery successfully.

The support of the uterus is essentially that of its cervix. The uterine cervix is intimately involved with the vaginal fornices, sharing integrated support structures. Thus prolapse of the uterus will inevitably be associated with prolapse of the upper vagina. Therefore, it should be called uterovaginal prolapse rather than the commonly used term uterine prolapse. Removing the prolapsed uterus without addressing vault support will result in vault prolapse. The surgeon should test for the presence of occult prolapse. Occult prolapse becomes apparent only when traction is applied on the cervix using tenaculum or ring forceps. This should be done routinely during vaginal hysterectomy, where maximum prolapse can be ascertained by pulling on the cervix until it stops descending. If the cervix descends to or beyond the hymenal ring this is considered as significant prolapse, and vault suspension should be considered. Cervical length should be assessed because cervical elongation is frequently associated with prolapse, while the uterine corpus may still lie in its normal location.

When there is uterine descent, hysterectomy is highly recommended; therefore, patients who are still in their reproductive years and desire fertility are advised to wait until they have completed their family before they undergo reconstructive pelvic surgery. In this case, the use of a pessary in the interim should be considered to relieve genital prolapse symptoms. Deciding on the route of hysterectomy is mainly a factor of adequate accessibility and experience. Where accessibility is not adequate because of uterine size or presence of adhesion, or in cases where accessibility includes accessibility not only to uterus but also to other structures as in cases of cancer staging or adnexal pathology, then the abdominal approach will be a wiser approach irrespective of the degree of genital prolapse. With laparoscopic availability, there is rarely an absolute contraindication to vaginal hysterectomy, because the laparoscope could potentially enable us to convert any abdominal surgery to a laparoscopic procedure or laparoscopic assisted vaginal procedure. This chapter discusses evaluation and management of vault prolapse with particular focus on sacrospinous vault suspension and abdominal colposacropexy.

Post-hysterectomy vault prolapse (PHVP)

In patients in whom the uterus has already been removed, descent of the vaginal apex below its normal position in the pelvis is referred to as post-hysterectomy vault prolapse (PHVP). When the vagina turns entirely inside out, the term "vaginal eversion" is used. It results from disruption to the endopelvic fascia and the pericervical ring of support and detachment of the uterosacral-cardinal ligament complex. The prolapsed vaginal apex that descends to within the lower one-third of the vagina with straining is considered a significant defect, and surgical repair and resuspension is indicated.

Extirpation of the uterus for uterovaginal prolapse without ensuring adequate vault support will result in PHVP. These patients need pelvic reconstructive procedures rather than an extirpative procedure. Similarly, an anterior and posterior colporrhaphy that is not accompanied by suspension of the vaginal apex will not cure the apical prolapse, and the problem remains uncorrected.

The prevalence of post-hysterectomy vault prolapse is largely dependent on the preoperative indication for hysterectomy. In an 11-year follow-up study of over 2000 patients. an overall incidence of 4.4% was noted [1].

There are three types of vault prolapse:

Type I	Enterocele only
	Low rectovaginal septum intact
Type II	Enterocele and rectocele
	Rectovaginal septum totally
	deficient
Type III	Total vaginal eversion
	Massive cystocele
	Rectovaginal septum totally
	deficient

Prolapse of the vaginal apex or uterus is invariably associated with enterocele. An enterocele is a hernia of the small intestine into the vagina. It happens when there is a defect in the attachment of the rectovaginal septum to the uterosacral–cardinal ligament complex. When the cul-de-sac loses its support, it becomes distended with the intestine, resulting in an outward bulge of the vaginal wall. It may follow vaginal or abdominal hysterectomy. It is classified as anterior or posterior depending on the relationship to the apex of the vagina, posterior enterocele being substantially more common. Other classifications of enterocele are traction, which is secondary to uterine prolapse, pulsion, which is due to increase in intra-abdominal pressure, and congenital, which is a rare inherent defect in vaginal support, often associated with other support defects such as rectal prolapse.

Enterocele extends from the apex of the vagina downward, and is sometimes evident as a bulge that overrides the more caudal rectocele. A careful inspection of the posterior vaginal wall with a speculum retracting the anterior wall can sometimes suggest that an enterocele is present. One way to detect an enterocele is by palpating the small bowel between the vagina and rectum during recto-vaginal examination with the patient straining so that the prolapse is protruding. To do this, the index finger is placed in the rectum and the thumb placed in the vagina. The examination can be repeated with the patient in the standing position. Then while the patient is straining, the rectovaginal space may be palpated to detect the bulge of the enterocele and the presence of small bowel, omentum or large bowel in this region. Magnetic resonance imaging and other imaging studies can be helpful in diagnosing enterocele [2], but it is considered investigational at this time. When pelvic reconstructive surgery is being contemplated it is important that the presence of enterocele as well as other vaginal defects be carefully and accurately assessed preoperatively and intraoperatively, so that appropriate correction can be achieved. Intraoperative evaluation should be done in all patients undergoing pelvic reconstructive surgery. This can be done before incising the posterior vaginal wall; by inserting the left index finger in the rectum, and bringing it forwards, while the right index finger is inserted vaginally, touching the rectal index finger and carefully sliding cranially and caudally to identify the enterocele sac. The sac can be seen after incising the posterior vaginal wall. With the left index finger in the rectum, a pickup or an Allis clamp can be used to identify the enterocele sac with its peritoneal fat. The latter is most helpful in the diagnosis of enterocele.

The difficult challenges facing the genitourinary and reconstructive pelvic surgeon is not only choosing the type of surgery to correct pelvic organ prolapse (POP) and/or incontinence but its route; abdominal, vaginal, laparoscopic or any combination thereof. With the rapidly growing technology and industry, and peer pressure, a number of new procedures, instruments, equipment and material are being used prior to undergoing full scientific testing and scrutiny. We have a duty as physicians to advocate for our patients and to evaluate what is in their best interest, and not to be carried away by our eagerness to try out new ideas or technology, and also to insist on evaluating these ideas and their results with properly designed double-blind randomized controlled trials.

Management of pelvic organ prolapse can be challenging. There is no single operative procedure, nor should there be one, that will correct all types of disorders associated with pelvic support systems. Several support defects often coexist; a summary of pelvic defects is presented in Table 39.1. Correction of one defect without proper correction of the other(s) may result in exaggeration of the other defect(s). For example, Burch colposuspension can worsen an enterocele, and sacrospinous vault suspension can exaggerate a cystocele.

Table 39.1 Clinical classification of pelvic organ prolapse (POP)

Anterior vaginal prolapse
  Urethrocele
  Cystourethrocele
  Cystocele
  Paravaginal defects
  Descent of urethrovesical junction
  Anterior enterocele
Apical vaginal prolapse
  Uterovaginal
  Vaginal vault (post hysterectomy)
  Enterocele
Posterior vaginal prolapse
  Enterocele[a]
  Rectocele
  Perineal descent

[a] Enteroceles usually involve the posterior vaginal fornix and posterior vaginal wall; they also may involve the apical, anterior and/or lateral vaginal walls.
Modified from ACOG technical bulletin [3].

The principles and goal of reconstructive pelvic surgery are to restore and maintain urinary and/or fecal continence, reposition pelvic structures to normal anatomical relationships, maintain ability to have normal coital function, correct any coexisting abnormal pelvic pathology, alleviate abnormal symptoms, and obtain a durable result. Table 39.2 summarizes the procedures involved in pelvic reconstructive surgery [4]. Reconstructive pelvic surgery deals with anatomy and function. Correcting defects and restoring anatomy does not guarantee restoration of function. This important

Table 39.2 Summary of pelvic reconstructive procedures

Reconstructive pelvic surgery includes:
Hysterectomy
Site-specific defect repair:
  Anterior colporrhaphy
  Paravaginal defect repair
  Posterior colporrhaphy
  Enterocele repair
  Perineorrhaphy
  Vault suspension
    Abdominal colposacropexy (ACSP)
    Uterosacral ligament colpopexy
    Sacrospinous vault suspension (SSVS)
    Other
Incontinence surgery
Obliterative surgery
  LeFort colpocleisis
  Colpectomy
Neovagina, neourethra reconstruction
Fistula repair
Bladder augmentation
Sphincter repair or replacement
Repair of rectal, bowel prolapse

fact should be carefully explained to patients prior to surgery.

Proper patient selection should be based on thorough history and physical examination, including meticulous neurological assessment. Urodynamic evaluation is essential in many cases to evaluate bladder function [5] and to rule out occult or potential incontinence, or voiding dysfunction, especially in patients with advanced genital prolapse or in those with mixed symptoms, and is mandatory after previous failed reconstructive surgery. In patients with advanced genital prolapse, the presence of potential or occult stress incontinence can be revealed by a cough stress test while reducing the prolapse without a speculum, both in lying and standing positions. The pessary test is a test involving fitting a pessary for a few days to reveal the existence of urinary incontinence. Urodynamics should be done with the prolapse reduced both with and without a pessary, measuring leak point pressure and urethral pressure profilometry. Ultrasound can be helpful in assessing bladder neck position and support [6]. Patients with significant anorectal symptoms and in particular fecal incontinence and/or rectal prolapse need a thorough investigation, which may include anorectal motility studies, defecography, anal ultrasound, pudendal terminal motor neuron latency studies and/or even colonoscopy prior to the decision for surgical correction.

Stress urinary incontinence can coexist with pelvic organ prolapse or can happen de novo after surgery. Additional surgery is occasionally needed for urinary stress incontinence correction [7]. Intraoperative measures to avoid excessive stretching on the upper anterior vaginal wall during surgical correction, support of urethrovesical junction, augmentation of urethral support with Kelly plication, buttressing sutures and/or urethral sling can help decrease this complication. The use of regional anesthesia can be helpful during surgery to allow the patient to cough during the procedure in order to check for the presence of stress urinary incontinence signs before and after surgical repair or to ensure accurate suture placement.

Conservative options should be offered to all patients prior to surgery. Non-surgical management involves addressing the underlying or risk factors such as chronic cough or obesity. Pelvic floor exercise, both active and passive, is very important not only as an effective conservative therapy especially in cases of stress urinary incontinence, fecal incontinence and constipation [8–10], but also in conjunction with operative treatment, and is essential to ensure long-term endurance of the repair. Pelvic floor exercise is helpful to the lower pelvic defects, but plays a limited role in improving apical vaginal prolapse. Estrogen should be offered to patients with hypoestrogenic, atrophic tissues if there are no contraindications [11]. The pessary is an effective alternative for patients who are not surgically fit, pregnant patients, and for patients who choose to defer or prefer not to have surgery. Patients should be involved in the decision-making process. The expectation for short- and long-term recovery and complications should be clearly outlined; including the need for suprapubic catheter, the risk of voiding dysfunction and retention, as well as the risk of failure.

The decision on who should be treated surgically should be individualized, depending on the size of the prolapse or the presence of symptoms. When the prolapse lies above the level of the hymenal ring, surgery should be performed only if definite symptoms are present and can be reliably attributed to the prolapse, as in the case of women with mild descent in the anterior vaginal wall with urethrovesical hypermobility who have stress incontinence. Women who experience difficulty voiding, and/or who need to reduce prolapse to help defecate "splinting to defecate", or who have symptomatic prolapse causing dragging discomfort, or who have backache caused by the genital prolapse should be considered for site-specific defect repair. Surgically fit patients in whom pessary use was not successful, or whose urinary incontinence symptoms were worsened by pessary use, should also be considered for surgical correction.

Indications for repair despite lack of symptoms includes recurrent urinary tract infection associated with an increased post-void residual urine volume caused by a large cystocele, and ureteral dilatation and hydronephrosis [12] caused by the prolapse (especially large prolapse), which may lead to an impairment of renal function. Evaluation should include excretory urography or intravenous pyelography (IVP) and renal function test. The ureteral obstruction or compression can be best illustrated when the IVP is done in the standing position.

In addition to the variables surrounding surgery such as the type, technique, sutures etc., several factors can affect the outcome of pelvic reconstructive surgery. Among these factors are:

- The patient's general condition and nutrition.
- Tissue characteristics, which are influenced by several extrinsic factors such as hormone status, presence of fibrosis and scarring from previous infection, surgery, or from radiation exposure.
- Intrinsic tissue qualities, such as the quantitative and qualitative types of collagen which may play a factor in pelvic organ prolapse, especially in

patients with recurrence of pelvic organ prolapse after previous repair [13].

- Recurrent pelvic stresses and increased intra-abdominal pressure as seen in such conditions as chronic cough, constipation, large intra-abdominal masses, repeated heavy weight lifting, and obesity.
- Rapid increase in intra-abdominal pressure as in pregnancy or ascites.
- The strength and integrity of pelvic musculature and its innervation.
- Smoking, which acts as a direct and indirect risk factor, causing a hypoestrogenic state in tissue and relative tissue anoxia, thus interfering with the tissue repair mechanism, as well as the chronic cough that some long-term smokers may suffer from.

Preoperative Preparation

For most patients, reconstructive pelvic surgery is an elective surgery; therefore the patient's condition has to be optimized prior to surgery. After proper selection of patients for surgery, patients with significant medical problems should be properly evaluated, treated and controlled prior to undergoing the procedure.

Estrogen can be used liberally to improve vaginal mucosa thickness, and its blood supply, if there are no contraindications. Local vaginal estrogen cream is often used in conjunction with systemic treatment to augment vaginal estrogenation. We often prescribe estrogen for postmenopausal women for a minimal duration of 4 weeks preoperatively.

Patients must be educated and counseled about the planned procedure, its expectation, the possibility of adding or modifying the procedure to address other defects or pathology, and the need for bladder rehabilitation, and catheterization. Patients must also be taught to perform Kegel exercises, and clean intermittent self-catheterization. Proper voiding habits must be enforced, and the patients must also be counseled on lifestyle changes such as smoking cessation, and avoidance of weight lifting. Nutritional advice and counseling should be given concerning supplements such as vitamin C, increase of dietary fiber if the patient is constipated and weight loss advice for obese women.

Patients should preferably receive full bowel preparation with magnesium citrate or Fleet's phospho-soda mixed with 4 oz (120 ml) of any clear liquid, immediately followed by 8–16 oz

(240–475 ml) of clear fluid at midday, the day before surgery. Enema to clear (i.e. there are no particulate matter in enema returns) is given that evening, and repeated the morning of surgery. Protective cream or ointments such as Anusol or dibucaine can be applied locally to the anus if needed to decrease discomfort. Patients must be put on clear fluid diet after breakfast, the day before surgery and then fasted after midnight.

In addition to the standard preoperative laboratory and radiological evaluation, urine must be obtained for culture, the week prior to surgery. Prophylactic antibiotics to cover both aerobic and anaerobic pathogens prior to surgery are highly recommended. Deep venous thrombosis prophylaxis should be considered for most patients undergoing major reconstructive surgery, particularly if they have other risk factors. Depending on utilization, it may be appropriate for the surgeon to consider preoperative autologous blood deposition in patients undergoing a major reconstructive gynecological repair procedure [14].

Vaginal Approach to Vault Suspension

Numerous techniques have been described for supporting the vaginal vault prolapse, both with or without enterocele repair, and with or without hysterectomy. Transvaginal culposuspension includes suspending the vaginal cuff to the iliococcygeus fascia [15,16]. The vault can also be suspended to the origin of the uterosacral and cardinal ligaments [17,18]. These procedures are typically done in association with obliteration of cul-de-sac [19], and restore the normal vaginal axis and depth, which potentially allows the patient to maintain normal sexual activity. Some surgeons found a strong anchor for the vaginal apex in incorporating the pubocervical fascia, uterosacral-cardinal ligament and the rectovaginal fascia done either vaginally or abdominally or laparoscopically [20,21]. The vaginal vault has also been suspended to other structures, such as Cooper ligaments [22], and innervated gracilis muscle graft [23].

Obliterative procedures such as partial (LeFort) colpocleisis [24], or colpectomy [25], or colpocervicectomy [26] are reserved for patients who are not and do not wish to become sexually active in the future, and patients who are not surgically fit to undergo major surgery, or in recurrent cases. The advantages of these procedures are; they carry a shorter operative time than reconstructive options,

are generally less morbid, have high success rates, which are comparable to or even exceed the reconstruction options.

Isolated perineoplasty can be undertaken to help the perineum retain a pessary in the vagina in surgically unfit patients with genital prolapse and poor perineal body. Such procedure can be performed under pudendal block, with local perineal anesthesia if needed.

Sacrospinous vault suspension (SSVS) is also called Richter operation [27]. SSVS results in satisfactory repair of the apical vaginal defect in 94% of cases [28]. Prophylactic SSVS can be considered if the vaginal vault still descends to the level of the ischial spines after routine vaginal hysterectomy. This can reduce the incidence of post-hysterectomy vault prolapse from 10% to 4% [29]. This finding was also supported by other investigators, where long-term analysis of primary SSVS at the time of hysterectomy reduced the rate of vault prolapse recurrence from 15.8% to 6.7% [30].

The SSVS Procedure and Related Anatomy

Sacrospinous ligament vault suspension (SSVS) is typically done unilaterally on the right side, theoretically to avoid the sigmoid. But in severe cases of genital prolapse, bilateral sacrospinous vault suspension can be considered [31]. During the procedure the surgeon must ensure that there is adequate vaginal mucosa, so that this bilateral suspension does not cause stricture in the rectum [32,33]. The repair should be done without tension. Alternatively, making a bridge from the sacrospinous ligament complex to the vaginal fornices bilaterally using a mesh or vaginal mucosa can avoid the risk of rectal stenosis in narrow vaginas.

The technique for SSVS involves opening the right pararectal space, then identifying the ischial spine, which is the lateral border of the coccygeus–sacrospinous ligament complex. The sacrospinous ligament is a strong ligament that extends on the gluteal or the posterior surface of this complex. Starting from the ischial spine, the index and middle fingers gently swipe medially across the muscle-ligament complex to its insertion on the sacrum; this bluntly dissects off the areolar tissue surrounding the rectum. The sacrospinous ligament complex is better felt than seen. Retractors such as Heaney or Briesky–Navratil retractors assist in displacing the rectum medially. Repeated rectal examinations are performed to ensure that the rectum was not inadvertently entered, and that the placed suture is well away from rectal mucosa.

With the rectum retracted medially, the suture is passed through the mid-portion of the muscle–ligament complex (not around the ligament complex), approximately one inch (2.5 cm) medial to the ischial spine. To ensure adequate suture placement, gentle traction on the suture will result in rocking the patient. Several needles and devices have been used to achieve this insertion. These needles include the Miya hook ligature carrier [34], Nichols–Veronikis ligature carrier [35], Long Deschamps ligature carriers, Capio (Laurus) needle driver, and EndoStitch [36–38]. Other devices such as a stapler [31], and the Vesica bone anchor kit [39] have also been used.

A thorough knowledge of anatomy is crucial prior to attempting sacrospinous vault suspension, in order to perform the procedure safely and correctly. Care must be taken not to injure the rectum medially, or the vascular plexus, or the nerves running superior, medial and lateral to the ligament complex. The coccygeus–sacrospinous ligament complex runs from the spine of the ischium to the sacrum. The sacrum is formed of fused five vertebrae, the ligament is attached to the posterolateral borders of vertebrae 2 to 5, and occasionally to the coccyx. The length of sacrospinous ligament complex correlates directly with the length of obstetric conjugate [40]. It converts the sciatic notches in the hip bones into the greater and lesser sciatic foramina. The sacrotuberous ligament is a stronger ligament and runs posterior and inferior to the sacrospinous ligament. The sacrotuberous ligament arises from the posterior surface of the sacrum and covers the posterior aspect of the hip bone down to the ischial ramus. The sacrotuberous ligament and the sacrospinous ligament join the sacrum to the ischium, and stabilize the inferior end of the sacrum, limiting its upward movement. Thus these ligaments provide resilience to the sacroiliac region during sudden weight increase. Because the sacrotuberous ligament is more inferior, posterior and lateral compared to the sacrospinous ligament, its use for vault suspension is not favored.

The coccygeus muscle, also called ischiococcygeus muscle, is on the internal or pelvic side of the coccygeus–sacrospinous ligament complex; it forms a small part of the pelvic diaphragm (pelvic floor) along with the levator ani. This muscle is well developed in animals; it flexes the coccyx and is used to wag their tails. It can be a very powerful muscle in some animals, but is rudimentary in humans.

Many major arteries run through the greater sciatic foramen, including the internal pudendal artery, inferior gluteal artery, and middle hemorrhoidal (or rectal) artery; these are direct branches of the anterior division of the internal iliac (or hypogastric) artery, and the lateral sacral artery is a branch of the posterior division of the internal iliac artery (Figure 39.1). There is also a rich hypogastric venous plexus. Avoiding looping around the sacrospinous ligament complex would decrease the risk of injury to these vessels or nerves.

[fig 39.1]

There is a large venous plexus both anterior and posterior to the sacrospinous ligament complex. The middle rectal veins run anterior to the sacrospinous ligament complex. The blood pressure in these venous plexus is around 4 to 15 mmHg. Care must be taken while dissecting the areolar tissue anterior to the sacrospinous ligament complex; but even then some injury to these vessels can be inevitable. After insuring good homeostasis and controlling bleeding from injured arteries or large veins, bleeding from small venules and capillaries can best be tamponaded by inserting vaginal packing, and leaving it in for 12–36 hours postoperatively. Hemorrhage from one of the large arteries can be controlled by clipping, cauterizing, or suturing these bleeds if possible. If bleeding becomes excessive and cannot be controlled by these measures, then large packing should be left in the vagina for prolonged pressure packing, for approximately 30 minutes, and immediate laparotomy can be performed with ligation of the internal iliac artery on that side. These measures are particularly helpful if bleeding arises from the internal pudendal artery. Arterial embolization is another alternative but with limited availability and experience.

During SSVS the structures vulnerable to injury are those that pass below (inferior to) the lower border of the periformis muscle which include the sciatic nerve, the posterior cutaneous nerve of the thigh, inferior gluteal nerve and the vessels, internal pudendal artery and vein, pudendal nerve, the nerve to obturator internus, and the nerve to quadratus femoris. The coccygeal branch of the inferior gluteal artery passes immediately behind the mid-portion of the sacrospinous ligament and pierces the sacrotuberous ligament in multiple sites. Therefore, the suture should not transgress the entire thickness of the sacrospinous ligament complex, but rather be inserted through the ligament complex. The artery that is most prone to injury if the suture was looped around the mid-portion of sacrospinous ligament complex is the inferior gluteal artery or its coccygeal branch. The pudendal complex and sciatic nerve travel posterior to the lateral third of the sacrospinous ligament [40]; therefore, insertion of suture in the lateral third of the sacrospinous ligament complex should be avoided.

Most of the reported injuries are those to the pudendal complex, which consists of the pudendal

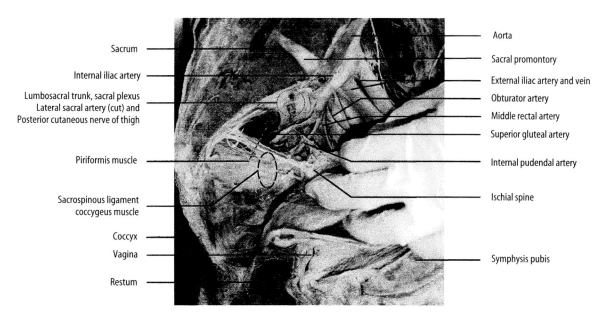

Sacrum

Internal iliac artery

Lumbosacral trunk, sacral plexus
Lateral sacral artery (cut) and
Posterior cutaneous nerve of thigh

Piriformis muscle

Sacrospinous ligament
coccygeus muscle

Coccyx

Vagina

Restum

Aorta

Sacral promontory

External iliac artery and vein

Obturator artery

Middle rectal artery

Superior gluteal artery

Internal pudendal artery

Ischial spine

Symphysis pubis

Figure 39.1 Female hemipelvis showing the anatomy of sacrospinous coccygeus muscle complex area.

nerve, internal pudendal artery, and veins. The pudendal complex runs in Alcock's canal. Alcock's canal is formed by duplication of the obturator internus fascia; it passes from the greater sciatic foramen crossing posterior to the ligament into the lesser sciatic foramen. The nerve to the obturator internus runs lateral to Alcock's canal, therefore it is at less risk of injury.

The pudendal nerve (PN) is composed of three roots derived from the 2nd, 3rd, and 4th anterior sacral rami (S 2,3,4). The roots may receive contribution from S1 and/or S5 [41]. The PN carries both motor and sensory fibers. The main branches of the pudendal nerve and internal pudendal vessels are: first, the inferior rectal or hemorrhoidal branch that supplies the anal region and sphincter ani externus with mainly motor and some sensory fibers; second, the perineal branches, which supply both sensory and motor fibers to the skin and muscles, both superficial and deep perineal muscles; third, the dorsal nerve of the clitoris (or penis), which carries only sensory fibers.

Injury to the pudendal nerve would result in denervation of the external anal sphincter, and damage to the perineal branches and the dorsal nerve of the clitoris. Compression of the pudendal Alcock's canal would result in the pudendal canal syndrome.

The nerve to obturator internus muscle runs lateral to Alcock's canal. Injury to this nerve causes paralysis of the obturator internus muscle and the gemellus muscle, affecting lateral rotation of the hip.

The obturator internus muscle also forms the lateral wall of the pelvis, and the obturator fascia forms the white line (arcus tendineus levator ani and arcus tendineus fasciae pelvis) which gives origin to the levator ani.

The sutures used in SSVS should be strong and long lasting. Two sutures are used; either permanent suture such as polypropylene (Prolene) or Gore-Tex, or long-acting absorbable suture such as polypropylene (PDS), polyglyconate (Maxon) monofilament sutures. Each suture is attached to the angle of the vaginal vault; either directly through the vaginal mucosa, if long-acting absorbable sutures are used, or buried submucosally with permanent suture [42]. when performing right SSVS, we typically pass two sutures through the sacrospinous ligament, 0.5–1 cm apart. The lateral suture is attached to the right lateral vaginal fornix and the medial suture is attached to the posterior fornix just off the midline to the right. By doing so, there would be no noticeable deviation of the vaginal vault, and no interference with coitus. The suture is attached firmly to the vault in a pulley manner, in order to leave no space between the suture and the ligament complex.

Advantages of the Vaginal Approach

The vaginal approach to the treatment of eversion of vagina has many advantages. It is associated with less morbidity and shorter hospitalization. It is proven to be safe and well tolerated even by aged women [43]. The vaginal procedures appear to be more appropriate when the abdominal approach is not otherwise indicated. The vaginal approach has a lower incidence of operative complications than the abdominal approach; it has the advantage of avoiding laparotomy. It facilitates other vaginal repairs during the same operation if needed, allowing the surgeon to correct coexistent cystocele and rectocele. SSVS is an effective procedure for repair of vaginal vault prolapse. SSVS can help cure pulsion enterocele and high rectocele [44]. It is effective in the treatment of vault prolapse and compares favorably with abdominal vault supporting procedures, preserving vaginal function and shortening the time necessary for anesthesia and surgery [42,45]. It seems to ensure a lower risk of recurrent cystocele than abdominal procedures even if simple and asymptomatic [46]. The overall initial satisfaction rate of SSVS is around 90% [47]. Improved bowel function after SSVS was reported in approximately 60% [47]. Improved sexual function after SSVS was reported in 50% [47,48]. SSVS can be used as an alternative treatment to vaginal hysterectomy in aged women with medical problems or for young women suffering from genital descent who desire fertility [45].

Complications of SSVS

SSVS has a reported failure rate of 2.4–12.5% [28,42,49,50]. The risk of recurrence of vaginal vault prolapse increases with time. In a review of 243 patients, Paraiso et al. observed that the rate of clinically significant defects, most commonly in the anterior segment, worsened with time, 11.7% at 1 year, 20.3% at 5 years, and 48.1% at 10 years, and 4.5% underwent subsequent surgery [45]. Other surgeons reported a 33% recurrence rate after SSVS [51]. In our experience, vaginal vault prolapse recurrence after SSVS was 2.4% [42].

Sciatic nerve damage has been reported; these cases are typically for a short duration with spontaneous recovery coinciding with suture absorption and nerve regeneration [52]. Sciatic neuralgia has been reported in 1.2% [50]. Buttock pain, (typically transient) has been reported [53]. Entrapment of the pudendal nerve following SSVS causes pudendal canal syndrome. Using non-absorbable suture can result in chronic pudendal neuropathy with perineal and/or buttock pain. It has been reported that removing these sutures even 2 years after the initial surgery would result in immediate relief of pain [54]. Retroversion and posterior fixation of the upper vagina predisposes the anterior fascial segment to excess pressure, and increases the incidence of cystocele above that which could be attributed to the effects of aging and menopause.

Ninety-two percent of 36 patients who had SSVS developed cystocele on their follow-up evaluation with a median follow-up of 42 months [55].

Hemorrhage, particularly from the internal pudendal artery [56], and hematoma formation has been reported [57]. Although some reports included no need for blood transfusion in their series, blood transfusion was required in 4.3% [50]. Therefore, preoperative autologous blood deposition in patients undergoing major reconstructive gynecological repair procedures should be considered [14]. Fever was reported in 8.1% [50]. Infection and febrile morbidity are the most common complications [58], ranging from urinary tract infection seen in approximately 10% [50] to cuff or pelvic cellulitis. Infection can be reduced with prophylactic preoperative antibiotics [59,60].

Ureteric complications, injury to bladder such as incidental cystostomy [56,57], and inadvertent entry to bowel or rectum [57] have been reported. Rectovaginal fistula after SSVS was diagnosed in 1.2% [50]. More serious complications such as massive evisceration after SSVS can probably be avoided by careful attention to surgical technique, good apposition of the vaginal vault to the sacrospinous ligament complex and adequate repair of enterocele [61].

SSVS is a successful procedure for repairing vault prolapse but does not repair the associated cystocele, enterocele, and rectocele or urinary incontinence; it may even worsen cystocele [62]. Additional procedures to address the additional defects were needed in virtually 100% of patients [37]. Therefore, these defects should be evaluated carefully pre and intra-operatively and repaired as needed. SSVS does not predispose to dyspareunia [55,63] unless the vagina has been narrowed [7,58]

Abdominal Approach for Vault Suspension

Various abdominal procedures have been described, such as plication and suspension of the vault to the uterosacral–cardinal ligament complex. This procedure is typically accompanied by obliteration of the cul-de-sac. Abdominal colposacropexy (ACSP) can be performed as a primary procedure for vaginal apex support, particularly in severe cases or cases associated with significant predisposing factors. ACSP is considered the procedure of choice for recurrent cases. ACSP is also recommended when an abdominal approach is needed for other indications. The abdominal approach was found to be more effective than the vaginal one for correction of significant pelvic prolapse [64]. ACSP was found to be safe to perform along with radical pelvic surgery for gynecologic cancer without an increase in intra or postoperative morbidity or mortality even in patients who require chemotherapy or radiation therapy after surgery [65]. Emergency ACSP can successfully and permanently repair post-hysterectomy ileal evisceration and intestinal occlusion following a complete rupture of an inverted vaginal vault prolapse, an extremely rare complication after hysterectomy [66].

It is preferable to remove the prolapsed uterus prior to suspending the vault. However, in young women who wish to remain fertile and who cannot wait until after child bearing, or women who choose not to have hysterectomy, suspension of genital prolapse with preservation of the uterus can be achieved using the Gore-Tex soft tissue patch or other material [67].

The ACSP Procedure and Related Anatomy

Colposacropexis is achieved by attaching the vaginal apex to the anterior longitudinal vertebral ligament overlying the sacrum with a suspensory hammock. This can be done by using synthetic or natural materials. The mesh can be laid posteriorly on the vault, or preferably on both anterior and posterior surfaces of the vagina in an inverted Y-shaped fashion, then gently laying the tail of the Y retroperitoneally into the hollow of the sacrum to allow the vagina to rest upon the upper anterior surface of the rectum in its normal anatomical position.

Because enterocele frequently coexists with vaginal vault prolapse, contemporary procedures such as ACSP must be combined with enterocele repair or culdoplasty such as Moschcowitz's procedure [68,69], or Halban culdoplasty [70]. To aid in identifying the prolapsed vaginal vault, a rectal dilator, or end-to-end anastomotic sizer or a similar instrument can be used vaginally to elevate the vaginal cuff during ACSP. A sponge on a stick can be used, but care must be taken not to suture the sponge to the vault; thus it should be checked after every suture application, to reduce the risk of retaining a foreign body; such a complication has been reported [71].

With the sigmoid colon adequately retracted laterally to the left, and the rectum and vaginal apex retracted anteriorly and inferiorly, the peritoneum is opened into the retroperitoneal presacral space at the level of sacral promontory. The peritoneum is tented and undermined. Meticulous blunt and sharp dissection is carried out through the retroperitoneal

fat and areolar tissue exposing the anterior longitudinal vertebral ligament. Care must be taken to avoid injury to presacral venous plexus, especially as the dissection is carried out caudally. The rectum starts, at the 2nd sacral piece (or vertebra), and above that is the terminal part of the sigmoid. The dissection should start paramedian; medial to the nerves of the anterior sacral foramina and pelvic sympathetic trunk. The pelvic sympathetic trunks run medial to the sacral foramina; one on each side. The lateral sacral artery and vein, which are branches of the posterior division of the internal iliac artery, run lateral to these nerves. The ureters run lateral to this area in the pelvic sidewall. The incision is made lateral to the median sacral artery, and gently swiped to the sides. The dissection is carried out inferiorly to the level of S3–4.

The median sacral artery is an unpaired artery, which typically arises from the posterior surface of the abdominal aorta just superior to its bifurcation. The median sacral artery represents the caudal end of the embryonic dorsal aorta that reduced in size as the tail of the embryo disappeared.

The tail of the Y-shaped mesh is best attached to the anterior longitudinal ligament at the level of S1–3, suspending the vagina with minimal tension, particularly anteriorly. If there is concomitant rectal prolapse, the Ripstein procedure can be performed [72]. The mesh from the rectal prolapse repair is attached to the sacrum at S2, S3 or S4 level below the mesh for the abdominal colposacropexy.

The mesh is retroperitonealized or extraperitonealized at the end of the procedure by suturing the peritoneum back together. Occasionally the serosa of the sigmoid colon is sewn to the peritoneum to avoid undue tension on the peritoneum, and decrease the risk of kinking the ureters. Attaching the mesh to the sacral promontory changes the normal axis of the vagina and may unmask latent stress urinary incontinence or predisposes the patient to stress urinary incontinence. To decrease the risk of mesh erosion into the vagina we attach the mesh to the vaginal mucosa over the peritoneum without dissecting it off the underlying endopelvic fascia.

A variety of synthetic and natural materials have been used to achieve this repair including: Marlex (polypropylene glycol) mesh [73], Prolene (polypropylene) mesh [74,75], Mersilene (polyester fiber) mesh [68], Teflon (polytetrafluoroethylene) mesh, Gore-Tex (expanded reinforced polytetrafluoroethylene) [46]; some authors prefer using Dacron graft prosthesis [76,77]. Natural material includes dura mater graft [78] and rectus fascia [79,80]. There are few studies comparing the use of different meshes; Occelli et al. in 1999 found that

Mersilene mesh was less likely to be rejected than Gore-Tex [69]. Generally, the choice of mesh depends mainly on personal preference and experience; other factors such as cost and availability may also be a role.

The presence of pelvic floor dysfunction can be managed at the time of surgery, after the patient has undergone the appropriate evaluation. If there is associated latent or overt stress urinary incontinence, this can be corrected simultaneously with either a Burch retropubic colpourethropexy or combined abdominal vaginal sling procedure [81,82], depending upon whether or not there has been previous incontinence surgery, and depending upon urethral closure pressures or leak point pressure.

Other defects should also be evaluated and addressed during the surgery. Perineal descent and low posterior vaginal defects can be repaired vaginally. If the apical vault of the vagina is very capacious, partial vaginectomy and/or internal anterior and/or posterior repair can be performed at the time of abdominal colposacropexy [83].

Advantages of the ACSP Procedure

The advantage of ACSP is that it is a robust repair, with the lowest failure and recurrence rate. The success rate is reported as 94–97% [84,85]. It preserves vaginal length [86], and sexual function [87]. It can also improve irritative bladder symptoms [87]. Dyschezia is improved, but does not relieve constipation [88].

Complications of ACSP

Intraoperative complications of ACSP are similar to those of other laparotomy procedures. Some of the complications that are specific to ACSP, although uncommon, can be life-threatening. Hemorrhage from presacral veins [89] can be a significant problem because of the communications with the adjacent pelvic veins, especially the left common iliac vein. Bleeding from this complex interlacing network of veins can be difficult to control because these veins can retract underneath the sacral periosteum and recede into the underlying channels of cancellous bone. The presence of the sacrum posteriorly makes it difficult to apply a homeostatic suture or metallic clips, but it can be attempted if the bleeding vessel is seen. Cautery has a limited role in controlling venous bleeding. Packing the presacral space may control bleeding temporarily, but care must be taken not to allow the pack to move or sweep to decrease the risk of causing more venous lacerations, and thus worsening bleeding. If bleed-

ing persists, this could be controlled with bone wax. Topical bone hemostatic agents, such as gelatin paste, microfibrillar collagen, fibrin glue and gelatin sponge soaked in thrombin, were found to be effective in reducing bleeding from cancellous bone, but there is limited experience in using them in gynecological surgeries [90–92]. If these measures are unsuccessful, stainless steel thumbtacks can be placed on the retracted bleeders. Preoperative autologous blood deposition may be appropriate in these patients since there is a high rate of usage of autologous blood and low postoperative hemoglobin in a significant proportion of patients [14].

Technical difficulty can be a factor preventing or limiting the extent of repair and increasing the risk of complications, such the presence of significant pelvic adhesion, or morbidly obese patients with deep pelves.

Febrile morbidity and wound infection was reported in 10%. Urinary tract infection is the most common complication, reported in 61.5% [84]. Administering preoperative prophylactic antibiotics can decrease pelvic infection and cellulitis [59,60]. Less common complications of ACSP include: vertebral osteomyelitis. It is usually polymicrobial osteomyelitis; the possible route of infection can be the contiguous spread from an infected mesh [93].

The development of voiding dysfunction was also found to be a common complication [94]. Stress urinary incontinence, either exacerbated or developing de novo, has been reported [42]. This complication can be caused or worsened by exerting tension in suspending the anterior vaginal wall to the sacrum.

Bowel complications, including enterotomy, proctotomy and sigmoid perforation, have also been reported [85]. One report described small bowel obstruction, caused by a trapped loop of ileum in a hole in the posterior peritoneum [78]. Other reported rare complications are nerve injury and ureteral damage kinking.

Long-term complications are mainly those related to the presence of the mesh, and to a lesser extent the failure rate. Persistent vaginal permanent suture or mesh erosion has been reported [77]. Persistent discharging sinus, sometimes necessitating removal of the mesh, was reported with both Mersilene mesh [94] and Gore-Tex mesh [95]. Partial removal of an exposed mesh eroding through the vaginal wall without proper débridement and approximation of healthy vaginal tissue can result in a persistent sinus tract from the vagina to the sacrum. Such cases require complete removal of all the mesh material and resection of the sinus tract [95]. Failure of ACSP and recurrence of vaginal vault prolapse has been reported in 1.3%, compared to 2.4% recurrence for SSVS [42].

Laparoscopic Approach for Vault Suspension

Laparoscopy has successfully replaced several of the open surgical procedures. Laparoscopy has been applied to many aspects of gynecologic surgery, including repair of vaginal vault prolapse and enterocele [96]. The vaginal vault has been suspended successfully to the deep layer of the uterosacral ligaments. This repair maintains the gross functional anatomy, and places the vagina in the midline with its proper parallel alignment to the rectum and re-constitution of proper relationship between the newly suspended vagina and pelvic viscera [97].

Colposacropexy can be done laparoscopically using staples, screw and endoscopic suturing [20,21,98]. In skilled hands and with the proper training, most laparoscopic procedures carry less morbidity and shorter hospital stay. There is, however, a learning curve, and therefore the level of expertise and outcome varies. The long-term efficacy and endurance are not yet evaluated. Details of laparoscopic procedures are explained in Chapter 35.

Conclusion

The successful treatment of vaginal vault prolapse with eversion continues to be an enigma to pelvic surgeons. The many surgical procedures that have been proposed testify to the fact that no single reliable procedure has been developed. Pelvic surgeons, however, should be well acquainted with the different procedures. A good knowledge of pelvic anatomy is crucial to achieve a safe and accurate repair. In choosing the best approach for the repair, it is essential to consider the patient's wishes, her general condition, pre-existent risk factors or presence of other pathology, the extent of the defects, intrinsic and extrinsic tissue factors. The experience of the surgeon, individualization of the repair to the patient, observing the goal of pelvic reconstructive surgery and addressing all the defects with a site-specific repair are important issues in insuring successful repair. Although vaginal repair carries less morbidity, emerging reports indicate that the abdominal approach results in a more durable repair, and thus should be considered in patients at high risk for recurrence, particularly if risk factors are not modifiable. Abdominal procedures should be considered for patients with specific indications for an abdominal approach.

References

1. Marchionni M, Bracco GL, Checcucci V, Carabaneanu A, Coccia EM, Mecacci F, Scarselli G. True incidence of vaginal vault prolapse. Thirteen years of experience. J Reprod Med 1999;44:679–84.
2. Comiter CV, Vasavada SP, Barbaric ZL, Gousse, Raz S. Grading pelvic prolapse and pelvic floor relaxation using dynamic magnetic resonance imaging. Urology 1999;54:454–7.
3. ACOG technical bulletin. Number 214. October 1995.
4. Drutz HP, Alnaif B Surgical management of pelvic organ prolapse and stress urinary incontinence. Clin Obstet Gynecol 1998;41:786–93.
5. Baker KR, Drutz HP: Retropubic colpourethropexy. Clinical and urodynamic evaluation of 289 cases. Int Urogynecol J 1991;2:196–200.
6. Bombieri L, Freeman RM. Recurrence of stress incontinence after vault suspension: can it be prevented? Int Urogynecol J Pelvic Floor Dysfunct 1998;9:58–60.
7. Backer MH Jr. Success with sacrospinous suspension of the prolapsed vaginal vault. Surg Gynecol Obstet 1992;175:419–20.
8. Weatherall M. Biofeedback or pelvic floor muscle exercises for female genuine stress incontinence: a meta-analysis of trials identified in a systematic review. BJU Int 1999;83:1015–16.
9. Ko CY, Tong J, Lehman RE, Shelton AA, Schrock TR, Welton ML. Biofeedback is effective therapy for fecal incontinence and constipation. Dis Colon Rectum 1997;40:821–6.
10. Rieger NA, Wattchow DA, Sarre RG, Cooper SJ, Rich CA, Saccone GT, Schloithe AC, Toouli J, McCall JL. Prospective trial of pelvic floor retraining in patients with fecal incontinence. Dis Colon Rectum 1997;40:821–6.
11. Mikkelsen AL, Felding C, Clausen HV. Clinical effects of preoperative oestradiol treatment before vaginal repair operation. A double-blind, randomized trial. Gynecol Obstet Invest 1995;40:125–8.
12. Delaere K, Moonen W, Debruyne F, Jansen T. Hydronephrosis caused by cystocele. Treatment by colpopexy to sacral promontory. Urology 1984;24:364–5.
13. Jackson SR, Avery NC, Tarlton JF, Eckford SD, Abrams P, Bailey AJ. Changes in metabolism of collagen in genitourinary prolapse. Lancet 1996;15:1658–61.
14. Wang C, Lau W, Herst R, Drutz H, Fernandes B. Preoperative autologous blood deposition in support of gynaecological repair procedures. Transfus Med 1998;8:23–7.
15. Peters WA 3rd, Christenson ML. Fixation of the vaginal apex to the coccygeus fascia during repair of vaginal vault eversion with enterocele. Am J Obstet Gynecol 1995;172:1894–900.
16. Inmon WB. Pelvic relaxation and repair including prolapse of vagina following hysterectomy. South Med J 1963;56:577.
17. Comiter CV, Vasavada SP, Raz S. Transvaginal culdosuspension: technique and results. Urology 1999;54:819–22.
18. Webb MJ, Aronson MP, Ferguson LK, Lee RA. Posthysterectomy vaginal vault prolapse: primary repair in 693 patients. Obstet Gynecol 1998;92:281–5.
19. McCall ML. Posterior culdoplasty. Surgical correction of enterocele during vaginal hysterectomy: a preliminary report. Obstet. Gynecol 1957;10:595–602.
20. Ross JW. Apical vault repair the cornerstone of pelvic vault reconstruction. Int Urogynecol J Pelvic Floor Dysfunct 1997;8:146–52.
21. Ross JW. Techniques of laparoscopic repair of total vault eversion after hysterectomy. J Am Assoc Gynecol Laparosc 1997;4:173–83.

22. Langmade CF, Oliver JA Jr, White JS. Cooper ligament repair of vaginal vault prolapse twenty-eight years late. Trans Pac Coast Obstet Gynecol Soc 1978;45:16–24.
23. Dibbell DG. Dynamic correction of intractable vaginal prolapse. Ann Plast Surg 1979;2:254–6.
24. Raz S, Nitti VW, Bregg KJ. Transvaginal repair of enterocele. J Urol 1993;149:724–30.
25. DeLancey JOL, Morley GW. Total colpocleisis for vaginal eversion. Am J Obstet Gynecol 176:1228,1997.
26. Rudigoz RC, Gonnet C, Rochet Y, Dargent D, Bremond A. Prolapse after hysterectomy. A study of 45 cases. J Gynecol Obstet Reprod (Paris) 1981;10:241–7.
27. Giuly J, Cravello L, D'Ercole C, Roger V Porcu G Blac B. Richter's spinofixation in vaginal prolapse. Chirurgie 1997;122:430–4.
28. Meschia M, Bruschi F, Amicarelli F, Pifarotti P, Marchini M, Crosignani PG. The sacrospinous vaginal vault suspension: Critical analysis of outcomes. Int Urogynecol J Pelvic Floor Dysfunct 1999;10:155–9.
29. Verhoest CR, Drutz HP. MacMillan JB. Prophylactic sacrospinous ligament fixation at the time of vaginal hysterectomy (abstract). Int Urogynecol J 1996;7:300.
30. Porges RF, Smilen SW. Long-term analysis of the surgical management of pelvic support defects. Am J Obstet Gynecol 1994;171:1518–26.
31. Febbraro W, Beucher G, Von Theobald P, Hamel P, Barjot P, Heisert M, Levy G. Feasibility of bilateral sacrospinous ligament vaginal suspension with a stapler. Prospective studies with the 34 first cases. J Gynecol Obstet Biol Reprod (Paris). 1997;26:815–21 [Article in French].
32. Pohl JF, Frattarelli JL. Bilateral SSVS. Bilateral transvaginal sacrospinous colpopexy: preliminary experience. Am J Obstet Gynecol 1997;177:1356–61.
33. Pohl JF, Frattarelli JL. Bilateral transvaginal sacrospinous colpopexy: preliminary experience. Am J Obstet Gynecol 1997 Dec;177(6):1356–61; discussion 1361–2.
34. Miyazaki FS. Miya hook ligature carrier for sacrospinous ligament suspension. Obstet Gynecol 1987;70(2):286–8.
35. Veronikis DK, Nichols DH Ligature carrier specifically designed for transvaginal sacrospinous colpopexy. Obstet Gynecol 1997;89:478–81.
36. Papasakelariou C. Sacrospinous ligament fixation simplified with a new endoscopic suturing device. Am Assoc Gynecol Laparosc 1996;3:S38.
37. Schlesinger RE. Vaginal sacrospinous ligament fixation with the Autosuture Endostitch device. Am J Obstet Gynecol 1997;176:1358–62.
38. Watson JD. Sacrospinous ligament colpopexy: new instrumentation applied to a standard gynecologic procedure. Obstet Gynecol 1996;88:883–5.
39. Shetty SD, Kirkemo AK. Bilateral bone anchor vaginal vault suspension: an initial report of a new technique. Tech Urol 1997;3:1–5.
40. Verdeja AM, Elkins TE, Odoi A, Gasser R, Lamoutte C. Transvaginal sacrospinous colpopexy: anatomic landmarks to be aware of to minimize complications. Am J Obstet Gynecol 1995;173:1468–9.
41. Shafik A, el-Sherif M, Youssef A, Olfat ES. Surgical anatomy of the pudendal nerve and its clinical implications. Clin Anat 1995;8:110–15.
42. Hardiman PJ, Drutz HP. Sacrospinous vault suspension and abdominal colposacropexy: success rates and complications. Am J Obstet Gynecol 1996;175:612–16.
43. Heinonen PK. Transvagianl sacrospinous colpopexy for vaginal vault and complete genital prolapse in aged women. Acta Obstet Gynecol Scand 1992;71:377–81.
44. Brieger GM, MacGibbon AL, Atkinson KH. Sacrospinous colpopexy. Aust NZ J Obstet Gynaecol 1995;35:86–7.
45. Ozcan U, Gungor T, Ekin M, Eken S. Sacrospinous fixation for the prolapsed vaginal vault. Gynecol Obstet Invest 1999;47:65–8.
46. Imparato E, Aspesi G, Rovetta E, Presti M. Surgical management and prevention of vaginal vault prolapse. Surg Gynecol Obstet 1992;175:233–7.
47. Hewson AD. Transvaginal sacrospinous colpopexy for posthtysterectomy vault prolapse. Aust NZ J Obstet Gynecol 1998; 38:318–24.
48. Paraiso MF, Ballard LA, Walters MD, Lee JC, Mitchinson AR. Pelvic support defects and visceral and sexual function in women treated with sacrospinous ligament suspension and pelvic reconstruction. Am J Obstet Gynecol 1996;175:1423–30.
49. Sauer HA, Klutke CG. Transvaginal sacrospinous ligament fixation for treatment of vaginal prolapse. J Urol 1995;154:1008–12.
50. Penalver MA, Angioli R, Mirhashemi R, Malik R. Management of early and late complications of ileocolonic continent urinary reservoir (Miami pouch). Gynecol Oncol 1998;69:185–91.
51. Sze EH, Miklos JR, Partoll L, Roat TW, Karram MM. Sacrospinous ligament fixation with transvaginal needle suspension for advanced pelvic organ prolapse and stress incontinence. Obstet Gynecol 1997;89:94–6.
52. Dellas A, Almendral AC. Surgical treatment of vaginal prolapse after hysterectomy. Geburtshilfe Frauenheilkd 1995;55:244–6.
53. Lind LR, Choe J, Bhatia NN. An in-line suturing device to simplify sacrospinous vaginal vault suspension. Obstet Gynecol 1997;89:129–32.
54. Alevizon SJ, Finan MA. Sacrospinous colpopexy: management of postoperative pudendal nerve entrapment. Obstet Gynecol 1996;88:713–15.
55. Holley RL, Varner RE, Gleason BP, Apffel LA, Scott S. Recurrent pelvic support defects after sacrospinous ligament fixation for vaginal vault prolapse. J Am Coll Surg 1995;180:444–8.
56. Hoffman MS, Harris MS, Bouis PJ. Sacrospinous colpopexy in the management of uterovaginal prolapse.
57. Halaska M. fixation of the prolapsed vagina to the sacrospinous ligament after hysterectomy- the Amreich II-Richter vaginal fixation operation. Ceska Gynekol 1997; 62:323–9.
58. Morley GW, DeLancey JO. Sacrospinous ligament fixation for eversion of the vagina. Am J Obstet Gynecol 1988;158:872–81.
59. Jennings RH. Prophylactic antibiotics in vaginal and abdominal hysterectomy. Antibiotics is helpful in reducing post op infection. South Med J. 1978;71:251–4.
60. Price SA, Polk HC Jr. Prophylactic and therapeutic use of antibiotics in pelvic surgery. J Surg Oncol 1999;71:261–8.
61. Farrell SA, Scotti RJ, Ostergard DR, Bent AE. Massive evisceration: a complication following sacrospinous vaginal vault fixation. Obstet Gynecol 1991;78:560–2.
62. Richter K, Albrich W. Long-term results following fixation of the vagina on the sacrospinal ligament by the vaginal rote (vaginaefixatio sacrospinalis vaginalis). Am J Obstet Gynecol 1981;141:811–16.
63. Holley RL, Varner RE, Gleason BP Apffel LA, Scott S. Sexual function after sacrospinous ligament fixation for vaginal vault prolapse. J Reprod Med 1996;41:355–8.
64. Benson JT, Lucente V, McClellan E. Vaginal versus abdominal reconstructive surgery for the treatment of pelvic support defects: a prospective randomized study with long-term outcome evaluation. Am J Obstet Gynecol 1996;175:1418–21; discussion 1421–2.
65. Patsner B Abdominal sacral colpopexy in patients with gynecologic cancer: report of 25 cases with long-term

follow-up and literature review. Gynecol Oncol 1999;
75:504–8.

66. Crespi C, De Giorgio AM. Prolapse of the vaginal vault complicated by ileal evisceration. Possible role of Dacron mesh in emergencies. Technical notes. G Chir 1991;12:498–500 [Article in Italian].

67. Van Lindert AC, Groenendijk AG, Scholten PC, Heintz AP. Surgical support and suspension of genital prolapse, including preservation of the uterus, using the Gore-Tex soft tissue patch (a preliminary report). Eur J Obstet Gynecol Reprod Biol 1993;50:133–9.

68. Addison WA, Livengood CH3rd, Sutton GP, Parker RT. Abdominal sacral colpopexy with Mersilene mesh in the retroperitoneal position in the management of post-hysterectomy vaginal vault prolpase and enterocele. Am J Obstet Gynecol 1985;153:140–6.

69. Occelli B, Narducci F, Cosson M, Ego A, Decocq J, Querleu D, Crepin G. Abdominal colposacropexy for the treatment of vaginal vault prolapse with or without urinary stress incontinence. Ann Chir 1999;53:367–77.

70. Halban J. Gynaklogische operationslerhre. Berlin: Urban and Schwarzenberg, 1932.

71. Hemelt BA, Finan MA Abdominal sacral colpopexy resulting in a retained sponge. A case report. J Reprod Med 1999;44:983–5.

72. Baker KR, Drutz HP, Stern HS, Deutsch A. Combining colposacropexy and Ripstein procedure for combined vaginal vault and rectal prolapse with and without retropubic colpourethropexy for stress urinary incontinence. Int Urogynecol J 1990;1:228–32.

73. Drutz HP, Cha LS Massive genital and vaginal vault prolapse treated by abdominal-vaginal sacropexy with use of Marlex mesh: review of the literature. Am J Obstet Gynecol 1987;156:387–92.

74. Baker KR, Beresford JM, Campbell C. Colposacropexy with Prolene mesh. Surg Gynecol Obstet 1990;171:51–4.

75. Schettini M, Fortunato P, Gallucci M. Abdominal sacral colpopexy with Prolene mesh. Int Uurogynecol J Pelvic Floor Dysfunct 1999;10:295–9.

76. Traiman P, De Luca LA, Silva AA, Antonini R, Dias R, Rodrigues JR. Abdominal colpopexy for complete prolapse of the vagina. Int Surg 1992;77:91–5.

77. Snyder TE, Krantz KE. Abdominal-retroperitoneal sacral colpopexy for the correction of vaginal prolapse. Obstet Gynecol 1991;77:944–9.

78. Lansman HH. Posthysterectomy vault prolapse: sacral colpopexy with dura mater graft. Obstet Gynecol 1984;63:577–82.

79. Maloney JC, Dunton CJ, Smith K. Repair of vaginal vault prolapse with abdominal sacropexy. J Reprod Med 1990;35:6–10.

80. Kauppila O, Punnonen R, Teisala K. Operative technique for the repair of posthysterectomy vaginal prolapse. Ann Chir Gynaecol 1986;75(4):242–4.

81. Drutz HP, Buckspan MB, Flaz S, Mackie L. Clinical and urodynamic re-evaluation of combined abdominovaginal Marlex sling operation for recurrent stress urinary incontinence. Int Urogynecol J 1990;1:70–3.

82. Spence-Jones C, DeMarco, Lemieux MC, Drutz HP. Modified urethral sling for the treatment of genuine stress incontinence and latent incontinence. Int Urogynecol J 1994;5:69–75.

83. Drutz HP, Baker KR, Lemieux MC. Retropubic colpourethropexy with tansabdominal anterior and or posterior repair for the treatment of genuine stress urinary incontinence and genital prolapse. Int Urogynecol J 1991;2:201–7.

84. Lecuru F, Taurelle R, Clouard C, Attal JP. Surgical treatment of genito-urinary prolapse by abdominal approach. Results in a continuous series of 203 operations. Ann Chir 1994;48:1013–19 [Article in French].

85. Lejeune V, Roullet-Audy JC, Guivarc'h M. Sigmoid perforation after colpopexy of the vaginal dome. J Gynecol Obstet Biol Reprod (Paris) 1994;23:931.

86. Given FT Jr, Muhlendorf IK, Browning GM. Vaginal length and sexual function after colpopexy for complete uterovaginal eversion. Am J Obstet Gynecol 1993;169:284–7; discussion 287–8.

87. Pilsgaard K, Mouritsen L. Follow-up after repair of vaginal vault prolapse with abdominal colposacropexy. Acta Obstet Gynecol Scand 1999;78:66–70.

88. Villet R, Morice P, Bech A, Salet-Lizee D, Zafiropulo M. Abdominal approach of rectocele and colpocele. Ann Chir 1993;47(7):626–30

89. Smith MR. Colposacropexy: an alternative technique. Am J Obstet Gynecol 1997;176:1374–5.

90. Harris WH, Crothers OD, Moyen BJ, Bourne RB. Topical hemostatic agents for bone bleeding in humans. A quantitative comparison of gelatin paste, gelatin sponge plus bovine thrombin, and microfibrillar collagen. J Bone Joint Surg 1978;60:454–6.

91. Malofsky H, Lopez AL. Application and assessment of microfibrillar collagen hemostat in heel spur surgery: a preliminary study. J Foot Surg 1985;24:445–7.

92. Spotnitz WD, Dalton MS, Baker JW, Nolan SP. Successful use of fibrin glue during 2 years of surgery at a university medical center. Am Surg 1989;55:166–8.

93. Cranney A, Feibel R, Toye BW, Karsh J. Osteomyelitis subsequent to abdominal-vaginal sacropexy. J Rheumatol 1994;21:1769–70.

94. Creighton SM, Stanton SL. The surgical management of vaginal vault prolapse. Br J Obstet Gynaecol 1991;98:1150–4.

95. Unger JB A persistent sinus tract from the vagina to the sacrum after treatment of mesh erosion by partial removal of a GORE-TEX soft tissue patch. Am J Obstet Gynecol 1999;181:762–3.

96. Paraosp MF, Falcone T, Walters MD. Laparoscopic surgery for enterocele, vaginal apex prolapse and rectocele. Int Urogynecol J Pelvic Floor Dysfunct 1999;10:223–9.

97. Osterzenski A. Laparoscopic colposuspension for total vaginal prolapse. Int J Gynaecol Obstet 1996;55:147–52.

98. Nezhat CH, Nezhat F, Nezhat C. Laparoscopic sacral colpopexy for vaginal vault prolapse. Obstet Gynecol 1994;84:885–8.

40 Repair of Posterior Vaginal Wall Prolapse

Margie A. Kahn and Abdul H. Sultan

Definition

Posterior vaginal wall prolapse is a hernia of intra-abdominal contents through the "fascia" or fibromuscular posterior wall of the vagina or its attachment to the perineal body. A rectocele involves only herniation of the rectum (Figure 40.1); a culdocele involves herniation of cul-de-sac contents (Figure 40.2) and comprises enteroceles, peritoneoceles, and sigmoidoceles.

Anatomy and Its Relationship to Surgery

Four anatomic abnormalities are described in association with posterior vaginal wall prolapse: disruption of the rectovaginal fascia, an abnormally deep cul-de-sac, widening of the levator hiatus, and attenuation of the anterior wall of the rectum.

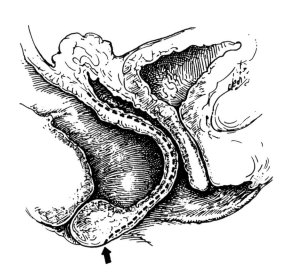

Figure 40.1 Lower vaginal and perineal rectocele. The arrow points to the beginning of the rectovaginal space. (From Nichols DH, Randall CL. Vaginal Surgery, Third edition, Baltimore: Williams & Wilkins.)

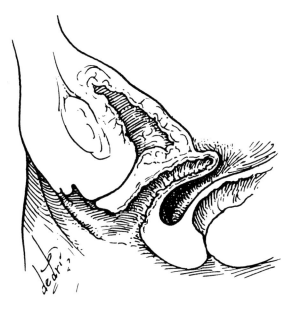

Figure 40.2 Culdocele. (From Nichols DH, Randall CL. Vaginal Surgery, Third edition, Baltimore: Williams & Wilkins.)

Fascia and Its Plication

The primary defects occur in the tough, shiny layer of tissue that is interposed between the rectum and the vagina. Often called the endopelvic fascia, vaginal fascia, rectovaginal septum or Denonvillier's fascia, this layer is believed by some authors to be simply the fibromuscular wall of the vagina [1–5]. In this chapter, we will refer to "fascia" for historical consistency, while recognizing that this issue is still hotly debated. Most descriptions of vaginal surgical repair refer to plication or reconstitution of this layer. However, it may be unwise to use a tissue with demonstrated incompetence for long-lasting surgical strength. Thus, some techniques reinforce this layer with an artificial mesh [6,7] or cadaveric tissue [8].

The Deep Cul-de-Sac and Its Obliteration

Nichols and Randall [9] recognize four types of enterocele. They hypothesize that the type associated with posterior vaginal wall prolapse is congenital, i.e. that during late fetal development, the anterior and posterior peritoneum of the cul-de-sac fail to fuse. Thus, obliteration of the cul-de-sac has been a mainstay of enterocele repair. However, a posterior enterocele may also result secondarily from herniation of the cul-de-sac through the rectovaginal fascia. In this case, again, fascial integrity must be restored.

Widening of the Levator Hiatus and Levator Plication

By levator myography, Berglas and Rubin [10] demonstrated widening of the levator hiatus in both

the anterior-posterior (Figure 40.3) and transverse diameter in patients with uterine prolapse. By vaginal examination or by ultrasound (Figure 40.4a and 40.4b), the measurement of the genital hiatus may increase in these same directions resulting in perineal descent and a "gaping introitus". The frequently debated "levator plication" part of the posterior colpoperineorrhaphy may have arisen in response to these observations. Because perineorrhaphy is often not distinguished from posterior colporrhaphy, it is

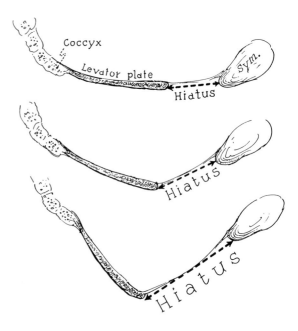

Figure 40.3 The relationship of genital hiatus length and perineal descent. (From Nichols DH, Randall CL. Vaginal Surgery, Third edition, Baltimore: Williams & Wilkins.)

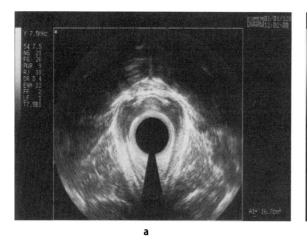

a

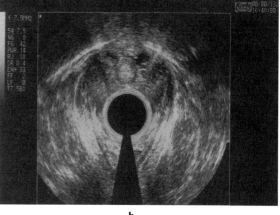

b

Figure 40.4 Vaginal ultrasounds of women without (**a**) and with (**b**) widening of the levator hiatus. (Courtesy of the Urogynaecology Unit at King's College Hospital, London, UK.)

not always clear whether the reconstitution of the perineal body performed in this part of the operation includes a few fibers from the puborectalis portion of the levator ani. This much smaller plication would very likely have different postoperative sequelae from extensive plication.

Attenuation of the Anterior Rectal Wall and Its Plication

Colorectal surgeons have observed that vaginal repair may not correct a ballooning anterior rectal wall and may plicate the excess from inside the rectum – a transanal or endorectal repair [11].

Etiology

Posterior vaginal wall prolapse is thought to be associated with similar neurogenic, mechanical and connective tissue abnormalities as cause other pelvic floor disorders. However, these abnormalities are associations and a clear cause and effect relationship is suggested, although not proven. Straining at stool with resultant perineal descent and pudendal neuropathy [12,13] is a common finding in these patients. Previous colposuspension [14] and prolapse surgery [15] predispose to rectocele formation, perhaps because of the change of the vectors of force applied to the vaginal axis. Probably the most important cause is childbirth, which is also associated with pubococcygeus denervation [16] and reinnervation [17] and can be directly traumatic to all of the supports of the pelvic floor, the rectum and the vagina. A congenitally deep cul-de-sac [18–20] or inadequate attention paid to reattachment of the uterosacral–cardinal ligament complex to the vaginal cuff and obliteration of the cul-de-sac at the time of hysterectomy are commonly implicated as causes of enteroceles, although such preventative measures have been shown to be effective only for vault prolapse [21,22].

Symptoms

Vaginal symptoms include awareness of a bulging mass in the vagina, perineal or lower abdominal pressure, slackness at intercourse or dyspareunia, and low back pain that worsens throughout the day and is relieved by lying down. Rectal symptoms for rectoceles include constipation, a feeling of incomplete emptying during defecation, the need to vaginally, rectally, or perineally digitate to effect evacuation, incontinence of feces, pain, and bleeding.

Although symptoms of impaired rectal emptying may be present with culdoceles, their obstructive nature is questionable. Extrinsic compression of the rectum by the hernia sac may create the sensation of a fecal bolus, even when the rectum is empty [23]. The cause and effect relationship of anorectal symptoms is not always clear because other colorectal disorders can cause similar symptoms [24] and the anatomic findings do not correlate with symptoms.

Signs and Classification

The diagnosis should be made in the unanesthetized patient in the lithotomy, Sims, sitting and/or standing [19] position with the patient bearing down or straining as if attempting to defecate. Because prolapse is dynamic, ask the patient if the demonstrated prolapse is at its worst.

Rectovaginal examination can help distinguish between rectocele and culdocele by the palpation of a sac dissecting between the rectum and vagina. Other distinguishing techniques utilize a bivalve speculum to visualize a secondary fold of vagina [25], transillumination of the rectovaginal space or observation of peristalsis in the posterior vaginal wall [26]. If the rectal vault is full of stool, an enema may allow a previously unidentified culdocele to become apparent. The location of the defect in the rectovaginal septum can be identified as high, mid, low or perineal [27]. However, the physical examination diagnosis is known to be frequently inconsistent with that identified at surgery.

Rectal examination also identifies other causes of impaired defecation or incontinence such as posterior rectocele, intussusception, poor anal sphincter or levator tone, skin tags and mucosal prolapse. The presence of stool in the rectum should be noted as well as the amount of perineal descent below the ischial spines during rest and while straining.

Numerous grading schemes have been proposed to quantify the size of the vaginal prolapse. The currently accepted international standard, the POP-Q (Pelvic Organ Prolapse Quantification) [28] incorporates direct measurements of the degree of vaginal prolapse in relation to the hymen (Figure 40.5). An adaptation of Baden and Walker's Halfway System [29], it provides more precise information than the traditional first /second/ third degree or mild/moderate/severe classifications. The stages in this system are identified as:

Stage 0: No prolapse identified
Stage I: The most distal portion of the posterior wall prolapse is >1 cm proximal to the hymen

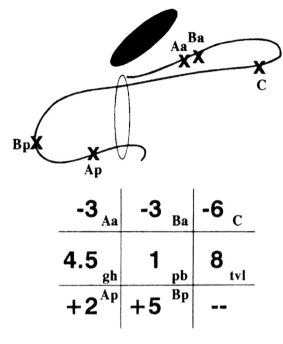

-3 Aa	-3 Ba	-6 C
4.5 gh	1 pb	8 tvl
+2 Ap	+5 Bp	--

Figure 40.5 Grid and line diagram of predominant posterior support defect. Leading point of prolapse is upper posterior vaginal wall, point Bp (+5). Point Ap is 2 cm distal to hymen (+2) and vaginal cuff scar is 6 cm above hymen (–6), Cuff has undergone only 2 cm of descent because it would be at –8 (total vaginal length) if it were perfectly supported. This represents stage III Bp prolapse. (From Bump et al. The standardization of female pelvic organ and prolapse and pelvic floor dysfunction. Am J Obstet Gynecol 1996;175:15.)

Stage II: The most distal portion of the prolapse is ≤ 1 cm proximal to or distal to the hymen

Stage III: The most distal portion of the prolapse is >1 cm distal to the hymen, but extends no farther than the total length minus 2 cm of the vagina, when its prolapse is reduced. Genital hiatus (anterior-posterior) and perineal body measurements are not staged in this system, but precisely measured.

Stage IV: Prolapse > stage III.

This system does not attempt to identify the structures behind the vaginal wall nor does it quantify the size of the rectocele from the rectal side. An objective clinical grading system for the rectal side does not exist.

The only grading system that quantifies culdoceles is the Baden and Walker Halfway System [29] in which each grade defines the maximum extent of the prolapse:

Grade 0:   Normal position
Grade 1:   Descent halfway to the hymen
Grade 2:   Descent to the hymen
Grade 3:   Descent halfway past the hymen
Grade 4:   Maximum possible descent

Before Surgery

Because the symptoms of posterior vaginal wall prolapse are not unique, it is important to search for other causes of the patient's symptoms:

1. Constipation. A patient who has one hard bowel movement per week may strain or digitate regardless of the presence of a rectocele. Indeed, if these are the only complaints, they may be resolved entirely by dietary changes alone. Before surgery, bowel habits must be normalized as much as possible by the use of bulking agents such as psyllium and osmotic expanders such as sorbitol or lactulose syrup. Bowel transit studies may be indicated in those in whom bowel frequency and consistency cannot be corrected. These patients are more apt to have postoperative continuation of bowel symptoms [30]; in addition, continued straining at stool may predispose to recurrent prolapse.

2. Incontinence. Fecal incontinence from rectoceles results from reflex relaxation of the anal sphincter when the rectum is overdistended by stool [31]. However, soiling may be caused by mechanical and neurological anal sphincter abnormalities, anal skin tags, rectal mucosal prolapse, and hemorrhoids. Diarrhea can overwhelm a borderline continence mechanism and may require testing for infection or malabsorption. Further investigation in patients with fecal incontinence should include anorectal physiological and imaging studies.

3. Bleeding. Rectal bleeding should be evaluated by colonoscopy or barium enema to diagnose malignancy.

4. Sexual dysfunction. Sexual problems can be caused by psychological factors, hypo-estrogenism, and partner impotency. The patient and her partner must understand that narrowing a lax genital hiatus may not restore neurological control of the pelvic floor and sexual sensation. Vaginal symptoms attributed to prolapse sometimes resolve with treatment of vulvovaginitis or atrophy.

The Operations

Posterior Colporrhaphy and Perineorrhaphy

History
Vaginal and perineal plastic surgery began in the sixteenth century with the repair of complete perineal tears following childbirth [32]. Simon of Heidelberg (1867) [32] is regarded by some as the originator of the present day operation and the term "posterior colporrhaphy".

Preoperative Preparation
Vaginal estrogen is advised, preferably for at least for 3 months. A phosphate enema is given the morning of surgery if the rectal vault is filled with stool. A second-generation cephalosporin is given intravenously in the holding area.

Technique
The patient is positioned in dorsal lithotomy position as for other vaginal surgery. The labia minora may be sutured laterally for better exposure. Serial Allis clamps are placed in the midline from the apex to 1–2 cm above the hymen. If a perineorrhaphy is to be performed, the future caliber of the vaginal introitus is estimated by placing Allis clamps bilaterally on the labia minora and approximating them in the midline. The final hiatus should admit three fingerbreadths easily to avoid postoperative constriction. One additional Allis clamp is placed in the midline between the hymen and the anus to mark the inferior extent of the perineorrhaphy. The diamond-shaped piece of vaginal mucosa and perineal skin marked by the four inferior Allises is excised by sharp dissection (Figure 40.6). A midline incision is made from the apex of the vagina to the top of this diamond. The vaginal mucosa is then freed laterally from the underlying fascia and rectal wall by a combination of blunt and sharp dissection with countertraction on the rectum until the puborectalis portions of the levator ani are reached. At the perineal body, the bulbocavernosus and transverse perineal muscles are also dissected free of the overlying vagina and perineum. Any enterocele sac or culdocele is obliterated by high concentric purse-string sutures. Using 00 or 0 delayed-absorbable sutures, the lateral rectovaginal fascia is plicated in the midline from the apex to the lower portion of the vagina. A finger may be placed in the rectum and curved toward the operator to help identify this tissue and to avoid placing sutures through the rectum. As the perineal body is approached, deep plication stitches may be placed in the puborectalis portions of the levator ani, taking care to avoid constriction of the vagina. Aggressiveness in this part of the operation is thought to cause postoperative dyspareunia [33]. Excess vaginal mucosa is trimmed bilaterally and the vaginal incision with a running locked stitch using 00 suture. For the perineorrhaphy, the perineal muscles are approximated with 0 deep sutures and the perineum is reconstituted beginning with the "crown" stitch as in episiotomy repair (Figure 40.7). The perineal skin is then closed with a subcuticular stitch. No vaginal pack is necessary if adequate hemostasis is obtained. Bladder drainage is usually necessary overnight because the most common immediate postoperative complication is urinary retention [34].

Postoperative Management
Patients are discharged with psyllium and sorbitol syrup to keep the stools as soft as toothpaste, forever, if possible. Sexual activity is encouraged after the 6-week check-up. Any vaginal stenosis is treated with dilators and liberal use of vaginal estrogen cream.

Long-term Results
The operation has long been recognized as a cause of postoperative vaginal scarring, stenosis, and dyspareunia [33,35] in approximately 20–27% [34,36,37] of women, greater than that caused by other vaginal operations alone. Most patients experience improvement in bowel symptoms [30], but many (48–62%) are left with some residual symptoms of

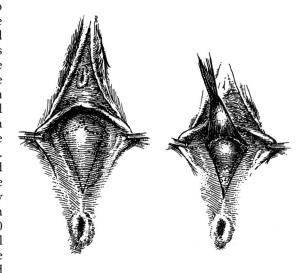

Figure 40.6 Diamond-shaped area of the vagina and perineum to be excised during the perineorrhaphy. (From Nichols DH, Randall CL. Vaginal Surgery, Third edition. Baltimore: Williams & Wilkins.)

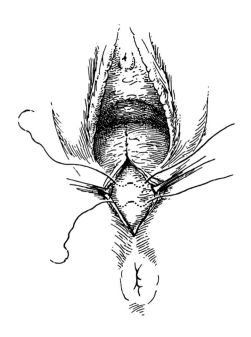

Figure 40.7 Deep perineal sutures that capture bulbocavernosus and transverse perineal muscles. (From Nichols DH, Randall CL. Vaginal Surgery, Third edition. Baltimore: Williams & Wilkins.)

impaired bowel emptying [30,34,37]. Prophylactic repair of an asymptomatic rectocele should be discouraged at the time of Burch colposuspension because the rectocele is more likely to recur [38].

Fascial Defect Repair

In 1993, Cullen Richardson described the directed fascial defect repair [39]. The operation differs from the one above in the fascial plication steps. Rather than universal midline plication, distinct defects are identified as breaks in the smooth, shiny layer of fascia that is identified by its ability to withstand traction by Allises. The most common defect is a low transverse disruption between the fascia and the perineal body. A high transverse defect is often associated with a culdocele. The direction of the reparative suture line conforms to the often irregular or curved shape of the defect as seen in Figures 40.8a–8d. Any residual breaks to be repaired are palpated with the rectal finger. Intuitively attractive, this technique has been only minimally evaluated. As with the traditional repair, most patients' rectal emptying improves, but 39–50% experience residual bowel symptoms [40,41] and 19% are left with dyspareunia [40]. It is not known whether repairing these discrete defects maintains adequate strength over time or whether additional plication of fascia or levators improves the longevity of the repair.

Reinforcement of the Rectovaginal Septum via Graft

Techniques that reinforce the rectovaginal septum developed in response to concerns about the intrinsic strength of this tissue.

In 1987, Øster and Astrup [42] described a technique of posterior colporrhaphy without levator plication for large rectoceles in which a dermis graft removed from the thigh is sutured into the rectovaginal space. Fifteen women were followed up for a mean of 2.6 years. Five patients suffered from constipation postoperatively, although the authors state that all 15 were cured of their defecatory and prolapse symptoms. Three patients experienced dyspareunia. Watson et al. [7] described placement of a Marlex mesh via a transperineal approach with levator plication in nine women who digitated to effect evacuation. Postoperatively, eight of the nine were cured of impaired bowel emptying. The mean symptom score for "vaginal lump" improved overall. One patient developed de novo dyspareunia. Lyons and Winer [6] followed 20 patients following laparoscopic placement of a polyglactin mesh in the rectovaginal space and reported an 80% success rate at one year. Unfortunately, these authors do not define success. An early report of cadaveric fascia used in 20 patients has shown promising results at 6 months. However, use of this material for suburethral slings has not been proven to be satisfactory as compared with autologous tissue [43].

Cul-de-Sac Obliteration

Repair of a culdocele normally involves its obliteration. Since the depth of the normal cul-de-sac is controversial [44,45], it is difficult to determine when prophylaxis becomes treatment.

Vaginal techniques of repair include the Torpin [46] or Waters [47] wedge excision of the enlarged cul-de-sac and vaginal wall. The McCall culdoplasty utilizes uterosacral ligament plication and suspension of the vaginal cuff to the lowest plication suture (Figure 40.9a). Given, in a 2- to 22-year follow-up of both techniques, reported only two failures and that in the McCall culdoplasty group [48]. Farrell reported a 2.5% incidence of ureteral obstruction and a 7.5% incidence of persistent granulation tissue or vault sutures for McCall culdoplasties [49].

Abdominal techniques include the Moschowitz [50] concentric purse-string closure (Figure 40.9b), which was originally devised for prolapse of the rectum, and the Halban technique [9,51]

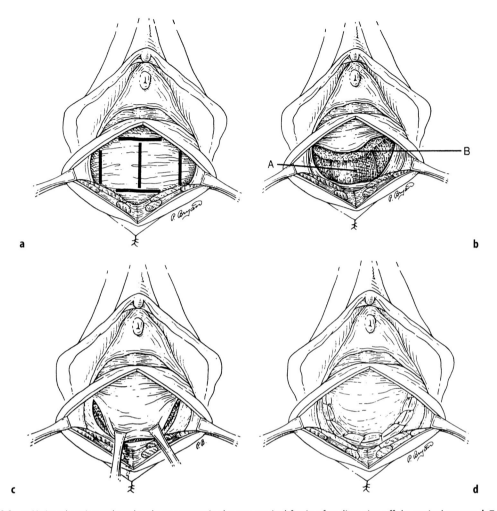

Figure 40.8 **a** Various locations where breaks may occur in the rectovaginal fascia, after dissecting off the vaginal mucosa. **b** Typical low transverse defect. A, rectum, B, rectovaginal fascia. **c** Fascial edges are approximated and (**d**) sutured together to reconstruct the rectovaginal septum. (From Richardson C. The rectovaginal septum revisited: Its relationship to rectocele and its importance in rectocele repair. Clin Obstet Gynecol 1993;36(4):980–1.)

(Figure 40.9c), which utilizes parallel longitudinal sutures. Both techniques incorporate only the visceral peritoneum and may be accompanied by uterosacral ligament plication to the vagina, essentially an "abdominal McCall", for further support (Figure 40.9d, 40.9e). Stanhope et al. [52] found culdoplasty sutures implicated in a small but significant proportion of postoperative ureteral obstructions. Bowel obstruction secondary to inadequate closure of the pouch of Douglas has also been reported from this technique [53].

Because the prevalence of enteroceles is low (0.1 to 16% of women undergoing gynecological surgical procedures [26]), the effectiveness of the various prophylactic and curative operations is difficult to determine. The are no randomized comparative studies.

Transanal Repair

History

In 1965, Redding [54] first noted that neglect of the rectocele resulted in failure of other anorectal surgery. Marks, in 1967, described anterior mucosal resection after vaginal repair [11]. Pitchford in 1967 [55] noted that in patients with anal ulcers or hemorrhoids, symptoms recurred unless concomitant posterior colporrhaphy was performed. Finally, Sullivan et al. [56] described a totally transrectal approach with transverse and longitudinal plication of the rectal wall following stripping of the anterior rectal mucosa, a modification of Delorme's operation for complete rectal prolapse [57]. Variations include plicating the rectal wall in two directions

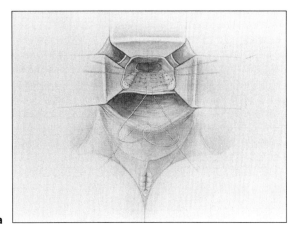

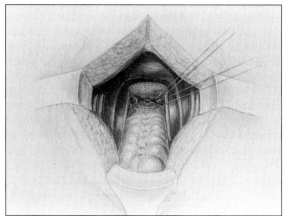

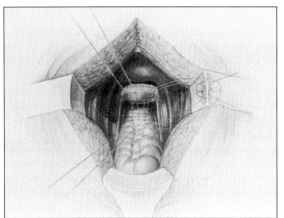

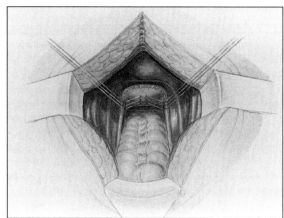

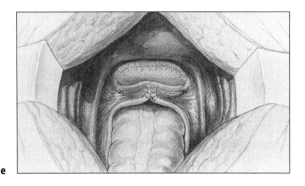

Figure 40.9 **a** McCall culdoplasty technique. **b** Moschowitz procedure. **c** Halban procedure. **d, e** Abdominal uterosacral ligament plication. (From Karram MM, Walters MD: Pelvic organ prolapse: enterocele and vaginal vault prolapse. In: Walters MD, Karram MM, editors. Clinical Urogynecology, St Louis: Mosby-Yearbook, 1993.)

[31,56,58–60], transversely only [61–63], longitudinally only [64], puborectalis plication through the rectum [56,58,61], or by imbrication of the rectal wall transversely without mucosal dissection [65,66]. Most techniques expose the inner circular muscle as seen in Figure 40.10a–10e.

Technique

The morning of surgery all women receive a phosphate enema. Prophylactic antibiotics of choice are given preoperatively. The patient is place in the prone jack-knife position with the buttocks sepa-

rated by adhesive tape. The anterior rectal mucosa is incised transversely, proximal to the dentate line, and dissected free of the underlying circular muscle to a distance 8–10 cm from the anal verge and extending laterally 180 degrees. The circular muscle is then plicated longitudinally with three or four parallel 0000 polypropylene sutures. The excess mucosa is excised and the defect closed with a running 000 polydioxanone suture. An iodine-soaked gauze roll is placed in the anus and removed the following morning. An intra-urethral catheter avoids the need for subsequent straight catheteriza-

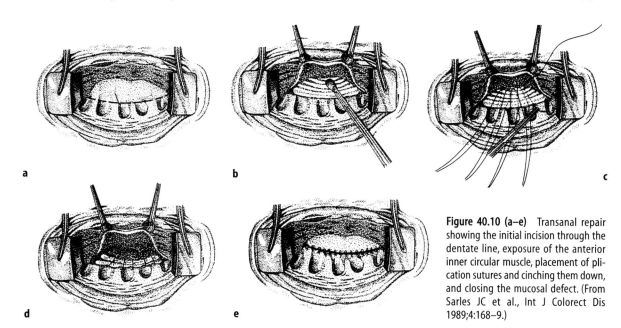

a   b   c

d   e

Figure 40.10 (a–e) Transanal repair showing the initial incision through the dentate line, exposure of the anterior inner circular muscle, placement of plication sutures and cinching them down, and closing the mucosal defect. (From Sarles JC et al., Int J Colorect Dis 1989;4:168–9.)

tion. Discharge is usually after the first bowel movement.

Results

As is the case for posterior colporrhaphy, most patients showed symptomatic improvement, but were left with some degree of anorectal complaint. The most recent study [62] relates historical data to postoperative improvement: The need for preoperative vaginal or perineal digitation was related to a good result ($p < 0.05$), while previous hysterectomy ($p < 0.01$) or the preoperative use of enemas, motor stimulants or several types of laxatives ($p < 0.05$) was related to a poor outcome. Rectal pain [34] and dyspareunia [67] appear to be less than for the vaginal repair.

Combined Vaginal/Transanal Repair

Sullivan et al. [56] originally abandoned the combined approach because of the need for re-operation in 21 of their 28 patients, which led to the development of the totally transanal approach. Recently, Van Dam et al. [68] prospectively studied 74 women who underwent posterior colporrhaphy and transanal repair together. All women had pre- and postoperative defecography with complete resolution of their rectoceles. Postoperatively 50% had marked defecatory disturbances and 18% had mild disturbances.

Conclusions and Recommendations

The results of surgical repair of the rectocele are variable. The small number of prospective studies, varying selection criteria, and variations in technique make comparison difficult, although postoperatively a large proportion of patients are left with some symptoms of impaired evacuation. Hence, conservative treatment with bulking agents and lactulose syrup are recommended as initial treatment for those with impaired defecation. Those women with fecal incontinence should be referred for anorectal studies. Women with long-standing constipation and less than two bowel movements per week will more likely have slow transit constipation and be less likely to benefit from surgery. Dyspareunia remains a complication in 11–27% [13,30,34,37] of patients.

Surgical repair of enterocele is difficult to evaluate because the prevalence in those undergoing gynecologic surgery ranges from 0.1 to 16% [26], so large numbers are needed to identify a difference in outcome. Postoperative prevention might be achieved by obliteration of the cul-de-sac, uterosacral plication, or careful fascial reapproximation at the time of hysterectomy.

Further investigations are needed to predict which patients will most likely benefit from surgery and to compare the risks and benefits of each technique.

References

1. Goff BH. Histological study of the perivaginal fascia in a nul-
    lipara. Surg Gynecol Obstet 1931;52:32–42.
2. Milley PS, Nichols DH. A correlative investigation of the
    human rectovaginal septum. Anat Rec 1968;163:443–4.
3. Ricci JV, Lisa, JR, Thom CH, Kron WL. The relationship of
    the vagina to adjacent organs in reconstructive surgery: a
    histologic study. Am J Surg 1947;74:387–410.
4. Ricci JV, Thom CH, Kron WL. Cleavage planes in reconstruc-
    tive vaginal plastic surgery. Am J Surg 1948;76:354–63.
5. Weber AM, Walters MD. What is vaginal fascia? AUGS
    Quarterly Report 1995;13(3).
6. Lyons TL, Winer Wl. Laparoscopic rectocele repair using
    polyglactin mesh. J Am Gynecol Laparosc 1997;4:381.
7. Watson SJ, Loder PB, Halligan S, Bartram CI, Kamm MA,
    Phillips RKS. l. Transperineal repair of symptomatic recto-
    cele with Marlex mesh a clinical, physiological and radio-
    logic assessment of treatment. J Am Coll Surg
    1996;183:257–61.
8. Kohli N, Karram MM. Use of cadaveric fascia in the treat-
    ment of posterior vaginal wall prolapse (abstract). In: 19th
    Annual Scientific Meeting of American Urogynecologic
    Society. Washington, DC, 1998.
9. Nichols DH, Randall CL. Enterocele. In: Vaginal Surgery.
    Baltimore: Williams & Wilkins, 1989; 318.
10. Berglas B, Rubin IC. Study of the supportive structures of the
    uterus by levator myography. Surg Gynecol Obstet
    1953;97:677–92.
11. Marks MM. The rectal side of the rectocele. Dis Colon
    Rectum 1967;10:387–8.
12. Kiff ES, Barnes PRH, Swash, M. Evidence of pudendal neu-
    ropathy in patients with perineal descent and chronic strain-
    ing at stool. Gut 1983;25:1279–82.
13. Siproudhis L, Dautreme S, Ropert A et al. Dyschezia and rec-
    tocele – a marriage of convenience? Physiologic evaluation
    of the rectocele in a group of 52 women complaining of
    difficulty in evacuation. Dis Colon Rectum 1993;36:1030–6.
14. Wiskind AK, Creighton SM, Stanton SL. The incidence of
    genital prolapse after the Burch colposuspension. Am J
    Obstet Gynecol 1992;167:399–405.
15. Virtanen HS, Mäkinen JI. Retrospective analysis of 711
    patients operated on for pelvic relaxation in 1983–1989. J
    Gynecol Obstet 1993;41109–2115.
16. Gilpin SA, Gosling JA, Smith JA. The pathogenesis of geni-
    tourinary prolapse and stress incontinence of urine. Br J
    Obstet Gynaecol 1989;96:15–23.
17. Allen RE, Hosker GL, Smith ARB, Warrell DW. Pelvic floor
    damage and childbirth: a neurophysiological study. Br J
    Obstet Gynaecol 1990;97:770–9.
18. Harrison JE, McDonagh JE. Hernia of Douglas' pouch and
    high rectocele. Am J Obstet Gynecol 1950;60:83–92.
19. Meigs JV. Enterocele or posterior vaginal hernia. Surg Clin
    North Am 1947;27:1226–30.
20. Phaneuf LE. Posterior vaginal enterocele. Hernia of the cul-
    de-sac of Douglas. Am J Obstet Gynecol 1943;45:490–6.
21. Borenstein R, Elchalal U, Goldchmit R et al. The importance
    of the endopelvic fascia repair during vaginal hysterectomy.
    Surg Gynecol Obstet 1992;175:551–4.
22. Hawksworth W, Roux JP. Vaginal hysterectomy. J Obstet
    Gynecol Br Emp 1958;65:214–28.
23. Halligan S, Bartram CI, Hall C, Wingate J. Enterocele
    revealed by simultaneous evacuation proctography and peri-
    toneography: does defecation block exist? Am J Roentgenol
    1996;167:461–6.
24. Mellgren A, Johansson C, Dolk A et al. Enterocele demon-
    strated by defaecography is associated with other pelvic
    floor disorders. Int J Colorect Dis 1994;9:121–4.
25. Waters EG. A diagnostic technique for the detection of ente-
    rocele. Am J Obstet Gynecol 1946;52:810–12.
26. Holley RL. Enterocele: a review. Obstet Gynecol Surv
    1994;49:284–93.
27. Nichols DH, Randall CL. Posterior colporrhaphy and perine-
    orrhaphy. In: Vaginal Surgery. Baltimore: Williams &
    Wilkins, 1989; 269–93.
28. Bump RC, Mattiasson A, Bo K et al. The standardization of
    terminology of female pelvic organ prolapse and pelvic floor
    dysfunction. Am J Obstet Gynecol 1996;175:10–17.
29. Baden W, Walker T. Surgical Repair of Vaginal Defects.
    Philadelphia: JB Lippincott, 1992.
30. Mellgren A, Anzen BV, Nilsson BY et al. Results of rectocele
    repair. A prospective study. Dis Colon Rectum 1995;38:7–13.
31. Janssen LWM, van Dijke CF. Selection criteria for anterior
    rectal wall prolapse. Dis Colon Rectum 1994;37:1100–7.
32. Jeffcoate TNA. Posterior colpoperineorrhaphy. Am J Obstet
    Gynecol 1959;77:490–502.
33. Goff BH. A practical consideration of the damaged pelvic
    floor with a technique for its secondary reconstruction. Surg
    Gynecol Obstet 1928;46:855–66.
34. Arnold MW, Stewart WR, Aguilar PS. Rectocele repair. Four
    years' experience. Dis Colon Rectum 1990;33:684–7.
35. Francis WJA, Jeffcoate TNA. Dyspareunia following vaginal
    operations. J Obstet Gynaecol Br Comm 1961;68:1–10.
36. Haase R, Skibsted L. Influence of operations for stress incon-
    tinence and/or genital descensus on sexual life. Acta Obstet
    Gynecol Scand 1988;67:659–61.
37. Kahn MA Stanton SL. Posterior colporrhaphy: its effects on
    bowel and sexual function. Br J Obstet Gynaecol
    1997;104:82–6.
38. Kahn MA, Stanton S L. Letter to the editor. Br J Obstet
    Gynecol 1997;104:972–3.
39. Richardson CA. The rectovaginal septum revisited. Its rela-
    tionship to rectocele and its importance in rectocele repair.
    Clin Obstet Gynecol 1993;36:976–83.
40. Cundiff GW, Weidner AC, Visco AG, Addison WA, Bump RC.
    An anatomic and functional assessment of the discrete
    defect rectocele repair. Am J Obstet Gynecol
    1998;179(6):1451–14571.
41. Pillai-Allen AV, Benson JT. Rectocele repair, defect
    approach, an early review [abstract]. 1994: AUGS 15th
    Annual Meeting.
42. Øster S, Astrup A. A new vaginal operation for recurrent and
    large rectocele using dermis transplant. Acta Obstet Gynecol
    Scand 1981;60:493–5.
43. Soergel T, Heit M. Suburethral slings utilizing rectus abdo-
    minis versus donor fascia lata: a retrospective study compar-
    ing objective cure rates. P27 at the AUGS 19th Annual
    Scientific Meeting, November 1998. 1998.
44. Kuhn RJP, Hollyhock VE. Observations on the anatomy of
    the rectovaginal pouch and septum. Obstet Gynecol
    1982;59:445–7.
45. Zacharin RF. Pulsion enterocele: review of functional
    anatomy of the pelvic floor. Obstet Gynecol 1980;55:135–40.
46. Torpin R. Excision of the cul-de-sac of Douglas, for the sur-
    gical care of hernias through the female caudal wall, includ-
    ing prolapse of the uterus. J Int Coll Surg 1955;24:322–30.
47. Waters EG. Vaginal prolapse: technique for correction and
    prevention at hysterectomy. Obstet Gynecol 1957;10:595–602.
48. Given, FT. "Posterior culdoplasty": revisited. Am J Obstet
    Gynecol 1985;153:135–9.
49. Farrell S, Sampson, Sheppard K. Perioperative and short-
    term complications of McCall's culdoplasty. P28 from the
    AUGS 19th Annual Scientific Meeting, November 1998.
50. Moschowitz AV. The pathogenesis, anatomy and cure of pro-
    lapse of the rectum. Surg Gynecol Obstet 1912;15:7–21.
51. Halban, J. Gynäkologische Operationslehre. Vienna: Urban
    and Scharzenberg, 1932, 171–3.

52. Stanhope CR, Wilson TO, Utz, WJ et al. Suture entrapment and secondary ureteral obstruction. Am J Obstet Gynecol 1991;164:1513–19.
53. Dicke JM. Small bowel obstruction secondary to a prior Moschowitz procedure. Am J Obstet Gynecol 1985;152:887–8.
54. Redding MD. The relaxed perineum and anorectal disease. Dis Colon Rectum 1965;8:279–82.
55. Pitchford CS. Rectocele: a cause of anorectal pathologic changes in women. Dis Colon Rectum 1967;10:464–6.
56. Sullivan ES, Leaverton GH, Hardwick CE. Transrectal perineal repair: an adjunct to improved function after anorectal surgery. Dis Colon Rectum 1968;11:106–14.
57. Delorme M. Sur le traitement des prolapsus du rectum totaux, par l'excision de la muqueuse rectale ou recto-colique. Cull Mem Soc Chir Paris 1900;24:499–518.
58. Sehapayak S. Transrectal repair of rectocele: an extended armamentarium of colorectal surgeons. A report of 355 cases. Dis Colon Rectum 1985;28:422–33.
59. Khubchandani IT, Sheets JA, Stasik JJ et al. Endorectal repair of rectocele. Dis Colon Rectum 1983;26:792–6.
60. Khubchandani IT, Clancy JP, Rosen L, Riether RD, Stasik JJ. Endorectal repair of rectocele revisited. Br J Surg 1997;84:89–91.
61. Capps WR. Rectoplasty and perineoplasty for the symptomatic rectocele: a report of fifty cases. Dis Colon Rectum 1975;18:237–44.
62. Karlbom U, Graf WG, Hilsson P, A[o]hlman SL. Does surgical repair of a rectocele improve rectal emptying? Dis Colon Rectum 1996;39:1296–302.
63. Murthy VK, Orkin BA, Smith LE, Glassman LM. Excellent outcome using selective criteria for rectocele repair. Dis Colon Rectum 1996;39:374–8.
64. Sarles JC, Srnoud, M, Selezneff I, Olivier S. Endo-rectal repair of rectocele. Int J Colorect Dis 1989;4:167–71.
65. Block IR. Transrectal repair of rectocele using obliterative suture. Dis Colon Rectum 1986;29:707–11.
66. Infantino A, Masin A, Melega E, Dodi G, Lise M. Does surgery resolve outlet obstruction from rectocele? Int J Colorect Dis 1995;10(97–199):97–100.
67. Kahn MA, Stanton SL, Kumar D. A randomized prospective trial of posterior colporrhaphy vs transanal repair of rectocele: preliminary findings. Int Urogynecol J 1997;8(4):246 (abstract 20a).
68. Van Dam JH, Ginai AZ, Gosselink MJ, Huisman WM, Bonjer JJ, Hop WCJ, Schouten WR. Role of defecography in predicting clinical outcome of rectocele repair. Dis Colon Rectum 1997;40:201–7.

8 Fistulas, Operative Trauma, Postoperative Problems

41 Urethral Fistulas and Diverticula

Raymond A. Lee

The female urethra is well protected and rarely injured except during childbirth, operation, or an automobile accident. As a result of the trauma, the patient may experience an avulsion of the urethra, generally in the area of the bladder neck. Less commonly, women may experience a penetrating wound as a result of being impaled while fence climbing or being struck by farming tools; such injuries frequently result in hematoma of the vulva and laceration of the urethra. Occasionally, injuries to the vagina, rectum, and urethra result from a disproportion between the size of the penis and that of the vagina. These usually result in disruption of the posterior vaginal wall and anal sphincter rather than trauma to the urethra or the base of the bladder.

Regardless of the cause, injury to the urethra and anterior vaginal wall usually consists of a linear laceration of the vaginal wall extending up the lateral fornix, but rarely is the urethra itself disrupted. We have seen four patients with disruption of the urethra at the bladder neck, and two of these injuries

occurred with vacuum extraction at the time of a primiparous delivery. Figure 41.1 shows a urethra traumatically disrupted from the bladder neck during operative vacuum extraction delivery. When catheterization is attempted, the catheter passes through the intact urethral meatus up the distal urethra, where it escapes into the vagina. Once the disrupted site is identified, the catheter can then be passed through the bladder neck into the bladder. Once the patient is stabilized, reconstruction is begun by developing a flap of vagina hinged posteriorly (Figure 41.2). Reconstruction of the urethra begins by reanastomosing the proximal end of the traumatized urethra to the bladder neck with an initial suture placed in the 3 o'clock position. Each delayed absorbable suture (3-0) is placed in an extramucosal position reanastomosing the urethra to the bladder neck (Figure 41.3). Once the urethra is firmly attached with the sutures, a vaginal flap is placed in such a way that it avoids overlying suture lines (Figure 41.4). A small urethral catheter (10 French) is left in place for 5–7 days, after

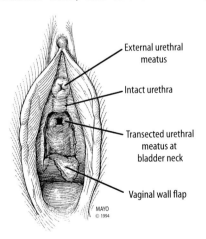

Figure 41.1 Vaginal flap exposing traumatic disruption of urethra. (By permission of Mayo Foundation.)

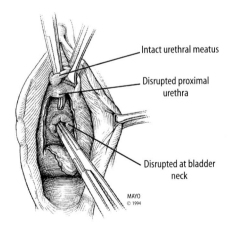

Figure 41.2 Disrupted proximal urethra with exposed bladder neck. (By permission of Mayo Foundation.)

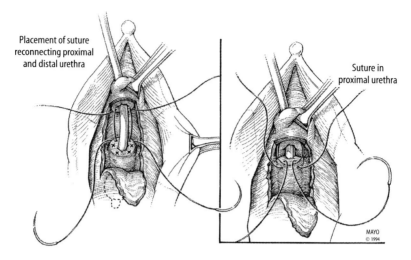

Figure 41.3 Initial urethral sutures placed in the 12 o'clock position with designated area for additional sutures in reconstruction of the urethra. Inset: Partially approximated urethra. (By permission of Mayo Foundation.)

which it is removed and spontaneous voiding occurs. If appropriate, at operation a suprapubic catheter can be placed and a small urethral catheter left in place as a stent for 48 hours. In the four cases of urethral disruption at the bladder neck, no urinary tract fistulas have developed and excellent urinary continence has been maintained.

Urethral Vaginal Fistula

Etiology

In less developed countries, prolonged labor continues to be a cause for destruction of the urethra and

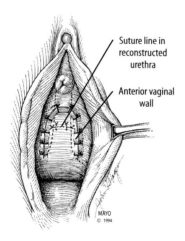

Figure 41.4 Reconstructed urethra deep to vaginal wall flap. (By permission of Mayo Foundation.)

the base of the bladder [1–3], whereas in the United States, elective vaginal operation is a leading cause of urethrovaginal fistula [4]. The excision of a friable, infected urethral diverticulum can be difficult and frequently leads to complications because of the underlying infection. Despite one's best efforts to reconstruct the urethral floor accurately, the combination of infection, edema, and hematoma formation leads to imperfect healing and fistula formation. Further, a high, tight plication of the urethra or the inadvertent intraluminal placement of a suture (vaginally or retropubically) may produce a fistula of the urethra or, of greater consequence, an actual slough of the floor of the urethra and the bladder neck [5]. In a review of 53 urethrovaginal fistulas treated at the author's institution, 16 followed anterior vaginal wall repair and 13 followed diverticulectomy [6]. Radiation therapy was an infrequent cause (six cases), and trauma or accident was responsible for even fewer (three).

Clinical Presentation

Patients who experience trauma to the urethra from forceps delivery or automobile accident have leakage immediately or within the first 24 hours after damage. If a urethral catheter is in place, after either delivery or trauma, removal of the catheter is generally followed promptly by leakage of urine. Patients who have undergone an operation generally have a catheter in place for 2–7 days. Some patients who have had an operation may have an unrecognized suture through the wall of the urethra; this generally results in necrosis of the tissue, possibly associated with hematoma formation and some degree of infection, the combination of which results in leakage of urine through a necrotic area of the urethra. The patient may initially be continent only to experience leakage 1–2 weeks postoperatively. Patients who have had irradiation generally note the leakage some time after the therapy, generally within 2–4 weeks after treatment.

Simple urethrovaginal fistula, depending on its location relative to the bladder neck, may not produce urinary incontinence and may not require operative repair (especially if located in the distal one-third of the urethra). A fistula located near the bladder neck may be technically more difficult to repair, and urinary continence cannot necessarily be ensured. Even after what appears to be a successful repair, the patient may experience urinary stress incontinence due to fibrosis or loss of contractility of the inherent urethral musculature. Although the fistula has been technically repaired, the patient's functional result is less than anticipated. A much more complex problem is presented by patients who have lost a major portion of the floor of the urethra, resulting in a linear loss, which may be especially difficult to repair if the bladder neck is involved.

Operative Repair

The basic phases of operative reconstruction consist of linear incision up the anterior vaginal wall, much as is accomplished with a Kelly–Kennedy anterior colporrhaphy (Figure 41.5). It is important that the vaginal wall be mobilized sufficiently far laterally, off the underlying cervicopubic fascia, to permit a tension-free closure of the fistula. This procedure must be accomplished in the proper bloodless tissue plane, exposing the critical endopelvic fascial supporting tissues. Once the vaginal walls are completely mobilized, the opening to the fistula is freshened, after which the urethra is reconstructed with fine 4-0 delayed absorbable sutures (Figure 41.6a). The first suture is placed distal to the fistula opening, and each suture thereafter is placed in an extramucosal position, approximating the edge of the fistulous tract, free of tension with perfect hemostasis. The presence of a small-caliber catheter within the urethra may assist in accurate placement of the sutures to close the fistulous tract. This initial suture line is imbricated with a second set of sutures, with the most distal suture being just distal to the initial closed suture line (Figure 41.6b). Snug application of the bladder neck by approximation, under the urethra of the so-called cervicopubic fascia, lateral to the urethra, promotes urinary control. A tension-free closure of the vaginal wall as the third layer (or when necessary for obliteration of dead space, the actual placement of the anterior vaginal wall with a pedicled-skin, fibrofatty labial graft) may be indicated. In each, it should be understood that a "second-stage" retropubic urethral vesical neck suspension may be undertaken for patients who have a good anatomical result with an apparent intact urethra but who nevertheless continue to have stress incontinence through an otherwise intact urethra. This may be required at a later date, but it is not predictable at the time of repair of the fistula.

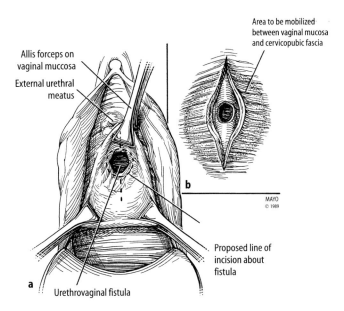

Figure 41.5 a Urethrovaginal fistula with proposed line of incision. b Urethrovaginal fistula with area to be mobilized deep to the cervicopubic fascia.

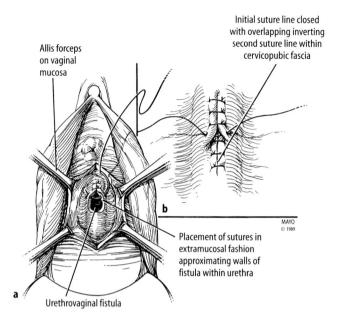

Figure 41.6   **a** Partial closure of urethrovaginal fistula showing extramucosal position of sutures. **b** Placement of second layer of sutures, inverting initial suture line closing the urethrovaginal fistula.

Linear Loss of the Floor of the Urethra

Patients who have a linear urethrovaginal fistula (loss of a major portion of the urethra) present a surgeon with one of the most challenging forms of genitourinary fistula. Various operative techniques can be undertaken to correct the anatomical defect (urethrovaginal fistula), but urinary continence rather than the anatomical result is the critical criterion of a successful operation. Regardless of the operative technique selected, the surgeon cannot anticipate successful restoration of urinary continence in all patients who have loss of a major portion of the urethra.

Operative Repair

A midline incision is made in the anterior vaginal wall and extended up and around the margins of the urethral defect (Figure 41.7a). The dissection is carried laterally to the descending pubic ramus, much as is done in a Kelly–Kennedy anterior colporrhaphy. With appropriate traction on the edges of the urethral wall, the urethra is mobilized sufficiently that a tension-free closure can be constructed. All adhesive bands of scar tissue that distort the urethra and the bladder neck must be dissected and released (Figure 41.7b). Usually a number 8 or 10 urethral catheter is placed in the

bed of the roof of the urethra; this permits accurate approximation of the freed edges of the floor of the urethra and reconstruction of the tube. The sutures are placed in an interrupted fashion with 4-0 delayed absorbable suture positioned extramucosally (Figure 41.8a). This initial suture line reconstruction of the urethra is inverted with a second layer approximating the periurethral tissues to aid in support of the initial suture line (Figure 41.8b). The third layer of sutures is placed in the cervicopubic fascia to plicate the urethra and bladder neck area further (Figure 41.8c).

Occasionally patients who have had a significant loss of the floor of the urethra also have lost a portion of the anterior vaginal wall, and thus approximation of the wall of the vagina cannot be accomplished without undue tension (Figure 41.9). In these cases, the size of the defect is accurately evaluated and an appropriate tongue of tissue from the labium majus is identified to be incised and swung into the vagina to replace the anterior vaginal wall (Figure 41.10). This fibrofatty bulbocavernosus flap is usually hinged anteriorly, but depending on the nature of the defect, it may be hinged posteriorly. The flap is developed, and the small venous bleeders in the subcutaneous tissues are suture ligated or cauterized as necessary. The most distal portion of the flap, that deepest in the vagina, is secured initially with full-

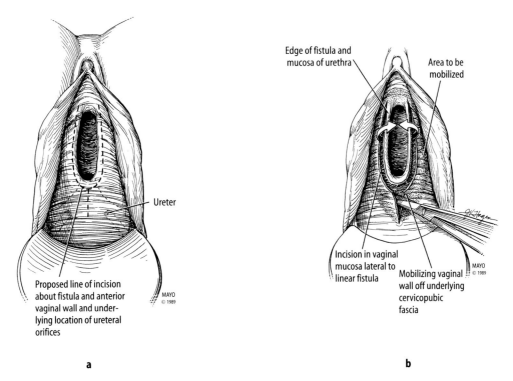

Figure 41.7 **a** Proposed line of incision about the fistula and anterior vaginal wall and underlying location of ureteral orifices. **b** Mobilized vaginal wall off underlying cervicopubic fascia joined with proposed closure of fistula.

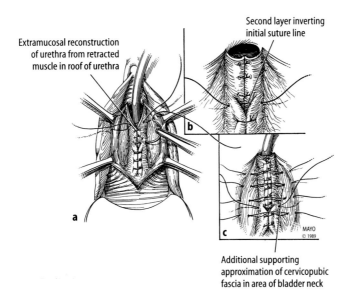

Figure 41.8 **a** Partial closure of urethrovaginal fistula with proposed placement of second layer inverting the initial suture line. **b** Reconstructed urethra showing proposed second layer inverting initial suture line. **c** Additional supporting tissues with approximation of cervicopubic fascia in the area of the bladder neck.

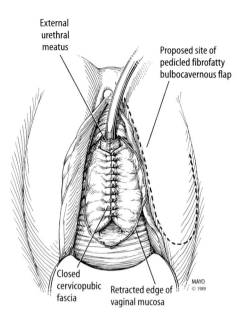

Figure 41.9   Reconstructed urethra with proposed site of pedicled fibrofatty bulbocavernosus flap.

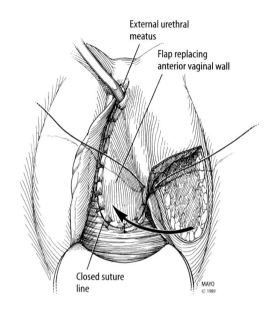

Figure 41.10   Placement of fibrofatty flap as a substitute for anterior vaginal wall.

thickness interrupted 3-0 delayed absorbable sutures (Figure 41.11). Care is taken to suture the vaginal flap to the edge of the vagina in an accurate way to promote primary healing. At the point at which the flap approximates the urethral meatus, it has a tendency to "hide" the meatus and may need to be tailored accordingly. The site of the graft is closed with an initial layer of subcutaneous sutures, which permits closure of the skin edges of the labium with 4-0 delayed absorbable sutures in a tension-free fashion. A small suction catheter may be placed under the labial graft between the graft and the reconstructed urethra. This is brought out through a stab wound laterally and usually is removed in 3 or 4 days.

Despite adequate vesical neck plication and satisfactory elevation and support to the reconstructed urethra, what appears to be an anatomically sound urethra may not provide total urinary control. Approximately 50% of patients undergoing repair of an extensive loss of the floor of the urethra will have urinary incontinence and require a second-stage Marshall–Marchetti–Krantz type of bladder neck elevation. Postoperatively, the patient receives appropriate antibiotic coverage. If a suprapubic catheter has been placed, it may be clamped on the 10th postoperative day, when voiding may be undertaken. Almost always, the patient is voiding within the first week that the catheter is clamped, and only 1 of our most recent 25 patients has required suprapubic drainage for more than 20 days. Obviously, the

goal of surgical correction is to construct a urethra that provides sufficient resistance to ensure good urinary continence; regrettably, a neourethra that appears to be anatomically sound, perfectly sup-

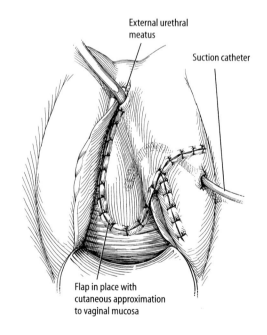

Figure 41.11   Closure of fibrofatty flap and site of its harvest.

ported, and in excellent position does not guarantee good urethral function and urinary control. A scarred, fixed, non-contractile urethra does not provide good urinary control regardless of the urethral angles or the apparent support.

Urethral Diverticulum

Diverticulum in the female urethra is a masquerading condition that causes untold misery in the patient [7]. Numerous investigative studies have been undertaken to clarify the cause and to emphasize its clinical presentation. Various innovative techniques have been suggested to improve the accuracy of diagnosis of this elusive condition. Surgical correction can be technically difficult and occasionally results in severe complications.

Etiology

Several theories have been advanced to explain the pathogenesis of urethral diverticulum. Huffman's [8] outstanding work aptly likened the urethra to a tree, from the base of which arise numerous stunted branches – the periurethral ducts and glands. They form a labyrinthine mass encircling the urethra on all sides, with ducts opening into the lateral, dorsal, and a few ventral urethral walls. Most agree that infection and obstruction of the periurethral glands result in the formation of retention cysts, which when infected rupture into the lumen of the urethra and give rise to a diverticulum. Other suggested etiologic causes are congenital, urethral trauma, catheterization, and childbirth.

Clinical Presentation

Although complaints vary, most patients experience urgency, frequency, dysuria, and dyspareunia. A history of recurrent urinary tract infections is common; hematuria, dribbling after voiding, and urinary stress incontinence are not infrequent. A palpable, tender, suburethral mass is found in approximately 60% of the patients that we have seen; actual protrusion of a diverticulum from the vaginal introitus is infrequent. The diagnosis is generally confirmed with cystourethroscopic examination or vaginal ultrasonography.

In our experience, 65% of diverticula are located in the proximal two-thirds of the urethra and bladder neck area, 20% have multiple sites of origin (most of which are in the mid-urethra with a second opening in the inner or outer segment), and only 15% are in the distal, external third of the urethra.

Operative Repair

A vertical incision is made in the anterior vaginal wall, exposing the underlying cervicopubic fascia (Figure 41.12). The vaginal walls are mobilized laterally to the descending pubic ramus. A similar incision is made in the fascia, which is mobilized laterally to expose the underlying diverticulum. The dissection must be sharp, accurate, and meticulously accomplished. Preoperative placement (coiling) of a ureteral catheter within the diverticulum to distend its walls, if it can be accomplished, may enhance the identification and dissection of the diverticulum. Not infrequently, the diverticulum is in immediate apposition to or even perforating the cervicopubic fascia and can be easily identified (and perhaps even inadvertently entered) during the dissection. Depending on the size of the diverticulum, it may have loculations containing various amounts of urine, purulent material, necrotic debris, and even small stones; such loculations or septa should be incised.

If the diverticulum is entered, on occasion I have found it advantageous to open the diverticulum and insert my left index finger within the diverticulum and place a broad Allis forceps on its rim, and gentle traction will assist in the dissection with scissors to ensure total excision (Figure 41.13). Occasionally, the sac of the diverticulum extends laterally and up and around the urethra. Rarely, it may extend into the retropubic space where the urethral orifice enters the roof of the urethra. In this instance, the dissection is continued as far superiorly as possible, at which time the neck of the diverticulum is simply

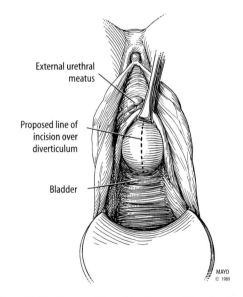

Figure 41.12 Proposed line of incision overlying diverticulum of urethra.

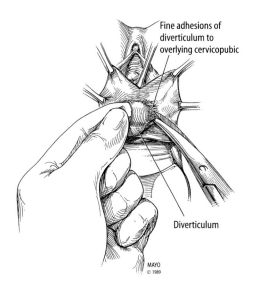

Figure 41.13 With surgeon's finger in the diverticulum, it is separated from the surrounding cervicopubic fascia.

transected and permitted to retract with no attempt made to close the defect. In some patients, the diverticulum is saddle-shaped, extending around the entire urethra or bladder neck; in these cases, extensive dissection of the lower trigone or even major part of the urethral floor is required.

The urethra is reconstructed in a linear direction over a number 10 Foley Silastic catheter, using interrupted 4-0 delayed absorbable sutures placed in

an extramucosal position (Figure 41.14). Occasionally, the opening of the urethra is more appropriately closed (to prevent tension on the suture line) in a transverse direction. The suture is inserted through the muscular coat of the urethra but does not penetrate or enter the urethral lumen. After the urethral defect is repaired, the cervicopubic fascia is imbricated in a side-to-side (vest-over-pants) fashion with interrupted 3-0 delayed absorbable sutures (Figure 41.15). By providing two additional supporting layers and avoiding superimposed suture lines, this method appears to diminish the possibility of fistula formation. In addition, it provides good support for the proximal urethra and the bladder neck. Complete hemostasis must be ensured as each layer is closed. This can be accomplished with fine interrupted sutures and judicious use of electrical cautery. The vaginal wall is closed with 3-0 delayed absorbable suture material (Figure 41.16). A urethral catheter is left in place for 4–7 days postoperatively. In some cases, the complexity of the repair may require that a catheter be retained longer or that a suprapubic catheter be used by itself or in combination with a urethral catheter.

Another operative approach reported by Spence and Duckett [9] is applicable to patients with the ostium of the diverticulum in the far distal urethra. The operative approach consists of a transvaginal marsupialization of the diverticulum with one blade of the scissors in the urethra and the other blade in the vagina. My concern with this approach is that, with menopause, atrophy of pelvic supports and

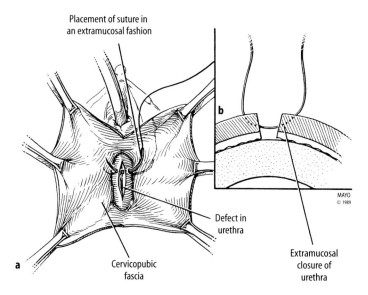

Figure 41.14 **a** Closure of urethra with extramucosal placement of sutures. **b** Proposed extramucosal position of sutures closing the urethra.

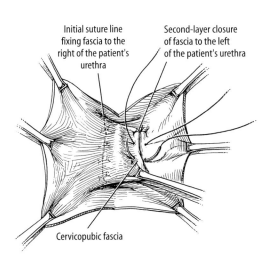

Initial suture line
fixing fascia to the
right of the patient's
urethra

Second-layer closure
of fascia to the left
of the patient's urethra

Cervicopubic fascia

Figure 41.15 Overlying cervicopubic fascia in repair of urethrovaginal fistula.

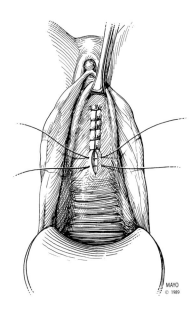

Figure 41.16 Primary closure of vaginal suture line overlying repair of diverticulectomy.

resultant loss of tone of the remaining smooth muscle may result in a significant incidence of urinary incontinence some years after what appears to be a successful marsupializing procedure.

Complications and Results

Prompt, complete, and long-lasting relief of symptoms usually is obtained after successful diverticulectomy. Urethroscopic examination demonstrates either a normal urethra or a shallow depression or a dimple at the operative site. We have seen no evidence of urethral stricture in patients who had diverticulectomy. More than 80% of patients remain asymptomatic and have not required postoperative medical or surgical management. A small number of patients may have persistent pain, dyspareunia, or recurrent urinary tract infection. In this group, cystourethroscopy and appropriate cultures of the urine should be re-evaluated. Rarely, a diverticulum of the urethra may recur in the same location or, presumably, a second diverticulum develops at another location. If it occurs in the same location, the original diverticulum may have been incompletely excised. A diverticulum that recurs elsewhere in the urethra may be a diverticulum that was overlooked at the original operative procedure or may represent the development of a second diverticulum.

We continue to favor transvaginal excision of the diverticulum, even though it is a more complex and tedious operation. Resection of the diverticulum has provided a relatively good long-term rate of cure

with an extremely low incidence of fistula and other serious complications. The operative area on the urethra is relatively small, the supporting tissues are of variable quality, and the wall of the urethra is thick. Given a sufficient blood supply, laceration, fistula, loss of the floor of the urethra, or diverticulum of the urethra can be reconstructed to form an intact and continent urethral tube.

Acknowledgments

Portions of this chapter were previously published in Lee RA (1991) Surgical management of genitourinary fistulas. In: Hurt WG, editor, *Urogynecologic Surgery*, Aspen Publishers, Gaithersburg, MD, pp 131–8. By permission of the publisher. Figures 41.5–41.16 are from Lee RA (1992) Atlas of Gynecologic Surgery. WB Saunders Company, Philadelphia. By permission of Mayo Foundation.

References

1. Hamlin RH, Nicholson EC. Reconstruction of urethra totally destroyed in labour. Br Med J 1969;i:147–50.
2. Shigui F, Qinge S. Operative treatment of female urinary fistulas. Report of 405 cases. Chin Med J (Engl) 1979;92:263–8.
3. Vanderputte SR. Obstetric vesicovaginal fistulae. Experience with 89 cases. Ann Soc Belg Med Trop 1985;65:303–9.

4. Gray LA. Urethrovaginal fistulas. Am J Obstet Gynecol 1968;101:28–36.
5. Symmonds RE, Hill LM. Loss of the urethra: a report on 50 patients. Am J Obstet Gynecol 1978;130:130–8.
6. Lee RA, Symmonds RE, Williams TJ. Current status of genitourinary fistula. Obstet Gynecol 1988;72:313–19.
7. Lee RA. Diverticulum of the female urethra: postoperative complications and results. Obstet Gynecol 1983;61:52–8.
8. Huffman JW. The detailed anatomy of the paraurethral ducts in the adult human female. Am J Obstet Gynecol 1948;55:86–101.
9. Spence HM, Duckett JW Jr. Diverticulum of the female urethra: clinical aspects and presentation of a simple operative technique for cure. J Urol 1970;104:432–7.

42 Ureterovaginal Fistula

Kathleen C. Kobashi and Gary E. Leach

Introduction

A ureterovaginal fistula (UVF) involves an abnormal communication between the ureter and the vagina. VanRoonhuyse is credited with the first UVF repair in 1672, in which he performed debridement of the edge of the fistula and closure using sharpened goose quills [1]. Joubert repaired a UVF with a labial skin flap in 1834.

The incidence of UVF following gynecologic procedures is reported to be 0.5% [2], making gynecologic surgery the most common cause of UVFs [3]. Amongst gynecologic procedures, total abdominal hysterectomy is the predominant cause of UVFs [4], although skeletonization of the ureter during radical hysterectomy [5], vaginal delivery [6] and ceserean section have also been reported as causes. The ureter passes beneath the uterine artery and vein (Figure 42.1), and ureteral injury during ligation of the uterine vessels is not uncommon. Urologic, colonic, and vascular surgeries also place a patient at risk for ureteral injury which can result in UVF. Preoperative radiation therapy increases the risk of UVF formation. However, postoperative radiation does not appear to be associated with an increased risk of UVF [7]. Other more rare causes of UVF include endometriosis and pelvic inflammatory disease [8]. Kumar reported on a case of UVF following extracorporeal shock wave lithotripsy [9].

Presentation and Evaluation

History

The presentation of a patient with a UVF usually varies according to the time of patient presentation in relation to surgery. In the immediate postopera-

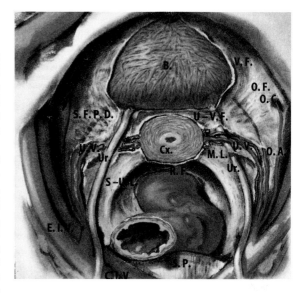

Figure 42.1 The proximity of the ureter to the uterine vessels is illustrated. The ureter actually passes beneath the vessels as it travels to the bladder. Reprinted with permission from F Hinman, et al. (Eds), *Atlas of Urologic Surgery*, 2nd edn. Philadelphia: WB Saunders, 1998; 258.

tive period, a patient may describe abdominal or flank pain, abdominal fullness, fever, or any combination of the above. Delayed presentation, days or weeks postoperatively, usually involves complaints of continuous urinary leakage, which the patient may or may not be able to discern is from the vagina. The volume of leakage may vary depending on the size of the fistula, with continuous urinary incontinence from large fistulas and a watery discharge from small fistulas. However, even small communications can result in extensive leakage. Patients typically void normally. Mandal et al. reported on 31 patients with UVF, most of whom were asymptomatic until 1 to 4 weeks postoperatively when they experienced a sudden onset of urinary incontinence [8]. This delay in presentation is perhaps due to the progression of the pathology. The ureteral wall is damaged, suffers ischemia, and then breaks down, making it possible for a fistula to develop.

Physical Examination

Physical examination may be completely normal. Abdominal examination may reveal nonspecific generalized tenderness, and costovertebral tenderness may be present. On vaginal examination, a mass or erythema of the vaginal wall may be visible.

Cystourethroscopy

Cystoscopy is performed to detect any erythema or evidence of a mass in the bladder. Insufflation of the vagina during cystoscopy may produce bubbles in the bladder [1]. Conversely, instillation of colored sterile water into the bladder with simultaneous speculum examination of the vagina may reveal a point of communication in the vagina.

Radiographic Imaging

A voiding cystourethrogram (VCUG) not only facilitates the detection of a vesicovaginal fistula (VVF), but can be helpful in the differentiation between a UVF and a VVF. However, it is imperative to keep in mind that a patient may have more than one type of fistula. Up to 10% of patients with VVFs may have a concomitant UVF. VCUG is also useful in assessment for vesicoureteral reflux, pelvic prolapse, or stress urinary incontinence, all of which could be corrected at the time of fistula repair.

Since most cases of UVF involve some degree of ureteral obstruction [4,10], an intravenous pyelogram (IVP) is an important study if UVF is suspected. Extravasation of contrast at any point along the course of the ureter suggests disruption of the continuity of the ureter. There may be variable visualization of the kidney secondary to ureteral obstruction. Additionally, an IVP will usually demonstrate a duplication of the collecting system if it is present.

The authors routinely perform retrograde pyelograms (RPG) in all patients suspected of having a UVF prior to surgical repair (Figure 42.2). An RPG is also performed in patients who cannot receive intravenous contrast secondary to allergy or impaired renal function or in cases in which the IVP is inconclusive.

Other Tests

Pad tests can help determine the location of the communication. Many variations of the pad test

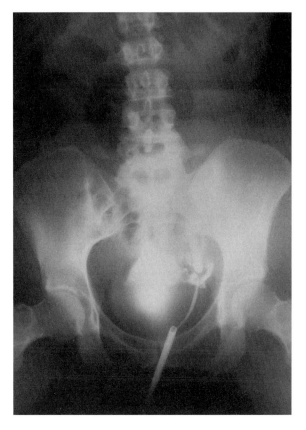

Figure 42.2 Retrograde pyelogram demonstrates extravasation of contrast in the distal ureter.

technique have been described. The algorithm used by the authors is illustrated in Figure 42.3. The pyridium test mentioned in the figure requires the patient to wear tampons and pads for 2–3 days while taking oral pyridium. The tampons and pads are examined by the clinician for staining pattern. Orange staining at the proximal aspect of the tampon is indicative of a UVF, while staining distally suggests a VVF. VVF is excluded by instilling blue dye into the bladder and performing simultaneous vaginal examination. Blue dye in the vagina confirms a VVF.

Treatment

General

Regardless of the therapeutic preference, the goals of treatment of UVFs are preservation of renal function, prevention of urosepsis [7], maintenance of hygiene, and alleviation of symptoms [10]. The timing of surgical intervention for UVFs is controversial. Early open repair decreases the risk of irre-

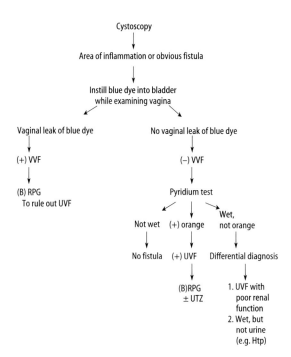

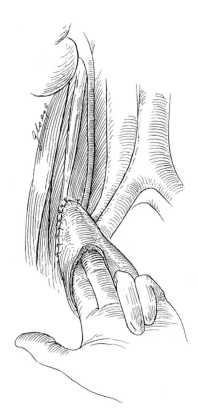

Figure 42.3 Algorithm for evaluation of suspected fistula. A suspected urinary tract–vaginal fistula is evaluated in a logical, stepwise fashion. The clinician must keep in mind that patients may have more than one communication site between the urinary tract and the vagina. VVF, Vesicovaginal fistula; (B)RPG, bilateral retrograde pyelogram; UVF, ureterovaginal fistula; UTZ, renal ultrasound; Htp, Hydrops tubae profluens.

Figure 42.4 A psoas hitch involves tacking of the bladder to the psoas tendon to minimize tension on the reimplanted ureter. Reprinted with permission from S Raz (Ed), Female Urology, 2nd edn. Philadelphia: WB Saunders, 1996; 517.

versible renal damage and avoids technical difficulty secondary to inflammation. Some authors suggest that if 2 weeks have passed since the injury, one should wait 3 months before attempting open repair [11]. Conservative therapy to provide drainage and facilitate ureteral healing with a retrograde ureteral stent is also an option advocated by many authors [12]. In those patients who are unable to undergo general or regional anesthetic or in whom a retrograde stent cannot be passed, percutaneous nephrostomy with or without antegrade ureteral stent placement is another alternative.

Open Surgery

Simple ureteroneocystotomy is the gold standard for treatment of UVFs. When ureteral length is short, mobilization of the kidney and ureteral reimplantation with a psoas hitch and/or Boari flap is usually possible. A psoas hitch is performed by tacking the mobilized bladder to the psoas major tendon. The psoas hitch is useful to decrease the tension on the reimplanted ureter (Figure 42.4). In cases in which the ureteral injury is so proximal that the tension is

not adequately relieved by a psoas hitch alone, a Boari flap can be created. Anticipation of the possible necessity for creation of a Boari flap is important when the cystotomy incision is made. In order for proper creation of a Boari flap, the cystotomy must be made in an oblique fashion (Figure 42.5). The flap is then tubularized, and the ureter is reimplanted into the distal portion of the tube (Figure 42.6). A psoas hitch is performed in conjunction with the Boari flap, again, to minimize tension on the reimplanted ureter. Up to 100% success rates are reported in some series (Table 42.1). Rarely, renal autotransplantation or construction of an ileal ureter is necessary. Historically, primary nephrectomy was performed, but this is now rare and is only considered in patients who have significant renal damage.

Endoscopic Management

Indications for endoscopic management of UVFs include presentation within 3 weeks of injury, <2 cm length of injury, with remaining ureteral continuity. Patel et al. suggest endoscopic techniques as a first-

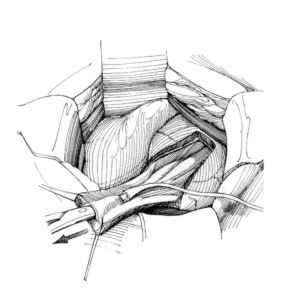 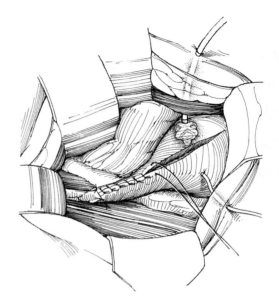

Figure 42.5   An oblique cystotomy should be made if the possibility of a Boari flap is anticipated to ensure maximal length and proper orientation of the flap. Reprinted with permission from F Hinman, et al (Eds), *Atlas of Urologic Surgery,* 2nd edn. Philadelphia: WB Saunders, 1998; 823.

Figure 42.6   The ureter is reimplanted into the tubularized Boari flap, and a psoas hitch is performed to decrease tension on the ureter. Reprinted with permission from F Hinman, et al (Eds), *Atlas of Urologic Surgery,* 2nd edn. Philadelphia: WB Saunders, 1998; 824.

Table 42.1   Results of ureteroneocystotomy for treatment of UVF

Author	Technique (n)	Follow-up Mean (range)	Complications (n)
Elabd et al. [13]	Direct (11) Boari w/psoas (2)	Unknown	Ureteral stricture (1)
Selzman et al. [14]	Direct (9)	5.3 years (1–8 years)	Mild hydronephrosis (2) Ureteral stricture (1)
Demirel et al. [15]	Direct (4) Boari (1)	Unknown	None reported
Yokoyama et al. [16]	Ureteroappendico-cystostomy (1) Psoas hitch (1)	4 months	None reported
Mandal et al. [8]	Direct (19) Boari (10)	Unknown	None reported
Murphy et al. [4]	Direct (9) Boari (2)	3–20 years	Distal ureteral slough (1) Renal failure (1)[a]

[a] Underwent secondary nephrectomy.

line method of treatment for benign, iatrogenic fistulas, but not in patients with malignancy or history of radiation therapy. Additionally, Patel et al. suggest that conservative management is unlikely to be successful in cases of complete ureteral transection [10]. In patients in whom endoscopic intervention is performed, renal ultrasound and urine cultures should be performed as frequently as every 2 weeks, to ensure that the ureter remains unobstructed [10]. This makes this approach a time-con-

suming and costly option; nonetheless, it can save the patient the trauma of open surgery. Urinary tract infection should be treated if present.

Conservative techniques include a retrograde ureteral stent, percutaneous nephrostomy, and antegrade ureteral stent placement. Selzman et al. treated 20 UVFs in 19 patients over 20 years with a mean follow-up of 5.3 years [14]. All the UVFs occurred secondary to gynecologic procedures. Seven patients were treated with internal stents

(5 retrograde, 2 antegrade) for 4–8 weeks with resolution of the fistula in all 7 patients. One patient had a complication of a ureteral stricture which was successfully treated endoscopically with follow-up IVP one year later showing no stricture.

For retrograde stent placement, cystoscopy is performed and a guide wire is placed. If a point of obstruction is unable to be traversed, rigid ureteroscopy may be helpful. Low flow irrigation should be used, and the wire is passed under direct vision. Inflamed, edematous ureters may tear, therefore, if the wire does not pass easily, the attempt should be aborted. When the wire passes, but the stent does not, the wire may be left in place and secured to a Foley catheter. A second attempt can then be made at a later date. Following successful stent placement, continuous bladder drainage should be maintained for a minimum of 5 days to prevent extravasation secondary to vesicoureteral reflux up the stent. Follow-up VCUG should be performed prior to discontinuation of the Foley catheter to ensure that the fistula has closed. Follow-up IVP should also be performed prior to discontinuation of the ureteral stent and 3–6 months later to document patency of the ureter.

In cases in which a stent cannot be placed retrograde or the patient is unable to undergo anesthesia, a percutaneous nephrostomy with or without antegrade stent placement is an option. Nephrostomy alone may allow spontaneous healing of a small fistula. Antegrade stents can obviate the need for external drainage, and the nephrostomy can be discontinued. As with retrograde stents, if a wire cannot be passed through a point of obstruction, the attempt should be discontinued, and the nephrostomy is left in place. Persistent attempts can result in tearing of the ureter and other problems, such as submucosal dissection and edema. Patel reported on antegrade wire placement with subsequent retrograde stent passage following unsuccessful attempts at antegrade passage of a stent over the wire [10]. Traction on the wire from above provided adequate tension for successful retrograde stent placement in 70% of patients [10].

Lingeman et al. successfully traversed a point of ureteral obstruction with a combined antegrade and retrograde "cut-to-light" technique in 13 patients [17]. Nine patients had associated fistulas, and 4 had no fistula. At a mean follow-up of 22 months, all patients had patent ureters without fistula recurrence.

Other

Occlusive techniques to provide total occlusion of the ureter proximal to the fistula with proximal percutaneous drainage have been described, but are not routinely recommended and are not advocated by the authors. Finally, percutaneous creation of a cutaneous ureterostomy [18] and renal embolization [19] have also been described in the literature.

Conclusions

Ureterovaginal fistulas are a relatively uncommon complication. However, a systematic evaluation is imperative to correctly and completely identify the problem. The clinician must be sure that all fistulas and any degree of ureteral obstruction are clearly identified.

Treatment options include minimally invasive endoscopic techniques and open surgery. Minimally invasive techniques may be costly and may require more frequent follow-up than a definitive open procedure, but they can save patients the morbidity of open surgery. Endoscopic or percutaneous approaches are especially useful in patients who are not surgical candidates or who have terminal illnesses and short life expectancies. Minimally invasive approaches are also beneficial patients who require temporizing until they are stable for surgery. Early open surgery is definitive and, in the right patient, can provide a solution with one procedure. Nonetheless, if minimally invasive techniques fail, one can always proceed to open surgery. In most cases, the decision regarding the optimal therapeutic approach is one that should be made by the clinician together with the patient. Regardless of the approach employed, the goal of treatment of a UVF is preservation of renal function and relief of symptoms. All logical treatment options should be presented to each patient, and the decision regarding therapy should be made by the clinician together with the patient.

References

1. Chapple CR. Lower urinary tract fistulae. In: Webster G, Kirby R, King L, Goldwasser B, editors. Reconstructive Urology. Oxford: Blackwell Scientific Publications, 1993; 561–71.
2. Mann WJ, Arato M, Patsner B, Stone BL. Ureteral injuries in an obstetrics and gynecology training program: etiology and management. Obstet Gynecol 1988;72:82.
3. Lee RA, Symmonds RE. Ureterovaginal fistula. Am J Obstet Gynecol 1971;109(7):1032–5.
4. Murphy DM, Grace PA, O'Flynn JD. Ureterovaginal fistula: a report of 12 cases and review of the literature. J Urol 1982;128(5):924–5.
5. Aronson MP, Sant GR. Urinary incontinence after pelvic surgery. In: O'Donnell PD, editor, Urinary Incontinence. St Louis: Mosby, 1997; 325–31.

6. Hosseini SY, Roshan YM, Safarinjehad MR. Ureterovaginal fistula after vaginal delivery. J Urol 1988;160(3 Pt 1):829.

7. McVary KT, Marshall FF. Urinary fistulas. In: Gillenwater JY, Grayhack JT, Howards SS, Duckett JW, editors. Adult and Pediatric Urology. St Louis: Mosby, 1996; 1355–77.

8. Mandal AK, Sharma SK, Vaidyanathan S, Goswami AK. Ureterovaginal fistula: summary of 18 years' experience. Br J Urol 1990;65(5):43–6.

9. Kumar RV, Kumar A, Banerjee GK. Ureterovaginal fistula: an unusual complication of stone fragments after extracorporeal shock wave lithotripsy in situ. J Urol 1994;152 (6 Pt 1):2096–7.

10. Patel A, Werthman PE, Fuchs GJ, Barbaric ZL. Endoscopic and percutaneous management of ureteral injuries, fistulas, obstruction, and strictures. In: Raz S, editor. Female Urology, 2nd edn. Philadelphia: WB Saunders, 1996; 521–38.

11. Marshall VF. Vesicovaginal fistulas on one urological service. J Urol 1979;121:25–9.

12. Chang R, Marshall FF, Mitchell S. Percutaneous management of benign ureteral strictures and fistulae. J Urol 1987;138:306.

13. Elabd S, Ghoniem G, Elsharaby M et al. Use of endoscopy in the management of postoperative ureterovaginal fistula. Int Urogynecol J Pelvic Floor Dysfunct 1997;8(4):185–90.

14. Selzman AA, Spirnak JP, Kursh ED. The changing management of ureterovaginal fistulas. J Urol 1995;153(3 Pt 1):626–8.

15. Demirel A, Polat O, Bayraktar Y, Gul O, Okyar G. Transvesical and transvaginal reparation in urinary vaginal fistulas. Int Urol Nephrol 1993;25(5):439–44.

16. Yokoyama M, Iio S, Iwata H, Takeuchi M. Bilateral ureterovaginal fistula treated by psoas hitch and ureteroappendicocystostomy. J Urol 1992;147(4):1102–4.

17. Lingeman JE, Wong MY, Newmark JR. Endoscopic management of total ureteral occlusion and ureterovaginal fistula. J Endourol 1995;9(5):391–6.

18. Smith AD, Moldwin R, Karlin G. Percutaneous ureterostomy. J Urol 1987;138:286–8.

19. Long MA, McIvor J. Renal artery embolization with ethanol and gelfoam for the treatment of ureteric fistulae with one year follow-up. Clin Radiol 1992;132:1134.

43 Vesicovaginal Fistula

Harold P. Drutz and Kevin R. Baker

Introduction

Genitourinary fistulas in women have existed since time immemorial. Derry [1] of Cairo, in 1935, while examining the Henhenit mummy, who was either a queen or dancer in the court of Mentuhotep of the eleventh dynasty, Egypt (circa 2050 BC), found an extensive urinary fistula and complete tear of the perineum – the result of difficult labor. Avicenna [2], the Perso-Arab physician of over a millennium ago, in his Al-Kanoon, warns the physician of the incurability and lifelong curse of fistulas. Reports of Van Roonhuyse [3] in 1663 and Fatio [4] in 1752 described early successes using quills. However, it was not until the nineteenth century and the pioneering work of James Marion Sims [5] in Montgomery, Alabama, that the first successful repair of vesicovaginal fistula (VVF) using "silver-wire sutures" was carried out, in 1849. This success set the stage for modern surgical techniques and earned Sims the title of "father of modern gynecology".

In 1890 Trendelenburg [6] described the suprapubic transvesical route, and in 1893 Von Dittel was the first to gain exposure transperitoneally [7]. In 1894, Mackenrodt [8] described the vaginal flap-splitting technique which we still advocate today.

Classification and Etiology of Genitourinary Fistulas

Classification [9] of genitourinary fistulas can be either: (1) anatomic (Table 43.1); (2) etiologic (Table 43.2); or (3) by surgical size as recommended by Waaldijk [10] for obstetrical fistulas in order to compare surgical techniques and results (Table 43.3).

As suggested by Waaldijk [10] the surgical technique becomes progressively more complicated from type I through type II Bb. The results of closure and continence worsen progressively from type I through type II Bb. It was felt that this classification would enable systematic comparison of different surgical techniques and an objective evaluation of results from different centers. We have recommended that etiologic classification (Table 43.2) is more useful and better explains the changing incidence [9].

Congenital fistulas [11] are often seen in hypospadias, in which the bladder opens directly into the vagina, or bladder extrophy and may be associated with defective ossification of the pubic bones and a bifid clitoris. It is generally accepted

Table 43.1 Anatomic classification of genitourinary tract fistulas in women [1]

Fistulas involving primary ureter
Ureterovaginal
Ureterocervical
Ureterovesicocervicovaginal
Fistulas involving primary urinary bladder
Vesicovaginal
Vesicouterine
Vesicourethrovaginal
Vesicopelvovaginal
Vesicocervicovaginal
Vesicoureterovaginal
Fistulas involving primary urethra
Urethrovaginal
Loss of urethra sloughed urethra
Urethrocervicovaginal
Fistulas of fixed or miscellaneous genitourinary structures
Combined fistulas

Table 43.2 Etiologic classification of genitourinary fistulas [9]

Congenital

Surgical
  Unrecognized incision in urinary structure
  Pressure necrosis (from hemostat, suture, ligature)
  Devascullarization

Obstetric
  Damage during course of labor
  Instrumentation during delivery
  Cesarean section

Malignant
  Primary from the lesion
  Secondary to treatment

Irradiation
  Primary due to "hot spots"
  Secondary

Infection   Primary, secondary
Traumatic   Intrinsic, extrinsic
Spontaneous or idiopathic

that surgical fistulas occur after (1) unrecognized incision in a urinary structure; (2) pressure necrosis (from a hemostat, suture or ligature); (3) devascularization; or (4) combination of these mechanisms. However, Meeks et al. [12] in a study using rabbits showed that suture placed through the bladder during closure of the vaginal cuff after transabdominal hysterectomy, as an isolated event, was not associated with formation of postoperative vesicovaginal fistula (VVF). The ureter's common danger points occur at the corners of the vaginal vault; at the points where the cardinal ligaments are anchored to the vagina; and at the base of the severed ovarian pedicle.

Obstetric fistulas occur because of (1) damage during the course of prolonged labor; (2) instrumentation during delivery (forceps or vacuum); or (3)

Table 43.3 Surgical classification for obstetric fistulas [10]

1. Type I   Fistulas not involving the urethral closing mechanism

2. Type II
  Fistulas involving the urethral closing mechanism
  (A) Without (sub)total urethral involvement
  (B) With (sub)total urethra involvement
    (a) Without a circumferential defect
    (b) With a circumferential defect

3. Type III   Involving ureter and other exceptional fistulas

consequences of cesarean section. When obstructed labor is unrelieved the presenting fetal part is impacted against the soft tissues of the pelvis and a widespread ischemic vascular injury develops that results in tissue necrosis and subsequent fistula formation. It has been suggested [13] that the obstetric fistula is the result of a "field injury" to a broad area and may result in multiple birth-related injuries to the woman that may include total urethral loss, stress incontinence, hydroureteronephrosis, renal failure, rectovaginal fistula formation, rectal atresea, anal sphincter incompetence, cervical destruction, amenorrhea, pelvic inflammatory disease, secondary infertility, vaginal stenosis, osteitis pubis, and foot-drop. In the developing world the "fistula victims" often develop serious social problems, including divorce, exclusion from religious activities, separation from their families, worsening poverty, malnutrition, and almost unendurable suffering. Isolated almost exlusively to the developing world, particularly Africa, this problem has not received the international attention that it deserves, from either a medical or a social standpoint.

In developed countries the increasing incidence of cesarean section has led to an increase in Youssef's syndrome [14] (cyclic menouria associated with a vesicouterine fistula) and a change in the etiology of this condition [15].

Incidence–Etiology–Prevention

The true incidence of genitourinary fistulas is not known. In the United States it has been estimated that serious injury to the urinary tract occurs in more than 8000 of the 700,000 patients who have hysterectomies performed each year. Several prospective studies of total abdominal hysterectomy (excluding radical operations) suggest that ureteral injury occurs in 0.5–2.5% of patients [16,17]. Some ureteral ligations are asymptomatic and may go undetected. Some small VVFs are difficult to recognize [18].

Urinary tract injuries can occur after pelvic surgery performed by even the most experienced surgeons. The key point, however, is that bladder and/or ureteral injuries recognized during an operation and repaired immediately rarely lead to fistula formation. Symmonds [19] reported that the incidence of fistulas can be kept to a minimum, in a study of 35,117 consecutive gynecologic operations (including radical pelvic procedures) reporting only 20 fistulas (0.05%). Nine of these fistulas occurred after post-irradiation radical hysterectomy. Of the 20 fistulas two healed spontaneously with catheter drainage.

The best form of prevention is having a high index of suspicion of potential injury to the genitourinary tract during an operative procedure, identification and immediate repair. The presence of pelvic disease (fibroids, pelvic inflammatory disease, endometriosis, gynecologic malignancy, ovarian masses, adhesions from previous surgery, etc.) that necessitates intricate dissection increases the risk of injury to the urinary tract. Appropriate exposure and adequate dissection (either vaginally, or abdominally via open or laparoscopic approach) either obviate the injury or promote its recognition, enabling prompt repair.

In patients with a history of previous pelvic surgery preoperative intravenous pyelography (IVP) or ultrasound of the kidneys and pelvis will identify abnormal positioning of the bladder or ureters and previous trauma (such as the silent trying off of a ureter) which may have gone unrecognized.

The use of methylene blue in the bladder during surgery will help recognize injury to the bladder. Intraoperative IVP or cystoscopy (either per urethra or via an abdominal approach and operative cystotomy) with the concomitant injection of intravenous indigo carmine or methylene blue will help to recognize injury to the ureter which can usually be repaired immediately with few abnormal long-term sequelae [20].

All pelvic surgeons will at one time or another find themselves in trouble. It is not getting into trouble but what you do when you are in trouble that can ultimately help to prevent such complications as fistula formation.

Diagnosis and Preoperative Evaluation

The postoperative finding of an elevation in temperature, an unusual degree of lower abdominal discomfort, flank pain, and an increased vaginal discharge can suggest the presence of a fistula. A watery vaginal discharge may be the only manifestation of a fistula. This discharge may appear within a few hours after the operation, suggesting that the fistula is secondary to actual laceration of the bladder or ureter, or it may not appear for 5–30 days, suggesting that it results from bladder injury, devascularization, tissue necrosis, or infection [21]. Two-thirds of fistulas may appear in less than 10 days, and 90% of fistulas appear in less than 30 days. Irradiation leads to devascularization (with or without prior surgery) and fistulas may appear from 30 days to 30 years after the treatment.

Table 43.4 outlines the principles of diagnosis and preoperative evaluation. Large genitourinary fistulas are easy to diagnose but, as the author and colleague

Table 43.4 Preoperative evaluation [9]

1. Diagnosis – number, location, condition
2. Freedom from local sepsis
3. Suitable timing of repair

[18] have reported, small fistulas may be unrecognized. Multiple fistulas may occur in up to 15–25% of cases and their location and condition are important. Diagnostic tests (Table 43.5) include the methylene blue test, which consists of the instillation of a solution of 1 ml of methylene blue per 100 ml of saline into the bladder via a urethral catheter and the insertion of a tampon or piece of gauze into the vagina. If the tampon becomes stained with blue, a vesicovaginal fistula is indicated. If the tampon is not dye stained another tampon is inserted in the vagina, followed by the intravenous administration of indigo carmine (5 ml of a 0.8% solution). If this tampon becomes stained with dye, a ureterovaginal fistula may be present. If neither tampon is stained a third tampon should be inserted into the vagina and the patient asked to cough while the external urethral meatus is being observed. Staining of the most distal tampon may indicate either stress urinary incontinence and/or a urethrovaginal fistula.

Infusion of CO_2 into the vagina, which may induce air bubbles when inspecting the bladder at cystoscopy, intravenous pyelography (IVP) and examination under anesthesia (EUA) are often required.

The position of the VVF with respect to proximity of the ureteric orifices needs to be assessed in determining whether an abdominal or vaginal route will be used in surgical correction. A biopsy of the edges of the fistula is mandatory when there is a history of pelvic neoplasm. A voiding cystourethrogram (VCUG) may rule out reflux and show associated prolapse or an open bladder neck. Underlying genuine stress urinary incontinence, which may coexist with a VVF should be documented both subjectively and objectively with urodynamics, and may be corrected at the time of fistula closure. The presence of more than one fistula (VVF and/or ureterovaginal (UVF)) has been reported in up to 25% of cases [22]. UVF in conjunction with VVF can be ruled out with bilateral retrograde bulb ureteropyelograms, which have lower false negative rates than IVP.

Table 43.5 Diagnostic tests

1. Methylene blue test with vaginally placed tampons
2. Intravenous indigo carmine
3. Infusion of CO_2 into the vagina
4. Cystoscopy and intravenous pyelography
5. Examination under anesthesia (EUA)

Freedom from local sepsis remains an ideal goal. It is important to treat any known urinary tract infection, but in post-irradiation or long-standing fistulas, this may not be feasible. Local skin infection of the vulva or perineum should be treated preoperatively.

Timing of Repair

Opinion regarding the timing of VVF repair remains controversial. Collins and associates [23] advocated the use of cortisone preoperatively, which allowed repair of the fistula within 10 days to 2 weeks of injury. However, accepting the dictum that the best time to cure a fistula is at the first operation, the results of early repair with preoperative steroids have never been as good as with waiting generally 3 months from the time of injury or recurrence. Recently Blaivas [24] reported a series of 24 consecutive patients 17 of whom were repaired at an average interval of 10.8 weeks with similar results to those repaired after a longer wait.

Generally for repeat operations or post-irradiation fistulas a minimum of a 6-month wait is required.

Method of Treatment

Table 43.6 outlines methods of treatment of vesicovaginal fistula. Spontaneous cure can occasionally be achieved for a small fistula (less than 3 mm) with the use of catheter drainage (either suprapubic or urethral) for a 3-week period. Falk and Orking [25] advocated the use of cautery for fistulas less than 3 mm followed by catheter drainage for 10 days. A number of cases referred to the senior author's (HPD) unit for repair of VVF have had attempted closure with cautery which was unsuccessful and if anything made the fistula bigger.

Because urologists are not primarily vaginal surgeons, they generally choose the suprapubic approach, and in reviewing the literature it is important to note from which type of center the report emanates. However, more recently, there have appeared urology reports advocating the vaginal approach to VVF [26,27]. Lee et al. [28] have suggested that the only indications for the abdominal approach to VVF are: (1) inadequate exposure because of a high or retracted fistula in a narrow vagina; (2) proximity of the fistula to the ureter; (3) associated pelvic pathology; and (4) multiple fistulas (cribriform type).

More recently a case of laparoscopic repair using techniques of videolaparoscopy, videocystoscopy, and operative laparoscopy [29], and also an endoscopic transvesico-transurethral approach [30] have been reported. At this point in time these isolated reports cannot be considered as generalized standard of care.

Principles of Surgical Repair

The principles of surgical repair of a vesicovaginal fistula are outlined in Table 43.7 [9]. Suitable equipment is essential as is good surgical assistance. Vaginal retractors (Sims, Bailey's, Chassar Moir's), tenaculum forceps (Allis, Stiles), and proper needle drivers (Lawrence, Halsted, Heaney) aid in the surgical repair. Sharp long-handled cutting instruments, strong small needles, and hooks are needed for repair of a high vaginal fistula and enable the surgeon to transfix the tissue by gentle "pull-back". Alternatively in our unit we have found that the use of a Fogarty biliary catheter or a small pediatric Foley catheter used in conjunction with four "Stay" sutures (4–0 vicryl) placed at the 12, 3, 6 and 9'oclock position at the edge of the fistula help bring the fistula into the vaginal operating field. Good lighting is important, and it is important to wash the bladder of clot at the end of the repair.

Adequate exposure during the surgery is provided through the standard or exaggerated lithotomy position, although often in developing countries the knee–chest position is preferred, especially for a large

Table 43.6 Methods of treatment of vesicovaginal fistulas

Spontaneous
Cautery
Operative approach
Vaginal
Transvesical extraperitoneal
Transabdominal (intraperitoneal)
Combined
Laparoscopic and endoscopic
Diversion

Table 43.7 Principles of surgical repair [9]

1. Suitable equipment and lighting
2. Adequate exposure during operation
3. Excision of fibrous tissue from edges of fistula (controversial)
4. Approximation of edges without tension
5. Use of suitable suture material
6. Efficient postoperative drainage of the bladder

circumferential fistula fixed and retracted behind the pubic bone. In the scarred vagina (long-standing fistula, radical or previous surgery, radiation, atrophic changes) the use of a Schuchardt releasing incision often improves exposure. Saline solution or a local anesthetic agent with or without eprinephrine injected into the vaginal wall around the fistulous tract is useful to separate the bladder from the vagina, especially when there is a lot of scar tissue. A vertical incision is made in the anterior vaginal wall with an elliptical incision around the VVF (Figure 43.1a). *Wide mobilization* by careful dissection is used to separate the bladder from the vagina without tension (Figure 43.1b). If the dissection proves difficult the fistulous tract edges can be inverted and do not necessarily need to be excised. This also cuts down on bleeding into the bladder. Absorbable 3-0, or 4-0 Dexon or Vicryl interrupted suture is used for the first layer (Figure 43.1c), and an interrupted layer of 2-0 or 3-0 similar suture, again *without tension* is used for the second layer (Figure 43.1d).

If there is any doubt about the strength of the closure, and certainly if: (1) a previous attempt at repair has failed, (2) there is marked scar of the anterior vaginal wall from previous surgery, radiation, or atrophic changes, it is best to cover the defective area with a Martius [31] pedicle graft of fibrofatty tissue from the labium majus (Figure 2a–c). Unilateral grafts generally are sufficient and they are relatively easy to do. The incision should be drained for the first 24–48 hours postoperatively with a Penrose, Jackson–Pratt, or Hemovac brought out through the inferior border or stab incision below the base of the incision. As the late Reginald Hamlin (with whom HPD had the privilege of working), the well-known fistula surgeon of Addis Ababa, Ethiopia used to say, "She is then better than the way she was created".

If the patient has a huge circumferential VVF, a urethrovesicovaginal fistula, or a sloughed urethra (Figure 43.3a) for which construction of a neourethra from the anterior vaginal wall

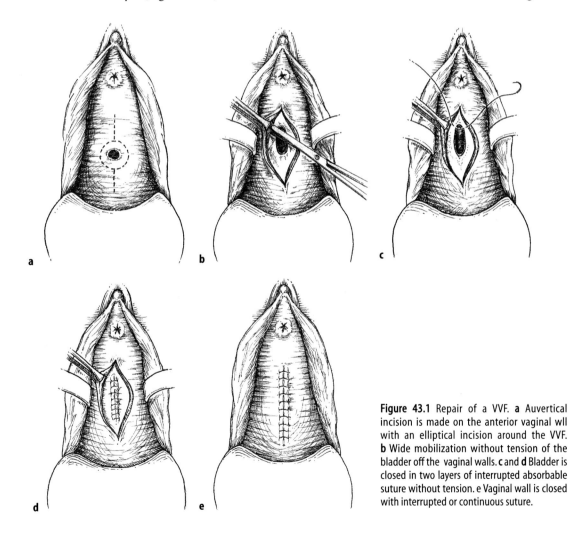

Figure 43.1 Repair of a VVF. **a** Auvertical incision is made on the anterior vaginal wll with an elliptical incision around the VVF. **b** Wide mobilization without tension of the bladder off the vaginal walls. **c** and **d** Bladder is closed in two layers of interrupted absorbable suture without tension. e Vaginal wall is closed with interrupted or continuous suture.

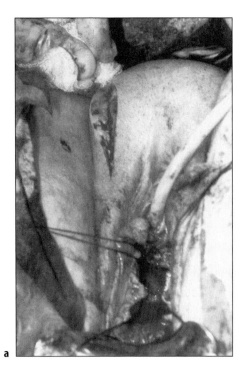

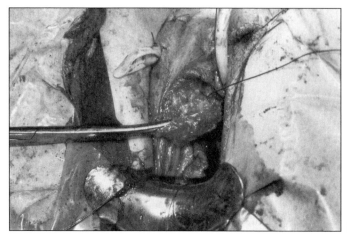

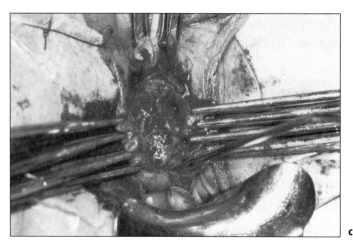

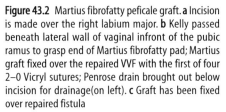

Figure 43.2 Martius fibrofatty peficale graft. **a** Incision is made over the right labium major. **b** Kelly passed beneath lateral wall of vaginal infront of the pubic ramus to grasp end of Martius fibrofatty pad; Martius graft fixed over the repaired VVF with the first of four 2–0 Vicryl sutures; Penrose drain brought out below incision for drainage(on left). **c** Graft has been fixed over repaired fistula

(Ward procedure)[32] (Figure 43.3a–c) is required it is necessary to cover the defect with either a Martius[31] or gracilis muscle graft[33] (Figure 43.4a–c). Reconstructive procedures can be carried out in conjunction with sling procedures using either synthetic[34] (Figure 43.3d) or autologous materials[35] in order to correct the sphincter weakness that coexists with the fistula.

In simple cases of repair of a VVF, after closing the bladder in two layers the anterior vaginal wall is closed using interrupted or running sutures of absorbable material (Figure 43.1e). It is feasible to use non-absorbable suture at this point but the sutures will have to be removed after 14 to 21 days and should be removed by the same operator.

In complex reconstructive cases after repair of the fistula and correction of any coexisting stress incontinence there may be no native anterior vaginal wall to close. Tissue can be obtained by using the medial half of the labia majora as a full-thickness pedicle graft, or alternatively a myocutaneous graft can be obtained from the medial surface of the thigh or even with a rectus abdominis myocutaneous flap[36].

Postoperative Drainage

Effective drainage during the postoperative period is best achieved with a suprapubic catheter, although this method may not work well if the patient has a small, shrunken bladder after irradiation or a long-standing fistula. Suprapubic catheters decrease the incidence of urinary tract infection, are more comfortable for the patient, and allow early mobilization. Drainage per urethra with a Foley catheter remains a common method, but if the fistula was at the base of the trigone or at the urethrovesical junction, it is best not to have the bulb of a Foley catheter sitting over the repair site.

If the patient has had a urethrovaginal fistula, sloughed urethra, or a urethral diverticulum repaired, a urethral stent is necessary in the postoperative period and should be left *in situ* for 10 to 14 days. The urethral catheter can be left in conjunction with a suprapubic catheter so that when the urethral stent is removed, repeated catheterizations will not be necessary if a normal voiding pattern is not established immediately.

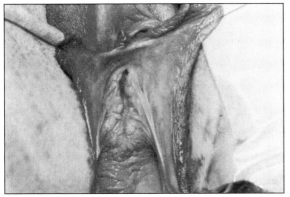
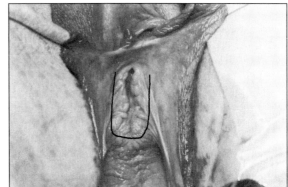

a

b

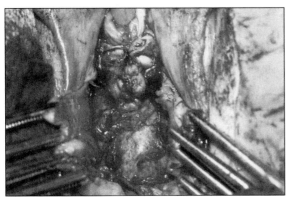
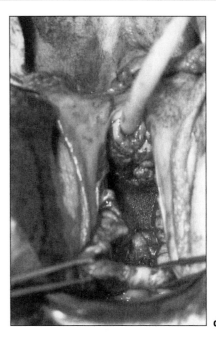

c

d

Figure 43.3 a Sloughed urethra following two anterior colporrhaphies. **b** "U" Shaped incision (Warp procedure [32]) for construction of neourethra. **c** Neouretha has been created in two layers. **d** modified urethra sling [34] using Marlex mesh.

Bladder irrigation need not be used routinely but should start at the first sign of any blockage in the system. Prophylactic antibiotics are not necessary if only a suprapubic catheter is present but should be considered when there is both a suprapubic catheter and a urethral stent. Documented urinary tract infection should be treated with the appropriate antibiotic.

On leaving the hospital, the patient should be instructed against the use of tampons, intercourse and douching for at least 6 weeks from the time of surgery and vaginal examination reveals adequate healing. For women wishing additional childbirth after successful repair of a VVF, cesarean section generally is recommended.

Conclusions

Genitourinary fistulas have become a less common entity in developed countries because of better obstetric care and more highly trained radical pelvic surgeons and radiotherapists. Surgical misadventure has emerged as the most common etiologic factor and is often associated with medicolegal issues. Nevertheless, problems with fistulas continue to occur and require the combined efforts and good clinical judgment of urogynecologists, general urologists, and general obstetrician-gynecologists in achieving permanent cures.

It remains the authors' opinion that the majority of VVF can be repaired successfully via the vaginal route.

Dedication

This chapter is dedicated to Catherine Hamlin and the memory of the late Reginald Hamlin of Addis Ababa, Ethiopia: superb surgeons, dedicated physicians, excellent teachers, cherished friends.

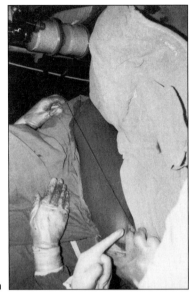
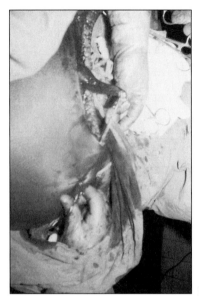

a   b

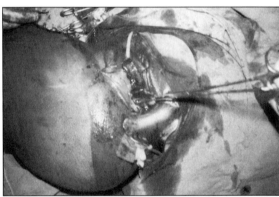

Figure 43.4 Gracilis muscle graft. **a** Landmarks
for incision are the inferior border of the
patella (Top) and the pubic tubercle (Bottom).
b Gracilis muscle is released from its insertion
to area where nerve and blood supply are and
then tunneled under the lateral vaginal wall.
c Gracilis fixed as a covering patch over the
repaired VVF.

c

References

1. Derry DE. J Obstet. Gynecol Br Emp 1935;42:490.
2. Avicenna. Al-Kanon, vol. 2. Cairo edition, p. 579 (in
   Typographica Medica, Romae, 1953, p. 580).
3. Van Roonhuyse H. Heelkonstige Aanmerikingebetr. de
   Gebrecken der Vrouwen. Amsterdam, 1663.
4. Fatio. Wehe-Mutter. Basel, 1762;284.
5. Sims JM. Am J Med Sci 1852;23:59.
6. Trendelenburg F. Volkmanns Samml Klive Vortr,
   1890;20:355.
7. Counselor VS, Welch JS. Classification and etiology of genitourinary fistulae. In: Youssef AF, editor. Gynecological
   Urology. Springfield, IL: Charles C Thomas, 1960;162–97.
8. Mackenrodt A. Zentralb Gynak 1894;18:180.
9. Drutz HP. Urinary fistulas. Obstet Gynecol Clin North Am
   1989;16(4):911–21.
10. Waaldijk K. Surgical classification of obstetric fistulas. Int J
    Gynecol Obstet 1995;49(2):161–3.
11. Rousseau T, Sapin E, Helardot PG. Congenital vesicovaginal
    fistula. Br J Urol 1996;77(5):760–1.
12. Meeks GR, Sams Jo 4th, Field KW, Fulp KS, Margolis MT.
    Formation of vesicovaginal fistula. The role of suture place-
    ment into the bladder during closure of the vaginal cuff
    after transabdominal hysterectomy. Am J Obstet Gynecol
    1997;177(6):1298–303.
13. Arrowsmith S, Hamlin EC, Wall LL. Obstructed labor injury
    complex: Obstetric fistula formation and gynecol survey
    1996;51(9):568–74.
14. Youssef AF. The syndrome of menouria after lower segment
    cesarean section (Youssef's syndrome). Am J Obst Gynecol
    1957;73:759.
15. Smith KM, Drutz HP. The changing etiology of uterovesical
    fistula. A case report and a literature review of the last
    century. Int Urogynecol J. Submitted for publications.
16. Freda VC, Tacchi D. Ureteral injury discovered after pelvic
    surgery. Am J Obstet Gynecol 1962;83(3):406–9.
17. Solomons E, Levin EJ, Bauman J et al. A pyelographic study
    of ureteric injuries sustained during hysterectomy for
    benign condition. Surg Gynecol Obstet 1960;111(1):41–48.
18. Drutz HP, Mainprize TC. Unrecognized small vesicovaginal
    fistula as a cause of persistent urinary incontinence. Am J
    Obstet Gynecol 1988;158:237.
19. Symmonds RE. Incontinence: Vesical and urethral fistulas.
    Clin Obstet Gynecol 1984;27(2):499–514.
20. Jabs CF, Drutz HP. The role of intraoperative cystoscopy in
    prolapse and incontinence surgery. Am J Obstet Gynecol
    2001;185(6):1368–71.
21. ACOG Technical Bulletin. Number 83. January 1985.

22. Ray H, Conger M, Ireland K. Ureteral obstruction in post-menopausal women with endometriosis. Urology 1985;26:577.

23. Collins CG, Collins JH, Harrison BR et al. Early repair of vesicovaginal vaginal fistula. Am J Obstet Gynecol 1971;111:524.

24. Blaivas JG, Heritz DM, Romanzi LJ. Early versus late repair of vesicovaginal fistulas: Vaginal and abdominal approaches. J Urol 1995;153(4):1110–12; discussion 1112–13.

25. Falk HC, Orking LA. Non-surgical closure of vesicovaginal fistulas. Obstet Gynecol 1957;9:538.

26. Zimmern PE, Hadley HR, Staskin D et al. Genitourinary fistulas: Vaginal approach for repair of vesicovaginal fistulas. Clin Obstet Gynecol 1985;12:403.

27. Dupont MC, Raz S. Vaginal approach to vesicovaginal fistula repair (Editorial). Urology 1996;48(1):7–9.

28. Lee RA, Symmonds RE, Williams TJ. Current status of genitourinary fistula. Obstet Gynecol 1988;72:313.

29. Nezhat CH, Nezhat F, Nezhat C, Rottenberg H. Laparoscopic repair of a vesicovaginal fistula: A case report. Obstet Gynecol 1994;83(5,Pt2):899–901.

30. Okamura K, Kanai S, Kurokawa T, Kondo A. Endoscopic transvesico-transurethral approach for repair of vesicovaginal fistula: Initial case report. J Endourol 1997;11(3):203–5.

31. Martius H. Zentralb Gynak 1928;52:480.

32. Ward GG. Surg Gynecol Obstet 1923;37:678.

33. Garlock JH: The cure of an intractable vesicovaginal fistula by the use of a pedicled muscle flap. Surg Gynecol Obstet 1928;47:225.

34. Spence-Jones C, DeMarco E, Lemieux MC, Drutz HP. Modified urethral sling for the treatment of genuine stress incontinence and latent incontinence. Int Urogynecol J 1994;5:69–75.

35. Ghoniem GM, Monga M. Modified pubovaginal sling and Martius graft for repair of the recurrent vesicovaginal fistula involving the internal urinary sphincter. Eur Urol 1995;27(3):241–5.

36. Viennas LK, Alonso AM, Salama V. Repair of radiation-induced vesicovaginal fistula with a rectus abdominis myocutanous flap. Plast Reconstr Surg 1995 Nov.;96(6):1435–7.

44 Rectovaginal Fistulas and Intraoperative Bowel Injury

Theodore M. Ross and Frederick D. Brenneman

Introduction

A rectovaginal fistula is an abnormal epithelium-lined communication between the rectum and vagina. There is nothing more physically and psychologically disabling than the aura of the incontinence of gas and fecal matter. There still remains controversy as to the best primary surgical corrective technique but an even more challenging decision is the approach to the patient who has failed corrective surgery. What is the role of a defunctioning stoma and when should more advanced surgical techniques be used? This section of the chapter outlines a practical and scientific approach to answer these difficult and controversial questions.

Table 44.1 Etiology of rectovaginal fistula

Congenital
Acquired

Traumatic:
  obstetric
  operative
  violence
  foreign body
  radiation

Inflammatory:
  infection
  inflammatory bowel disease

Neoplastic

Etiology

A rectovaginal fistula may be congenital or acquired (Table 44.1). Congenital fistulas will not be addressed in this chapter.

Although there is variation within most surgical series, traumatic fistulas are the most commonly seen. Amongst these fistulas, those of obstetrical etiology are most frequent [1]. These develop from an unrecognized injury, an inadequately repaired fourth degree tear or a repair which has been disrupted by infection. Venkatesh and associates found fistulas of obstetrical etiology to be a rare occurrence since they found only 25 fistulas developed following 22 050 vaginal deliveries (0.1%) [2].

Operative trauma from rectal or vaginal procedures can result in a fistula either because of direct injury or because of postoperative sepsis which decompresses through the rectovaginal septum. A high fistula may follow pelvic operations, whereas a low fistula may occur after low anterior resection or ileoanal pouch anastomosis for ulcerative colitis. Other traumatic fistulas can be caused by violence or foreign bodies.

Radiation for treatment of pelvic carcinoma may result in a fistula, 6 months to 2 years after treatment [3]. Radiation proctitis may progress to ulceration and in a small proportion may progress to fistula formation. The incidence depends upon the dose of radiation and predisposing conditions including diabetes mellitus and hypertension.

Inflammatory fistulas may be secondary to diverticulitis, Bartholin's abscess or inflammatory bowel disease. Crohn's disease is complicated by rectovaginal fistulas more commonly than is ulcerative colitis. In fact, Bandy reported an 11% incidence of Crohn's disease in his series of rectovaginal fistulas, whereas none had ulcerative colitis [4].

Colorectal or gynecological neoplasms, either primary or recurrent, can also result in a fistula.

Classification

In addition to etiology, a fistula may be described as low, middle or high. A low fistula is located at or above the dentate line. A high fistula is defined as one where the vaginal opening is near the cervix and a middle fistula lies in between.

In attempting to rationalize a practical approach to these fistulas, Tsang and Rothenberger described a classification of simple and complex fistulas by incorporating location and etiology [5].

A simple fistula is one that is low, small (<2.5 cm) and caused by trauma or infection. A complex fistula is large, high and caused by inflammatory bowel disease, radiation, malignancy or results from multiple failed repairs.

Clinical Symptoms

The most disabling symptoms are those of the involuntary passage of gas and fecal matter into the vagina. This may be associated with a fecal odor or recurrent vaginal infections. When patients describe incontinence of stool, one must clarify whether this is due to the rectovaginal fistula or to an associated sphincter injury.

Investigations:

A proper evaluation results in:

1. Establishing the underlying etiology of the rectovaginal fistula.
2. Defining the presence and site of the fistula.
3. Identifying a concomitant sphincter deficit.

A detailed history will often establish the etiology of the fistula as it relates to obstetrical injury, anal suppurative disease, inflammatory bowel disease, radiation or trauma.

Physical examination first begins with inspection of the perineum for other fistulas. Rectal examination and palpation of the rectovaginal septum will often identify the fistula tract. Vaginal speculum examination and proctosigmoidoscopy will often confirm the presence and location of the fistula. In addition, they will establish that the rectal and vaginal mucosa are non-edematous and free of underlying disease. In fact, Allen-Mersh and colleagues reported that over a third of radiation-induced fistulas are malignant [6].

Obscure fistulas may be identified by inserting a vaginal tampon after giving a methylene blue enema. Staining of tampon after 15 minutes will often confirm the presence of a fistula.

If the fistula cannot be identified, a radiologic evaluation by Hypaque enema is often helpful. If the patient remains symptomatic but the fistula is still not clearly identified then an examination under anesthesia is performed. Careful probing of the rectovaginal septum or instillation of air transrectally with vaginal speculum examination will usually identify the site. If the site remains obscure, instillation of water into the vagina with rectal air insufflation is sensitive to identify a small hole.

The third goal of investigation is to establish whether there is an anal sphincter deficit since this will modify the surgical approach. Although clinical examination is helpful, endorectal ultrasound is an important addition to the evaluation tools. It should be performed when there has been a traumatic injury and when history and clinical evaluation suggest but do not clearly identify a deficit. Anal manometry and pudendal nerve terminal latency testing are not essential preoperatively but may allow the surgeon to assess the success of postoperative continence objectively.

Timing of the Operative Procedure

The correct timing of a repair is controversial but can be simplified by determining two essential factors. The first is a determination of the overall nutritional health of the patient, which may be a significant issue when a fistula is secondary to inflammatory bowel disease, malignancy or radiation. The second relates to the health of the local tissues, which must be soft, pliable, non-edematous and uninvolved with active inflammatory bowel disease. Immediate repair may not satisfy the above criteria and may not allow a small fistula to heal spontaneously. The above criteria may be used to determine if a repair should be immediate or requires a delay of several months.

Surgical Repairs

Repairs can be performed through a rectal, vaginal, perineal or transabdominal approach. A summary of the alternative repairs is found in Table 44.2. All patients should have a mechanical and an antibiotic bowel preparation. For most local repairs, diet is restricted to clear fluids for 24 hours followed by bulk stool softeners postoperatively. The commonly used approaches will be addressed.

Table 44.2 Operative repairs of rectovaginal fistulas

Rectal:
  mucosal advancement flap
  layered closure

Vaginal:
  layered closure
  inversion of fistula

Perineal:
  conversion to complete laceration with layered closure
  sphincteroplasty

Muscle interposition:
  gracilis
  bulbocavernosus
  other

Abdominal:
  anterior resection
  coloanal
  other

Diversion:
  ileostomy
  colostomy

Rectal Approach

Mucosal Advancement Flap
First described by Noble in 1902, this repair has been modified by Lowry et al. such that a flap of rectal mucosa and internal sphincter is used for the repair [7] (Figure 44.1). The patient is placed in the prone jackknife position. The fistula is identified and the intersphincteric plane is infiltrated with a 1:200 000 epinephrine solution. The flap is initiated just distal to the fistula, 1–1.5 cm in diameter at its apex to include mucosa and internal sphincter. The dissection proceeds in a cephaled direction with extreme care at the level of the fistula to re-enter the correct plane above the fistula so as not to enlarge its size. The dissection is carried 3–5 cm above the fistula while one gradually widens the base of the flap to 3–4 cm. The vaginal opening may be left open for drainage if small (<5 mm) but if larger is usually fully or partially closed by interrupted 3-0 absorbable sutures. The rectal mucosa is gently separated from the cut edge of the internal sphincter. The repair is fashioned with interruped 3-0 absorbable sutures which reappose the internal sphincter. The flap is then drawn down, the ischemic rectal site of the fistula is excised and the flap closed with running and interrupted 3-0 absorbable sutures. Success rates for endorectal advancement flap vary from 29 to 100%. Lowry reported a 78% success rate in 56 patients. The success of this repair

seems to depend upon patient selection and the number of previous attempted repairs.

Rectal Approach – Layered Closure
This repair involves total excision of the fistula. The rectal mucosa is dissected free for 2 cm. The vaginal mucosa and rectovaginal septum are closed followed by advancement of the rectal mucosa distal to the deeper repair prior to closure (Figure 44.2). Hoexter and associates reported that 35 patients were successfully repaired without recurrence after a 4-year follow-up [8].

Vaginal Repairs

Excision of Fistula with Layered Closure
The fistula is elliptically excised followed by layered closure of the rectum and vagina with absorbable suture. Tancer reported 100% success in 10 patients using this technique [9].

Inversion of Fistula
A circular incision is made around the rectovaginal fistula. The vaginal mucosa is elevated around the margins of the fistula and two purse-string sutures are placed to invert the fistula into the rectum. The vaginal mucosa is subsequently closed.

Perineal Approach

The approach converts a rectovaginal fistula into a fourth degree tear (Figure 44.3). The inflamed fistula tissue, sphincter muscle and perineal body are debrided and the repair is closed anatomically. The rectum is closed in one layer, the sphincter is reapposed with interrupted sutures and the vaginal mucosa is closed last. Tancer reported success in all 34 repairs using this method [9].

Sphincteroplasty

When there is a sphincter deficit as well as a fistula demonstrated by clinical evaluation and endoanal ultrasound, a sphincteroplasty is the surgical treatment of choice. In these circumstances clinical evaluation often demonstrates a loss of the perineal body and sphincter anteriorly. There may be a fibrotic band anteriorly with a rectovaginal fistula. The technique involves initially positioning the patient in the prone jackknife position (Figure 44.4). If present the fibrotic band is divided. Dissection is initiated horizontally and then curved around the anus to protect the pudendal nerves as they enter posterolaterally. The dissection is carried in a cephaled direction separat-

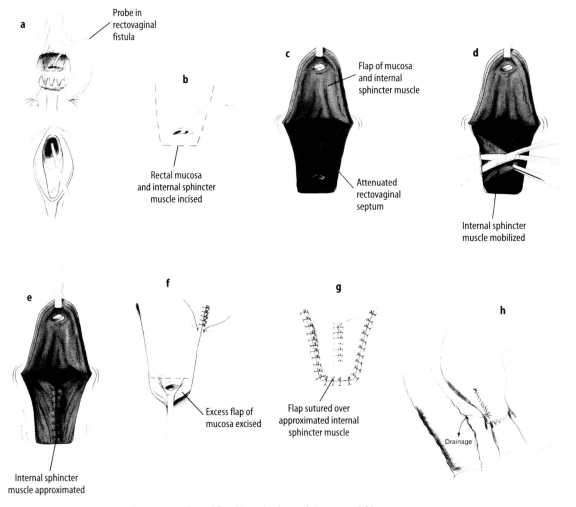

Figure 44.1   a–H Endorectal advancement of rectal flap. (From Gordon and Nivatvongs [3].)

ing the rectum from the vagina. The ends of the divided external and internal sphincter are identified and the fibrotic ends are preserved. If the injury involves the deep external sphincter, levatoroplasty may be added. The sphincter is reconstructed by overlapping the ends and securing the repair with horizontal mattress 2-0 absorbable sutures. The rectal mucosa is repaired and advanced to the anal verge. The vaginal mucosa is similarly closed. Skin coverage may require a local advancement flap. A small drain is left in place and diet is slowly advanced over 3 to 4 days. In separate series, Lowry and MacRae reported excellent results with sphincteroplasty [7, 10].

Muscle Interposition

Gracilis Muscle Interposition
The gracilis muscle can be mobilized from the right leg, providing a bulk of vascularized tissue to interpose between the rectum and vagina (Figure 44.5).

Following mobilization based on the proximal blood and nerve supply, the muscle is divided at the knee and tunneled subcutaneously. A transverse incision is made between the rectum and vagina and carried above the level of the fistula. The fistula tract is debrided and the rectum and vagina are closed prior to interposition of the gracilis muscle. The muscle is then fixed to the left ischial tuberosity (Figure 44.5).

Bulbocavernosus Fat Flap
An incision is made over the labia majora from the level of the mons pubis to the level of the posterior fourchette. The fat and fibromuscular content of the labia retain their vascular supply by the pudendal vessels. Through a subcutaneous tunnel the pedicle is drawn to the site of the fistula to be covered. As with a gracilis interposition, the fistula is debrided and closed in layers prior to placement of the bulbocavernosus flap.

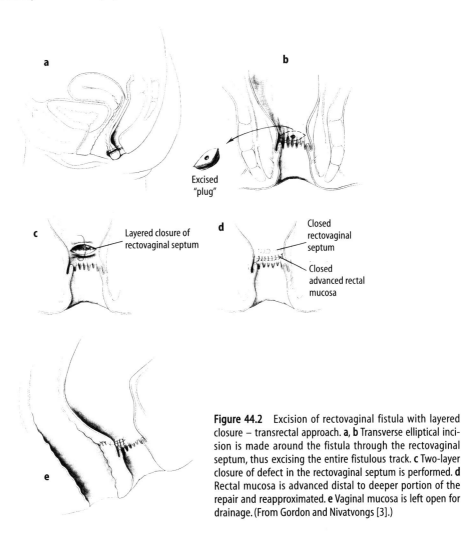

Figure 44.2 Excision of rectovaginal fistula with layered closure – transrectal approach. **a, b** Transverse elliptical incision is made around the fistula through the rectovaginal septum, thus excising the entire fistulous track. **c** Two-layer closure of defect in the rectovaginal septum is performed. **d** Rectal mucosa is advanced distal to deeper portion of the repair and reapproximated. **e** Vaginal mucosa is left open for drainage. (From Gordon and Nivatvongs [3].)

Transabdominal Repairs

This approach is indicated for a high fistula or when a low fistula repair has failed, or when a low fistula is secondary to radiation or a neoplasm. In principle, the rectum and vagina are separated at the site of the fistula. A portion of the rectum usually must be resected and an anastomosis is accomplished by low anterior resection or a handsewn coloanal anastomosis. If possible, an omental pedicle is interposed between the new anastomosis and the closed vagina. When a radiation-induced fistula is approached, a coloanal sleeve anastomosis as described by Parks et al. has been successfully used [11] (see radiation-induced fistula, below).

Selection of Surgical Approach

The algorithm for management of simple and complex fistulas is presented in Figure 44.6.

Simple Fistula

This is by definition a low fistula that has developed in a well-nourished patient or one that has developed in a patient with controlled inflammatory bowel disease. These simple fistulas rarely require a defunctioning stoma or a muscle interposition graft. The selection of the best primary repair may depend upon the individual surgeon's experience and preference, but there are potential advantages of each of the techniques.

A rectal approach by a mucosal advancement flap offers several potential advantages over other repairs. Hoexter, Labow and Moseson have pointed out that a rectal approach provides the best exposure to the high pressure side of the rectovaginal fistula [8].

In addition, there are theoretical advantages to the staggered suture lines in a mucosal advancement flap. When there is an intact anal sphincter, repairs which do not disrupt the sphincter mechanism may have a better functional result (mucosal advancement flap, layered rectal or vaginal repairs).

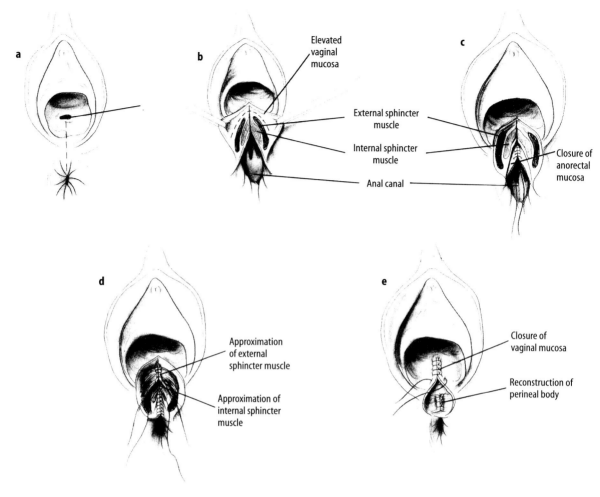

Figure 44.3   Conversion of rectovaginal fistula to complete perianal laceration and layer closure – transvaginal approach. **a** Entire rectovaginal fistulous track, including the sphincters and perineal body is incised. **b** Vaginal wall is dissected from remnants of the perineal body. **c** Layered repair of rectal mucosa and external and internal sphincter muscles is begun. **d, e** Perineal body is reconstructed and vaginal epithelium is approximated. (From Gordon and Nivatvongs [3].)

If a sphincter deficit is identified preoperatively, an anterior sphincteroplasty should be performed.

With the high success rate of the alternative repairs, the selection of the approach will ultimately depend upon the surgeon.

Complex Fistula

This is by definition a high fistula or one that has developed after a failed primary repair. It may have developed as a result of uncontrolled Crohn's disease or as a result of radiation. Because of the diversity of disease states resulting in complex fistulas, the best approach may be determined by etiology.

Recurrent or Failed Low Traumatic Fistulas
Decision analysis should incorporate the answers to the following questions:

1. Should the same type of repair be repeated?
2. Does the patient need a stoma?
3. Should a muscle interposition be added to the repair?

Lowry et al. have noted that the success rate of a mucosal advancement flap dropped from 88% to 85% when used as a second repair, but success was significantly poorer when used as a third procedure (55%). MacRae et al. reported a success rate of only 44% for a second repair with an advancement flap, but an 85% success rate with sphincteroplasty [10]. In view of this, an alternative local repair to the initial failed approach should be seriously considered. A loop-ileostomy should be deferred unless this second attempt fails. Any subsequent attempt should include a defunctioning stoma which may be combined with a further local repair, gracilis muscle

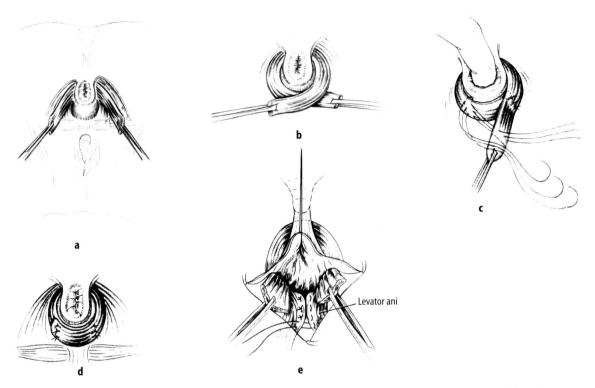

Figure 44.4 Sphincteroplasty. **a** External sphincter widely dissected from its bed to the ischiorectal fat. **b** Overlapping of the sphincter preserving the severed ends of the muscle. **c** Horizontal mattress sutures are placed to achieve desired degree of tightness. **d** Sutures are tied securely but not so tight as to cause muscle ischemia. **e** If the injury is more severe, plication of the levator ani is performed prior to overlapping sphincteroplasty. (From Rothenberger DA, Goldberg SM. Surgery of the Colon, Rectum and Anus. Oxford: Butterworth-Heinemann, 1993.)

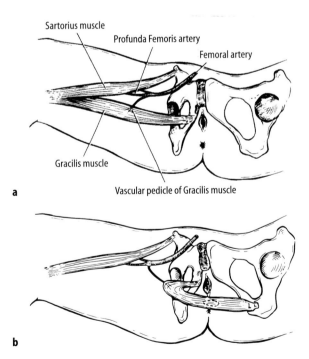

Figure 44.5 **a** Anatomy of the gracilis muscle. **b** Mobilization of the gracilis muscle, interposition between the rectum and vagina and fixation to left ischial tuberosity. (From Gorenstein et al. [12].)

interposition or alternatively a transabdominal approach with coloanal anastomosis.

Crohn's Disease

The decision to repair a fistula with underlying Crohn's disease depends upon the general activity of the disease, patient nutrition and the activity of the local rectal disease. If the rectum is not actively involved and the patient's disease is under good control, any primary repair without stoma creation may be attempted. If circumstances are not ideal (as described above) improved medical control of the disease followed by loop-ileostomy and primary repair can be attempted. If the fistula causes minimal symptoms, it may be left alone; if there is severe rectal disease, a proctectomy may have to be considered.

Anastomotic Vaginal Fistula

These fistulas may follow a low anterior resection for a carcinoma of the rectum or an ileo-anal pouch for ulcerative colitis. Once the fistula is recognized, the patient requires a defunctioning ileostomy or colostomy. If the fistula is due to incorporation of the vaginal suture line in the anastomosis, this may require laparotomy and separation of the rectum (pouch) from the vagina with reanastomosis.

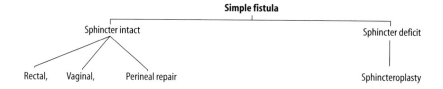

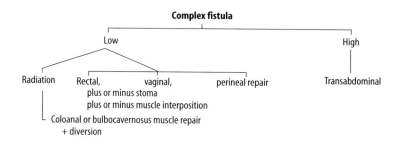

Figure 44.6 Algorithm for management of simple and complex fistulas.

Alternatively, local procedures including mucosal advancement flap or a gracilis muscle interposition can be successful, as described by Gorenstein, Boyd and Ross [12].

Radiation-induced Fistula

Local repair of these fistulas is fraught with failure and therefore uninvolved vascularized tissue must be used for repair.

Parks described a transabdominal approach where the rectum is transected below the level of the fistula [11]. The rectum and involved sigmoid colon are resected. Through a perineal approach the distal rectal mucosa is stripped and the uninvolved descending colon anastomosed by hand at the level of the anal canal. Nowacki et al. reported good results in 11 of 15 patients using this technique [13]. Bricker's on-lay patch anastomosis or Boronow's flap of bulbocavernosus muscle and labial fat have also been successfully used [14,15].

Conclusion

The myriad of techniques available for repair of a rectovaginal fistula is testimony to the difficult problem that it presents to surgeons. A knowledgeable, rational, organized approach combined with meticulous surgical technique will minimize failure and provide relief from the disabling symptoms.

Intraoperative Bowel Injury

Intraoperative bowel injury is an issue that all surgeons who perform a laparotomy must be able to manage, whether general surgeons, urologists, or gynecologists. Ideally, injury to the bowel should be avoided. However, when it occurs, the management depends on a number of factors. The first step is to recognize that such an injury has occurred, as missed bowel injuries carry with them a significant degree of morbidity and a risk of mortality. This section of the chapter will divide intraoperative bowel injuries anatomically and discuss specific considerations that are similar and unique to each portion of the bowel.

Prevention of Bowel Injury

Many bowel injuries occur as a result of previous surgery and subsequent intra-abdominal adhesions. Adhesions may also be caused by previous peritonitis or radiation. No well-accepted method has been developed to prevent post-surgical adhesions, although various solutions instilled at the time of laparotomy closure have been tried. One method to prevent the bowel from adhering to an anterior abdominal wall incision is to interpose omentum between the bowel and the abdominal wall. However, some patients have very little omentum, or the omentum is removed therapeutically as in the surgical treatment of ovarian cancer. Great care must be taken during the initial stages of a laparotomy, so that the abdominal cavity is safely entered without inflicting a bowel injury. Similarly, during the course of the laparotomy, adhesions must be dissected with care to avoid serosal and full-thickness tears to the bowel wall, and injury to other intra-abdominal organs. Overaggressive retraction of the bowel for exposure of other organs may cause an injury to the bowel wall or to the mesentery.

The timing of a repeat laparotomy may be crucial in avoiding bowel injury. Early adhesions tend to be quite vascular and more adherent to the bowel, while adhesions that are at least 3 months old (from the time of the previous laparotomy) are more mature, less vascular, and more readily dissected free from the bowel. Waiting for at least 3 months for subsequent surgery, when feasible, often makes for more "friendly" adhesions and less risk of bowel injury.

Small Bowel Injury

Injury to the small bowel can be classified as either injury to the bowel wall or injury to the small bowel mesentery and vascular structures. One type of injury to the bowel wall is a serosal tear, usually easily managed with Lembert-style suture repair. Minor serosal tears may not require any treatment whatsoever. Intramural hematomas will usually heal spontaneously and do not require exploration. Full-thickness defects will require either primary repair or resection and primary anastomosis, depending on the extent of injury to the bowel. If primary repair is chosen, the surgeon

must be careful not to narrow the lumen of the bowel. A transverse direction of the suture or staple line is advocated to avoid this complication (Figure 44.8).

Mesenteric injuries may or may not involve the blood supply to the involved segment of bowel. If the blood supply remains intact after hemostasis is achieved, then the only consideration is to close any mesenteric defect to avoid subsequent internal herniation. A mesenteric vascular injury results in either a mesenteric hematoma or a laceration and mandates careful assessment of the bowel for viability. All segments of small bowel that are not viable require wide resection followed by primary anastomosis. An injury to the proximal superior mesenteric artery is more serious, and may require the assistance of a vascular surgeon and arterial reconstruction. Exposure of the proximal superior mesenteric artery is best achieved either through the lesser sac or with medial visceral rotation on the left side.

Large Bowel Injury

The treatment of intraoperative colon injuries is often more controversial than treatment of small bowel injuries. The unprepared colon has a high fecal content and, as such, more potential for septic complications following full-thickness injury. Fortunately, intraoperative colon injuries during elective surgery often occur in favorable conditions. The presence of a preoperative mechanical bowel preparation and lavage decreases the bacterial content of the colon and allows for safer primary repair and resection with anastomosis. The blood supply to the colon is not quite as extensive as that

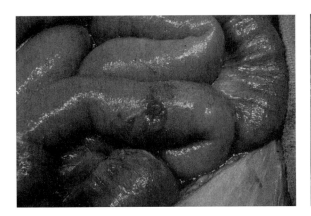

Figure 44.7 "Blow out" type of small bowel injury secondary to blunt trauma.

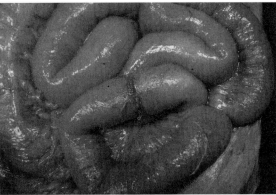

Figure 44.8 The staple repair of small bowel injury in a transverse fashion.

to the small bowel. A good blood supply is one of the most important factors in the successful healing of a repair or anastomosis of the bowel.

The management of intraoperative colon injuries can be formulated from the experience found in the trauma literature. Historically, the treatment of colon trauma evolved to include mandatory colostomy after better results were achieved with the use of colostomy in World War II in comparison to primary repair [16]. In fact, the Surgeon General of the Armed Service Forces of the United States made colostomy the standard of care for large bowel trauma in 1943 [17]. More recently, the pendulum has swung back to the side of primary repair for penetrating colon injuries. Stone published the first prospective randomized clinical trial that showed better outcomes with the use of primary repair in patients with favorable criteria including the absence of shock, few associated injuries, minimal fecal contamination and a short time (less than 8 hours) from injury to repair [18]. More liberal selection criteria were employed in later studies, to include right and left colon injuries and even injuries that were extensive enough to warrant resection. These subsequent prospective trials have advocated primary repair or resection and anastomosis for most colon injuries resulting from penetrating trauma [19–22]. A further consideration is the not insignificant morbidity (5–55%) associated with colostomy closure at a later date [23–25]. This evidence has resulted in most contemporary trauma surgeons performing primary repair of penetrating colon injuries, including resection and anastomosis of unprepared bowel [26].

Rectal Injury

The treatment of an injury to the rectum in the setting of trauma includes rectal wound repair, a diverting colostomy with distal colorectal washout, and occasionally presacral drainage [27]. In contrast, an intraoperative rectal injury during elective surgery may be treated with primary repair without a proximal colostomy if a preoperative bowel preparation was used. However, in the context of unprepared bowel, strong consideration should be given to a defunctioning loop colostomy to decrease the chance of postoperative pelvic sepsis. A Hartmann's procedure should be used for extensive rectal injuries.

References

1. Hibbard LT. Rectovaginal fistulas and complete perineal tears. Am J Obstet Cynecol 1978; 130:139–141.
2. Venkatesh KS, Ramanyam PS, Larson DM, Haywood MA. Anorectal complications of vaginal delivery. Dis colon Rectum 1989; 32:1039–41.
3. Gordon PH, Nivatvongs S. Principles and Practice of Surgery for the Colon, Rectum and Anus. Quality Medical Publishing 1992;361–82.
4. Bandy LC, Addison A, Parker RT. Surgical management of rectovaginal fistulas in Crohn's disease. Am J Obstet Gynecol 1983;147:359–63.
5. Tsang CB, Rothenberger DA. Rectovaginal fistulas. Therapeutic options. Surg Clin North Am 1997;77(1):95–114.
6. Allen-Mersh TG, Wilson ET, Hope-Stone HF, Mann CV. The management of radiation induced rectal injury after treatment of carcinoma of the uterus. Surg Gynecol Obstet 1987;164:521–4.
7. Lowry AC, Thorson AG, Rothenberger DA et al. Repairs of simple rectovaginal fistula. Influence of previous repairs. Dis Colon Rectum 1988;31:676–8.
8. Hoexter B, Labow SB, Moseson MD. Transanal rectovaginal fistula repair. Dis Colon Rectum 1985: 28:572–5.
9. Tancer ML, Lasser D. Rosenblum N. Rectovaginal fistula or perineal and anal sphincter disruption, or both, after vaginal delivery. Surg Gynecol Obstet 1990;171:43–6.
10. MacRae HM, McLeod RS, Cohen Z, Stern H, Reznick R. Treatment of rectovaginal fistula that has failed previous repair attempts. Dis colon Rectum 1995;38:921–5.
11. Parks AG, Allen CLO, Frank JD et al. A method of treating postirradiation rectovaginal fistulas. Br J Surg 1978;65:417–21.
12. Gorenstein L, Boyd JB, Ross TM. Gracilis muscle repair of rectovaginal fistula after restorative proctocolectomy; Report of two cases. Dis Colon Rectum 1988;31:730–4.
13. Nowacki MP, Szawlowski AW, Borkowski A. Parks' coloanal sleeve anastomosis for treatment of postirradiation rectovaginal fistula. Dis Colon Rectum 1986;29:817–20.
14. Bricker EM, Johnston WD. Repair of postirradiation rectovaginal fistula and stricture. Surg Gynecol Obstet 1979; 148:499–506.
15. Boronow RC. Repair of the radiation-induced vaginal fistula utilizing the Martius technique. World J Surg 1986;10:237–48.
16. Ogilvie WH. Abdominal wounds in the western desert. Surg Gynecol Obstet 1944;78:225–38.
17. Office of the Surgeon General, Circular Letter No. 178, October 28, 1943.
18. Stone HH, Fabian TC. Management of perforating colon trauma: randomization between primary closure and exteriorization. Ann Surg 1979;190(4):430–6.
19. Chappuis CW, Frey DJ, Deitzen SD, Panetta TP, Buechter KJ, Cohn Jr. IC. Management of penetrating colon injuries: a prospective randomized trial. Ann Surg 1991;213(5):492–8.
20. George Jr. SM, Fabian TC, Voeller GR, Kudsk KA, Mangiante EC, Britt LG. Primary repair of colon wounds: a prospective trial in nonselected patients. Ann Surg 1989;209(6):728–34.
21. Sasaki LS, Allaben RD, Golwala R, Mittal VK. Primary repair of colon injuries: a prospective randomized study. J Trauma 1995;39(5):895–901.
22. Gonzalez RP, Merlotti GJ, Holevar MR. Colostomy in penetrating colon injury: is it necessary? J Trauma 1996;41(2):271–5.
23. Yajko RD, Norton LW, Bloemendal L, Eiseman B. Morbidity of colostomy closure. Am J Surg 1976;132:304–6.
24. Sola JE, Bender JS, Buchman TG. Morbidity and timing of colostomy closure in trauma patients. Injury 1993;24(7):438–40.
25. Berne JD, Velmahos GC, Chan LS, Asensio JA, Demetriades D. The high morbidity of colostomy closure after trauma:

further support for the primary repair of colon injuries. Surgery 1998;123(2):157–64.

26. Eshraghi N, Mullins RJ, Mayberry JC, Brand DM, Crass RA, Trunkey DD. Surveyed opinion of American trauma sur- geons in management of colon injuries. J Trauma 1998;44(1):93–7.

27. Ivatury RR, Licata J, Gunduz Y et al. Management options in penetrating rectal injuries. Am Surg 1991;57:50.

45 Intraoperative Management of Injury to the Lower Urinary Tract

Said A. Awad and Philip Scott Bagnell

Introduction

Intraoperative injuries to the lower urinary tract are uncommon, but potentially troublesome problems. Early recognition and repair of a damaged bladder or urethra can significantly improve outcome and limit postoperative morbidity. The increase in the number of "minimally invasive" procedures in recent years such as laparoscopic and vaginal surgery has created the potential for more bladder and urethral injuries at time of surgery since they have been shown to have a higher incidence of lower urinary tract injuries when compared to transabdominal pelvic surgery. Nevertheless, a large percentage of these procedures are still carried out through an abdominal incision. A recent study of urinary tract injuries following hysterectomy in Finland from 1990 to 1995 showed that 75% of all hysterectomies were still being carried out transabdominally (95% in 1990) [1]. Also, a number of operations for urinary stress incontinence are still performed through an abdominal incision. Obviously, the surgical approach selected is dependent not only on the surgeon's preference but also on the nature of the patient problem and preoperative factors.

This chapter will focus on injuries to the bladder and urethra during abdominal, vaginal and transurethral surgery. We will focus on incidence, prevention and management of these problems. Clearly, there is no substitute for prevention of these types of injury; also these injuries are far easier to deal with at time of primary surgery and become much less traumatic to the patient.

Abdominal Surgery

The abdominal approach is associated with lower incidence of damage to the bladder or urethra when compared to the other approaches. Nevertheless, it is not without its own unique problems and potential for injury. Many of the patients requiring an abdominal incision have extensive pathology and are poor candidates for minimally invasive surgery because of multiple previous abdominal and/or pelvic surgery or have a disease process that requires a more invasive approach (e.g. endometriosis, pelvic inflammatory disease or malignancy) [2,3].

The relation of the bladder dome to the lower abdominal wall puts it at risk for damage upon entering the abdominal cavity. A laceration of the dome of the bladder is usually identified easily and repaired. These injuries are usually sustained when the bladder is not emptied prior to entering the abdomen and are quite easily prevented. The extent of the surgery, presence of adhesions, existing pathology, and any significant bleeding distorting tissue planes contribute to the potential for further damage to the bladder [4]. Patients with a past history of endometriosis, pelvic radiation, pelvic inflammatory disease, cesarean section, or prior surgery are at significantly increased risk of damage to the lower urinary tract. Usually, the base of the bladder and trigone are the site of damage. These injuries occur primarily as the bladder is dissected away from the cervix and upper vagina [5]. Aggressive, blunt or sharp dissection in the wrong tissue plane is usually the cause. Most can be avoided through caution and careful identification of correct tissue planes, especially when dissection is carried out through areas of scar tissue or adhesions. This is particularly important when faced with a pelvis that has been irradiated in the past or preoperatively. The incidence of bladder injury rises significantly in these patients. Insertion of a Foley catheter in these patients preoperatively can aid in identifying the trigone and urethra. If there is any question of damage; saline, methylene blue, or intravenous indigo carmine solution may be injected to rule out a possible leak. Preoperative ureteric stenting is recommended in any surgery that has high risk of injury to the trigone or ureters. Obviously, these problems are only compounded by the limited exposure afforded by laparoscopic surgery. The CREST study [3] compared the number of bladder injuries in total abdominal hysterectomies versus vaginal hysterectomies prospectively, between 1978 and 1981. Bladder damage was sustained in 0.3% versus 1.4% respectively. These results are supported by more recent literature. Laparoscopic hysterectomies have an incidence of approximately 1–1.2% of bladder injuries [6].

Management

In the event that the bladder is injured by either dissection or a clamp "crush" type injury, the damaged tissue should be excised and the bladder closed in two layers. The normal bladder is quite vascular and should heal quite well with adequate tissue approximation and catheter drainage for 7–10 days. With an irradiated bladder, or whenever the bladder tissue is tenuous or has poor blood supply, a pedicled graft of omentum should be added to the closure, thus separating the bladder from the vagina and enhancing healing because of the rich omental blood supply. Depending on the extent of the injury a suprapubic catheter in addition to the Foley catheter may be advisable. Proper postoperative bladder drainage is absolutely crucial to ensure healing.

Vaginal Surgery

The majority of surgery carried out from a vaginal approach consists of anterior repairs, needle suspensions, sling procedures and simple hysterectomies. Surgery for urinary stress incontinence places both the urethra and bladder at risk of possible injury, especially if these patients have undergone multiple operations. They may have poor tissue, perivesical scarring, or the bladder may be stuck to the lateral wall of the pelvis from prior

pelvic surgery. A potentially thin bladder wall increases the risk of complication. Controlled, sharp dissection of the bladder base and trigone during the reflection of the vaginal flaps will limit the chance of injury. A Foley catheter will delineate the path of the urethra, identify the location of the bladder neck, and keep the bladder empty.

Management

Any lacerations identified should be closed in two layers immediately to avoid extension of the injury. Control of any bleeding should be attained quickly and a labial flap (Martius) may have to be used to separate the bladder suture line from the vagina and enhance healing by the rich blood supply of the labial fat [7].

Accidental Penetration of the Bladder

Another complication unique to urinary stress incontinence surgery is the accidental penetration of the bladder by needles or sutures through the full thickness of the bladder wall. This usually occurs as a result of inadequate mobilization of the bladder away from the lateral pelvic wall and is easily recognized endoscopically. If missed, the resultant tissue damage may produce a cellulitis in the space of Retzius due to leakage of urine and later development of vesicovaginal fistula and possibly bladder stones around the suture. This, could also result in further scarring and fixation of the bladder neck and there have been reported cases of fixation of vesical wall to the periosteum of the pubis resulting in osteitis pubis.

A few techniques can be employed to avoid or recognize these injuries. The presence of a Foley catheter provides an excellent landmark. Also careful introduction of the needles immediately behind the pubic bone and finding a plane between the bladder and the lateral pelvic wall is important. This is even more important in sling procedures where a Kelly forceps is sometimes used to develop this plane, since a tear from the forceps will be far more extensive. Cystoscopy following placement of the Stamey needles or Kelly forceps is absolutely essential and will identify any bladder penetration.

Management

Immediate removal and proper repositioning of the Stamey needle or Kelly forceps once it has been shown to have penetrated the bladder should be carried out. Rarely, if the bladder tear is large, a transabdominal repair needs to be carried out as described below.

Urethral Injuries

Injuries to the urethra during vaginal surgery occur more frequently than with abdominal surgery although, relatively speaking, they are still rare. The location of the female urethra in the anterior vaginal wall, and the very thin perivaginal tissue that separates the two, predisposes it to injury during vaginal surgery. The most common sources of injury are anterior colporrhaphy and stress incontinence surgery. Previous surgery or radiation increases the risk. Careful, gentle dissection when faced with such situations reduces the chance of injury.

Management

The principles of repair of urethral injuries are similar to those for the bladder. A two-layered, water-tight closure is essential for proper healing. Once again, a labial fat graft (Martius flap) may need to be used. Care must be taken to ensure that the sphincter mechanism of the urethra is not damaged by the repair. Proper bladder drainage must be accomplished using a Foley catheter and, if necessary, a suprapubic catheter.

Transurethral Surgery

Bladder perforation during transurethral surgery is encountered most frequently during bladder tumor resection. Such a complication is avoidable with careful surgical technique such as maintaining good visibility during the resection by controlling bleeding, being aware that the bladder wall in women is often thin and avoiding bladder overdistension. In the past, bladder perforation also occurred occasionally during lithopaxy when mechanical lithotrites were often used. With the new technology available today, such as electrohydraulic or holmium laser lithotripsy, such a complication is rare. Bladder perforation may also rarely occur during forceful manual bladder distension instead of hydrostatic distension by gravity in patients with severe interstitial cystitis.

Management

Intraoperative cystogram should be carried out whenever bladder perforation is suspected to confirm the diagnosis and to rule out intraperi-

toneal extravasation. Once bladder perforation has been identified, the procedure should be discontinued immediately after ensuring that there is no significant bleeding. The 20 French catheter inserted for the cystogram will be used to provide free urinary drainage postoperatively. In cases where the perforation was shown to be intraperitoneal on the cystogram, or if catheter drainage alone in extraperitoneal extravasation is felt to be inadequate because of the size or location of the perforation, abdominal exploration with bladder repair and placement of a suprapubic catheter is advisable. Adequate bladder drainage should be maintained postoperatively for 7–10 days with antibiotic coverage.

Conclusion

It is clear from all the studies that there is no substitute for prevention of these injuries. However, if identified immediately and dealt with at time of surgery these injuries are rarely troublesome. The same cannot be said of undiagnosed bladder or urethral injuries resulting in a variety of problems with long-term morbidity. The risk of injury to the lower urinary tract increases for a given patient population when minimally invasive procedures are performed. It is important, under these circumstances, to keep these potential problems in mind and maintain a high index of suspicion.

References

1. Harkki-Siren Paivi, Sjoberg J, Tiitinen A. Urinary tract injuries after hysterectomy. Obstet Gynecol 1990;92:113–18.
2. Schmidbauer C, Hadley R, Staskin D, Simmern P, Leach G, Raz S. Complications of Vaginal Surgery. Semin Urol 1986;4:51–62.
3. Dicker R, Greespan J, Strauss L, Cowart M, Scally M, Peterson H, Destefano F, Rubin G, Ory H. Complications of abdominal and vaginal hysterectomy among women of reproductive age in the United States, the collaborative review of sterilization. Am J Obstet Gynecol 1982;144:841–9.
4. Symmonds RE. Loss of the urethral floor with total urinary incontinence. Am J Obstet Gynecol 1969;103:664.
5. Mattingly R, Borkowf H. Acute operative injury to the lower urinary tract. Clin Obstet Gynecol 1979;5:123–47.
6. Harris W, Daniell J. Early complications of laparoscopic hysterectomy. Obstet Gynecol Surv 1996;51(9):559–66.
7. Martius H. Supplementary surgery with bulbocavernosus fat flap. In: McCall ML, Bolton KA, editors. Martius' Gynecological Operations. Boston, Toronto: Little Brown, 1956; 322–34.

46 Postoperative Voiding Dysfunction

J. Barry MacMillan and Harold P. Drutz

An often overlooked and minimized aspect of anti-incontinence and pelvic reconstructive reparative procedures is the problem of postoperative voiding dysfunction and urinary retention. The focus of most surgical research centers around continence. How many patients are dry and for how long remains the mainstay of our discussions about surgical success. The prospect of ongoing urinary retention with chronic catheterization is difficult to contemplate, even for patients with severe urinary incontinence. It has been suggested that some patients may prefer the use of intermittent catheterization over urinary incontinence [1]. Most patients are not quite so accepting. True surgical success is judged by the return of normal voiding function along with long-lasting continence. The type of surgery performed is critical to such success. One of the mechanisms of success for anti-incontinence procedures is urethral obstruction through elevation of the posterior urethral vesical angle. Some procedures are more obstructive than others, leading to a greater chance of urinary retention. This is the case with many sling operations. To some extent, improvement in continence rates may occur at the risk of more postoperative voiding dysfunction. Appropriate patient and surgical selection are paramount to the prevention of this problem.

Once voiding dysfunction has occurred, there are many treatment options available. This chapter will address postoperative voiding dysfunction from expected incidence and pathophysiology to appropriate diagnosis, treatment and management.

Incidence

The incidence of postoperative voiding dysfunction varies based upon the procedure performed.

Urinary retention can follow any surgical procedure. Most studies show a rate of 7–35% following various types of surgery [2–4]. Orthopedic [5,6], upper abdominal [3] and cardiovascular (thoracotomy) [2] surgery can precipitate urinary retention. Even laparoscopic procedures such as herniorrhaphy [7,8] can be complicated by urinary retention that prolongs hospital stay or delays recovery. Procedures that are undertaken in close proximity to the bladder have the highest urinary retention risk postoperatively. Orthopedic operations, such as hip arthroplasties, and rectal operations for bowel carcinoma, such as low anterior or abdominoperineal resections, pelvic pouch procedures, proctectomies, and diversions, are particularly troublesome [9,10]. Both immediate and long-term urinary retention is very commonly reported. The etiology of retention following these types of surgeries is likely multifactorial, but interference to pelvic neuroanatomy plays a major role.

All gynecological procedures may be associated with postoperative urinary retention and various other types of voiding dysfunction. The actual incidence is procedure specific with certain operations being notable for the problem. About 50% of patients require catheterization for urinary retention following hysterectomy [11]. Up to 35% may need catheterization for several days before effective bladder emptying is restored [4]. With routine hysterectomy and other common gynecological procedures not associated with bladder neck suspension, the urinary retention is usually temporary. An example is rectocele repair, with urinary retention being the most common postoperative complication, occurring in about 13% of cases [12]. Resolution usually occurs within days, but occasionally can extend hospitalization. Bladder suspension procedures and radical pelvic surgery for gynecological malignancies represent high risk procedures for both immediate and long-term voiding dysfunction.

Pathophysiology

The causes of postoperative voiding dysfunction are quite varied (Table 46.1). Pain is perhaps the most common immediate cause of postoperative urinary retention. The endogenous release of catecholamines in association with a pain or stress response can lead to alpha-adrenergic stimulation of the urethral musculature [13]. Increased urethral tone or pressure creates a functional outlet obstruction. Adequate pain relief is an important aspect of effective postoperative care, with narcotic analgesics being the most common method of pain control. Such pain control must be undertaken with care, as opiate analgesics are also responsible for urinary retention [14,15]. Use of PCA (patient-controlled analgesia) opiates may be particularly problematic [16]. Opiate analgesics can blunt the normal sensation to void, leading to bladder overdistension. Excessive enlargement of the bladder leads to injury at the muscle fiber layer. Actin and myosin fibers become separated and effective contractile function inhibited [17].

Epidural and spinal anesthetics probably lead to voiding problems through a similar mechanism to that described above with opiate analgesics. Nerve sensation blockade and detrusor relaxation coupled with vigorous intravenous hydration can create a loss of normal sensation to void. Acute bladder overdistension and resultant injury may lead to a prolonged inability to void. Pregnancy is the most common clinical situation in which this mechanism of voiding

Table 46.1   Causes of postoperative urinary retention

Pain
Opiate analgesics
Anesthetic agents
Epidural and spinal anesthetics
Edema of the bladder neck and urethra
Bladder neck dislocation
Inhibition to void
Pre-existing bladder problems
Neuropathic
Disk protrusion
Multiple sclerosis
Diabetes
Other drugs
Cholinergic
Adrenergic
Muscle relaxants
Age

dysfunction may be pertinent. Debate rages as to the management of bladder emptying during labor – particularly with concomitant use of epidural analgesia [18]. Whether indwelling catheterization or intermittent catheterization is used, care must be taken to avoid bladder overdistension.

Anesthetic agents can cause a central inhibitory effect to normal voiding sensation, through decreased sensibility of the thalamocortical pain tracts [19]. Other anesthetic agents may have adrenergic and cholinergic interactions that can lead to functional bladder neck obstruction. Examples include atropine, neuroleptics, selective muscle relaxants and ketamine.

Pre-existing bladder problems may represent a major cause of postoperative voiding dysfunction. Some studies have suggested that a preoperative detailed urological history is important to avoid such postoperative difficulties [2]. Patients with neurological disease, multiple sclerosis, diabetes and vertebral disc disease may be at particular risk. Increased age has been identified as a risk factor for post operative voiding dysfunction [2,20]. Bladder complaints and other medical conditions increase with age and may confound age alone as a risk factor. Curiously, young women aged 21–40 seem to be susceptible as well [3]. Especially strong sympathetic tonus due to psychic inhibition is felt to be the cause.

The role of patient inhibition to void is often hard to quantify as a cause and should only be considered as an explanation after other causes have been ruled out. There is no question that some patients exhibit a psychological inhibition likely due to discomfort with voiding in hospital. The use of a bedpan, unfamiliar bathroom facilities or shared facilities in hospital wards will create varying degrees of anxiety in patients. Anxiety may lead to adrenergic stimulation that is enough to cause a functional urethral obstruction and urinary retention.

Procedures carried out in close proximity to the bladder neck, and in particular anti-incontinence procedures, can cause direct functional and even anatomical bladder neck obstruction. Excessive bladder neck elevation or surgical overcorrection is a potential complication of any bladder suspension operation. Urodynamically these patients demonstrate a high intravesical pressure in combination with a slow or absent flow [21]. Postoperative edema in the upper vagina or periurethra can directly obstruct urine outflow or interfere with parasympathetic nerve supply to the bladder and urethra.

Pelvic parasympathetic nerve supply for the bladder originates at sacral nerve roots S2 to S4. These nerves pierce the parietal fascia over the piriformis muscle and pass to the pelvic parasympathetic plexus located close to the anterolateral aspect of the lower rectum, near the anorectal junction. The nerves then form a mesh along the upper third of the vagina and extend into the bladder base (Figure 46.1). The nerves lie in close proximity to the inferior vesical arteries, veins and lymphatics [22]. Most of the pelvic parasympathetic nerves are located below the level of the cardinal ligaments, making direct nerve injury unlikely with routine hysterectomy. Radical hysterectomy with excision of the upper vagina can directly injure this nerve supply. Abdominal-perineal bowel resections, especially for malignancy, can also injure the pelvic parasympathetic nerve supply through direct excision and traction injury. Clinical experience with high rates of urinary retention following both of these procedures confirms what is found anatomically [10,23].

Voiding Dysfunction Following Radical Pelvic Surgery

The risk of postoperative voiding dysfunction increases proportionally with the radicalness of the pelvic surgery for malignancy. Manzl reviewed various types of radical hysterectomies for cervical cancer, comparing immediate and 1-year rates of incontinence and decreased sensation with voiding [24]. Standard Wertheim hysterectomy was associated with incontinence in 10% of patients immediately and 4% at 1 year following the surgery. With an ultraradical cuff resection (Latzko technique), the incidence increased substantially to 21% and 27% immediately, and at 1 year respectively. Similarly, immediately following surgery, 27% of patients described decreased sensation with voiding following standard Wertheim hysterectomy while 90% had

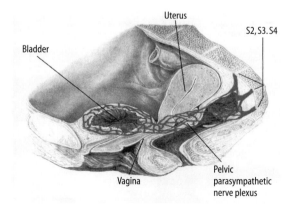

Figure 46.1 Pelvic parasympathetic nerve supply and innervation of the bladder base.

such complaints following a Latzko radical hysterectomy. These reported rates decreased substantially by 1 year following surgery to 18% and 45%, but the increased risk of problems associated with the more radical procedure was still clearly apparent

Urodynamic changes following radical hysterectomy provide some quantification of this voiding dysfunction. Ralph [25] studied 40 patients urodynamically before, and up to 1 year following radical hysterectomy for stage Ib or IIb cervical cancer. At 2 weeks following surgery, all patients were found to have small, spastic bladders. Bladder capacity, functional urethral length, urethral closure pressure and intraurethral pressure were all reported to decrease in these patients. There was an increase in intravesical pressure and post-void residual urine volume. All patients reported decreased sensation with voiding. At 1 year after surgery, residual urine volumes returned to normal and 63% still reported impaired sensation with voiding. There was a decrease in urine flow rate and prolongation of voiding times. Most patients (85%) adapted by developing a Valsalva or abdominal voiding technique to empty the bladder effectively. Urodynamic evidence of stress urinary incontinence was also increased from 35% preoperatively to 55% at 1 year after surgery.

Other authors have reported similar bladder abnormalities following radical hysterectomy [26–29]. The initial injury appears to manifest as a hypertonic but poorly contracting bladder. Late findings include ongoing decreased sensation, altered voiding technique and urinary incontinence. Up to 3% of patients having such operations may sustain chronic bladder atony, and never have satisfactory voiding again [30].

The suspected mechanism of voiding dysfunction following these radical gynecological operations is direct pelvic nerve plexus injury. This injury is often intentional and can occur at two anatomical sites. Excision of a wide vaginal cuff may be necessary for adequate removal of central cervical cancer. The wider the cuff, the greater the interruption to and excision of direct parasympathetic supply to the bladder. Various types of radical hysterectomy involve complete excision of the cardinal ligaments along with parametrial tissue following isolation and mobilization of the ureters. Some have suggested that complete cardinal ligament excision is not necessary [31]. Less radical hysterectomies involve taking the cardinal ligaments at the midpoint between the cervical and pelvic sidewall. The presumed risk with this technique is that of incomplete removal of lymphatic channels containing possible tumor spread. The parasympathetic nerves are definitely located in the bases of the cardinal ligaments and thus directly interrupted [22]. Occasionally, unintentional injury to the urinary tract also occurs. Not the least of such injuries is that of postoperative genitourinary fistulas. Alteration of regional blood flow with ischemic nerve injury, local edema from lymph node dissection and direct tissue trauma are likely associated factors, compounding nerve conduction to the bladder and causing the various bladder abnormalities described.

Management of this very common postoperative complication varies from use of indwelling catheters for long time periods to intermittent self-catheterization. Forney [32] showed that voiding dysfunction was related to the extent of cardinal ligament resection. Patients voided satisfactorily in 20 days following partial cardinal ligament dissection, at radical hysterectomy, but not for 51 days on average if full cardinal ligament resection was done. Hence, suprapubic catheters are often placed prophylactically. Anticipation of long-term voiding difficulties and avoidance of urinary tract infection as seen with urethral catheters are cited as reasons for this approach. Teaching the patient to void using a Valsalva or Credé maneuver has also been advocated. It is hard to know which approach is the best. Subjective success may be acceptable with many approaches as various clinicians have streamlined their own effective management protocols. Despite individual management differences, most seem to agree on the importance of recognizing this problem and avoiding the additional complications associated with overdistension injury to the bladder. Experience has dictated how dramatically acute overdistension can impair timely bladder rehabilitation.

Voiding Dysfunction Following Routine Hysterectomy

The issue of voiding dysfunction following hysterectomy of a routine nature, for non-malignant indications, has been debated extensively through the literature. It is interesting to note that few investigators have attempted to answer this question in an appropriate fashion. This is true, despite the common practice of hysterectomy throughout the world and the importance of providing patients with full disclosure of the potential complications of surgery.

Since Hanley [33] reported voiding dysfunction as a late complication following hysterectomy there have been many studies that have approached this problem [34–47]. These studies are summarized in

Table 46.2. Several of these studies used a retrospective postoperative questionnaire of patients that had undergone hysterectomy [44,45]. Few studies used control groups [42,43,46]. Urodynamic assessments were used in some studies, but sample sizes were usually small.[35,36,39–42] Several studies are quite notable and have influenced some aspects of clinical practice [37].

Parys et al. [40,42] have carried out both retrospective and prospective approaches to answering this question. The first retrospective review studied a group of 126 women presenting for urological consultation with bladder complaints that the patient related to have onset following simple hysterectomy. All of the patients had urodynamic abnormalities, with 47% showing detrusor instability, 37% having urethral obstruction and 25% stress incontinence. Comparison was made to a group of 20 age-matched neurologically normal women who were awaiting hysterectomy. There was a significantly lower incidence of urological complaints among the control group. A subsequent study provided a prospective investigation of 42 women undergoing simple hysterectomy [40]. Urinary symptoms, urodynamic findings and sacral reflex latencies were assessed pre- and postoperatively. The incidence of all of these parameters increased postoperatively. Specifically, urinary symptoms increased from 58% pre- to 75% postoperatively, and actual urodynamic findings were altered in 31% of patients. Of those with urodynamic changes postoperatively, 73% had evidence of pelvic neuropathy on sacral reflex latencies. Assessments were carried out at 3 and 6 months following hysterectomy.

These studies provide the strongest evidence for the negative impact of hysterectomy on normal voiding function. Other studies are not supportive of these findings, and some actually reported a decrease in the incidence of urinary incontinence following hysterectomy [36,43]. Hansen et al. [47] showed such a decrease with 35 study patients having pre- and postoperative urodynamics. Over 50% of patients studied did have evidence of stress urinary incontinence and urge incontinence prior to surgery. Griffith-Jones et al. [43] used a pre- and postoperative questionnaire among 80 patients having hysterectomy and 78 patients having dilatation and curettage. The response rate was only 60–67% but no differences were found between these groups with respect to urinary symptoms other than the incidence of stress urinary incontinence, which actually decreased following total abdominal hysterectomy. Wake [35], Vervest et al. [41] and Langer et al. [39] have all shown a lack of clinically significant urodynamic changes or urinary incontinence following hysterectomy with studies

Table 46.2 Voiding dysfunction following hysterectomy: summary of studies

Author	Study	No. of patients	Urodynamic assessment	Control group	Results
Jequir (1976) [34]	Prospective (questionnaire)	104	No	No	Equivocal
Wake (1980) [35]	Prospective	27	Yes (Pre/Postop)	No	Equivocal
Hansen et al. (1985) [47]	Prospective	35	Yes (Pre/Postop)	No	Unpredictable (high incidence of denied preoperative urodynamic proven SUI or urge UI)
Lalos and Bjerle (1985) [36]	Prospective	35	Yes (Pre/Postop)	No	Decrease in SUI postoperatively (50% had UI on preoperative study)
Kilkku (1985) [37]	Retrospective (postoperative UI questionnaire)	212	No	No	Decrease in sensation of residual urine and postoperative UI in subtotal hysterectomy group
Farghaly et al. (1986) [38]	Retrospective	98	No	No	Increase in bladder symptoms postoperatively
Langer et al. (1989) [39]	Prospective	16	Yes (Pre/Postop)	No	No difference in urodynamic parameters
Parys et al. (1989) [40]	Prospective	42	Yes (Pre/Postop)	No	31% increase in urinary symptoms 6 months postoperatively
Vervest et al. (1989) [41]	Prospective	32	Yes	No	No difference in SUI or DI; decrease in bladder complaints postoperatively
Parys et al. (1990) [42]	Retrospective	126	Yes (Postop)	Yes (20 "matched" controls)	Only patients with urinary complaints after hysterectomy studied
Griffith-Jones et al. (1991) [43]	Prospective (questionnaire)	158	No	Yes (28 patients post D&C)	decreased SUI in hysterectomy group (65% response)
Milsom et al. (1993) [44]	Postal questionnaire	10 000 patients (75% response)	No	No	Prevalence of urinary incontinence higher in patients with prior hysterectomy (p < 0.05)
Brown et al. (1996) [45]	Cross-sectional study (retrospective questionnaire)	7949	No	No	Hysterectomy is risk factor for UI (post operatively) in older women – average age 77
Demirci et al. (1999) [46]	Prospective study of bladder neck mobility	39 TAH patients (30 SUI controls)	Perineal ultrasound to assess bladder neck	Yes	Hysterectomy did not weaken urethral support or increase SUI

UI, urinary incontinence; SUI, stress urinary incontinence; DI, detrusor instability; D&C, dilatation and curettage. TAH, total abdominal hysterectomy.

that had each used prospective pre- and postoperative urodynamics. Demirci et al. [46] used perineal ultrasound to assess the bladder neck before and one year after hysterectomy in 39 patients. A control group of 30 patients having dilatation and curettage was used for comparison. The bladder neck was significantly lower at rest postoperatively in the study group, but stress urinary incontinence was not significantly different between the groups after one year. It was concluded that hysterectomy did not weaken urethral support or contribute to an increase in urinary incontinence.

Perhaps the most widely quoted and poorly understood study of postoperative voiding dysfunction and the type of hysterectomy performed is that of Kilkku [37]. This study looked at subtotal versus simple hysterectomy with reference to subjective bladder symptoms and incontinence. A questionnaire was used for 212 patients to compare urinary symptoms following either subtotal or total hysterectomy. There was a significant decrease in the "sensation of residual urine" and postoperative incontinence in the subtotal hysterectomy group. The sensation of residual urine was a subjective complaint on the patient questionnaire and was not correlated with objective incomplete bladder emptying. There was no randomization as the incidence of preoperative voiding dysfunction was actually higher in the subtotal hysterectomy group. This study, in combination with some understanding of pelvic parasympathetic neuroanatomy, has led to the suggestion of preferential use of subtotal hysterectomy over total hysterectomy. Careful analysis indicates the severe limitations of this study in its subjective and non-randomized method of data collection. The anatomical studies of Mundy [22] have clearly shown that most of the parasympathetic nerve supply to the bladder is located below the cardinal ligaments and should not be disrupted with simple hysterectomy, regardless of whether or not the cervix is removed. Additional studies also cast some doubt on the conclusions of the Kilkku study. Lalos and Bjerle [36] reported that, with pre- and postoperative urodynamic testing, there were no differences between 22 patients undergoing subtotal or total hysterectomy.

Brown et al. [45] carried out an interesting cross-sectional population study to assess risk factors for urinary incontinence in older women. Almost 8000 women aged 69–101 participating in an osteoporotic fractures study were surveyed with a questionnaire and limited physical examination. Previous hysterectomy was identified as one of various independent associations for urinary incontinence in these patients. Other risk factors included increased age, obesity, stroke, poor health, chronic obstructive pulmonary disease and diabetes. There was a non-significant trend with increasing parity. Attributable risk for urinary incontinence was calculated at 14% for hysterectomy and 16% for obesity. Multivariate logistic regression analysis was used to control for confounding variables and to determine independent risk factors for urinary incontinence. Milsom et al. [44] also carried out a large postal questionnaire of 10 000 Swedish women age 46–86 to assess the effects of age, parity, duration of previous oral contraceptive use, menopause and hysterectomy on the prevalence of urinary incontinence. The response rate was about 75%. The patients were divided into seven birth cohorts between 1900 and 1940. Urinary incontinence was linearly related to increased age (p < 0.001), with the prevalence increasing from 12.1% to 24.6% through the increasing birth cohorts. Urinary incontinence increased with increasing parity, described in 5.5% of nulliparous women within the 1940 birth cohort and increasing to 10.6% in women with one prior delivery and 16.4% in women having had three or more pregnancies. Hysterectomy was associated with a higher prevalence of urinary incontinence, being reported by 20.8% of patients who had undergone this procedure versus 16.4% who had not (p<0.05). Menopause and prior oral contraceptive use did not appear to be associated with urinary incontinence. There are some concerns with these study methods, including selection bias, use of a subjective questionnaire, and a lack of clinical and physical examination correlation. Nonetheless, the information presented warrants serious consideration, especially given the large sample size studied.

The association between urinary incontinence or long-term voiding dysfunction following hysterectomy remains unclear. It is likely that routine simple hysterectomy carries no significant increased risk for the development of postoperative urinary incontinence. Subtotal hysterectomy does not represent a superior technique for the avoidance of subsequent urinary problems. A definitive study capable of answering this question has yet to be carried out. Conclusions that can be drawn from the information collected to date include: (1) recognition of the common coincidence of urinary complaints in patients undergoing hysterectomy; (2) appreciation for the proximity of the pelvic parasympathetic nerve supply to the resection margins in a simple hysterectomy; and (3) the possibility that some patients may develop transient urinary complaints following hysterectomy.

Voiding Dysfunction Following Anti-incontinence Surgery

Voiding dysfunction following procedures for the correction of urinary incontinence can be classified into two categories: (1) recurrent urinary incontinence and (2) postoperative urinary retention (Table 46.3). Recurrent urinary incontinence is usually regarded as a marker of surgical failure, but de novo detrusor instability has also been described after 6–27% [48,49] of anti-incontinence procedures. Detrusor instability may be related to postoperative urinary retention and bladder neck obstruction. Bladder neck surgery itself may compromise normal bladder innervation, facilitating irritability [48]. Recurrent stress urinary incontinence can be due to ongoing urethral hypermobility, urethral sphincter deficiency or even a genitourinary fistula. These two aspects of postoperative outcome will be dealt with elsewhere as part of the management of failed anti-incontinence surgery.

Recurrent Urinary Incontinence

Postoperative detrusor instability can become a significant problem, occasionally resulting in urinary incontinence of a similar or even greater extent to that which existed preoperatively. Although the precise mechanism by which this occurs is poorly understood, a possible explanation is through increased outflow resistance from excessive bladder neck elevation and urethral compression [49]. In turn, raised intravesical pressure lowers the

Table 46.3 Voiding dysfunction following anti-incontinence surgery classification

1. *Postoperative urinary incontinence* De novo detrusor instability Recurrent stress urinary incontinence Overflow incontinence 2. *Postoperative urinary retention* Immediate Early Late

threshold of normal bladder compensatory compliance, resulting in an uncontrolled detrusor contraction. A possible analogous situation is seen in men with prostatic hypertrophy. Urinary incontinence secondary to detrusor instability is seen in these patients and relieved by treatment of the urethral obstruction [50]. Bump et al. [51] showed that high urethral pressure transmission ratios occurred in patients who developed postoperative detrusor instability, but not in patients with detrusor instability unrelated to anti-incontinence surgery. This supports a theory of overcorrection or bladder outlet obstruction causing de novo detrusor instability and also underscores the importance of establishing appropriate, but not excessive urethral pressure transmission ratios with anti-incontinence procedures. Despite this supportive evidence, changes in peak flowrate, maximum voiding pressure and maximum urethral closure pressure are sometimes not seen after anti-incontinence procedures in women [49,52], leaving the explanation for postoperative detrusor instability still somewhat unclear. Langer et al. [49] actually found that preoperative detrusor instability could be corrected in many patients with colposuspension surgery. Although this is an interesting finding, most would actually regard preoperative detrusor instability as a relative contraindication to anti-incontinence surgery [53,54]. Other causes for postoperative detrusor instability may include postoperative cystitis, recognized or unrecognized bladder injury or perivesical edema with disruption of parasympathetic nervous control. Another common and perhaps related complaint is that of increased urinary urgency and frequency following many anti-incontinence procedures [55–57]. Such symptoms are often quite transient, requiring reassurance only. Resolution usually occurs within weeks to months following surgery. Symptom persistence may indicate a need for investigation.

The management of de novo detrusor instability following anti-incontinence surgery should be based on the extent of the problem. Urine infection is common and needs to be ruled out by urine culture.

Antibiotic treatment of culture-proven urinary infection and may alleviate suspected detrusor instability. In the absence of infection, bladder irritability immediately following surgery may be treated with antispasmodics. Buscopan can be used for temporary relief and need not be continued long term. Ongoing difficulties may require urodynamic reassessment and use of oxybutynin, flavoxate , tolterodine or other similar medications. Generally, these treatments would be given over courses ranging from weeks to months. If detrusor instability is due to a relative bladder neck obstruction from over-elevation or sling placement at the bladder neck, it may not be permanent if good bladder emptying can be accomplished. Therefore, consideration needs to be given to cessation of these medications following a reasonable period of symptomatic relief. If improvement is not forthcoming with medical treatment and refractory postoperative detrusor instability develops, then active consideration needs to be given to urethrolysis or surgical revision of the anti-incontinence procedure.

It is important to document appropriate bladder emptying prior to initiation of antispasmodic treatment postoperatively, as high post-void residuals can increase, leading to an escalating problem of bladder distension and overflow incontinence. Overflow incontinence [58] postoperatively can present like detrusor instability or recurrent stress urinary incontinence and feigns surgical failure. A post-void catheterization for residual urine or ultrasound assessment of post-void residual can be easily carried out in an office setting and will clearly help guide appropriate treatment decisions. It may even be necessary to carry out multiple measurements of post-void residual volumes for diagnosis. Management may require catheter placement for temporary bladder drainage or intermittent self-catheterization patient teaching.

Recurrent stress urinary incontinence will likely persist and may occur immediately or long after any anti-incontinence procedure. All of the procedures have established failure rates over time. Repeat urodynamic assessment is imperative for such situations. As already mentioned, other types of urinary incontinence such as detrusor instability or overflow incontinence can only be elucidated by careful clinical and investigative reassessment. Subsequent treatment will be based on the results of reinvestigation. Kegel exercises, behavior modification, medical or surgical management may be required, with the understanding that repeat operations usually carry a higher morbidity and lower overall success rates [59].

Genitourinary fistulas represent a potential complication following anti-incontinence operations [60]. Fistulas usually present as immediate severe or total urinary incontinence following surgery and catheter removal. Some fistulas present later or in a much more subtle fashion. Clinical suspicion must remain high for this problem. Diagnosis may be made simply by pelvic examination and recognition of urine draining from a sinus tract into the posterior fornix of the vagina. A methylene blue dye test using two or three vaginal tampons may be necessary for diagnosis when pelvic examination is not helpful. (i.e. filling the bladder with 200–300 ml of methylene blue stained normal saline while placing two or three tampons in the vagina. The patient is usually asked to walk around for 20–30 minutes and then the tampons are removed and checked for blue staining. The location of staining can often help to localize the fistula tract in the vagina.) If a more complicated fistula such as urethrovaginal or ureterovaginal communication is suspected, more extensive imaging techniques such as an IVP (intravenous pyelogram) or lateral voiding cystogram may be required. Intravenous indigo carmine or oral pyridium in combination with placement of vaginal tampons may help to identify a ureterovaginal fistula when the methylene blue dye test is negative. Timely investigation, diagnosis and treatment with indwelling catheterization may result in resolution of small genitourinary fistula. A larger or long-standing fistula will likely require surgical repair.

Postoperative Urinary Retention

Voiding dysfunction, in the form of urinary retention, following anti-incontinence procedures is actually not an uncommon event. The incidence has been reported at between 2.5% and 25% [1,60–71] depending on the type of procedure performed. As a general rule, sling operations tend to have a higher incidence of significant postoperative urinary retention than do retropubic bladder neck suspensions or needle suspensions, but this is not always the case. Some authors have suggested that the opposite is true [72], creating an inconsistent and sometimes confusing picture. Specifically, the original Marshall–Marchetti–Krantz procedure involved placement of sutures in the proximal urethral wall [73]. This was felt to predispose to urethral obstruction. Later modifications of this technique have resulted in a lesser incidence of postoperative urinary retention (about 3.6%) [60]. The original description of the Burch retropubic colpourethropexy specifically outlines placement of the supportive sutures in perivaginal fascia lateral to the urethral and bladder neck with a resultant lower incidence of postoperative urinary retention [74,75].

Other bladder neck suspensions, including endoscopic needle suspensions, also rely on suture placement in supportive tissue lateral to the urethra and bladder neck and tend to be associated with a lower incidence of long-standing urinary retention [76]. Few studies exist comparing anti-incontinence procedures from the perspective of postoperative voiding dysfunction. Of note, Colombo et al. [77] did prospectively compare the Burch colposuspension and modified Marshall–Marchetti–Krantz urethropexy for the treatment of primary genuine stress urinary incontinence in a group of 80 women. They reported a faster resumption of normal spontaneous voiding (8.5 versus 13.8 days, p = 0.002) in patients who had the Burch procedure. Only one patient in the study, modified Marshall–Marchetti–Krantz group, had prolonged voiding difficulties, clouding the significance of the early voiding differences between the procedures. What does seem certain is that postoperative voiding dysfunction is difficult to clarify due to an absence of standard definition, identification and treatment.

What actually constitutes postoperative voiding dysfunction? Obviously, an inability to void at all following surgery seems an obvious example of urinary retention, but when is this regarded as a problem and not just an expected part of routine recovery? The literature is not clear on this issue. Voiding challenges with catheter removal are initiated from immediately following certain anti-incontinence operations, to days or weeks after others. The differences in postoperative management are not only procedural, but often colloquial or individual, varying between hospitals and surgeons. The differences can be significant. Nilsson et al. [78] report that effective and almost immediate bladder emptying can be achieved in 96% of patients within hours following the tension-free vaginal tape (TVT) procedure. Similarly, Bergman, Ballard and Koonings [52] found, in their randomized trial, that the mean number of days of postoperative bladder drainage before resumption of normal spontaneous voiding (post-void residuals less than 50 ml) was almost identical following anterior repair, Pereyra bladder suspension and the Burch retropubic colpourethropexy. All groups had an average length of postoperative catheter use of around 4 days, and there were no patients with long-term voiding dysfunction over 3 weeks. Yet Beck [1] reported that the average length of catheter use until successful voiding (no significant residual urine greater than 100 ml) was 59.6 days in 170 patients who underwent a fascia lata sling procedure.

These very different voiding dysfunction rates are individually regarded as acceptable by the involved authors. This obvious inconsistency of definition for postoperative voiding dysfunction makes treatment even more confusing. What one surgeon may regard as a voiding problem, another may consider to be normal or an expected part of recovery from a bladder suspension operation. The situation becomes even more clouded when additional voiding dysfunction symptoms are considered. For example, subjective complaints of irritative or obstructive voiding symptoms, with or without objective evidence of incomplete bladder emptying (post-void residual greater than 100 ml), recurrent urinary tract infections and even recurrent urinary incontinence from suspected de novo urinary urgency or detrusor instability are often considered as important clinical manifestations of underlying postoperative urinary retention secondary to presumed bladder outlet obstruction [79]. Relief of these symptoms can often be achieved with urethrolysis surgery.

Attempts have been made to establish criteria for the diagnosis of bladder outlet obstruction. Massey and Abrams [80] proposed that two or more of the following four urodynamic parameters should be present to secure the diagnosis: flow rate less than 12 ml per second, detrusor pressure at peak flow greater than 50 cm water, urethral resistance (detrusor pressure at maximum flow rate divided by the square of the maximum flow rate) greater than 0.2 or significant residual urine in the presence of high pressure or resistance. Farrar et al. [81] suggested that only low flow rates were necessary for the identification of urethral obstruction, as low flow (less than 15 ml per second) in the presence of normal or low detrusor pressures may be associated with relative obstruction. Conversely, peak flow greater than 15 ml per second with a normal uroflometry curve and no significant residual urine volume essentially rules out significant outlet obstruction. Applying these criteria to patients following anti-incontinence surgery in a standardized fashion is difficult, as all bladder neck elevations tend to cause increases in outflow resistance [82,83], even though urodynamic correlation may be lacking [49,51]. An increase in detrusor work and voiding pressure also occurs, but is felt to equilibrate over the weeks following surgery in most patients. Bhatia [84] reported that decreased preoperative flow rates (i.e. non-detrusor voiders) needed prolonged catheterization following bladder neck suspensions. Lose et al. [61] found that 25% of patients had voiding difficulties immediately after the Burch colposuspension. These patients were found to have preoperative low pressure voiding with detrusor pressures less than 15 cm water. Another 20% of patients developed late voiding dysfunction

defined as persistent strangury and urodynamic evidence of impaired bladder emptying at follow-up. Preoperative increased urethral resistance was a predisposing factor in this late group.

These reports highlight the lack of standards in the classification of voiding difficulties following anti-incontinence surgery. Delay of normal micturition is common following most bladder suspension operations, but when should it be considered pathologic? Treatment options will also differ depending on the timing of voiding difficulties after surgery. Given the inconsistency of standard definitions, it seems practical to categorize voiding dysfunction following anti-incontinence procedures into immediate, early and late subgroups. Such a classification will facilitate the review and understanding of the treatment of postoperative voiding dysfunction (Figure 46.2).

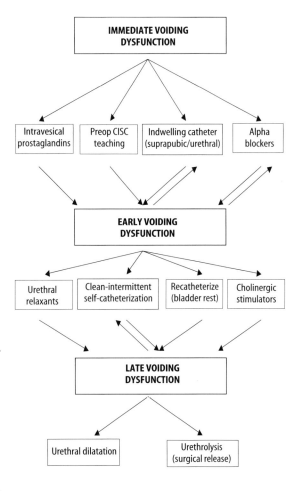

Figure 46.2 Postoperative voiding dysfunction: treatment algorithm.

Treatment of Immediate Postoperative Voiding Dysfunction

Immediate postoperative voiding dysfunction is demonstrated by an inability to establish effective bladder emptying once a voiding challenge is initiated. This could occur immediately after surgery or when dependent catheter drainage is stopped several days following an operation. Catheterization is the standard method of treatment for such immediate difficulties. It is suggested that urethral catheters should only be used short term owing to the increased risk of urinary tract infection with prolonged use greater than 72 hours [85]. To reduce this infection risk, suprapubic catheters are often used [86]. Suprapubic catheterization is also felt to have the advantage of better patient tolerance due to the avoidance of trauma and discomfort from urethral recatheterizations. Assessment of post-void residuals is also facilitated without the need for further catheterization.

For those patients in which a particularly long return to normal voiding is suspected, consideration must be given to preoperative teaching in clean intermittent self-catheterization (CISC) [87]. This technique obviously requires some degree of patient manual dexterity and dedicated nursing education, but it does have benefits over both urethral and suprapubic catheters. These advantages include a reduction in the incidence of urinary tract infection and increased patient autonomy with regard to management of voiding dysfunction. This also reduces the need for ongoing nursing catheter care. Intermittent catheterization has demonstrated its effectiveness in elderly patients following orthopedic procedures [5,6] and its usefulness after anti-incontinence operations seems empiric.

Pharmacological treatments have been used in the immediate postoperative period to reduce voiding dysfunction and urinary retention, with varying success. Intravesical prostaglandins (i.e. PGF_{2a} and PGE_2) have been shown in vivo to induce detrusor muscle contractions through a direct contractile effect [88]. They act without the need for an intermediate neurotransmitter mediator. Jaschevatzky et al. [89] showed a significant decrease in postoperative urinary retention among patients having vaginal hysterectomy and repairs with the use of intravesical PGF_{2a}. In this study, 102 patients were randomized to the use of PGF_{2a} or intravesical saline. Similarly, Tammela et al. [90] found that 10 mg of intravesical PGF_{2a} significantly improved bladder emptying in a group of 18 patients following anti-incontinence procedures. A control group of 18 patients received placebo with no such improvement. Wagner et al. [91] studied 28 patients with documented urinary retention postoperatively, and administered three different doses of PGE_2 and placebo intravesically. The post-void residual volumes dropped in all the groups, resulting in no clinically significant improvement from the intravesical prostaglandin use. The small numbers in this study likely contributed to these results. Grignaffini et al. [92] showed that PGE_2 enhanced bladder function after hysterectomy and cystourethropexy for moderate to severe genital prolapse. A total of 110 patients were studied. Fifty received 1.5 mg of PGE_2 intravesicular solution on postoperative day 4, just prior to catheter removal. The other 60 patients comprised the control group, receiving no PGE_2. The treated group had a significant reduction in urinary retention compared to the control group (10% versus 27%, $p < 0.05$). Regardless of their apparent effectiveness in the reduction of immediate postoperative urinary retention, intravesical prostaglandins remain a cumbersome method of treatment. Their therapeutic activity is local and temporary. Repeated treatments require monitoring and catheter reinsertion. Needless to say, they have not gained any form of widespread use.

Alpha-adrenergic blockade has also been proposed as a means of improving immediate postoperative voiding after many surgeries, including bladder suspension procedures [13]. Prazosin, terazosin and phenoxybenzamine have all been shown to decrease urethral resistance. These medications also appear to reduce postoperative urinary retention in a variety of clinical circumstances, including anti-incontinence surgery. Livne et al. [93] randomized a group of 99 patients to placebo or treatment with an alpha blocker following vaginal and abdominal hysterectomy and found a significant reduction in urinary retention in the treated group. Tammela [94] randomized 160 patients with unexpected postoperative retention to treatment with an alpha blocker (phenoxybenzamine), carbachol or placebo. The results were significant, with only 17% of the alpha blocker group, versus 49% of the carbachol group and 57% of the placebo group, experiencing recurrent urinary retention. Lose and Lindholm [95] reported that prophylactic alpha-blockade with phenoxybenzamine significantly improved bladder emptying, reduced time to spontaneous voiding and reduced postoperative residual urine volumes in patients following vaginal reparative surgery for genital prolapse. A case report has indicated that the serotonin antagonist ketanserin can also promote bladder emptying in acute urinary retention due to benign prostatic hypertrophy, presumably through alpha receptor blockade

[96]. It is theorized that alpha-adrenergic blockers help to overcome an immediate surgical stress-induced sympathetic overstimulation. Caution must be exercised in the use of these medications in elderly and hypertensive patients, owing to their primary vascular and hemodynamic effects (i.e. hypotension).

Treatment of Early Postoperative Voiding Dysfunction

Many of the treatments mentioned above are actually administered to prevent or minimize early postoperative urinary retention. Voiding dysfunction that persists despite such treatments and lasts for days to weeks following an anti-incontinence procedure can be classified as early.

Perhaps the simplest form of management for early urinary retention is recatheterization and ongoing bladder rest. This needs to be carried out carefully and with the understanding that recurrent and complicated urinary tract infections can result. Clean intermittent self-catheterization can be taught at this stage and maintained for months as bladder function recovers. Surgical intervention should be avoided as many patients will improve simply with the support of some form of bladder drainage and a "tincture of time". Urine culture needs to be carried out and infections appropriately treated. One must be supportive and clinically confident during the care of patients with these difficulties, as patient anxiety is common and serves only to worsen the situation.

Urethral relaxants and cholinergic medications may be considered to promote bladder emptying. Benzodiazepines, although nonspecific urethral striated muscle relaxants, tend to be well tolerated and are safer than alpha blockers. The main side effect of these medications is sedation due to their principal action on the central nervous system. Stanton et al. [97] actually found that oral diazepam was more effective than oral phenoxybenzamine, oral bethanechol chloride or intravesical prostaglandin E_2 in reducing time to spontaneous voiding following colposuspension surgery. Bethanechol chloride has been shown to relieve postoperative urinary retention in many old studies [98]. Regrettably, most of the studies using bethanechol are uncontrolled and do not provide any standards of drug dose. More recent studies are conflicting in their conclusions, with some indicating prevention of postoperative urinary retention [99] and others suggesting no such effect [100]. There appears to be a tremendous anecdotal experience with bethanechol, which transcends a rigorous assessment of its efficacy and

propagates ongoing use. Finkbeiner [98] published an extensive literature review on the clinical effectiveness of bethanechol for the promotion of bladder emptying. Despite the widespread use of bethanechol, there is little objective evidence to support its use. Bethanechol appears to be pharmacologically active as evidenced by patients experiencing cholinergic side effects with administration, but clinical reports indicating a clear benefit to effective bladder emptying are lacking. It appears that oral doses of 10–100 mg are pharmacologically ineffective for the treatment of urinary retention. Oral doses of 50 mg four times per day must be used. Obviously, cholinergic side effects are worse with higher doses, thus limiting therapeutic usefulness. Subcutaneous and parental routes of administration have been shown to be more effective, but also run the risk of a greater side-effect profile. Lastly, bethanechol definitely causes an increase in intravesical pressure, but there is no indication that it promotes a detrusor contraction, relaxes urethral resistance or helps to improve actual bladder emptying. In normal bladder subjects, it increases discomfort and a subjective need to void, but does not necessarily help to empty the bladder. Regardless of this information, bethanechol will likely continue to be used for postoperative urinary retention and, as acknowledged by Starr and Ferguson [101], if it is not well tolerated – and not helping the patient – it can easily be stopped with complete resolution of the side effects.

Treatment of Late Postoperative Voiding Dysfunction

Eventually there will be some patients who fail to empty their bladders properly for weeks to months following an anti-incontinence procedure. Fortunately, complete long-standing urinary retention is quite rare. If one also includes patients with persistent irritative voiding symptoms, asymptomatic incomplete bladder emptying, de novo detrusor instability and recurrent urinary tract infections, then the incidence of late voiding dysfunction clearly increases. For the purposes of this classification, late postoperative voiding dysfunction is defined as that which persists for months, despite the treatments instituted at an earlier stage. There is no exact point at which the line is crossed, as some patients will tolerate urinary retention better than others. Some patients may even prefer the option of ongoing clean intermittent self-catheterization over any operation to undo a "successful" anti-incontinence operation [1]. This tolerance clearly needs to be explored with each patient preoperatively and during the initial postoperative management of urinary retention. The decision to reoperate for the purpose of release of an anti-incontinence operation (i.e. urethrolysis) must not be taken lightly or carried out prematurely. A thorough urodynamic and cystoscopic reassessment is often recommended.

Cystoscopy with urethral dilatation has been widely used for the treatment of women with voiding dysfunction. Massey and Abrams [80] have shown that urethral dilatation can resolve up to 76% of voiding dysfunction caused by intramural urethral problems. The efficacy of this method of treatment for postoperative urinary retention remains in question, but it is still commonly used. Prior to a urethrolysis, it seems quite practical to recommend cystoscopic examination of the chronically obstructed bladder to rule out new pathology or lesions, trabeculations, high retropubic urethral fixation and foreign bodies. Urethral dilatation carried out concomitantly may also be therapeutic. If this fails then urodynamic studies should be done, especially if recurrent incontinence or irritative bladder symptoms accompany the urinary retention. Foster and McGuire [72] suggested that urodynamic assessment may not always be necessary before proceeding with urethrolysis. The urodynamic diagnosis of bladder neck obstruction is often hard to establish. A clinical and pelvic examination which demonstrates urinary retention and incomplete emptying with a fixed retropubic urethra is often enough to warrant surgical treatment.

Urethrolysis has been described using a vaginal or abdominal route, and both with or without immediate bladder neck resuspension. Webster and Kreder [102] carried out retropubic takedown procedures or urethrolysis through sharp retropubic

dissection, with obturator shelf repair (Figure 46.3) in a group of 15 patients presenting with voiding dysfunction 2–24 months following anti-incontinence procedures. These original operations included 6 Marshall–Marchetti–Krantz procedures, 6 Stamey operations, 2 Pereyra needle suspensions and 1 Burch colpourethropexy. All patients had extensive preoperative video-urodynamic studies before urethrolysis. None of the patients had evidence of recurrent stress urinary incontinence, but 13 had evidence of bladder instability felt to be secondary to urethral obstruction and 7 had urinary retention requiring clean intermittent catheterization. The retropubic takedown procedure and obturator shelf repair was successful in 14 of the 15 patients (93%), with one requiring ongoing intermittent catheterization for urinary retention. Two patients developed intrinsic sphincter deficiency recurrent stress urinary incontinence. All patients with detrusor instability symptoms were cured. Obturator shelf repair was felt to be necessary for proper anatomical positioning of the urethrovesical unit. Omentum was often used to fill the retropubic dead space. Others argue that a transvaginal urethrolysis, without resuspension, is sufficient for correction of urethral obstruction.

Foster and McGuire [72] performed transvaginal urethrolysis in 48 patients presenting with urethral obstruction following one ore more prior anti-incontinence operations (including needle suspensions, retropubic urethropexies and slings). The original bladder suspension operations occurred from 2 months to 35 years before the urethrolysis procedure. These patients also had a combination of urinary retention and irritative voiding symptoms before urethrolysis. The urethrolysis was carried out through a suburethral inverted U-shaped incision in the vaginal mucosa, with sharp and blunt dissection

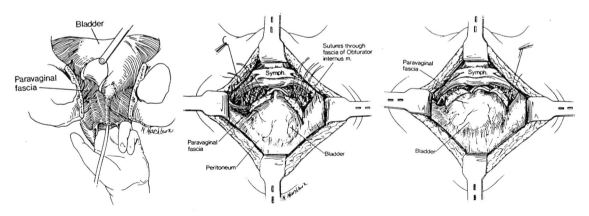

Figure 46.3 Obturator shelf repair following urethrolysis for postoperative voiding dysfunction. Webster GD, Kreger KJ. Voiding dysfunction following cystourethropexy: Its evaluation and management. *J Urol* 1990; 144:670–3. [102]

being used to release and mobilize the urethra bilaterally from adhesions to the undersurface of the symphysis pubis (Figure 46.4). Concomitant bladder neck resuspension was not felt to be necessary and therefore not carried out. Normal voiding was restored in 65% of the patients. Ten patients required more than one urethrolysis procedure. With no major complications being reported, this technique was felt to be a safe and effective means of urethrolysis. A later study by McGuire [103] reports a resolution of symptoms in 85% of 39 patients presenting with postoperative urethral obstruction and having the same type of transvaginal urethrolysis. Similarly, Goldman et al. [104] found a success rate of 77–84% in patients having transvaginal urethrolysis without concomitant resuspension. Regrettably, 19% of patients did end up with recurrent stress incontinence.

Raz [79,105] has advocated a similar transvaginal approach to the urethrolysis, but with concomitant resuspension using a modified needle suspension approach. Polypropylene sutures were placed in the endopelvic fascia and vaginal wall lateral to the bladder neck and delivered suprapubically with long needles. The sutures were then tied separately over the midline and rectus muscle. Curiously, the patients reported in this study had urethral obstruction with or without recurrent stress urinary incontinence. Of the 41 patients treated, 71% returned to normal voiding, 1 had persistent stress urinary

incontinence and 20% continued to self-catheterize for urinary retention.

Carr and Webster [82] compared outcomes in 51 women who underwent 54 urethrolysis procedures. Their preferred treatment changed over time, eventually favoring transvaginal urethrolysis over a retropubic approach due to better patient tolerance and lower morbidity with the vaginal technique. An infrapubic approach was used in four of the patients where there was restricted vaginal access and suspected extensive retropubic fibrosis. Routine resuspension was not carried out; instead bladder neck mobility was reassessed once the urethrolysis was completed. If hypermobility was found in conjunction with urinary loss during an intraoperative Credé maneuver, resuspension was carried out vaginally using the Raz technique. A Martius fat pad was often interposed between the urethra and symphysis pubis after transvaginal urethrolysis to avoid recurrent fibrosis and fixation of the urethra to the posterior symphysis. All patients having a retropubic urethrolysis underwent a concomitant obturator shelf repair. Successful outcomes with resolution of urinary retention and voiding dysfunction were reported in 86% of retropubic, 73% of transvaginal and 25% of infrapubic approaches to urethrolysis. Lastly, in view of the limitations of preoperative urodynamic criteria for urinary retention, the only absolute selection criterion for offering urethrolysis was a clear temporal relationship between the onset

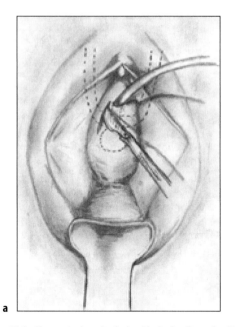

a

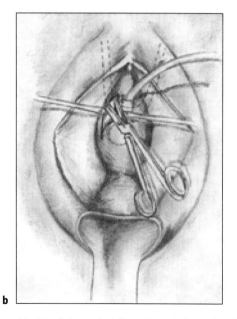

b

Figure 46.4 Tranvaginal urethrolysis. **a** Vaginal unilateral or U-shaped suburethral incision. **b** Periurethral dissection and release of synthetic sling, sutures or adhesions.

of voiding dysfunction symptoms and a prior anti-incontinence procedure. A waiting period of at least 3 months before urethrolysis was recommended for anticipated spontaneous symptom resolution.

Although bilateral urethrolysis is often necessary following retropubic bladder neck suspensions and needle urethropexies, a unilateral transvaginal release without resuspension may be preferred by some following sling operations. Such an approach has not been studied, but may prove to be beneficial through release of a fixed urethral obstruction without completely removing the support and bladder neck elevation provided by the original procedure. Clearly, avoidance of recurrent urinary incontinence is a major concern, as patients who end up with this problem following urethrolysis may have no other treatment options remaining other than periurethral collagen injections.

Conclusions

Perhaps the most important lesson to be learned from a review of the complexities of voiding dysfunction following anti-incontinence surgery is the value of a thorough preoperative urodynamic assessment. Understanding a given patient's voiding function before surgery goes a long way to predicting, understanding and treating the difficulties that may be encountered after surgery. The patient can often be counseled more appropriately with respect to expected outcomes as they pertain not only to surgical success, but also to potential complications. Surgical procedures can be tailored to the patient urodynamic profile with the hope of avoiding problems. Patients can be preoperatively taught to manage catheters or voiding dysfunction. Different types of and timing for catheterization may be chosen to make the postoperative recovery much more tolerable – even in the event of complications.

Aside from preoperative urodynamic assessment, one must establish a well-organized and systematic approach to postoperative voiding dysfunction once it is established. A stepwise treatment plan, as is outlined above, helps the patient and physician see their way through what can be a frustrating cloud of "what-ifs". This creates clinical confidence and builds the patient–physician relationship, as both work towards the common goal of a restoration of normal continent bladder function.

References

1. Beck RP, McCormick S, Nordstrom L. The fascia lata sling procedure for treating recurrent genuine stress incontinence of urine. Obstet Gynecol 1988;72:699–703.

2. Tammela T, Konturri M, Lukkarinen O. Postoperative urinary retention 1. Incidence and predisposing factors. Scand J Urol Nephrol 1985;20:197–201.

3. Shapiro J, Hoffman J, Jersky J. A comparison of suprapubic and transurethral drainage for postoperative urinary retention in general surgical patients. Acta Chir Scand 1982;148:323–7.

4. Stanton SL, Cardozo LD, Chaudhury N. Spontaneous voiding after surgery for urinary incontinence. Br J Obstet Gynaecol 1978;85:149.

5. Smith N, Morrant J. Postoperative urinary retention in women: Management by intermittent catheterization. Age Ageing 1990;19:337–40.

6. Skelly JM, Guyatt GH, Kalbfleisch R, Singer J, Winter L. Management of urinary retention after surgical repair of hip fracture. Can Med Assoc J 1996;146(7):1185–9.

7. Sayad P, Hallak A, Ferzli G. Laparoscopic herniorrhaphy: review of complications and recurrence. J Laparoendosc Adv Surg Tech A 1998;8(1):3–10.

8. Velasco JM, Vallina VL, Esposito DJ, Theodore S. Laparoscopic herniorrhaphy in the geriatric population. Am Surg 1998;64(7):633–7.

9. Zaheer S, Reilly WT, Pemberton JH, Ilstrup D. Urinary retention after operations for benign anorectal diseases. Dis Colon Rectum 1998;41(6):696–704.

10. Zaheer S, Pemberton JH, Farouk R, Dozios RR, Wolff BG, Ilstrup D. Surgical treatment of adenocarcinoma of the rectum. Ann Surg 1998;227(6):800–11.

11. White SC, Wartel LJ, Wade ME. Comparison of abdominal and vaginal hysterectomies. Obstet Gynecol 1971;37:530.

12. Arnold MW, Stewart WR, Aguilar PS. Rectocele repair: Four years' experience. Dis Colon Rectum 1990;33(8):684–7.

13. Drutz HP. Neurophysiology and neuropharmacology of the lower urinary tract. Int Urogynecol J 1990;1:91–9.

14. Picard P, Bazin JE, Conio N, Ruiz F, Schoeffler P. Ketorolac potentiates morphine in postoperative patient controlled analgesia. Pain 1997;73(3):401–6.

15. Silvasti M, Rosenberg P, Seppala T, Svartling N, Pitkanen M. Comparison of analgesic efficacy of oxycodone and morphine in postoperative intravenous patient-controlled analgesia. Acta Anaesthesiol Scand 1998;42(5):576–80.

16. Petros JG, Mallen JK, Howe K, Rimm EB, Robillard RJ. Patient-controlled analgesia and postoperative urinary retention after open appendectomy. Surg Gynecol Obstet 1993;177(2):172–5.

17. Tammela T, Autio-Harmainen H, Lukkarinen O, Sormunen R. Effect of distension on function and nervous ultrastructure in the canine urinary bladder. Urol Int 1987;42(4):265–70.

18. Fedorkow DM, Drutz HP, Mainprize TC. Characteristics of patients with postpartum urinary retention. Int Urogynecol J 1990;1:136–8.

19. Pertek JP, Haberer JP. Effects of anesthesia on postoperative micturition and urinary retention. Ann Fr Anesth Reanim 1995;14(4):340–51.

20. Wynd CA, Wallace M, Smith KM. Factors influencing postoperative urinary retention following orthopaedic surgical procedures. Orthop Nurs 1996;15(1):43–50.

21. Coptcoat MJ, Shah PJR, Cumming J, Charig C, Worth PHL. How does the bladder function change in the early period after surgical alteration in outflow resistance? preliminary communication. J R Soc Med 1987;80:753–4.

22. Mundy AR. An anatomical explanation for bladder dysfunction following rectal and uterine surgery. J Urol 1982;54:501–504.

23. Gertensberg TC, Nielsen ML, Clausen S, Blaabjerg J, Lindenberg J. Bladder function after abdomino-perineal resection of the rectum for anorectal cancer. Ann Surg 1980;191:81–6.

24. Manzl J, Marberger F, Hetzel H, Klammer J, Geir W, Dapunt O. Funktionelle Storungen des unteren Harntraktes nach Radikaloperationen des Kollumkarzinoms. Geburtsh Frauenheilk 1981;41:145–50.
25. Ralph G, Tamussino K, Lichtenegger W. Urodynamics following radical abdominal hysterectomy for cervical cancer. Arch Gynecol Obstet 1988;243:215–20.
26. Seski JC, Diokno AC. Bladder dysfunction after radical abdominal hysterectomy. Am J Obstet Gynecol 1977;128:643–51.
27. Lewington W. Disturbances of micturition following Wertheim hysterectomy. J Obstet Gynaecol Br Emp 1956;63:861–4.
28. Fraser AC. The late effects of Wertheim's hysterectomy of the urinary tract. Br J Obstet Gynaecol 1966;73:1002–7.
29. Barclay DI, Roman-Lopez JJ. Bladder dysfunction after Schauta hysterectomy. Am J Obstet Gynecol 1975;123:519–26.
30. Low J, Mauger G, Carmicheal J. The effect of Wertheim hysterectomy upon bladder and urethral function. Am J Obstet Gynecol 1981;139:826.
31. Piver M, Rutledge F, Smith J. Five classes of extended hysterectomy for women with cervical cancer. Obstet Gynecol 1974;44:265.
32. Forney JP. The effect of radical hysterectomy on bladder physiology. Am J Obstet Gynecol 1980;138:374.
33. Hanley HG. The late complications of total abdominal hysterectomy. Br J Urol 1969;41:682–4.
34. Jequir AM. Urinary symptoms and total hysterectomy. Br J Urol 1976;48:437–41.
35. Wake CR. The immediate effect of abdominal hysterectomy on intravesical pressure and detrusor activity. Br J Obstet Gynecol 1980;87:901–2.
36. Lalos O, Bjerle P. Early and late effects of suprapubic and total abdominal hysterectomy on bladder function. Arch Gynecol Suppl 1985;237:140.
37. Kilkku P. Supravaginal uterine amputation versus hysterectomy with reference to subjective bladder symptoms and incontinence. Acta Obstet Gynecol Scand 1985;64:375–9.
38. Farghaly SA, Hindmarsh JR, Worth PHL. Post-hysterectomy urethral dysfunction: Evaluation and management. Br J Urol 1986;58:299–302.
39. Langer R, Neuman M, Ron-El R, Golan A, Bukovsky I, Caspi E. The effect of total abdominal hysterectomy on bladder function in asymptomatic women. Obstet Gynecol 1989;74:205–7.
40. Parys BT, Haylen BT, Hutton JL, Parsons KF. The effects of simple hysterectomy on vesicourethral function. Br J Urol 1989;64:594–9.
41. Vervest HAM, Van Venrooij GEPM, Barents JW, Haspels AA, Debruyne FMJ. Non-radical hysterectomy and the function of the lower urinary tract. Acta Obstet Gynecol Scand 1989;68:221–35.
42. Parys BT, Woolfenden KA, Parsons KF. Bladder dysfunction after simple hysterectomy: Urodynamic and neurological evaluation. Eur Urol 1990;17:129–33.
43. Griffith-Jones MD, Jarvis GT, McNamara HM. Adverse urinary symptoms after total abdominal hysterectomy – fact or fiction? Br J Urol 1991;67:295–7.
44. Milsom I, Ekelund P, Molander U, Arvidsson L, Areskoug B. The influence of age, parity, oral contraception, hysterectomy and menopause on the prevalence of urinary incontinence in women. J Urol 1993;149:1459–62.
45. Brown JS, Seeley DG, Fong J, Black DM, Ensrud KE, Grady D. Urinary incontinence in older women: Who is at risk? Obstet Gynecol 1996;87:715–21.
46. Demirci F, Ozden S, Alpay Z, Demirci ET. The effects of abdominal hysterectomy on bladder neck and urinary incontinence. Aust NZ J Obstet Gynecol 1999;39(2):239–42.
47. Hansen BM, Bonnesen T, Hvidberg JE, Eliasen B, Nielsen K, Frimodt-Moller C. Changes in symptoms and colpo-cystourethrography in 35 patients before and after total abdominal hysterectomy: A prospective study. Urol Int 1985;40:224–6.
48. Cardozo LD, Stanton SL, Williams JE. Detrusor instability following surgery for genuine stress incontinence. Br J Urol 1979;51:204–7.
49. Langer R, Ron-El R, Newman M, Herman A, Caspi E. Detrusor instability following colposuspension for urinary stress incontinence. Br J Obstet Gynaecol 1988;95:607–10.
50. Turner-Warwick RT, Whiteside CG, Worth PHL, Milroy EJG, Bates CP. A urodynamic view of the clinical problems associated with bladder neck dysfunctions and its treatment by endoscopic incision and trans-trigonal posterior prostatectomy. Br J Urol 1973;45:44–59.
51. Bump RC, Fantl JA, Hurt WG. Dynamic urethral pressure profilometry pressure transmission ratio determinations after continence surgery: understanding the mechanism of success, failure and complications. Obstet Gynecol 1988;72:870–7.
52. Bergman A, Ballard CA, Koonings PP. Comparison of three different surgical procedures for genuine stress incontinence: Prospective randomized study. Am J Obstet Gynecol 1989;160:1102–6.
53. Stanton SL, Cardozo L, Williams JE, Ritchie D, Allan V. Clinical and urodynamic features of failed incontinence surgery in the female. Obstet Gynecol 1978;51:515–20.
54. Arnold EP, Webster SR, Loose H, Brown ADG, Turner-Warwick RT, Whiteside CG, Jequier AM. Urodynamics of female incontinence. Factors influencing the results of surgery. Am J Obstet Gynecol 1973;117:805–13.
55. Tegerstedt G, Sjoberg B, Hammarstrom M. Clinical outcome of abdominal urethropexy – colposuspension: A long-term follow up. Int Urogynecol J 2001;12:161–5.
56. Morgan JE. A sling operation using Marlex polypropylene mesh for treatment of recurrent stress incontinence. Am J Obstet Gynecol 1970;106(3):369–77.
57. Horbach NS, Blanco JS, Ostergard DR, Bent AE, Cornella JL. A suburethral sling procedure with polytetrafluoroethylene for the treatment of genuine stress urinary incontinence in patients with low urethral closure pressure. Obstet Gynecol 1988;71:648–52.
58. Richardson D. Overflow incontinence and urinary retention. Clin Obstet Gynecol 1990;33(2):378–81.
59. McGuire EJ. Urodynamic findings in patients after failure of stress incontinence operations. Prog Clin Biol Res 1981;78:351.
60. Mainprize TC, Drutz HP. The Marshall-Marchetti-Krantz procedure: A critical review. Obstet Gynecol Surv 1988;43(12):724–9.
61. Lose G, Jorgensen L, Mortensen SO, Molsted-Pedersen L, Kristensen JK. Voiding difficulties after colposuspension. Obstet Gynecol 1987;69:33–37.
62. Spencer JR, O'Conor VJ, Schaeffer AJ. A comparison of endoscopic suspension of the vesical neck with suprapubic vesicourethroplasty for treatment of stress urinary incontinence. J Urol 1987;137:411.
63. Mundy AR. A trial comparing the Stamey bladder neck suspension with colposuspension for the treatment of stress incontinence. Br J Urol 1983;55:687.
64. McDuffie RW, Litin RB, Blundon KE. Urethrovesical suspension (Marshall-Marchetti- Krantz). Experience with 204 cases. Am J Surg 1981;141:297.
65. Spence-Jones C, DeMarco E, Lemieux M-C, Drutz HP. Modified urethral sling for the treatment of genuine stress incontinence and latent incontinence. Int Urogynecol J 1994;5:69–75.
66. Rost A, Fiedler U, Fester C. Comparative analysis of the results of suspension-urethroplasty according to Marshall-

Marchetti-Krantz and of urethrovesicopexy with adhesive. Urol Int 1979;34:167.

67. McLaren HC. Late results from sling operations. J Obstet Gynaecol Br Cwlth 1968;75:10–13.

68. Iosif CS. Sling operation for urinary incontinence. Acta Obstet Gynecol Scand 1985;64:187–90.

69. Stanton SL, Brindley GS, Holmes DM. Silastic sling for urethral sphincter incompetence in women. Br J Obstet Gynaecol 1985;92:747–50.

70. Bryans FE. Marlex gauze hammock sling operation with Cooper's ligament attachment in the management of recurrent urinary incontinence. Am J Obstet Gynecol 1979;133:292–4.

71. Morgan JE, Farrow GA, Stewart FE. The Marlex sling operation for the treatment of recurrent stress urinary incontinence: A 16-year review. Am J Obstet Gynecol 1985;151:224–6.

72. Foster HE, McGuire EJ. Management of urethral obstruction with transvaginal urethrolysis. J Urol 1993;150:1448–51.

73. Marshall VF, Marchetti AA, Krantz KE. The correction of stress incontinence by simple vesicourethral suspension. Surg Gynecol Obstet 1949;88:509.

74. Burch JC. Urethrovaginal fixation to Cooper's ligament for correction of stress incontinence, cystocele and prolapse. Am J Obstet Gynecol 1961;81(2):281–90.

75. Burch JC. Cooper's ligament urethrovesical suspension for stress incontinence. Nine years' experience – results, complications, technique. Am J Obstet Gynecol 1968; 100:764–74.

76. Karram MM, Angel O, Koonings P, Tabor B, Bergman A, Bhatia N. The modified Pereyra procedure: a clinical and urodynamic review. Br J Obstet Gynaecol 1992;99:655–8.

77. Colombo M, Scalambrino S, Maggioni A, Milani R. Burch colposuspension versus modified Marshall-Marchetti-Krantz urethropexy for primary genuine stress urinary incontinence: A prospective, randomized trial. Am J Obstet Gynecol 1994;171:1573–9.

78. Nilsson CG, Kuuva N, Falconer C, Rezapour M, Ulmsten U. Long-term results of the Tension-Free Tape (TVT) procedure for surgical treatment of female stress urinary incontinence. Int Urogynecol J 2001;(Suppl 2):S5–S8.

79. Nitti VW, Raz S. Obstruction following anti-incontinence procedures: Diagnosis and treatment with transvaginal urethrolysis. J Urol 1994;152:93–8.

80. Massey JA, Abrams PH. Obstructed voiding in the female. Br J Urol 1988;61:36.

81. Farrar DJ, Osborne JL, Stephenson TP, Whiteside CG, Weir J, Berry J, Milroy EJG, Turner-Warwick RT. A urodynamic view of bladder outflow obstruction in the female: factors influencing the results of treatment. Br J Urol 1975; 47(7):815–22.

82. Carr LK, Webster GD. Voiding dysfunction following incontinence surgery: Diagnosis and treatment with retropubic or vaginal urethrolysis. J Urol 1997;157:821–3.

83. Pope AJ, Shaw PJR, Coptcoat MJ, Worth PHL. Changes in bladder function following a surgical alteration in outflow resistance. Neurourol Urodyn 1990;9:503.

84. Bhatia NN, Bergman A, Karram M. Changes in urethral resistance after surgery for stress urinary incontinence. Urology 1989;34(4):200–4.

85. Kass EH, Sossen HS. Prevention of infection of the urinary tract in presence of indwelling catheters. JAMA 1959;169:1181.

86. Sethia KK, Selkon JB, Turner CM, Kettlewell MG, Gough MH. Prospective randomized controlled trial of urethral versus suprapubic catheterization. Br J Surg 1987; 74:624–5.

87. Lapides J, Diokno AC, Silber SJ, Lowe BS. Clean intermittent self-catheterization in the treatment of urinary tract disease. J Urol 1972;107:458–61.

88. Bultitude MI, Hills NH, Shuttleworth KED. Clinical and experimental studies on the action of prostaglandins and the synthesis inhibitors on detrusor muscle in vitro and in vivo. Br J Urol 1976;48:631–7.

89. Jaschevatzky OE, Anderman S, Shalit A, Ellenbogen A, Grunstein S. Prostaglandin F2a for prevention of urinary retention after vaginal hysterectomy. Obstet Gynecol 1985;66:244–6.

90. Tammela T, Kontturi M, Kaar K, Lukkarinen O. Intravesical prostaglandin F2a for promoting bladder emptying after surgery for female stress incontinence. Br J Urol 1987;60(1):43–6.

91. Wagner G, Husslein P, Enzelsberger H. Is prostaglandin E2 really of therapeutic value for postoperative urinary retention? Results of a prospectively randomized double-blind study. Am J Obstet Gynecol 1985;151:375–9.

92. Grignaffini A, Bazzani F, Bertoli P, Petrelli M, Vedora E. Intravesicular prostaglandin E2 for the prophylaxis of urinary retention after colpohysterectomy. J Int Med Res 1998;26(2):87–92.

93. Livne PM, Kaplan B, Ovadia Y, Servadio C. Prevention of post-hysterectomy urinary retention by alpha-adrenergic blocker. Acta Obstet Gynecol Scand 1983;62:337–40.

94. Tammela T. Prevention of prolonged voiding problems after unexpected postoperative urinary retention: comparison of phenoxybenzamine and carbachol. J Urol 1986;136(6):1254–7.

95. Lose G, Lindholm P. Prophylactic phenoxybenzamine in the prevention of postoperative retention of urine after vaginal repair: a prospective randomized double-blind trial. Int J Gynecol Obstet 1985;23(4):315–20.

96. Horby J, Gyrtrup HJ, Frimodt-Moller C, Mathieson FR. The effect of a serotonin antagonist on acute urinary retention. Scand J Urol Nephrol 1989;23:121–2.

97. Stanton SL, Cardozo LD, Kerr-Wilson R. Treatment of delayed onset of spontaneous voiding after surgery for incontinence. Urology 1979;13(5):494–6.

98. Finkbeiner AE. Is bethanechol chloride clinically effective in promoting bladder emptying? A literature review. J Urol 1985;134:443–9.

99. Gottesman L, Milsom JW, Mazier WP. The use of anxiolytic and parasympathomimetic agents in the treatment of postoperative urinary retention following anorectal surgery. A prospective randomized, double-blind study. Dis Colon Rectum 1989;32(10):867–70.

100. Burger DH, Kappetein AP, Boutkan H, Breslau PJ. Prevention of urinary retention after general surgery: a controlled trial of carbachol/diazepam versus alfuzosine. J Am Coll Surg 1997;185(3):234–6.

101. Starr I, Ferguson LK. Beta-methylcholine-urethane. Its action in various normal and abnormal conditions, especially post-operative urinary retention. Am J Med Sci 1940;200:372.

102. Webster GD, Kreder KJ. Voiding dysfunction following cystourethropexy: Its evaluation and management. J Urol 1990;144:670–3.

103. Cross CA, Cespedes RD, English SF, McGuire EJ. Transvaginal urethrolysis for urethral obstruction after anti-incontinence surgery. J Urol 1998;159(4):1199–201.

104. Goldman HB, Rackley RR, Appell RA. The efficacy of urethrolysis without re-suspension for iatrogenic urethral obstruction. J Urol 1999;161(1):196–8.

105. Zimmern PE, Hadley HR, Leach GE, Raz S. Female urethral obstruction after Marshall-Marchetti-Krantz operation. J Urol 1987;138:517–20.

9 Training Guidelines

47 Guidelines for Training in Urogynecology and Reconstructive Pelvic Surgery (URPS)

International Urogynecological Association

Introduction

The Education Committee of IUGA (Chairman, Professor Drutz) was first established in 1995 at the annual meeting of IUGA held in Kuala Lumpur. Although a number of members of IUGA expressed initial interest in participating in this Committee, the seven members listed below remained as the Committee's active members, and were responsible for the preparation of the final drafts as they were proposed in Rome in October 2000. Professor Riss became Chairman of the Education Committee in 1999.

After reviewing existing guidelines and policy statements, at the IUGA meeting in Denver (August 1999), the Education Committee decided to prepare three sets of guidelines:

1. Guidelines for General Medical Training
2. Guidelines for Residency Training
3. Guidelines for Postgraduate and Subspecialty Training

On April 29, 2000, the Education Committee of IUGA met in Vienna, Austria. The aim of this meeting was to complete the drafts of the educational guidelines. These guidelines were then submitted to the executive and members of IUGA via the IUGA Website for all members to have an opportunity to provide input. A final discussion of the guidelines took place at a special Educational Workshop at the IUGA annual meeting in Rome (October 2000). After additional input was incorpo- rated into the FINAL guidelines, the Executive Board of IUGA voted on the guidelines and they were considered ready for publication.

In the opinion of the Educational Committee, the guidelines represent a consensus of IUGA and provide minimum standards of knowledge and skills in Female Pelvic Medicine and Reconstructive Pelvic Surgery (FPMRPS) at the three levels. It is the obligation of national societies and licensing bodies to use the guidelines and adapt them to national and regional needs.

The Education Committee recognizes that the practice of health care in women in general, and of female pelvic health, varies widely throughout the world, and is dependent on cultural, socio-economic and professional circumstances. However, the Education Committee feels that there is a need for minimum standards for training in FPMRPS at all levels of medical education in order to ensure quality assurance purposes. Finally the Committee recognizes the need for regular review of these guidelines.

Committee members:

1. Harold P. Drutz, Toronto, Canada, Chairman Coordinating Committee
2. Paul A. Riss, Moedling/Vienna, Austria, Chairman Education Committee
3. Michael Halaska, Prague, Czech Republic
4. Engelbert Hanzal, Vienna, Austria
5. Vik Khullar, London, UK
6. Heinz Koelbl, Halle, Germany
7. Harry Vervest, Tilburg, Netherlands

1. Guidelines for General Medical Training Programs in Urogynecology and Reconstructive Pelvic Surgery

Background

It is recognized that Urogynecology and Reconstructive Pelvic Surgery (URPS) is an integral part of general medical training. Every student and every licensed physician has to be familiar with the relevant aspects of urogynecology, and has to acquire the necessary knowledge and skills for his or her own practice. Therefore, all accredited medical training programs should provide access to meet these teaching objectives.

The International Urogynecological Association (IUGA), as the leading organization in this field, wishes to establish guidelines that will be universally acceptable to allow governing boards and licensing bodies on national levels to establish educational objectives.

IUGA is aware of the fact that there are important national or regional differences in the organization and structure of medical undergraduate training (university or medical school) and postgraduate training leading to a license to practice medicine (usually general practitioner or family practitioner). By publishing universal guidelines IUGA tries to promote a high and global standard for the care of women with pelvic floor disorders, to enhance scientific knowledge, and to encourage international dialogue between all health care providers involved with female pelvic health.

Scope of these Guidelines

The guidelines in this paper provide standards for general medical training programs (pre- and post-graduate) leading to a general license to practice medicine. However, actual guidelines may differ between countries, depending on national laws and regulations.

Objectives for URPS in General Medical Training Programs

The following objectives are formulated for general medical training programs:

- To improve the quality of care of women with pelvic floor disorders.
- To improve knowledge, practice, teaching and research.
- To promote knowledge and clinical skills relating to female pelvic health.

Definition

A student is a person attending university or medical school. In his or her training – leading usually to a degree of MD – the student should acquire knowledge in urogynecology and reconstructive pelvic surgery. Postgraduate training provides theoretical and practical training necessary for a general practitioner. Since these two components of general medical training vary widely in different countries they are considered together for the purpose of these guidelines.

Specialists in obstetrics/gynecology will have undertaken appropriate training in the field of URPS according to universal guidelines proposed by IUGA for residency training.

Subspecialists in Urogynecology and Reconstructive Pelvic Surgery (URPS) are defined as obstetricians/gynecologists or urologists who, having undertaken appropriate additional higher training, are recognized to have special expertise in the field of URPS.

General Requirements

Since medical school curricula and the specifics of general training programs vary widely the present guidelines focus on knowledge and skills every physician with a license to practice medicine should have. It is the responsibility of local academic, professional and government institutions to incorporate the aims of the guidelines in program curricula.

Training Program and Guide to Learning

Theoretical Aspects
The following knowledge should be acquired:

The Urinary Tract and Pelvic Floor

- Embryology
- Anatomy
- Physiology
- The urinary tract in pregnancy

Lower Urinary Tract Dysfunction

- History and physical examination
- Urodynamic evaluation
- Urinary incontinence – general considerations
- Genuine stress incontinence

- Detrusor instability
- Voiding abnormalities
- Urinary tract infections
- Urethral disorders
- Intraoperative injuries
- Urinary tract fistulas
- Neoplasia
- Psychological impact of genitourinary disorders

Genital Prolapse

- Pathophysiology
- Diagnosis
- Treatment

Anal Incontinence and Rectal prolapse

- Pathophysiology
- Diagnosis
- Treatment

Clinical Expertise

On the basis of the learning objectives listed above the physician must have clinical expertise and skills in the following areas (specific skills are listed in appendix 2).

Diagnostic Techniques The student must understand the indications for, the technique of, and the interpretation of results of diagnostic techniques used in the differential diagnosis of urinary incontinence, pelvic floor and anorectal disorders.

Clinical Skills Objectives The student should have acquired a high degree of clinical competence and skills to be able to understand pelvic floor disorders, to counsel patients and to make basic management decisions.

Community Care The student will understand and interact with the role of the community nurse in the detection and management of urinary and fecal incontinence and other pelvic floor disorders in the community. A knowledge of health care economics and resource availability within the community together with the provision of facilities must be obtained.

Appendix 1: Knowledge and Understanding

Mandatory

- Differential diagnosis of incontinence
- Normal and pathologic micturition
- Pelvic floor and urinary tract anatomy

Encouraged

- Principles of proctology
- Principles and interpretation of multichannel urodynamics
- Fistulas
- Effect of pelvic tumors on the urinary tract
- Anatomy and physiology of fecal incontinence
- Operations for incontinence and pelvic floor relaxation
- Postoperative care after surgery for incontinence and prolapse

Appendix 2: Skills

Mandatory

- Detailed history
- Urinalysis
- Clinical examination including evaluation of pelvic floor function

Encouraged

- Cystoscopy
- Evaluation of the upper urinary tract (ultrasound, X-ray)
- Single channel cystometry
- Clinical stress test
- Fitting and management of pessaries

2. Guidelines for Resident Training Programs and Educational Objective for Resident Training in Urogynecology and Reconstructive Pelvic Surgery

Background

It is recognized that Urogynecology and Reconstructive Pelvic Surgery (URPS) is an integral part of residency training (RT) in obstetrics and gynecology (OB/GYN). The physician in training has to become familiar with all relevant aspects of urogynecology, and has to acquire the necessary knowledge and skills for his or her practice. Therefore, all accredited RT programs in OB/GYN should provide access to meet these teaching objectives.

The International Urogynecological Association (IUGA), as the leading organization in this field, wishes to establish guidelines that will be universally acceptable to allow governing boards and licensing bodies on national levels to establish educational objectives. By publishing universal guidelines IUGA tries to promote a high and global stadard for care to women with pelvic floor disorders, to enhance scientific knowledge, and to encourage international dialogue between all health care providers involved with female pelvic health.

Scope of These Guidelines

The guidelines in this paper provide standards for RT programs. However, these requirements may differ between countries, depending on national laws and regulations. Each national organization or association in URPS, government or licensing body may adjust these requirements to their national situation or law.

Objectives for URPS in Residency Training Programs

The following objectives are formulated for RT in URPS.

- To improve the quality of care of women with pelvic floor disorders.
- To improve knowledge, practice, teaching and research.
- To promote specialized expertise, special facilities and clinical material that will be of considerable benefit to some patients and hence improve the quality of their care.
- To encourage coordinated management of relevant clinical services throughout a region

Definition

Specialists in obstetrics/gynecology will have undertaken appropriate training in the field of URPS according to universal guidelines proposed by IUGA for residency training.

Obstetrician/Gynecologists trained according to IUGA Guidelines will have a detailed knowledge of the anatomy and physiology of the pelvis, the contained viscera and the pathological processes affecting their function. They will have defined skills and knowledge in the investigation and treatment of disorders of lower urinary tract function, pelvic floor disorders and other benign pelvic conditions in women. They should be in a position to perform

basic examinations and to direct conservative treatment in patients with urinary incontinence and pelvic floor disorders and should know when to refer women with complicated urinary and pelvic floor problems to a URPS subspecialist.

Requirements for Trainees

In order to start an RT program in URPS the following requirements are mandatory:

- Trainees should be qualified physicians.
- The minimum requirements for entry into an RT program in Obstetrics/Gynecology is dependent on national laws and regulations.

Length of Training and Registration

The length and scope of specialty training is dependent on national laws and regulations. It is encouraged that a formal period is dedicated to URPS training.

In order to qualify as a specialist in OB/GYN the trainee should meet skills in URPS as outlined in these objectives.

Requirements for Residency Training Programs

Special Requirements

An accredited residency training program in OB/GYN should

- have access to a service for the referral and transfer of patients with urogynecological problems, with close collaboration with other gynecologists, family physicians, urologists, geriatricians, colorectal surgeons, or other primary care providers, within and outside the center, and
- have access to a urodynamic laboratory including cystometry, urethral function tests, uroflowmetry, ambulatory equipment, cystourethroscopy, ultrasound, and videourodynamics.

General Requirements

In addition to these special requirements the following general requirements must be met:

- have established close collaboration with other obstetricians and gynecologists within and outside the center, including major regional roles in continuing education and training, research advice and coordination, and audit;
- have a program director who will coordinate the training program, accept the main responsibility

for its supervision and be actively involved in it; when more than one center provides the program, there must be a supervisor at each center, with one having overall responsibility as director;

- have adequate medical staff to enable the trainee to be engaged in his/her field on a full-time basis (or in the case of a part-time trainee, during all of his/her normal working hours); participation in emergency and on-call work outside normal working hours is not excluded;
- have adequate library, laboratory and other resources to support training.

Training Program and Guide to Learning

Theoretical Aspects
The following knowledge should be acquired.

The Urinary Tract and Pelvic Floor

- Embryology
- Anatomy
- Physiology
- The urinary tract in pregnancy

Lower Urinary Tract Dysfunction

- History and physical examination
- Urodynamic evaluation
- Urinary incontinence – general considerations
- Genuine stress incontinence
- Detrusor instability
- Voiding abnormalities
- Urinary tract infections
- Urethral disorders
- Intraoperative injuries
- Urinary tract fistulas
- Neoplasia
- Psychological impact of genitourinary disorders

Genital Prolapse

- Pathophysiology
- Diagnosis
- Treatment

Anal incontinence and Rectal Prolapse

- Pathophysiology
- Diagnosis
- Treatment

Clinical Expertise
On the basis of the learning objectives listed above (section 8.1) the resident must develop clinical expertise and skills in the following areas (specific skills are listed in appendix 2).

Diagnostic Techniques The trainee must understand the indications for, the technique of, and the interpretation of results relating to the items listed in appendix 1.

Clinical Skills Objectives The trainee should have acquired a high degree of clinical competence and skills to be able to make a clinical diagnosis, plan appropriate management and treat women with the clinical problems listed in appendix 2.

Medical Therapy and Surgical Skills The trainee must be fully conversant with the indications for, techniques of and complications surrounding the items listed in appendix 3.

Community Care The obstetrician/gynecologist will understand and interact with the role of the community nurse, community advisor and general practitioner in the detection and management of urinary and fecal incontinence and other pelvic floor disorders in the community. A knowledge of health care economics and resource availability within the community together with the provision of facilities such as caregivers commodes, enuresis alarms and laundry services must be understood.

It is to be recognized that specific skills necessary for the practice of urogynecology will vary in different parts of the world. The educational committee of IUGA acknowledges these regional differences and encourages regional boards to develop detailed guidelines tailored to the needs of the population served.

Appendix 1: Knowledge and Understanding

Mandatory

- Principles and interpretation of multichannel urodynamics
- Differential diagnosis of incontinence
- Normal and pathologic micturition
- Fistulas
- Effect of pelvic tumors on the urinary tract
- Pelvic floor and urinary tract anatomy

- Anatomy and physiology of anal incontinence and rectal prolapse
- Operations for incontinence and pelvic floor relaxation
- Postoperative care after surgery for incontinence and prolapse

Encouraged

- Evaluation and management of anorectal disorders

Appendix 2: Skills

Mandatory

- Detailed history
- Urinalysis
- Clinical examination including evaluation of pelvic floor function
- Clinical stress test
- Fitting of pessaries
- Management of pessaries

Encouraged

- Cystoscopy
- Evaluation of the upper urinary tract (ultrasound, X-ray)
- Basic urodynamics

3. Guidelines for Postgraduate Training Programs and Educational Objectives for Subspecialty Training in Urogynecology and Reconstructive Pelvic Surgery

Background

In order to improve the care given to women with disorders of the pelvic floor, to enhance medical knowledge and to enhance scientific research, several Boards and Colleges around the world have estalished guidelines for subspecialization in Urogynecology and Reconstructive Pelvic Surgery (URPS).

The International Urogynecological Association (IUGA), as the leading organization in this field, wishes to establish guidelines that will be universally acceptable to allow governing boards and licensing bodies on national levels to establish educational guidelines. By publishing universal guidelines IUGA tries to promote a high and global standard for care to women with pelvic floor disorders, to enhance scientific knowledge, and to encourage international dialogue between all health care providers involved with female health care.

Publications Used in this Paper

Guidelines for subspecialization in Urogynecology and Reconstructive Pelvic Surgery of the following Boards and Colleges were used in this paper: Royal College of Obstetricians and Gynaecologists (RCOG), German Society of Urogynecology, Society of Obstetricians and Gynaecologists of Canada (SOGC), American Board of Obstetrics and Gynecology (ABOG) and Royal Australian College of Obstetricians and Gynaecologists (RACOG).

In this paper the joint proposal for General and Special Requirements for the new subspecialty of Female Pelvic Medicine and Reconstructive Pelvic Surgery from the American Board of Obstetrics and Gynecology and American Board of Urology has been incorporated.

Committee Members

The following IUGA Education Committee members participated in the preparation of this paper: Dr Harry Vervest (The Netherlands), Dr Harold Drutz (Canada), Dr Paul Riss (Austria), Dr Heinz Koelbl (Germany), Dr Vic Khullar (United Kingdom), Dr Michael Halaska (Czech Republic), Dr Engelbert Hanzal (Austria). The first draft has been prepared by Dr John Bergstrom (USA), the final draft by Dr Harry Vervest.

Scope of These Guidelines

These guidelines provide optimal standards for subspecialization. However, they may differ between countries, depending on national laws and regulations. Each national organization or association in Urogynecology and Reconstructive Pelvic Surgery, government or licensing body may adjust these requirements to their national situation or law.

The guidelines will be updated or revised on a regular basis.

Objectives for Subspecialization in URPS

The following objectives are formulated for subspecialization in URPS.

- To improve the quality of care of women with pelvic floor disorders.

- To improve knowledge, practice, teaching and research.
- To promote the concentration of very specialized expertise, special facilities and clinical material that will be of considerable benefit to some patients and hence improve the quality of their care.
- To establish a close understanding and working relationship with other disciplines involved in the field of URPS.
- To encourage coordinated management of relevant clinical services throughout a region.
- To accept a major regional responsibility for higher training, research and audit in the subspecialty fields.

These objectives may vary from country to country.

Definition

Subspecialists in Female Pelvic Medicine, Urogynecology and Reconstructive Pelvic Surgery (URPS) are defined as obstetricians/gynecologists or urologists who, by virtue of education and training, are prepared to provide consultation and comprehensive management of women with complex benign pelvic conditions, lower urinary tract disorders, and pelvic floor dysfunction. Comprehensive management includes those diagnostic and therapeutic procedures necessary for the total care of the patient with these conditions and complications resulting from them.

Subspecialists in URPS will have a detailed knowledge of the anatomy and physiology of the pelvis, the contained viscera and the pathological processes affecting their function. They will have clinical competence in the investigation and treatment of the disorders of function of the lower urinary tract in women, pelvic floor and anorectal function. They should be in a position to establish and maintain a URPS unit and should provide a referral service for women with complicated urinary and pelvic floor problems. They should be active in research and teaching and concerned with the management of women with intractable urinary and/or fecal incontinence, and persistent pelvic floor dysfunction.

Requirements for Trainees

In order to start a subspecialization in URPS the following requirements are mandatory:

- Trainees should be qualified physicians, certified by their national Board as having successfully completed general residency training in obstet-

rics and gynecology, urology, or colorectal surgery.
- The minimum requirements for entry into the clinical subspecialty of URPS are dependent on national laws and regulations.

Length of Training and Registration as Subspecialist in URPS

- The length of subspecialist training is dependent on national laws and regulations. It is encouraged that this period is at least two years and must include scientific research leading to peer-reviewed publication.
- The minimum requirements for recognition as a subspecialist in URPS are dependent on national laws and regulations, which may include Board examination and certification.
- In order to register as a subspecialist in URPS the trainee should be able to demonstrate his or her skills by means of a list of performed diagnostic and therapeutic procedures, scientific publications and have the approval of the director of the training program to be recognized as subspecialist.

Requirements for Training Centers in URPS

To be eligible for subspecialty training in URPS a center must adhere to the following special and general requirements.

Special requirements

- Provide a service for the referral and transfer of patients with urogynecological problems, with close collaboration with other gynecologists, family physicians, urologists, geriatricians, colorectal surgeons, or other primary care providers, within and outside the center.
- Have an sufficient clinical workload1. The center should have a wide range of urogynecological problems.
- Have a well-equipped urodynamic laboratory which includes cystometry, urethral function tests, uroflowmetry, ambulatory equipment, and cystourethroscopy.
- There must be easy access to neurophysiological equipment, ultrasound, videourodynamics and cystourethrography, and anorectal function studies.
- Have close collaboration, including cross-referral of patients, with a consultant urologist, a consul-

tant for medicine of the elderly, a colorectal surgeon, a neurologist, a continence nurse advisor, and an appropriately trained physiotherapist, all with definite commitments to the management of urogynecological, pelvic floor, sexual problems and pelvic pain.

- Have close support from, and close collaboration with, a medical physics service.
- Have an active research program in urogynecology for the trainee to access.

General Requirements

In addition to these special requirements the following general requirements must be met:

- Have established close collaboration with other obstetricians and gynecologists within and outside the center, including major regional roles in continuing postgraduate education and training, research advice and coordination, and audit.
- Have a program director who will coordinate the training program, accept the main responsibility for its supervision and be actively involved in it; when more than one center provides the program, there must be a supervisor at each center, with one having overall responsibility as director. Directors and supervisors will be consultants with special experience in URPS, and with the eventual development of subspecialization the directors and supervisors will themselves be trained and accredited subspecialists.
- Have adequate medical staffing to enable the trainee to be engaged in his/her subspecialty field on a full-time basis (or in the case of a part-time trainee, during all of his/her normal working hours); participation in emergency and on-call work outside normal working hours is not excluded, subject to approval by the National Subspecialty Committee (applications for approval of training program should include an outline of the on-call commitments etc., but all trainees must have suitable experience of emergency and on-call work relevant to their subspecialty.
- Have adequate library, laboratory and other resources to support subspecialty work, training and research.

Certification

Certification of training centers in URPS is carried out by the national government or the national licensing body, dependent on the national regulations or law. It is encouraged that approved programs be reviewed periodically, but not less frequently than every five years.

Training Program and Guide to Learning

Theoretical Aspects

The following advanced knowledge and skills should be acquired:

- Anatomy and embryology
  the bony pelvis
  all pelvic viscera
  the pelvic floor and endopelvic fascia
  the development of the urogenital system including congenital malformations
- Physiology
  A detailed knowledge of the physiology of the urinary tract, lower gastrointestinal tract, pelvic floor and genital viscera
- Pharmacology
  the principles of pharmacology
  the pharmacology of chemical substances which act upon the pelvic organs
- Pathophysiology
- The effects of pregnancy, parturition, menopause and aging upon the pelvis and its organs. The effects of disease, both mental and physical, upon the pelvic organs. The effects of surgery, trauma, and radiotherapy upon the pelvic organs.

Clinical Expertise

Diagnostic Techniques The trainee must understand the indications for, the technique of, and the interpretation of results relating to the items listed in appendix 1.

Clinical Skills Objectives The trainee should have acquired a high degree of clinical competence and skills to be able to make a clinical diagnosis, plan appropriate management and treat women with the clinical problems listed in appendix 2.

Medical Therapy and Surgical Skills The trainee must be fully conversant with the indications for, techniques of and complications surrounding the items listed in appendix 3.

In order to obtain these skills a modular attachment to other departments including Colorectal and Care of the Elderly in the same or another hospital are to be encouraged. A modular attachment to Urology must occur. The details of these modular attachments will vary depending upon national or local circumstances.

Community Care The URPS subspecialist will understand and interact with the role of the community nurse, community advisor and general practitioner in the detection and management of urinary and fecal incontinence and other pelvic floor disorders in the community. A knowledge of health care economics and resource availability within the community together with the provision of facilities such as caregivers commodes, enuresis alarms and laundry services must be understood.

Other Related Skills and Expertise

Epidemiology and Research The trainee should be familiar with the basics of epidemiology and statistics in order to interpret scientific literature and in order to design research trials that will encourage evidence-based medicine.

Scientific Meetings The trainee should have the opportunity to attend and present their own research at appropriate scientific meetings of the training center and national meetings. Trainees should be encouraged to attend the annual meetings of the International Urogynecological Association, the International Continence Society, the American Urogynecologic Society and other relevant societies.

Teaching The trainees should gain experience in teaching which will include:

- some responsibility for teaching medical students, interns, core residents, junior staff, general practitioners, nursing staff and midwives in their subspecialty area;
- full participation in the unit's postgraduate program with some administrative responsibility for organization of teaching in their subspecialty, to include scheduled teaching rounds and journal clubs;
- participation in the undergraduate teaching program;
- gain experience of appraisal and assessment techniques.

Ethical and Legal Aspects The trainee should be able to discuss the ethical and legal aspects of the clinical practice of this subspecialty within the scope of their national law and regulations.

Administration The trainee should be given some administrative experience and responsibility which will allow the development of skills relevant to the future provision and organization of clinical services. Types of relevant knowledge and experience are listed below:

- Attendance at a management course.
- An understanding of health service organization and administrative and advisory structures.
- An understanding of the mechanisms of health care purchasing, provision of care, resource allocation and contractual issues relevant to the clinical service.
- Be cognizant of the need for regional referral systems and role of tertiary service in health care provision.
- The system for managing hospital complaints.
- Know how to review a service and formulate a business plan.

Training Assessment

It is recommended that trainees keep a record of their training in a Training Assessment Record Book. It is furthermore recommended that periodically (i.e. every six months) the training is evaluated by the supervisor or the program director.

Certification

Designing and certification of the training program is carried out by the national government or the national licensing body, dependent of the national regulations or law. These international guidelines are designed to assist the individual national groups (or bodies).

Appendix 1: Diagnostic Techniques (Section 8.2.1)

- Subjective assessment including quality of life measurement(s) (QoL)
- Clinical assessment of the patient including the pelvic organs, a prolapse grading system, pelvic floor tone and strength, an appropriate neurological examination, and a mobility/mental state assessment
- Determination of residual urine
- Urinalysis and cytology of urine and the microbiology of the urogenital tract
- Frequency-volume charts
- Quantification of urine loss by pad or ambulatory studies
- Uroflowmetry (simple and pressure/flow/EMG)
- Cystometry – filling and voiding phases (simple and subtracted)
- Ambulatory cystometry
- Urethral function tests including urethral pressure profilometry, electrical conductance test, Q tip, and leak point pressures
- Perineometry
- Anal sensation and manometry
- Imaging techniques
  ultrasound (transabdominal including upper tracts, transvaginal, perineal, introital, endo-anal)

radiological (micturating cystograph, IVU, video cystourethroscopy, pelvic barium studies (defecograph), image intensification, urethrogram, MRI, CT) nuclear medicine – isotope bowel transit studies cystourethroscopy including biopsy
- Electrophysiological studies
- Electromyography
- Nerve conductant studies

Appendix 2: Clinical Skills Objectives (Section 8.2.2)

- Urinary incontinence due to genuine stress incontinence, detrusor instability, mixed incontinence, trauma and congenital abnormalities
- Voiding disorders and urinary retention
- Urinary frequency and urgency
- Pelvic pain
- Lower urinary tract and lower gastrointestinal tract fistulas
- Genital tract prolapse, both primary and recurrent
- Chronic inflammatory conditions of the lower urinary tract
- Sensory disorders of the lower urinary tract
- Urethral lesions, e.g. diverticula
- Effects of pelvic surgery and irradiation on the lower bowel urinary tract and pelvic floor
- Urinary disorders in pregnancy
- Evaluation and care of the elderly
- Lesions of the central nervous system affecting urinary, fecal control and pelvic floor
- Difficult defecation
- Disorders of lower gastrointestinal tract function including incontinence and motility
- Urinary disorders in childhood
- The physically or mentally handicapped
- Sexually transmitted diseases
- Emotional and behavioral disorders
- Hormone deficiency states
- Urinary problems secondary to medical disorders and drugs
- Sexual problems related to URPS

Appendix 3: Medical Therapy and Surgical Skills (Section 8.2.3)

Management options

- catheterization (urethral, suprapubic and clean intermittent self-catheterization)
- devices (mechanical and electronic)
- aids, appliances, pants and pads

Non-surgical treatment

- urinary and GI tract disorders including incontinence
- physiotherapeutic techniques and aids including biofeedback
- electrical and magnetic therapy
- behavioral therapy including bladder and bowel retraining and acupuncture
- role of pharmacologic agents to treat pelvic floor disorders
- role of hormonal therapy

Surgical procedures

- urethral dilatation
- urethrotomy
- suprapubic cystotomy
- bladder neck buttress, TVT
- vaginal repair of genital tract prolapse including anterior colporrhaphy, posterior colpoperineorrhaphy, vaginal hysterectomy and repair, enterocele repair, Manchester repair, sacrospinous fixation, iliococcygeal fixation, paravaginal repairs
- vaginal and abdominal repair of recurrent prolapse including sacrocolpopexy, rectopexy, uterosacral ligament complication, sacrohysteropexy, Moscowitz procedure colposuspension and similar suprapubic suspension operations (both open and through minimal invasive techniques)
- sling procedures
- long needle suspension procedures
- para- and transurethral injection procedures
- vaginal plastic surgery
- implantation of artificial urinary sphincter
- repair of vesicovaginal, ureterovaginal, urethrovaginal, and rectovaginal fistulas
- Martius graft technique
- augmentation cystoplasty
- urinary diversion and undiversion
- urethral diverticulectomy and excision of paraurethral cysts
- urethral reconstruction
- urethral closure techniques
- rectal mucosal prolapse surgery (abdominal Ripstein procedure, and rectal approach)
- post-anal repair
- anal sphincter repair – primary and secondary
- sacral nerve stimulation and implantation
- dynamic gracilis plasty

- recognition and treatment of intraoperative bladder and bowel injuries

Conclusion

The Final Draft of these Guideline Proposals will be distributed to international and national societies, organizations, and governing boards in Obstetrics and Gynecology and other related specialties for their input and suggestions within a specified timeframe. The *International Urogynecology Journal* will publish the final guidelines.

Index